THE
NEUROSCIENCES
AND THE
PRACTICE OF AVIATION MEDICINE

Experience is never limited, and it is never complete;
it is an immense sensibility, a kind of huge spider web of the finest silken
threads suspended in the chamber of consciousness, and catching every
air-borne particle in its tissue.

The Art of Fiction
Henry James
(1843–1916)

Dedication

Centre of Human and Aerospace Physiological Sciences
School of Biomedical Sciences
King's College London

The
Neurosciences
and the
Practice of Aviation Medicine

Edited by
ANTHONY N. NICHOLSON

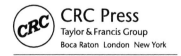

CRC Press
Taylor & Francis Group
Boca Raton London New York

CRC Press is an imprint of the
Taylor & Francis Group, an **informa** business

Readers are advised to consult the most recent publications of Pharmaceutical Companies before prescribing any of the drugs cited in this book, particularly with respect to their appropriateness, dose, frequency and duration of administration.

CRC Press
Taylor & Francis Group
6000 Broken Sound Parkway NW, Suite 300
Boca Raton, FL 33487-2742

First issued in paperback 2017

© 2011 by Anthony N. Nicholson
CRC Press is an imprint of Taylor & Francis Group, an Informa business

No claim to original U.S. Government works

ISBN 13: 978-1-138-11622-1 (pbk)
ISBN 13: 978-0-7546-7292-0 (hbk)

Visit the Taylor & Francis Web site at
http://www.taylorandfrancis.com

and the CRC Press Web site at
http://www.crcpress.com

CONTENTS

❖

LIST OF FIGURES

LIST OF TABLES

FOREWORD

The Rt Hon. the Lord Owen CH MA MB BChir FRCP
Fellow, King's College London

The importance of the neurosciences, both physiological and clinical, to occupational medicine is very evident throughout this book. Some occupations involve exposure to a hostile environment, and assessing the nature of the stress and the significance of its effects demands both physiological and clinical expertise. But this is particularly so for aviation medicine.

This book brings together physiologists with expertise in aviation medicine and clinicians with expertise in neurological disorders. Although the chapters dealing with the environment are directed specifically toward the aviation environment, the clinical chapters have a broad application to occupational medicine. In particular, they emphasize diagnoses and prognosis – often the most difficult aspects of the decision-making process as it affects the individual working in a stressful environment.

I cannot claim any up-to-date expertise in the areas covered in this book. Yet I found the different contributions both fascinating and comprehensible.

House of Lords
Westminster, London
2011

PREFACE

Aviation medicine, *par excellence*, is a discipline that calls for equal consideration of the physiological effects of the domain and of the clinical status of those involved, and so making possible an understanding of how aircrew can cope with such a demanding environment. In this context the integrity of the nervous system is paramount. Aircrew have to be protected, at least partially, from the hypoxia of altitude and the hypotension of increased gravitational stress, understand the disorientation inherent in being airborne and manage the disturbed sleep that arises from the displacement of the circadian rhythm from the alternation of day and night. Even so, in such a complex environment, responsiveness, both accurate and timely, must be preserved.

These are the stresses that may be encountered by aircrew, day by day, and that can easily impair the ability to operate effectively. However, clinical disorders, not necessarily infrequently encountered and likely to be subtle in nature, may also lead to impaired responsiveness. Epilepsy, syncope, hypoglycaemia, headache and migraine, mild head injury and excessive daytime sleepiness are episodic or transient disturbances that can impair responsiveness and prejudice effectiveness, while disorders of the vestibular, oculomotor and visual systems and of hearing have implications for the ability of aircrew to handle the complexities of the aviation task.

These thoughts in mind, based on experience gained over many years in the postgraduate teaching of aviation medicine at King's College London, have led to the present volume. The content reflects the areas of the neurosciences, both physiological and clinical, that are of particular relevance to the practice of aviation medicine. The book has brought together much expertise from the physiological and clinical neurosciences, and its primary purpose is to explore the ways in which responsiveness may be impaired and the relevance of the prognosis of clinical disorders that may also prejudice this skill.

It has been a singular privilege to participate in this publication. The process, over a few years, provided the opportunity to work with distinguished colleagues who have made notable contributions to the neurosciences that have, in turn, influenced the current practice of occupational medicine, and so that of aviation medicine. I am, indeed, grateful to all the authors who without exception expressed enthusiasm to take part in this venture, even though demands on their time weighed heavily. Their appreciation of the occupational aspects of medicine and their interest in applying their knowledge to a demanding environment have created a text that highlights the importance of the neurosciences to the practice of aviation medicine as well as to other occupations involving demanding environments.

The publication of this work gives me the opportunity to place on record my indebtedness to King's College London. For many years I directed the postgraduate courses for medical practitioners concerned with the day-to-day well-being of air personnel, and the present work was planned and prepared while holding the appointment of a Visiting Professor. I would also place on record the excellent editorial support provided by the Ashgate Publishing organization.

Lord Owen, Fellow of King's College London, kindly agreed to write the foreword to this work and I am indebted for the interest he has shown in this endeavour.

Anthony N. Nicholson
Lately, Visiting Professor (Aviation Medicine)
School of Biomedical Sciences
King's College London
2011

AUTHORS AND AFFILIATIONS

Thomas C. Britton MA MD FRCP
Consultant Neurologist, King's College
Hospital, London

Adolfo M. Bronstein MD PhD FRCP
Professor of Clinical Neuro-otology,
Centre for Neurosciences, Imperial
College London

Consultant Neurologist, National
Hospital for Neurology and
Neurosurgery, Charing Cross Hospital,
London

John H. Coote DSc PhD FSB FRGS
Emeritus Professor of Physiology,
Formerly, Head and Bowman Professor
of Physiology, College of Medical
and Dental Sciences, University of
Birmingham

Visiting Professor in Cardiovascular
Medicine, University of Leicester

Royal Air Force Civil Consultant in
Applied Physiology

**Garth S. Cruickshank BSc MBBS
PhD FRCS (Edinburgh and London)**
Professor of Neurosurgery, College of
Medical and Dental Sciences, University
of Birmingham

Honorary Consultant in Neurosurgery,
Queen Elizabeth Hospital, Birmingham

**Andrew R. C. Cummin MA DM
FRCP**
Consultant in Pulmonary Medicine,
Charing Cross Hospital, London

Honorary Senior Lecturer in
Respiratory Diseases, Imperial College
London

Civil Consultant in Respiratory
Physiology, Royal Air Force

Formerly, Senior Medical Officer
(Research), Royal Air Force Institute
of Aviation Medicine, Farnborough,
United Kingdom

**Nicholas J. Cutfield BMedSc
MBChB FRACP**
Lately, Clinical Research Fellow
in Neuro-otology, Centre for
Neurosciences, Imperial College
London

Now, Consultant Neurologist,
Department of Neurology, Dunedin
Hospital, New Zealand

Clinical Senior Lecturer, Department
of Medicine, University of Otago, New
Zealand

Russell G. Foster BSc PhD FRS
Professor of Circadian Neuroscience,
and Senior Fellow Brasenose College,
University of Oxford

Head, Nuffield Laboratory of
Ophthalmology, Medical Sciences
Division, University of Oxford

Simon R. Heller BA DM FRCP
Professor of Clinical Diabetes,
University of Sheffield

Honorary Consultant Physician,
Sheffield Teaching Hospitals
Foundation Trust

**The late Ronald Hinchcliffe BSc
MD PhD FRCP (Edinburgh and
London)**
Emeritus Professor of Audiological
Medicine, University College London

David A. Low BSc PhD
Research Fellow, Department of
Medicine, St Mary's Hospital, Imperial
College London

**Linda M. Luxon CBE BSc MBBS
FRCP**
Professor of Audiovestibular Medicine,
University College London Ear Institute

Consultant Neuro-otologist,
Department of Neuro-otology,
National Hospital for Neurology and
Neurosurgery, London

**Christopher J. Mathias DSc MBBS
DPhil FRCP**
Professor of Neurovascular Medicine,
Department of Clinical Neuroscience,
St Mary's Hospital, Imperial College
London

Consultant in Neurology, National
Hospital for Neurology and
Neurosurgery, London

**James S. Milledge MD FRCP
(London and Edinburgh)**
Honorary Professor, Department of
Physiology, University College London

Formerly, Consultant Physician and
Scientific Member, Medical Research
Council, Northwick Park Hospital,
London

Member, Silver Hut Expedition (1960–
1961)
American Medical Research Expedition
to Mount Everest (1981)

**Anthony N. Nicholson OBE DSc
MBChB PhD FRCP (Edinburgh and
London) FRCPath FRAeS**
Formerly, Head (Commandant) and
Director of Research, Royal Air
Force Institute of Aviation Medicine,
Farnborough, United Kingdom

Visiting Professor (Aviation Medicine),
School of Biomedical Sciences, King's
College London

Lately, Visiting Professor (Medicine),
National Heart and Lung Institute,
Imperial College London

Michael D. O'Brien MD FRCP
Emeritus Physician for Nervous
Diseases, Department of Neurology,
Guy's Hospital, London

Consultant Adviser in Neurology, United
Kingdom Civil Aviation Authority

Gordon T. Plant MA MD FRCP FRCOphth
Consultant in Neurology and Neuro-ophthalmology, National Hospital for Neurology and Neurosurgery

Moorfields Eye Hospital and St Thomas' Hospital, London

Honorary Senior Lecturer, Institute of Neurology, University College London

Michael B. Spencer BA MSc
Formerly, Principal Statistician, Royal Air Force Institute of Aviation Medicine, Farnborough, United Kingdom

J. R. Rollin Stott MA MBBChir MRCP DIC DAvMed (RCP)
Formerly, Senior Medical Officer (Research), Royal Air Force Institute of Aviation Medicine, Farnborough, United Kingdom

Honorary Senior Lecturer in Aviation Medicine, Centre of Human and Aerospace Physiological Sciences, School for Biomedical Sciences, King's College London

Aeromedical Examiner, United Kingdom Civil Aviation Authority

Matthew C. Walker MA MBBChir PhD FRCP
Professor of Neurology, Department of Clinical and Experimental Epilepsy, Institute of Neurology, University College London

Honorary Consultant in Neurology, National Hospital for Neurology and Neurosurgery, London

Jane Ward BSc MBChB PhD
Senior Lecturer in Physiology and, Deputy Director (Postgraduate Courses in Aviation Medicine), Centre of Human and Aerospace Physiological Sciences, School for Biomedical Sciences, King's College London

Chapter 1

WAKEFULNESS, AWARENESS AND CONSCIOUSNESS

Anthony N. Nicholson

Understanding impaired responsiveness in aircrew demands familiarity with the aviation domain and with relevant aspects of the neurosciences, both physiological and clinical. The manifestations of the adverse effects of the aviation environment and of some clinical disorders have much in common. Wakefulness may be impaired when aircrew have difficulty in coping with irregularity of their rest and activity, and excessive daytime sleepiness occurs with some disorders of sleep. Impaired awareness can lead to illusions or the loss of orientation. Awareness is prejudiced by excessive arousal, by inadequate or incorrect sensory information linked mainly to the visual and vestibular systems, and by incorrect or inadequate processing of the information as in coning of attention and errors of expectancy (Benson, 1999). Consciousness may be impaired during exposure to positive accelerations as well as by hypoxia, by trauma and by various transient and episodic disorders of the nervous system.

States of Responsiveness

The states of wakefulness, awareness and consciousness are crucial to the aviator. Wakefulness is an enabling state (Rees *et al.*, 2002) that underpins vigilance (a state of keeping watch for possible difficulties – Oxford English Dictionary). It involves the physiological event of arousal. It is a state that can be impaired by disturbed sleep. Awareness and consciousness are less well defined and the terms are used varyingly in different disciplines. It is, therefore, useful to explore what can be meant by awareness and consciousness, and how these states relate to the aviation domain.

Awareness involves perception and in aviation it is especially concerned with the appreciation of the spatial environment. It involves the sense of location in relation to the immediate and the remote surroundings. Awareness facilitates the sensory input essential to orientation and, when impaired, leads to disorientation. However, awareness (with perception) is not necessarily concerned with the interpretation of information.

The interpretation of what is perceived in the wakeful state is a higher nervous function – consciousness. Awareness does not create consciousness, though it modulates the process that leads to the conscious state. The nature of consciousness itself is uncertain, and attempts to understand consciousness involve the disciplines of philosophy and neuroscience.

In summary, as far as aviation is concerned, vigilance (watching for possible difficulties) is dependent on the wakeful state and may be impaired by disturbed sleep and circadian dysfunction, while orientation is prejudiced by loss of awareness. Clearly, both vigilance (dependent on the wakeful state) and orientation (dependent on awareness) have much relevance to air safety. The operational significance of consciousness, though little understood in itself, is obvious. Hypotension during increased gravitational stress (positive acceleration) and hypoxia during exposure to altitude are potent threats to the integrity of a phenomenon that involves sensory, central (introspective) and purposeful motor functions.

The identification of the anatomical substrates for these states of responsiveness and understanding the physiological basis of wakefulness, awareness and consciousness are of much interest in the neurosciences. It would appear that central structures of the nervous system are pivotal. The activities of the peripheral sensory systems do not create wakefulness, awareness or consciousness – they modulate pre-existing states. Initially, as far as sleep and wakefulness were concerned, the importance of the sensory input was much emphasized. However, in the middle of the twentieth century, studies concerned with the physiological basis of this continuum shifted the emphasis from a primarily

sensory process to one involving central structures in the brainstem and, in due course, studies implicated the midbrain and projections toward the cortex.

Similarly, during the latter part of the same century and to date, studies on spatial awareness are shifting the emphasis of the processing of information from the sensory organs to structures within the medial temporal lobe with possible projections to the parietal cortex. As far as consciousness is concerned, recent studies have raised the possibility that the thalamocortical system is involved, and the confirmation of the neural substrate for consciousness would set aside forever the myth of dualism.[1] There may well be a long way to go before responsiveness is adequately understood, but it is worthwhile to review briefly the present state of knowledge and the possibilities opened up by recent research.

Wakefulness

Due to the efforts of experimental and clinical neurophysiologists throughout most of the twentieth century and onwards to this day, there is now a reasonable understanding of the physiological basis of the sleep–wakefulness continuum. Present-day understanding of the wakeful state originated with the studies of Bremer (1935, 1938). Continuous sleep was observed in animals with transection of the brain at the boundary between the brainstem and the cerebrum (Figure 1.1a), and it was considered that this state was due to the loss of the sensory input to the cortex (Figure 1.1b). That interpretation was in keeping with generally held views on the nature of sleep at the turn of the nineteenth

---

1   Separation of mind and body was advocated by Descartes (1591–1650) and Spinoza (1632–1677). Of recent years, dualism was strongly advocated by Eccles (1970, 1994) – the distinguished neurophysiologist and Nobel Laureate (Curtis and Andersen, 2001).

century, and even from ancient times.[2] The observations provided experimental evidence for the importance of the brainstem in the control of sleep and wakefulness. However, as the transection was at the boundary between brainstem and cerebrum, the brain was not entirely devoid of sensory input and so there were difficulties with the emphasis that was placed on sensory input.

Reticular Activating System

The solution emerged when Moruzzi and Magoun (1949) identified the reticular activating system within the brainstem. Awakening was not impaired if sections at the level of the brainstem similar to those used by Bremer (1935, 1938) were limited to the sensory pathways (Figure 1.1c). It was the section of the central core of the brainstem that led to sleep (Figure 1.1d), and it was the ascending influences arising from the reticular formation that were responsible for wakefulness. These, and later studies (Batini *et al.*, 1958), indicated that neurons located in the anterior part of the upper third of the pons were predominantly responsible for wakefulness while neurons of the lower third of the brainstem dampened the process of wakefulness and could actively induce sleep.

The reticular activating system within the brainstem is an essential network,

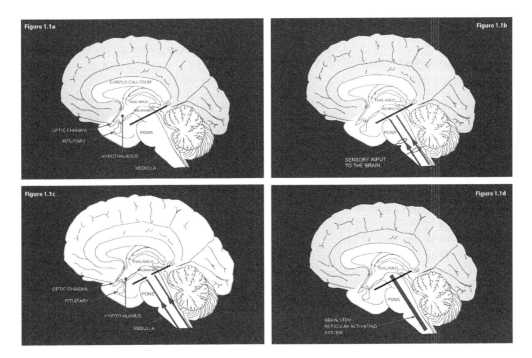

Figure 1.1   Schematic depiction of the studies by Bremer (1935, 1938) and Moruzzi and Magoun (1949) (see colour section)

Source: Nicholson, A.N. 1998. *The Neurosciences and Aviation Medicine: A Century of Endeavour. International Academy of Aviation and Space Medicine,* Auckland: Uniprint (L.J. Thompson (ed.) with permission from the Academy).

---

2   A scholarly account of the history of the deafferentation hypothesis of sleep from the days of Epicurus (341–270 BC) and Lucretius (99–55 BC) to the middle of the twentieth century is given by Moruzzi (1964).

though not the unique structure, as far as the generation of sleep and wakefulness is concerned. It has now been established that structures concerned with the control of sleep and wakefulness extend well into the cerebrum. The anterior part of the pons, the midbrain, posterior hypothalamus and basal forebrain structures are concerned with wakefulness while the lower brainstem (nucleus tractus solitarius), anterior hypothalamus and the basal forebrain are involved with sleep promotion. Studies have also shown that spindles and slow-wave activity during sleep are dependent on the activity of the thalamocortical system (Steriade, 2001) and that such activity is generated between the thalamus and the cortex and modulated by the systems of the brainstem, hypothalamus and basal forebrain (Steriade and Deschenes, 1984; McCormick and Bal,1997; Amzica and Steriade, 1998).

Circadian System

The full manifestation of the sleep–wakefulness continuum involves not only the arousal system projecting from the brainstem, but also the circadian system. A circadian influence in humans was anticipated by the observation of Fulton and Bailey (1929) working in the surgical clinic of Harvey Cushing (1869–1939). They observed that the rhythm of sleep and wakefulness was disturbed in a young woman with a tumour just above the pituitary. Minnie had experienced transient attacks of drowsiness for several years. She was even unable to stay awake to have her photograph taken (Figure 1.2) and she would often drop off to sleep in the company of friends even when the conversation was said to be animated. The attacks of drowsiness became progressively more severe

and more prolonged, and somnolence became almost continuous. She died at the age of 24 years.

It was patients like Minnie that encouraged discussion on the rhythmic nature of sleep and wakefulness during the early part of the twentieth century. The paper by Fulton and Bailey (1929) contained almost a prophecy: 'It was, perhaps, erroneous to speak of a sleep centre in the brain, but tumors above the pituitary gland may disturb the rhythm of sleep and wakefulness.' This appears to be the first suggestion in the clinical literature that the alternating pattern of sleep and wakefulness was somehow related to a specific part of the brain, and, in turn, that whatever may be involved in the control of sleep and wakefulness there was a rhythmic input.

It is now well established that a pacemaker exists near to the pituitary gland, the suprachiasmatic nucleus, and that it receives input from the eyes through the retinohypothalamic tract. The emerging complexities of the physiology and pharmacology of the circadian system are dealt with

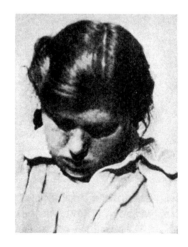

Figure 1.2   Minnie

Source: Fulton, J.F. and Bailey, P. 1929. Tumors in the region of the third ventricle: their diagnosis and relation to pathological sleep, 69, 1–25. (With permission from Wolters Kluwer Health).

in Chapter 2 (Circadian System and Diurnal Activity). As far as aviation is concerned, the potential significance of the circadian system to the efficiency of aircrew was explored initially by Klein *et al.* (1970), and its implications to the work of aircrew, together with those of the sleep–wakefulness continuum, are dealt with in Chapter 3 (Aircrew and Alertness).

Electroencephalography

Over the same years that progress was being made in understanding the anatomy and physiology of sleep and wakefulness, there was an increasing interest in the human electroencephalogram and its relation to the behavioural manifestations of the sleep–wakefulness continuum. The electrical activity of the brains of animals had been recorded in the nineteenth century (Caton, 1875), but the first recordings in humans were made by Berger (1929). Adrian and Matthews (1934a, 1934b) then explored the variations and abnormalities of the waves in the electroencephalogram and showed that the alpha rhythm disappeared when the individual was attentive or in deep sleep.

Later, Loomis *et al.* (1937) described the changes in the electroencephalogram with the states of sleep, and that led to the manual published by the National Institutes of Neurological Diseases and Blindness (Rechtschaffen and Kales, 1968), since revised by the American Academy of Sleep Medicine (Iber *et al.*, 2007). These manuals provide definitions for the identification of wakefulness, drowsiness, various stages of sleep and arousals, and have been supplemented by recordings of peripheral activities relevant to the assessment of sleep disorders. A brief description of these recordings, intended to introduce

the aeromedical practitioner to polysomnography, is given in Chapter 10 (Investigation of Sleep and Wakefulness in Aircrew).

The potential of electroencephalography for clinical medicine was soon appreciated. Electroencephalography is now an essential feature of the assessment of neurological disorders that prejudice responsiveness, and so are particularly relevant to the practice of aviation medicine. These are considered in Chapter 11 (Excessive Daytime Sleepiness: Clinical Considerations) and Chapter 12 (The Diagnosis of Epilepsy). Sleep electroencephalography has also proved to be a useful tool for the investigation of disturbed sleep in aircrew as it has enabled the accurate measurement of wakefulness in relation to rest periods. Such studies are described in Chapter 3 (Aircrew and Alertness).

Awareness

Awareness facilitates perception and is dependent on the wakeful state. It is a state wherein information becomes accessible. However, awareness does not imply that what is perceived is adequately interpreted. Interpretation demands higher nervous activity when the individual is 'aware of being aware', and that state is consciousness. Awareness makes perception possible and what is perceived may modify pre-existing consciousness, but awareness does not create consciousness. It must also be appreciated that there are limitations to the usefulness of studies on perception, such as binocular rivalry and blindsight, in understanding consciousness as opposed to awareness, as such studies are carried out in individuals who are already conscious (Searle, 2007). Essentially, consciousness embodies what is implied by 'the awareness of awareness', in that what is perceived is interpreted. However, for a discussion of the possible meanings of consciousness related to the practice of clinical neurology, the reader is referred to the paper by Zeman (2001).

Clinical Neurology

Awareness can have many meanings that are dependent on the discipline in which they are being used. It may imply perception without interpretation of the information gained or an activity that is synonymous with consciousness. The distinction between functions that can be ascribed to awareness and consciousness may not always be clear. Some authors, from time to time, may use awareness in the sense of consciousness, though they are cognizant of, and indeed contribute to, the complexity of the arguments that centre around the distinctiveness of awareness and consciousness (Zeman, 2001).

It is useful to regard wakefulness, awareness and consciousness as discrete functions of the nervous system, though with subtle interactions (Portas et al., 1998). For example, there may be no evidence of a sleep–wake cycle in the coma that can result from diffuse hemispheric or focal brainstem and/or thalamic injury (Plum and Posner, 1982; Plum, 1991; Schiff and Plum, 2000; Zeman, 2001), but the alternation of sleep and wakefulness may be preserved or regained in the vegetative state (Jennett and Plum, 1972; Zeman et al., 1997). It is accepted that the vegetative state may lack unambiguous signs of conscious perception and deliberate action, but the position with regard to awareness is less certain. With the preservation, at least in part, of the sleep–wakefulness continuum, it is possible that a degree

of awareness, though not consciousness, may exist. Indeed, whether those in the vegetative state are inevitably unaware has been questioned (Zeman, 2001).

These profound neurological disorders emphasize the complexity of responsiveness, but impairment of awareness is also relevant to many other aspects of clinical medicine and in turn significant to the practice of aviation medicine. Impaired responsiveness may arise from head injury (Chapter 16), and from disorders of the visual (Chapter 17), vestibular (Chapter 18) and cochlear (Chapter 19) systems as well as from transient and episodic disorders – in particular, epilepsy (Chapter 12), syncope (Chapter 13), hypoglycaemia (Chapter 14) and headache (Chapter 15). These disorders highlight the importance of the integrity of sensory systems to awareness, but also emphasize the part played by the central nervous system in the integration of awareness with the states of wakefulness and consciousness.

Spatial Awareness

As far as aviation is concerned, the issue of awareness is most importantly concerned with the spatial environment. Over the years, the discipline of aviation medicine has contributed significantly to the understanding of awareness in this domain. The physiology of spatial orientation is dealt with in Chapter 4 (Spatial Orientation and Disorientation). It is of interest that recent work has implicated the hippocampus and the entorhinal cortex in the central processing of spatial orientation (O'Keefe, 1976; Morris et al., 1982; Taube et al., 1990; Best et al., 2001), and it could well be that similar central mechanisms will be established as far as other senses are concerned. This is somewhat intriguing as it recalls the increased emphasis that was placed on brainstem mechanisms, as opposed to sensory input, in the control of sleep and wakefulness by the studies carried out by Moruzzi and Magoun (1949). It would appear possible that responsiveness in humans, as in the states of wakefulness and spatial awareness, involves discrete and intricate central neurophysiological networks. Perhaps this will also prove to be the case with the neurological substrates of consciousness.

Consciousness

The discipline of philosophy has had a significant impact on present-day understanding of consciousness, and its deliberations are consistent with the emerging understanding of its neural substrate. For critical discourses concerned with the part played by the discipline of philosophy in understanding consciousness, the reader is referred to the text *Thinking about Consciousness* by Papineau (2002) and the commentaries by Searle listed in the references (1999, 2000, 2007, 2009).

The Philosophical Dimension

Consciousness, like wakefulness and awareness, is a property of the brain. It is a highly developed evolutionary system that functions most obviously in the wakeful state when the individual is attuned to the environment and, possibly, during rapid eye movement sleep when dreaming. However, the conscious state implies far more, and the discipline of philosophy has been much concerned with the analysis of these attributes. It is evident that consciousness uses sensory information, though, significantly, consciousness is not entirely dependent on sensory input. Consciousness can exist in situations where there is little, if any, perceptual input, and perception is not an essential process for consciousness. The conscious state also displays physical attributes as with the initiation of bodily movement. It is also concerned with subjective feelings such as hunger, thirst and pain, though these may also have objective manifestations. Indeed, it is the totality of phenomenological and physical attributes that sets consciousness apart from all other neural systems.

The subjective attributes of consciousness raise the most intriguing question in the neurosciences. How can subjective phenomena arise from a physical process such as the activity of neurons? It is often claimed, though without any apparent evidence, that something that is subjective cannot be caused by neuronal activity. Yet it is beyond discussion that the brain is essential for consciousness, even though it is not clear how consciousness is generated by neural processes. Unfortunately, the subjective attributes of consciousness have in some minds tended to preserve dualism, and encouraged others to conclude that the nature of consciousness is beyond objective scientific analysis. Only a few years ago there was a similar assertion that it was not possible to explain the 'livingness' of living things by the action of molecules (Crick and Koch, 1998).

Consciousness is, indeed, a mystery, but its subjective attributes do not necessarily preclude a neural basis, and as conscious states can influence bodily movements it is reasonable to infer that the conscious state must have physical properties (Searle, 2000; Papineau, 2002). At this moment in time the causal link between neuronal activity and the subjective aspects of consciousness has not been established, but the search for the physiological characteristics and the neural substrate of consciousness is no longer outside the realm of scientific endeavour. Indeed, it is the remit of the discipline of neuroscience to solve this problem.

Neurophysiological Considerations

It is possible to extend the discussion on the physiology of consciousness by further consideration of the phenomenon. It is evident that the initiation of body movements, such as raising an arm, must arise from a mental event and, as a bodily movement involves synaptic processes, mental events must have physical properties. Consciousness is, therefore, a real phenomenon dependent on processes within the brain and possessing causal properties. At present, the anatomical substrate of consciousness is far less certain than those of wakefulness and even those of spatial awareness. There is the tendency to formulate neural models on the observed activity of single neurons. However, it is increasingly appreciated that the global activity of the brain is dependent on the interactions of many structures and cannot be inferred from the activity of isolated neurons that do not take into consideration the influence of the activity of neurons in other structures (Steriade, 2001).

It must be emphasized that the intrinsic activity of neurons is modulated by the activity of synaptic networks, and it is synaptic activity that relates to behavioural states. Further, it is the activity of neuronal networks such as those that involve the thalamus and cortex that generates brain rhythms rather than the intrinsic properties of neurons. This position is consistent with the philosophical analysis of the genesis of consciousness. For the purposes of discussion, Searle (2007) distinguishes between the 'building block' model involving sensory systems and the concept that conscious states are part of a unified field of brain activity. The former implies that consciousness is, essentially, made up of sensory activity, but the difficulty with this approach is that the subject must already be conscious to experience these sensory inputs. What needs to be established, in the first place, is how the brain creates consciousness and that suggests a unified function of the brain.

It has been proposed that certain neurons in the visual cortex (Crick and Koch, 1998) are specifically concerned with awareness, with the implication that the activity of these neurons is closely involved (possibly synonymous) with consciousness. However, Steriade (2001) has pointed out that it has been an undue reliance on studies concerned with the activity of individual neurons that has led to the idea that consciousness may result from the activity of limited sets of neurons, and that it is difficult to accept such a role for neurons whose activity is not, in any case, unique. Cortical areas outside those primarily linked to the visual system may also be involved in the process (Rees *et al.*, 2002), but it is, nevertheless, still difficult to reduce conceptually an even more complex function than wakefulness to the local firing of cortical neurons or even to associated widespread cortical areas.

A pervasive system that involves ascending and descending integrative systems along the long axis of the brain together with widespread cortical structures and their sensory and motor connections may be implicated in the physiological basis of consciousness. The reader is referred again to the paper by Moruzzi (1964) on the history of the deafferentation hypothesis for sleep. It was not until the middle of the twentieth century, some 2,000 years after the writings of Lucretius in the first century BC, that the role of the midline structures was established beyond discussion. Perhaps a similar story is evolving as far as consciousness is concerned, but it is to be hoped that its neurological basis will be solved in less than two millennia after the writings of Descartes on dualism.

The Neural Substrate

Adopting an unequivocal neural approach to the basis of consciousness naturally encourages curiosity for the search for an anatomical substrate with appropriate physiological characteristics. In that search it is useful to recall that the conscious state can initiate motor activity and that sensory experiences can influence its subjective manifestations. As the forebrain is involved in sustaining wakefulness and in awareness, it is, therefore, reasonable to propose that forebrain structures should also be capable of supporting consciousness (Villablanca, 2004). The property of consciousness may well involve midbrain systems, while the ability to initiate motor activity and its responsiveness to sensory experiences indicate the involvement of cortical structures and of their afferent and efferent connections. It is the possibility of the widespread involvement of neural networks in consciousness that has given rise to the concept of the global workspace (Baars, 1989; Dehaene and Naccache, 2001; Dehaene, 2009).

Of crucial significance to the search for the neural basis of consciousness is that the conscious state is not necessarily dependent on sensory input. That would imply that the substrate for consciousness involves intrinsic neuronal activity. There is tentative evidence for an integrative forebrain system with intrinsic neuronal activity independent of, though supported by, sensory inputs. The evidence comes from the studies on the intrinsic activity of neurons and on the activity of neuronal networks (Llinás et al., 1998; Llinás and Ribary, 2001; Llinás and Steriade, 2006). The substrate for consciousness would involve the corticothalamocortical system with neurons within that system possessing intrinsic activity. The input from the cortex to the thalamus exceeds that from the peripheral sensory systems, and it is proposed that consciousness arises from a continuous dialogue between the thalamus and cortex (Llinás, 1990; Llinás and Ribary, 2001). Such an approach suggests intrinsic neuronal activity within neural systems that are known to be concerned with responsiveness.

Aeromedical Perspective

Throughout the years that aviation has flourished, there has been the need to understand the nature of the threats to responsiveness that exist within the domain and to develop means that would help the aviator to cope. During the early years the skills of the respiratory and the cardiovascular physiologist were to the fore, and their work led to personal equipment that ameliorated the effects of exposure to altitude and positive accelerations. Essentially, the efforts of these physiologists were directed at preserving the integrity of the nervous system by ensuring, as far as possible, that alveolar and arterial gas exchange and blood pressure at head level respectively were as near normal as possible.

However, the solution to threats such as impaired wakefulness and disorientation and the possibility of mitigating the effects of hypoxia and hypotension on consciousness will depend on advances in the understanding of the reactivity of the central nervous system itself. Wakefulness, spatial awareness and consciousness are of obvious significance to the aviator, but each system is complex and preserving their activity presents a considerable challenge. The systems involve interactions between sensory and central systems. The central systems involve ascending structures from the brainstem to the thalamocortical projections and structures that include the entorhinal and neocortex.

What, then, have the neurosciences achieved that is of practical significance to the aviator in the twenty-first century? Advances in clinical neurology, as detailed in the later chapters of this book, have improved the accuracy of diagnosis and so the reliability of prognosis, and this is important in a domain that can involve disorders of wakefulness, awareness and consciousness. Defining the electroencephalographic correlates of sleep and wakefulness has made possible field studies on the quality of the sleep of aircrew operating worldwide. Understanding circadian desynchrony, together with sleep disturbance, has influenced the scheduling of aircrew and minimized the potentially adverse effects of sleep disturbance. Studies on spatial awareness and the dissemination of that knowledge have had a significant effect on air safety.

As far as the environment is concerned, studies on hypoxia have determined the pressures of the cabins of transport aircraft compatible with acceptable levels of cognition of the aircrew, though the advent of non-stop flights that exceed 20 hours in duration may lead to a revision of the current maximum cabin altitude.[3] Other studies concerned with the environment have involved the adaptation and acclimatization of the nervous system to hypoxia, including the behavioural sequelae and neuropathology of exposures to extreme altitude that could be encountered in decompressions in transport aircraft and space capsules. In that context, studies on mountaineers have provided the link in understanding the spectrum of effects from those of mild to profound hypoxia, and helped to determine the profiles of exposure to hypoxia that lead to permanent brain damage.

Impaired Consciousness

Impaired consciousness related to hypoxia and hypotension remains a hazard. Consciousness is concerned with introspection, memory and subjectivity, as well as the integration of perception and movement. These discrete functions are critical to the day-to-day effectiveness of aircrew. What is implied by 'time of useful consciousness' during exposure to a hypoxic environment is not all that clear. What is 'useful'? What is understood by 'loss of consciousness' during positive accelerations? Indeed, what is 'lost'? It has to be accepted that the physiological basis of consciousness is little understood and that the possibility of, at least, ameliorating an imminent state of unconsciousness, whether induced by hypoxia or by hypotension, is a considerable challenge. Little is known about the way in which the nervous system attempts to cope with impending unconsciousness, though that issue is considered later with respect to hypotension (Chapter 5: Cerebral Circulation and Gravitational Stress).

---

3   The Aerospace Medical Association (2008) has concluded that there are insufficient data to recommend a change in the currently accepted *maximum* cabin altitude of 8,000 feet. However, the *maximum* cabin altitude may be reduced to 6,000 feet in some transport aircraft under development. This development may be particularly appropriate for long-range transport aircraft involving sector lengths around 20 hours. It is claimed that this change, together with enhanced air quality and raised cabin humidity, will lead to improved well-being of aircrew and passengers.

It is possible that understanding the physiology of consciousness could lead to interventions that would extend the 'time of (so-called) useful consciousness' in an hypoxic environment and delay the onset of (so-called) 'loss of consciousness' during acute and profound hypotension. Progress in the pharmacology of neuroprotection directed toward the amelioration of a pathological state due to hypoxia or ischaemia has been disappointing (Johnston, 2006; O'Collins *et al.*, 2006; Endres *et al.*, 2008), but impaired consciousness due to a transient stress is presumably a reversible event and so may be responsive to pharmacological agents. In that context, the knowledge gained from research related to cerebral ischaemia may yet prove to be useful.

In any case, as far as hypotension is concerned, future advances in aeronautical engineering will lead to stresses that are far beyond an antidote that the flight of the imagination of the acceleration physiologist could concoct. This implies unmanned aircraft in the air superiority role, and manoeuvres could involve accelerations far exceeding those that could ever be tolerated by aircrew, even when supported by pressure garments and pressure breathing. Unmanned systems could afford a significant advantage in air-to-air combat.

However, autonomous systems sustaining G forces way beyond those experienced in manned aircraft in the air superiority role would still need to operate with split-second responsiveness. This would involve highly developed on-board artificial intelligence independent of the delays in decision making inherent in ground control. It is considered by the engineering fraternity that such developments could be achieved by the middle of the twenty-first century. The simulation of human cognition with the ability to solve problems would be the immediate requirement.

One day, probably not within the twenty-first century, the neurosciences will provide an understanding of the peculiarities of consciousness and of its manifestations in the same way that knowledge of the sleep–wakefulness continuum and of spatial awareness has been gained and the implications of disorders of the central nervous system for responsiveness have been explored. Understanding wakefulness and spatial awareness as states of the nervous system has proved to be of day-to-day relevance to the aviator, and understanding the conscious state itself will be critical to the emergence of machine consciousness.[4]

Conclusion

It has to be accepted that, in years to come, there will be limitations to the contribution that the neurosciences will be able to make to the amelioration of impaired responsiveness in aircrew. However, over the coming decades, both experimental and clinical neurosciences will play an important part in ensuring the integrity of aircrew in such a demanding environment.

Many hazards that lead, or could lead, to impaired responsiveness remain to be solved. They include impaired wakefulness in transport aircrew operating worldwide, disorientation in

---

4   Perhaps machine consciousness (or artificial consciousness) is far beyond even the foreseeable future, but machine consciousness has become an emerging discipline in recent years with its own journal – *International Journal of Machine Consciousness* (World Scientific Publishing Company). A technologically based simulation of the human brain may be possible, but the uncertainty of the emergence of machine consciousness appears to rest with conceptual limitations of consciousness itself. Perhaps it will be the understanding of consciousness itself that will, in turn, determine progress in the engineering world. The long-term prospects are discussed by Holland (2009), and the article provides a useful introduction to the subject. Further, Cleeremans (2009) has discussed briefly the conflict between unlimited computational ability and dysfunctional behaviour as experienced by Commander Data (*Star Trek: The Next Generation*).

aircrew operating in a three-dimensional environment, the possible adverse effects of prolonged exposure to mild hypoxia in ultra-long-range transport aircraft and the possibility of ameliorating to a limited extent the adverse effects of hypoxia. Further, though advances in aeronautical engineering are leading toward unmanned aircraft, G-induced loss of consciousness is a current problem (Lyons *et al.*, 2004; Green and Ford, 2006; Goodman *et al.*, 2006) and will remain so for many years.

Such hazards, together with the inevitability of clinical disorders involving the nervous system, will, for the foreseeable future, present challenges to the practice of aviation medicine. As far as the neurosciences are concerned, the ultimate challenge is to unlock the mystery of consciousness. When that is achieved, the door will be open to the incorporation of consciousness into autonomous systems (Nicholson, 2011).

References

Adrian, E.D. and Matthews, B.H.C. 1934a. The interpretation of potential waves in the cortex. *Journal of Physiology*, 81, 440–71.

Adrian, E.D. and Matthews, B.H.C. 1934b. The Berger Rhythm: Potential changes from the occipital lobes in man. *Brain*, 57, 355–85.

Aerospace Medical Association. 2008. Cabin cruising altitudes for regular transport aircraft. *Aviation, Space, and Environmental Medicine*, 79, 433–9.

Amzica, F. and Steriade, M. 1998. Electrophysiological correlates of sleep delta waves. *Electroencephalography and Clinical Neurophysiology*, 107, 69–83.

Baars, J.A. 1989. *A Cognitive Theory of Consciousness*. Cambridge: Cambridge University Press.

Batini, C., Moruzzi, G., Palestini, M., Rossi, G.F. and Zanchetti, A. 1958. Persistent patterns of wakefulness in the pretrigeminal midpontine preparation. *Science*, 128, 30–32.

Benson, A.J. 1999. Spatial Disorientation – General Aspects. In: J. Ernsting, A.N. Nicholson and D.J. Rainford (eds) *Aviation Medicine – Third Edition*. London: Arnold, Ch. 31.

Berger, H. 1929. Ueber das Elektrenkephalogram des Menschen. *Archive für Psychiatre und Nervenkrankheiten*, 87, 527–70.

Best, P.J., White, A.M. and Minai, A. 2001. Spatial processing in the brain: The activity of hippocampal place cells. *Annual Review of Neuroscience*, 24, 459–86.

Bremer, F. 1935. Cerveau 'isole' et physiologie du sommeil. 1935. *Comptes-rendus des Séances de la Societe de Biologie*, 118, 1235–41.

Bremer, F. 1938. L'activité électrique de l'écorce cérébrale et le problème physiologique du sommeil. *Bollettino-Societa Italiana Biologia Sperimentale*, 13, 271–90.

Caton, R. 1875. The electric currents of the brain. *British Medical Journal*, 2 (765), August 28, 278.

Cleeremans, A. 2009. Spock. In: T. Baine, A. Cleeremans and P. Wilken (eds) *Oxford Companion to Consciousness*. Oxford: Oxford University Press, 611–2.

Crick, F. and Koch, C. 1998. Consciousness and neuroscience. *Cerebral Cortex*, 8, 97–107.

Curtis, D.R. and Andersen, P. 2001. John Carew Eccles. *Biographical Memoires of Fellows of the Royal Society*, 47, 159–87.

Dehaene, S. 2009. Neuronal Global Workspace. In: T. Baine, A. Cleeremans and P. Wilken (eds) *Oxford Companion to Consciousness*. Oxford: Oxford University Press, 466–70.

Dehaene, S. and Naccache, L. 2001. Towards a cognitive neuroscience of consciousness: Basic evidence and a workspace framework. *Cognition*, 79, 1–37.

Eccles, J.C. 1970. *Facing Reality: Philosophical Adventures by a Brain Scientist*. Berlin: Springer-Verlag.

Eccles, J.C. 1994. *How the Self Controls its Brain*. Berlin: Springer-Verlag.

Endres, M., Engelhardt, B., Koistinaho, J., Lindvall, O., Meairs, S. *et al.* 2008. Improving outcome after stroke: Overcoming the translational roadblock. *Cerebrovascular Disease*, 25, 268–78.

Fulton, J.F. and Bailey, P. 1929. Tumors in the region of the third ventricle: Their diagnosis and relation to pathological sleep. *The Journal of Nervous and Mental Disease*, 69, 1–25.

Goodman, L.S., Grosman-Rimon, L. and Mikuliszyn, R. 2006. Carotid sinus pressure changes during push-pull maneuvers. *Aviation, Space, and Environmental Medicine*, 77, 921–8.

Green, N.D.C. and Ford, S.A. 2006. G-induced loss of consciousness: Retrospective survey results from 2259 military aircrew. *Aviation, Space, and Environmental Medicine*, 77, 619–23.

Holland, O. 2009. Machine Consciousness. In: T. Baine, A. Cleeremans and P. Wilken (eds) *Oxford Companion to Consciousness*. Oxford: Oxford University Press, 415–7.

Iber, C., Ancoli-Israel, S., Chesson, A. and Quan, S.F. (eds) 2007. *Manual for the Scoring of Sleep and Associated Events: Rules, Terminology and Technical Specifications*. Westchester, IL: American Academy of Sleep Medicine.

Jennett, B. and Plum, F. 1972. Persistent vegetable state after brain damage. *Lancet*, 1, 734–7.

Johnston, S.S. 2006. Translation: Case study in failure. *Annals of Neurology*, 59, 447–8.

Klein, K., Bruner, H., Holtman, H., Rehrne, H., Stolze, J., Steinhoff, W.D. and Wegmann, H.M. 1970. Circadian rhythm of pilot's efficiency and effects of multiple time zone travel. *Aerospace Medicine*, 41, 125–32.

Llinás, R.R. 1990. Intrinsic electrical properties of mammalian neurons and CNS function. In: *Fidia Research Foundation Neuroscience Award Lectures*. New York, NY: Raven Press, 40, 1–10.

Llinás, R. and Ribary, U. 2001. Consciousness and the brain: The thalamocortical dialogue in health and disease. *Annals of the New York Academy of Sciences*, 929, 166–75.

Llinás, R., Ribary, U., Contreras, D. and Pedroarena, C. 1998. The neuronal basis for consciousness. *Philosophical Transactions of the Royal Society of London Series B – Biological Sciences*, 353, 1841–9.

Llinás, R. and Steriade, M. 2006. Bursting of thalamic neurons and states of vigilance. *Journal of Neurophysiology*, 95, 3297–308.

Loomis, A.L., Harvey, E.N. and Hobart, G.A. 1937. Cerebral states during sleep, as studied in human brain potentials. *Journal of Experimental Psychology*, 21, 127–44.

Lyons, T.J., Davenport, C., Copley, G.B., Binder, H., Grayson, K. and Kraft, N.O. 2004. Preventing G-induced loss of consciousness: 20 years of operational experience. *Aviation, Space, and Environmental Medicine*, 75, 150–53.

McCormick, D.A. and Bal, T. 1997. Sleep and arousal: Thalamocortical mechanisms. *Annual Review of Neuroscience*, 20, 185–215.

Morris, R.G.M., Garrud, P., Rawlins, J.N.P. and O'Keefe, J. 1982. Place navigation impaired in rats with hippocampal lesions. *Nature*, 297, 681–3.

Moruzzi, G. 1964. The historical development of the deafferentation hypothesis of sleep. *Proceedings of the American Philosophical Society*, 108, 19–28.

Moruzzi, G. and Magoun, H.W. 1949. Brain stem reticular formation and activation of the EEG. *Electroencephalography and Clinical Neurophysiology*, 1, 455–73.

Nicholson, A.N. 2011. The neurosciences and air capability. *Aviation, Space, and Environmental Medicine*, 82, 574–5.

O'Collins, V.E., MacLeod, M.R., Donnan, G.A., Horky, L.L., van der Worp, B.H. and Howells, D.W. 2006. 1,026 experimental treatments in acute stroke. *Annals of Neurology*, 59, 467–77.

O'Keefe, J. 1976. Place units in the hippocampus of the freely moving rat. *Experimental Neurology*, 51, 78–109.

Papineau, D. 2002. *Thinking about Consciousness*. Oxford: Clarendon Press.

Plum, F. 1991. Coma and Related Global Disturbances of the Human Conscious State. In: A. Peters and E.G. Jones (eds) *Cerebral Cortex*. New York, NY: Plenum Press, 359–425.

Plum, F. and Posner, J.B. 1982. *The Diagnosis of Stupor and Coma – Third Edition*. Philapelphia, PA: F.A. Davis.

Portas, C.M., Rees, G., Howseman, A.M., Josephs, O., Turner, R. and Frith, C.D. 1998. A specific role for the thalamus in mediating the interaction of attention and arousal. *Journal of Neuroscience*, 18, 8979–89.

Rechtshaffen, A. and Kales, A. (eds) 1968. *A Manual of Standardized Terminology, Techniques and Scoring System for Sleep Stages of Human Subjects*. Washington, DC: United States Public Health Service, Government Printing Office.

Rees, G., Kreiman, G. and Koch, C. 2002. Neural correlates of consciousness in humans. *Neuroscience*, 3, 261–70.

Schiff, N.D. and Plum, F. 2000. The role of arousal and 'gating' systems in the neurology of impaired consciousness. *Journal of Clinical Neurophysiology*, 17, 438–52.

Searle, J.R. 1999. The future of philosophy. *Philosophical Transactions of the Royal Society of London Series B – Biological Sciences*, 354, 2069–80.

Searle, J.R. 2000. Consciousness. *Annual Review of Neuroscience*, 23, 557–78.

Searle, J.R. 2007. Dualism revisited. *Journal of Physiology – Paris*, 101, 169–78.

Searle, J.R. 2009. Biological Naturalism. In: T. Baine, A. Cleeremans and P. Wilken (eds) *Oxford Companion to Consciousness*. Oxford: Oxford University Press, 107–9.

Steriade, M. 2001. Impact of network activities on neuronal properties in corticothalamic systems. *Journal of Neurophysiology*, 86, 1–39.

Steriade, M. and Deschenes, M. 1984. The thalamus as a neuronal oscillator. *Brain Research Reviews*, 8, 1–63.

Taube, J.S., Muller, R.U. and Ranck, J.B. Jnr, 1990. Head direction cells recorded from the postsubiculum in freely moving rats. I. Description and quantitative analysis. *Journal of Neuroscience*, 10, 420–35.

Villablanca, J.R. 2004. Counterpointing the functional role of the forebrain and of the brainstem in the control of the sleep-waking system. *Journal of Sleep Research*, 13, 179–208.

Zeman, A. 2001. Consciousness. *Brain*, 124, 1263–89.

Zeman, A., Grayling, A.C. and Cowey, A. 1997. Contemporary theories of consciousness. *Journal of Neurology, Neurosurgery and Psychiatry*, 62, 549–52.

Chapter 2

CIRCADIAN SYSTEM AND DIURNAL ACTIVITY

Russell G. Foster

Our lives are ruled by time and we use time to tell us what to do. But the alarm clock that instructs us to wake or the wristwatch that tells us that it is time for lunch are unnatural clocks. Our bodies answer to another more persistent beat that probably started to tick shortly after life evolved. Embedded within the genes of humans, and almost all life on earth, are the instructions for a biological clock that marks the passage of approximately 24 hours. Biological clocks or 'circadian clocks' drive or alter our sleep patterns, alertness, mood, physical strength, blood pressure and every other aspect of our physiology and behaviour. Under normal conditions we experience a 24-hour pattern of light and dark, and our circadian clock uses this signal to align biological time to the day and night. The clock is then used to anticipate the differing demands of the 24-hour day and 'fine-tune' physiology and behaviour in advance of the changing conditions. Body temperature drops, blood pressure decreases, cognitive performance falls and tiredness increases in anticipation of going to bed. Then, before dawn, metabolism is geared up in anticipation of increased activity when we wake.

Historical Background

The constant adjustment of physiology by an internal clock is at odds with the original concept of homeostasis proposed by Claude Bernard (1813–1878) and Walter Cannon (1871–1945). For these physiologists, and the several generations that followed, constancy was everything, and deviations away from a 'set-point' represented a breakdown in homeostatic mechanisms rather than an adaptive response to a changing environment (Mrosovsky, 1990). Medical practice has been dominated by the concept of an unchanging internal environment, and students have been expected to learn a vast range of physiological parameters that describes the 'average human' over a narrow temporal range. However, blood pressure shows a substantial variation over the 24-hour day. It is considered in a healthy individual to be around 120 mm

Hg (systolic) and 80 mm Hg (diastolic), yet in the early hours of the morning it can drop by a third in healthy individuals (Millar-Craig *et al.*, 1978). Similarly, body temperature is not always set at 37 degrees centigrade. It reaches its peak around 20:00 hours and then falls by about a degree centigrade between 04:00 and 06:00 in the morning.

Certain hormones, such as melatonin and growth hormone, have low plasma levels during the day but these are elevated at night, while the incidence of epileptic seizures also increases at night. Such changes provide critical information relating to the potential health and performance of our species. In his pioneering studies on human biological rhythms, Aschoff (1981) made the point that not only is an awareness of these changes important for the practice of medicine, but it should also be used to help gauge the likelihood of accidents and performance-related mistakes in groups as diverse as night-shift workers, nurses and aircrew.

After almost a century of detailed investigation, the study of biological clocks has come of age and the clock-driven changes in physiology are being incorporated into mainstream teaching. Circadian biology – chronobiology – has not yet been entirely embraced by medical practice, but clock-driven changes are no longer ignored. The concept of time-dependent variables is replacing the 'fixed set-points' of former years. This knowledge is welcomed, although the practice of medicine has become even more demanding as yet another dimension has to be taken into consideration, that of body time. This chapter provides an overview of the mechanisms that regulate, generate and coordinate circadian rhythms. Although the study of circadian rhythms has its origins in the eighteenth century, it is only within the last 20 years that

a fundamental understanding of the neurobiology and molecular substrate of rhythms has been gained.

The first person to study biological rhythms in an experimental context was the French astronomer Jean-Jacques d'Ortous de Mairan (1678–1771). His interest in the rotation of the Earth led him to ask why the leaves of plants move up and down during each day in time with the 24-hour rotation of the Earth. In 1729 he placed mimosa plants in a cupboard and isolated them from the daily light and dark cycle. He noted that the plants still moved their leaves such that they drooped when it was night and were raised up during the day, even though the plants had no direct contact with the light and dark cycle. He suggested that these plants had to have some internal or endogenous knowledge of the time of day. A century later, in 1832, the Swiss botanist Augustin Pyramus de Candolle (1778–1841) made the observation that, under constant darkness, the period of leaf movement was not exactly 24 hours, and that it varied slightly between different plants.

This early work was pioneering, but the rigorous investigation of biological rhythms began in Germany with the studies of Erwin Bünning (1906–1990). In the 1930s Bünning worked on the bean plant, phaseolus, and showed that leaf movement oscillated with a mean period of 24.4 hours in constant darkness. He established one of the critical properties of all circadian clocks, that, when isolated from environmental cues, they persist with a period close to, but never exactly, 24 hours. This near 24-hour oscillation under constant conditions is the 'free-running' rhythm of the clock. Free-running rhythms close to 24 hours were then demonstrated in many different animals and plants, so that a collective term was needed to describe such phenomena.

It was Halberg who suggested that they should be called circadian rhythms. However, circadian rhythms are not the only biological clock-driven rhythms observed in nature. Other rhythms have been defined on the basis of their period under constant conditions and relatedness to environmental cycles. For example, circannual rhythms have periods of approximately one year and have been best described in hibernating mammals such as the golden-mantled ground squirrel. There are also circalunar or circatidal rhythms that have periods of approximately 30 days and are found in many intertidal organisms (Foster and Kreitzman, 2004). In parallel with the demonstration of free-running rhythms, Karl von Frisch (1886–1982), who studied bees, and Gustav Kramer (1910–1959), working on migratory birds, showed that animals must use an internal clock. Both studied time-compensated sun compass navigation. Bees and birds orientate their movements by using the sun as a navigational reference point. Bees will forage for nectar and locate different plants at specific times of the day, and birds will migrate at different times of the year. On average the sun moves across the sky at 15 degrees per hour, and both groups of animals consult an internal clock to compensate for this movement. In the case of birds migrating north in the spring, they will orientate so that the sun is 90 degrees to the left at 09:00, straight ahead at 12:00 and 90 degrees to their right at 15:00 (Foster and Kreitzman, 2004).

Circadian Rhythmicity

By the mid-twentieth century the stage was set for a more formal description of circadian rhythmicity. Pittendrigh (1993) pioneered the study of circadian rhythms in the fruit fly (*drosophila*) and applied his reasoning to a broad range of different animal models. He examined the nature of free-running rhythms, but his major contribution was that he went on to characterize and identify the fundamental properties of all circadian clocks, temperature compensation and entrainment.

Temperature Compensation

Biological clocks are temperature-compensated; that is, their period is more or less constant irrespective of environmental temperatures. The clock of ectotherms would be useless if it were not. Circadian clocks do not obey the Q_{10} rule as a rise of 10 degrees centigrade does not double the period of the oscillation. This issue of temperature compensation was a major point of controversy in the early days of biological clock research. It was argued that that no biological process could possibly act independently of temperature, and the constancy of the circadian period under different temperature conditions must mean that these rhythms were driven by some unknown environmental factor related to the Earth's rotation. However, Pittendrigh *et al.* (1973) showed that *drosophila* would always emerge from their pupal case (eclosion) at dawn, irrespective of the environmental temperature. This observation has been duplicated in many different species using multiple circadian outputs, but an understanding of how temperature compensation is brought about is little more than guesswork.

Entrainment

By contrast, the mechanisms that adjust biological clock time to environmental time (entrainment) are far better understood. A biological clock is only of any use if internal clock time is adjusted to environmental time. The classic example of a mismatch between biological and environmental time is 'jet-lag'. In the natural environment many factors could set or 'entrain' circadian rhythms to a specific phase of the 24-hour rotation of the Earth. Light, temperature, food availability or even social contact could indicate the time of day. However, only those factors that provide the most reliable indicator have been selected by evolution to entrain circadian clocks, and, for most species, the 24-hour change in the quality of light at dawn and dusk provides this signal or *zeitgeber* (Roenneberg and Foster, 1997). In the absence of light, other signals such as temperature or food can act as *zeitgebers*, but if animals are exposed to conflicting signals such as light and temperature, light will invariably be selected (Aschoff, 1981; Dunlap *et al.*, 2004).

Pittendrigh (1981) was one of the first to make a systematic study of entrainment. He explored the effects of short pulses of light on free-running rhythms in a variety of animals, including *drosophila*, maintained in constant darkness. He showed that light had different effects on the clock at different phases of the circadian cycle. As the animals were kept under constant darkness, he used the phase of activity of the animal to determine the position of the clock. In a nocturnal species, activity onset was considered to indicate the beginning of the night and designated circadian time CT (circadian time) 12. The subjective night would span CT 12–24, whilst in a diurnal species the start of activity was considered to signal dawn and designated CT 0 with the subjective day spanning 0–12. Pittendrigh (1981) observed that light pulses given to free-running animals during their subjective day would have no marked effect on the

clock, whilst light during the first half of the night (CT 12–18) would delay the clock. The animal would become active later the next day. By contrast, light given during the second part of the night (CT 18–24) would advance the clock, and activity would start earlier the next day.

A range of both nocturnal and diurnal species has been studied (Pittendrigh and Daan, 1976; Pittendrigh, 1981). Remarkably, all have shown the same basic 'phase response curve' to light (Figure 2.1), though the precise shape varies between species. In all organisms studied to date, including humans, light around dusk will delay the clock, and light around dawn will advance the clock, and in this way activity is broadly aligned to the expanding and contracting light–dark cycle throughout the year. The phase response curve (PRC) model of entrainment has been helpful in searching for entrainment mechanisms and the molecular components of the circadian system. However, it does

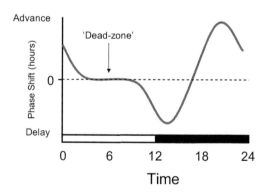

Figure 2.1   Generalized phase response curve of the circadian system

Illustrates the response to light administration at different phases of the circadian cycle. Advances correspond to an earlier activity onset (e.g. getting-up earlier the following day after the light exposure), whereas delays correspond to a later activity onset (e.g. getting-up earlier the following day after the light exposure). The 'dead zone' represents a period of relative insensitivity to light. Under normal circumstances morning light (0/24h) advances the clock whilst evening light (Dusk ~ 12h) delays the clock. In this manner circadian activity is appropriately aligned to the dawn/dusk cycle.

not provide a complete description of entrainment. It is not fully understood how light intensity, wavelength, the phase of exposure, the length of the free-running period, the magnitude of the advances and delays or even how photic and non-photic cues might interact to generate stable entrainment (Foster and Helfrich-Forster, 2001).

Figure 2.1 illustrates the response to light administration at different phases of the circadian cycle. Advances correspond to an earlier activity onset (for example, getting up earlier the following day after the light exposure), whereas delays correspond to a later activity onset (for example, getting up earlier the following day after the light exposure). The 'dead zone' represents a period of relative insensitivity to light. Under normal circumstances, morning light (0/24h) advances the clock whist evening light (dusk ~ 12h) delays the clock. In this manner circadian activity is appropriately aligned to the dawn/dusk cycle.

The 'Master' Clock

The existence of circadian rhythms and their basic properties of persistence under constant conditions, temperature compensation and entrainment were established by the 1970s, and interest began to shift to more mechanistic questions. If there is a clock, where is it? How does it work? How does light synchronize the clock to local time? Is there just one clock? How did clocks evolve? Progress in answering these questions over the past few years has been spectacularly rapid, and currently there is perhaps no better example of how patterns of gene expression and protein interactions generate a specific set of behaviours. An attempt to summarize some of the major findings is given below.

Early on in the hunt for circadian mechanisms, a conceptual framework emerged that placed the circadian system of all organisms into three basic elements. These were the input or entrainment pathway, the core circadian oscillator and an output pathway (Figure 2.2). Whilst this depiction has turned out to be overly simplistic, largely because different molecules often span an input/oscillator or oscillator/output function (Foster and Lucas, 1999; Roenneberg and Merrow, 2001), it has, nevertheless, provided a valuable model to develop experimental questions and define the various elements of the circadian system. The identification of the master circadian pacemaker of the mammalian circadian system has followed the classical approach in the neurosciences, starting with anatomy, followed by lesions, then transplantation to restore function, and finally *in vitro* and *in vivo* analysis. One of the major goals of neuroscience is to identify the anatomical substrates of specific behavioural control systems. This has proven frustratingly difficult in many cases, but the achievement of locating the mammalian master pacemaker is one of the success stories.

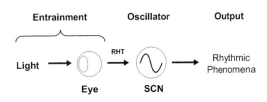

Figure 2.2 Schematic depiction of the key components of the mammalian circadian system

Light-entrainment signals detected by the eye provide an input to the suprachiasmatic nuclei (SCN) oscillator via the retinohypothalamic tract (RHT), and the SCN coordinating circadian patterns of physiology and behaviour.

Suprachiasmatic Nucleus

The seminal contribution of Richter (1967, 1971) to chronobiology was to help find the location of the mammalian clock. He conducted an extensive series of experiments, first of all, to confirm that it was the brain that housed the clock and, second, to try to establish where exactly it was in the brain. He removed adrenals, gonads, pituitary, thyroid, pineal, pancreas. It was only when he turned to the brain that he was able to destroy endogenous 24-hour rhythms. He made more than 200 studies investigating what happened if he damaged the rat brain, in which he measured the effect of the lesion on locomotion, feeding and drinking behaviours. He reported that lesions in the front part of the hypothalamus of the brain eliminated multiple behaviour rhythms, but he could not get any closer. However, Stephan and Zucker (1972a, 1972b) linked together the observations that the oestrus cycle was dependent on a small part of the brain in the anterior hypothalamus and that there was circadian control in the timing of hormone release. By careful lesions in the frontal part of the hypothalamus, they identified a small paired cluster of cells known as the suprachiasmatic nuclei (SCN) as critical elements in organizing rhythms of behaviour such as drinking and locomotion.

Retinohypothalamic Tract

At the same time, Moore (Moore and Lenn, 1972; Moore and Eichler, 1972) was using a different approach to finding the clock. Many studies had shown that there was an intimate relationship between the clock and light. The approach was to follow the light path as it came in through the eye. Moore and his co-workers injected radioactive amino acids into the eyes of rats. They followed the tracer molecules as they travelled from the eye, through the optic nerves, and concentrated in the suprachiasmatic nucleus (SCN) as well as the known visual structures. The newly found pathway from the eye to the SCN was called the retinohypothalamic tract (RHT). When the SCN was lesioned, there was a loss of the circadian rhythm of the hormone corticosterone. Essentially, Richter, Moore, Stephan and Zucker had established that removing the whole of the SCN (but not just a part of it) destroyed circadian rhythms in both behavioural and endocrine outputs. Just 20,000 or so cells seemed to be responsible for controlling the timing of the endogenous rhythms of mammals. Confirmation came from studies on the metabolism of the SCN. Schwartz and Gainer (1977) injected 2-deoxyglucose, and found that the SCN was metabolically active during the light phase of a 12h:12h light–dark cycle and relatively inactive during the dark phase. Significantly, no other brain region showed such a dramatic rhythm.

Transplantations: Tau Mutation

By the middle of the 1980s, several laboratories had shown that circadian activity rhythms in SCN-lesioned adult rats and hamsters could be restored by transplanting a foetal SCN. The final proof that the SCN contained the 'master clock' came from the chance discovery of a mutant golden hamster. One of the hamsters in a routine shipment of animals had a circadian activity period of 22 hours, which was far below anything seen before. This hamster was named the Tau mutation, and subsequent breeding experiments showed that this was a single gene defect and that two alleles of the Tau gene resulted in a 20-hour circadian period (Ralph and Menaker, 1988). Menaker and colleagues then used these animals as a tool to see whether the SCN was indeed the key oscillator. They asked the critical question. If the SCN was taken from a 20-hour mutant and transplanted into a wild-type SCN-lesioned host, would the recipient show a circadian period of the donor (20 hours) or of the recipient (24 hours)? The results were unambiguous. In every case the restored rhythm showed a period close to 20 hours. Likewise, when the transplantation was done the other way round, from normal to mutant, again it was the period of the donor that was restored (Ralph *et al.*, 1990). This specificity of the period was the unambiguous proof needed to satisfy even the severest sceptic. The hypothesis that the SCN contained a circadian oscillator was correct.

Soon after the Tau mutant transplantation studies, other researchers found that even individual cells in the SCN showed a circadian rhythm. An SCN was placed into culture and the individual cells were then dissociated from each other while supported on a multi-electrode array. SCN neurons fire at a frequency between 0.3 and 9.9 Hz. However, the overall firing rate of the rat SCN neurons showed a marked circadian rhythmicity averaging 24.35 hours, with peak rates of firing occurring during the subjective day (Welsh *et al.*, 1995; Herzog *et al.*, 1998). So not only was the SCN the anatomical site of the oscillator, but it was composed of individual cells that themselves oscillated and somehow co-coordinated their individual firing to give an overall rhythm. The hunt for the master circadian pacemaker of mammals dominated chronobiology for about 80 years, and establishing a central role for this structure represents one of the major achievements in the field. But,

as discussed below, the view of a master clock within the mammalian SCN simply driving peripheral rhythmicity in physiology and behaviour, as depicted in Figure 2.2, is an oversimplification. It is now clear that most tissues of the body possess the ability to generate a circadian oscillation independently of the SCN. The uniqueness of the SCN, however, is that it coordinates the clocks in other tissues and it alone is the only part of the brain able to restore rhythmicity when transplanted into an SCN-lesioned host.

Circadian Activity and Sleep

Appreciating the interaction between the circadian and sleep systems is fundamental to solving the problems experienced by aircrew who have to cope with time-zone changes and with irregularity of rest and activity. Sleep appears to be generated by two broadly opposing mechanisms: the homeostatic drive for sleep and the circadian system that regulates wakefulness (Figure 2.3). Together they interact to consolidate sleep. The homeostatic drive describes a process whereby the drive for sleep increases the longer an individual has been awake. In contrast with the established anatomical location of the circadian clock within the SCN, the brain structures regulating the homeostatic sleep drive remain unclear. Studies suggest that a build-up of adenosine, a breakdown product of adenosine triphosphate, in specific brain regions could provide the molecular basis for sleep pressure (increased sleepiness) during wakefulness (Basheer *et al.*, 2004; Wigren *et al.*, 2007; Landolt, 2008). The basal forebrain has been implicated in this process, whilst other brain regions such as the amygdala, hippocampus and cerebral cortex appear not to be involved

(Zeitzer *et al.*, 2006; Christie *et al.*, 2008; Krueger *et al.*, 2008).

The sleep–wake cycle is generated by two broadly opposing mechanisms involving the circadian system and a wake-dependent homeostatic build-up of sleep pressure (Figure 2.3). The circadian pacemaker located within the suprachiasmatic nuclei (SCN) coordinates a circadian rhythm of wakefulness throughout the day and sleep during the night. This is opposed by the homeostatic drive for sleep, whereby the sleep pressure increases during wake and dissipates during sleep. This process has been described as an 'hourglass oscillator'. The brain structures regulating the homeostatic sleep drive remain unclear. The circadian and

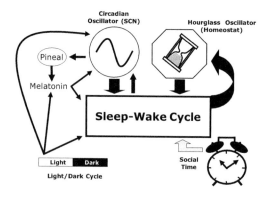

Figure 2.3   Diagram illustrating the key components in the generation and maintenance of sleep

The sleep/wake cycle is generated by two broadly opposing mechanisms involving the circadian system and a wake-dependent homeostatic build-up of sleep pressure. The circadian pacemaker located within the suprachiasmatic nuclei (SCN) coordinates a circadian rhythm of wakefulness throughout the day and sleep during the night. This is opposed by the homeostatic drive for sleep, whereby the sleep pressure increases during wake and dissipates during sleep. This process has been described as an 'hourglass oscillator'. The brain structures regulating the homeostatic sleep drive remain unclear. The circadian and homeostatic drivers regulate the multiple neurotransmitter and brain systems involved in sleep and arousal. Sleep-wake behaviour in-turn feeds back upon the circadian pacemaker and homeostat. These components are modulated by light which acts to entrain the circadian pacemaker to the environmental light/dark cycle, acutely suppresses melatonin production from the pineal and acutely elevates or suppresses levels of arousal. Finally, social activities such as meal times or forced awakening by an alarm clock will drive sleep-wake activity.

homeostatic drivers regulate the multiple neurotransmitter and brain systems involved in sleep and arousal. Sleep–wake behaviour in turn feeds back upon the circadian pacemaker and homeostat. These components are modulated by light which acts to entrain the circadian pacemaker to the environmental light–dark cycle, acutely suppresses melatonin production from the pineal and acutely elevates or suppresses levels of arousal. Finally, social activities such as mealtimes or forced awakening by an alarm clock will drive sleep–wake activity.

Sleep pressure acts upon a mutually inhibitory interaction between sleep-promoting and arousal-promoting systems. Sleep-promoting neurons localized in the ventrolateral preoptic area and median preoptic nucleus exert gabaergic and galaninergic inhibitory control over arousal-promoting cell groups localized in multiple arousal centres in the upper brainstem and diencephalon (Fuller *et al.*, 2006). Non-rapid eye movement sleep occurs as a consequence of the activation of neurons within the ventrolateral preoptic area and the progressive decrease in the firing rate of aminergic and cholinergic arousal-promoting neurons resulting from increased release of γ-aminobutyric acid (GABA). Both the activation of the neurons and the GABA release increase proportionally with growing sleep depth. After an adequate amount of sleep, wakefulness occurs at a circadian time during the transition from night to day (Fuller *et al.*, 2006). It is the circadian system that determines the timing of sleep propensity and wakefulness and is often defined as the wake-promoting system (Borbély 1982; Borbély and Achermann, 1999). In the absence of the circadian component, after an SCN lesion, sleep will still occur, but it becomes highly fragmented and is expressed as a continuous series of relatively short sleep episodes promoted by the homeostatic drive alone (Cohen and Albers, 1991).

Core Body Temperature

Core body temperature and/or plasma melatonin (the principal hormone of the pineal gland) also appear to be important in the consolidation of the sleep of humans and other diurnal mammals (Figure 2.3). A circadian rhythm in melatonin synthesis is regulated by a multisynaptic pathway that originates in the SCN. The rhythm in pineal melatonin is aligned to the 24-hour day so that melatonin is always released at night. It rises shortly after dusk and falls in anticipation of dawn. Melatonin synthesis is acutely inhibited by light. In humans, sleep is normally initiated during the rising phase of melatonin release and the falling phase of core body temperature (Arendt, 2005; Claustrat et al., 2005). Attempts to sleep during the declining phase of melatonin and the rising phase of core body temperature, as with night-shift workers, usually results in a shorter and less well-consolidated sleep episode (Dijk et al., 1999). If exogenous melatonin is taken during the day, it can induce sleepiness and produce an impairment of cognitive performance. Numerous experiments have shown that people can become sleepy between half an hour and two hours after taking melatonin (0.5–5.0 mg), but not everyone is similarly affected. And, not surprisingly, it does not have a hypnotic effect in nocturnal rodents. The SCN has high concentrations of melatonin receptors, and melatonin is particularly effective in suppressing the electrical activity of the SCN around dawn and dusk (Stehle et al., 1989).

The Molecular Clock

Forward and reverse genetics have been used to identify the components of the mammalian molecular clock. Forward genetics represents the classical approach for identifying gene function, and typically starts with an abnormal phenotype and attempts to isolate the gene responsible. By contrast, reverse genetics starts with a gene of interest (often due to homology) and investigates the effects of mutations or deletions. Forward genetic approaches in circadian biology were originally thought to be impossible in mammals due to the intensive nature of screening programmes. However, it was, in fact, a forward genetics approach that isolated the first clock gene (Clock) in mammals after the screening of only 25 animals (Vitaterna et al., 1994). Despite this success, the majority of the mammalian clock genes have been identified using reverse genetic approaches and understanding the molecular clock in drosophila. The success of this approach highlights the remarkable conservation of clock components between insects and mammals. Please note below: by convention, a gene is usually referred to in lower case (for example, PER) and the protein product of the gene in upper case (for example, PER).

Interacting Feedback Loops

The mammalian molecular clock appears to be the emergent product of multiple interacting transcriptional–translational feedback loops, comprising both positive and negative elements. The following is an attempt to summarize a current model of how all these interactions fit together to yield the molecular mechanism that enables the mammalian clock to tick (Figure 2.4).

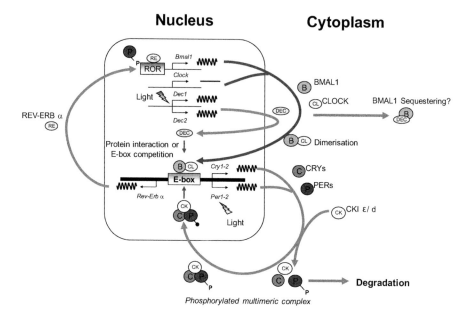

Figure 2.4   Mammalian molecular clock (see colour section)

The mammalian molecular clock is based upon a transcriptional drive produced by CLOCK:BMAL1 heterodimers. Clock is constitutively expressed, whereas Bmal1 is rhythmically expressed. The CLOCK:BMAL1 heterodimers bind to E-box enhancers in the Period and Cryptochrome promoters, producing rhythmic Per and Cry expression. Per1 and Per2 have a well-documented role in this feedback loop, whilst Per3's role is less clear. The resulting PER proteins are phosphorylated by CK1ε/δ and interact with CRY proteins to form a phosphorylated multimeric complex. This complex enters the nucleus and produces a negative feedback by inhibiting CLOCK:BMAL1-mediated transcription. An additional loop is produced via Rev-erbα, which also possesses an E-box enhancer activated by CLOCK:BMAL1. Rev-erbα acts via a ROR element in the Bmal1 promoter to inhibit Bmal1 transcription, thus feeding back to remove the positive drive produced by CLOCK and BMAL1. As the PER/CRY/CK1ε/δ complex re-enters the nucleus and inhibits the CLOCK:BMAL1 drive on the E-box, Rev-erbα expression is also reduced. This leads to a disinhibition (activation) of Bmal1, thus restarting the molecular cycle. The newly identified components Dec1 and Dec2 may modulate the CLOCK:BMAL1 drive by competing for E-box binding or sequestering BMAL1. Light detection by photosensitive retinal ganglion cells (pRGCs) ultimately alters the expression levels of Per1–2 and possibly Dec1. Altered levels of these proteins act to advance or delay the molecular feedback loops and so aligns the molecular clock to the light/dark cycle.

The driving force of the mammalian oscillator appears to be the rhythmic transcriptional enhancement provided by CLOCK:BMAL1 heterodimers. Bmal1 transcription yields rhythmic BMAL1 protein that heterodimerizes with constitutively expressed CLOCK. The CLOCK:BMAL1 complex binds to E-box enhancers driving rhythmic transcription of the Per1–3 and Cry1–2 genes. The PER and CRY proteins form homo- and heterodimers and translocate back to the nucleus, where CRY forms the negative limb of the clock by interacting with CLOCK and/or BMAL1 to inhibit Per and Cry transcription (Kume *et al.*, 1999; Okamura *et al.*, 1999; Shearman *et al.*, 1999 and 2000; Yu *et al.*, 2002).

A positive drive also occurs and, indeed, may be an essential component for sustained rhythmicity, providing the instability required for sustained oscillations. PER2 has been suggested to provide a positive drive on Bmal1 transcription (Shearman *et al.*, 2000), and *in vitro* assays have revealed that transcription of Bmal1 is enhanced by both CRYs and PER2, but is repressed by CLOCK:BMAL1, suggesting the presence of both positive and negative drives on Bmal1 transcription (Yu *et al.*, 2002).

These findings can be explained, at least in part, by the action of a nuclear orphan receptor Rev-Erbα (Reppert and Weaver, 2002). As well as driving the expression of PERs and CRYs, CLOCK:BMAL1 also enhances expression of Rev-Erbα via an E-box, and thus REV-ERBα protein synthesis. REV-ERBα then feeds back to inhibit Bmal1 transcription by acting through ROR response elements in the Bmal1 promoter (Preitner *et al.*, 2002; Ueda *et al.*, 2002). The inhibition produced by REV-ERBα is removed by the CRY negative feedback loop on the CLOCK:BMAL1 heterodimer, which leads to a disinhibition (activation) of Bmal1. The central drive of the clock may in turn be modulated by DEC1 and DEC2, as these proteins are capable of inhibiting CLOCK:BMAL1-mediated transcriptional activation *in vitro*, through either direct protein–protein interactions or competition for E-box binding (Honma, *et al.*, 2002). Light detection by the eye triggers a cascade of events that ultimately increases the expression levels of Per1–2 (Albrecht *et al.*, 1997; Shearman *et al.*, 1997; Shigeyoshi *et al.*, 1997; Takumi *et al.*, 1998; Zylka *et al.*, 1998) and Dec1 (Honma *et al.*, 2002). Altered levels of these genes and their protein products acts to advance or delay the molecular feedback loops and so aligns the molecular clock to the light–dark cycle.

Whilst translational delays are expected to occur between mRNA and protein synthesis (especially with post-transcriptional modification of large polyintronic mRNAs), these delays by themselves appear insufficient to provide a cycle of 24 hours. The discovery of a range of post-translational mechanisms that affect nuclear entry, protein interactions, phosphorylation states and degradation of the clock proteins will all build time delays into the molecular mechanism to produce the 24-hour output. For example, as the mutation in Ck1ε in the Tau mutant hamster results in a shortened circadian period and diminished rate of phophorylation of PER *in vitro* (Lowrey and Takahashi, 2000), phosphorylation has been proposed as one mechanism for providing time delays. In addition, the degree of phosphorylation of PER has been shown to affect its cytoplasmic retention, possibly by masking nuclear localization signals (Vielhaber *et al.*, 2000). Furthermore, the half-life of human PER1 is reduced by phosphorylation (Keesler *et al.*, 2000), and phosphorylation of PER1 and PER3 by CK1 results in rapid degradation via the ubiquitin–proteasome pathway (Akashi *et al.*, 2002).

The Whole Body is a Clock

Whilst early studies recognized the expression of clock genes outside of the SCN, the finding was ignored due to the essential role of the SCN in providing rhythmicity. SCN-lesioned animals lose their 24-hour rhythms. However, it has become clear over the last decade that the broad expression patterns of the clock genes in many, if not all, tissues appear to reflect oscillatory mechanisms that are independent of the SCN (Buijs and Kalsbeek, 2001; Balsalobre, 2002). The field of chronobiology was stunned when Schibler (1998) found that a cell line of fibroblasts cultured for about 30 years could be induced to show a 24-hour pattern of clock gene expression. He was able to induce 24-hour cycles of expression by simply treating the cultured cells with serum. Somehow, one of the many ingredients in the serum (or a combination) was capable of initiating a 24-hour oscillation of clock gene expression for a few cycles before the oscillation flattened and damped out. The rhythm could be induced once again with a further exposure to serum (Balsalobre *et al.*, 1998).

The possibility of peripheral oscillators made sense of a range of somewhat anomalous findings. Early studies had shown that, when food was available only for a limited time each day, rats increased their locomotor activity two to four hours before the onset of food availability. Critically, this anticipatory behaviour persisted after their SCN had been destroyed by a lesion. More recent work has shown that circadian rhythms of clock genes within the liver can function independently of both the SCN and the light and dark cycle (Stokkan *et al.*, 2001). Providing food for a four-hour period in the middle of the subjective day had little effect on the general nocturnal behaviour of the rat, but it showed increased locomotor and clock gene expression in the period before feeding. This suggests that food intake in itself generates an entraining signal for the liver and perhaps other digestive organs, and suggests that the hierarchical method is still at least partially valid. The SCN does generate rhythmic neural and hormonal signals that influence rhythms in other brain areas, in peripheral endocrine organs such as the pineal and in behaviour. Nevertheless, circadian oscillations in the liver (and perhaps in other peripheral organs) may respond more directly to the environment. This revised view of mammalian circadian organization emphasizes the possible role of behaviour in maintaining internal temporal structure (Stokkan *et al.*, 2001).

Hierarchy of Multiple Oscillators

The view of the circadian system in mammals has changed from a central clock driving all outputs to a hierarchy of multiple oscillators that include tissues such as the liver, heart, spleen, kidney, lung and testes. As such, the differences between central and peripheral oscillators have remained difficult to clarify. Synchronization of these oscillators may represent an inevitable consequence of multiple oscillatory phenomena, whereby any stimuli capable of transferring temporal information from one oscillator to another may function as a potential synchronizer. The importance of the SCN may simply reflect its privileged position of receiving light input from the retina, and its ability to modulate peripheral rhythms directly via hormonal and autonomic outputs, as well as indirectly through driving locomotor activity. Many years after Richter started to study endogenous activity in the rat, there is a return to one of his central themes. He showed that an animal maintains its internal stability through its general behaviour as well as through specific and automatic physiological processes. The recent studies on food restriction and liver activity suggest that there is a possible role for behaviour in maintaining internal temporal structure. Thus, models for circadian organization in mammals should include feedback loops from outputs, such as feeding, which may act as *zeitgeber* signals to assist in the overall regulation of the circadian system.

Photoreceptors and the Circadian System

A clock is not a clock unless it can be set to local time. So how is the master pacemaker in the SCN regulated by light? Loss of the eyes, like constant darkness, results in free-running rhythms in all mammals studied, including humans. However, claims have been made from time to time that mammals have non-ocular photoreceptors. There has even been a suggestion that humans have photoreceptors behind the knee as bright light shone in this region apparently shifted human circadian rhythms (Campbell and Murphy, 1998). It was an entertaining thought, but the findings could not be replicated (Wright and Czeisler, 2002).

All the experimental evidence shows that the circadian system of mammals is entrained exclusively via photoreceptors within the eye (Foster, 1998). The assumption, of course, was that the same light-sensitive cells within the eyes that are used for vision, the rods and cones, are also used to adjust the clock. This assumption, however, was incorrect. Until the late 1990s it seemed inconceivable to most vision biologists that there could be an unrecognized class of photoreceptor within the vertebrate eye. After all, the eye was the most understood part of the central nervous system. A century and a half of research had explained how humans see. Photons are detected by the rods and cones, and their graded potentials are assembled into an 'image' by inner retinal neurons followed by advanced visual processing in the brain.

The eye and the brain are connected via the retinal ganglion cells (RGCs) whose topographically mapped axons form the optic nerve (Figure 2.5).

This representation of the eye left no room for an additional class of ocular photoreceptor. However, mice homozygous for gene defects (retinal degeneration; *rd/rd*) and with undetectable visual responses were studied to determine the impact of rod/cone loss on photoentrainment. Mice (*rd/rd*) lacking all their rods and most cones were able to regulate their circadian rhythms with the same sensitivity as fully sighted animals (Foster *et al.*, 1991). These, and a host of subsequent experiments including studies in humans with genetic defects of the eye (Czeisler *et al.*, 1995; Lockley *et al.*, 1997), showed that the processing of light information by the circadian and classical visual systems must be different, and raised the possibility that the eye might contain an additional non-rod, non-cone photoreceptor. These data were far from conclusive, however, because there remained the possibility that only small numbers of rods and/or cones are necessary for normal photoentrainment.

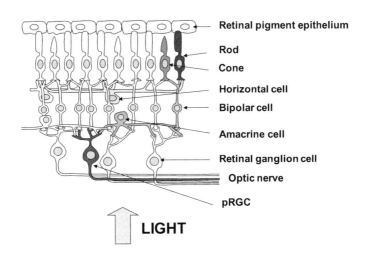

Figure 2.5   Cellular structure of the retina (see colour section)

As a result, a mouse was engineered in which all rods and cones were ablated (*rd/rd* cl). Remarkably, the loss of all types of known photoreceptor had little effect on photoentrainment, although loss of the eyes abolished this capacity completely (Freedman *et al.*, 1999). Mammals had to possess another ocular photoreceptor.

Retinal Ganglion Cells

These cells had been implicated as the photoreceptors, but the final link came from two independent approaches, one in rats and the other with *rd/rd* cl mice. Both showed that the retina contains a small number of photosensitive retinal ganglion cells (pRGCs) (Figure 2.5). In rats, a subpopulation of retinal ganglion cells was labelled by retrograde dye injected into the SCN. The retina was removed and the electrical activity of individually labelled RGCs monitored by intracellular recording. These cells responded to bright light. This in itself was no surprise, because the rods and cones were present in the retina. However, light-evoked depolarizations persisted in the presence of a cocktail of drugs considered sufficient to block all retinal intercellular communication, and even persisted in RGCs that were micro-dissected from the surrounding retinal tissue (Berson *et al.*, 2002).

The second approach exploited the *rd/rd cl* mouse retina in combination with calcium (Ca^{2+}) imaging. This technique is capable of detecting small changes in the concentration of intracellular Ca^{2+} in large numbers of individual living cells across the entire retina. The use of the *rd/rd cl* mouse meant that pharmacological or surgical isolation of ganglion cells from the rod and cone photoreceptors was unnecessary. This study demonstrated that approximately 3 per cent of the neurons in the retinal ganglion cell layer responded to light, but, after blocking gap junctions, the number of RGCs responding to light dropped to about 1 per cent. These results showed that there exists an extensive network of photosensitive RGCs that can be uncoupled by application of gap-junctional blockers. Furthermore, three types of light-evoked Ca^{2+} influx were observed in these neurons: a sustained, a transient and a repetitive response. Collectively, the studies in *rd/rd cl* mice identified a heterogeneous coupled syncytium of pRGCs (Sekaran *et al.*, 2003).

Melanopsin

The photopigment of the pRGCs was defined in the first instance by action spectroscopy. This approach rests upon the fact that a photopigment has a characteristic absorbance spectrum or profile, which describes the likelihood of photons being absorbed at different wavelengths. Thus, a description of the spectral sensitivity profile (action spectrum) of any light-dependent response will describe the absorbance spectrum of the photopigment upon which the response is based. All vitamin-A-based photopigments have a characteristic absorption spectrum. This means that although the peak sensitivity of the pigment may vary widely across the visible spectrum (ultraviolet at 360 nanometres to deep red at 750 nanometres), all these pigments have the same basic shape – rather like a bell-shaped curve. The first full action spectrum to define the nature of the photopigment of the pRGCs again came from *rd/rd cl* mice. Lucas *et al.* (2001) described a previously uncharacterized, opsin/vitamin-A-based photopigment with peak sensitivity in the 'blue' region of the spectrum near 480 nanometres (opsin photopigment/OP[479]). It remains unclear what selective advantage this wavelength might confer on such diverse species. One possibility is that the pRGCs are tuned to the dominant wavelength of light at twilight. When the sun is close to the horizon, there is relative enrichment of 'blue' light in the dome of the sky because of the preferential scattering of short wavelengths of light passing obliquely through the atmosphere.

Although the photopigment of the pRGCs had been described, the molecular identity of the opsin gene remained unknown. Melanopsin soon emerged as the strongest candidate. The melanopsin gene family, also designated Opn4, was first identified in *Xenopus* photosensitive pigment cells (melanophores – hence the name melanopsin), and then orthologues were isolated from other vertebrate classes including zebrafish and several mammalian species including humans and mice (Provencio *et al.*, 2000). Melanopsin was immediately implicated as the photopigment as it is expressed in pRGCs, and ablation of the melanopsin gene abolishes the pRGC responses to light (Berson *et al.*, 2002; Sekaran *et al.*, 2003). Furthermore, mice in which rods, cones and melanopsin have all been ablated fail to show circadian or pupillary responses to light, arguing that these three classes of photoreceptor can fully account for all light detection within the eye (Hattar *et al.*, 2003). Although highly suggestive, the melanopsin knock-out data could not demonstrate that melanopsin was the photopigment of the pRGCs. Gene ablation alone can only indicate that a gene is important, and biochemistry on the protein product is usually required to define its function. This critical issue was finally resolved independently by three different groups using heterologous expression of either human or murine melanopsin in Neuro2A cells (Melyan *et al.*, 2005), HEK293 cells (Qiu *et al.*, 2005) and *Xenopus* oocytes (Panda *et al.*, 2005). In each expression system, melanopsin expression was fully sufficient to convert a non-photosensitive cell into a photoreceptor.

It is now clear that the retina contains a population of melanopsin-based pRGCs that are used to measure environmental irradiance and entrain the circadian system. The initial assumption was that there would be little functional overlap between pRGCs and the rods and cones. It is now known that there is cross-talk between these image- and non-image-forming ocular photoreceptors. For example, the loss of melanopsin in the pRGCs alone does not abolish circadian photosensitivity, but attenuates circadian responses to light. It seems that under these circumstances the rods and/or cones can partially compensate for pRGC loss of function. Additional evidence for rod, cone and pRGC interaction come from recent studies on the macaque. Intracellular recording from melanopsin pRGCs has shown that the short-wavelength (S) cones (λ_{max} ~ 435 nm) attenuate the light responses of pRGCs, whilst the inputs from the rods, medium (M) (λ_{max} ~ 530 nm) and long (L) (λ_{max} ~ 560 nm) wavelength cones provide an excitatory input (Dacey *et al.*, 2005). The explanation for this opponent interaction remains unclear, but may relate to the complex task of twilight detection or the adaptive responses of the eye to differing levels of environmental illumination.

Aeromedical Implications

Although much may remain to be understood concerning the physiology and pharmacology of the circadian system, it is evident that the retinohypothalamic pathway plays a crucial part in the integration of circadian activity and the sleep–wakefulness continuum. The interplay of the neurological networks that support these systems determines vigilance, and in the aviation domain this crucial attribute is much at risk as aircrew have to cope with displacement of their body clock from that of the environment and with irregularity of their rest and activity inherent in operating worldwide. The current approach to the management of aircrew is based on present-day understanding of the circadian and sleep–wake systems, and this is dealt with in Chapter 3 (Aircrew and Alertness). However, it is evident that recent discoveries of the class of melanopsin-based ocular photoreceptors suggest much complexity in the organization and control of circadian activity. Unravelling this may one day indicate how circadian rhythmicity can be modulated pharmacologically and make possible the amelioration of the adverse effects of the repeated time-zone changes experienced by aircrew.

References

Akashi, M., Tsuchiya, Y., Yoshino, T. and Nishida, E. 2002. Control of intracellular dynamics of mammalian period proteins by casein kinase I epsilon (CKIepsilon) and CKIdelta in cultured cells. *Molecular and Cellular Biology*, 22, 1693–703.

Albrecht, U., Sun, Z.S., Eichele, G. and Lee, C.C. 1997. A differential response of two putative mammalian circadian regulators, mper1 and mper2, to light. *Cell*, 91, 1055–64.

Arendt, J. 2005. Melatonin: Characteristics, concerns, and prospects. *Journal of Biological Rhythms*, 20, 291–303.

Aschoff, J. 1981. Freerunning and Entrained Circadian Rhythms. In: J. Aschoff (ed.) *Handbook of Behavioral Neurobiology: Biological Rhythms*. New York, NY, and London: Plenum Press, 81–94.

Balsalobre, A. 2002. Clock genes in mammalian peripheral tissues. *Cell and Tissue Research*, 309, 193–9.

Balsalobre, A., Damiola, F. and Schibler, U. 1998. A serum shock induces circadian gene expression in mammalian tissue culture cells. *Cell*, 93, 929–37.

Basheer, R., Strecker, R.E., Thakkar, M.M. and McCarley, R.W. 2004. Adenosine and sleep-wake regulation. *Progress in Neurobiology*, 73, 379–96.

Berson, D.M., Dunn, F.A. and Takao, M. 2002. Phototransduction by retinal ganglion cells that set the circadian clock. *Science*, 295, 1070–73.

Borbély, A.A. 1982. A two process model of sleep regulation. *Human Neurobiology*, 1, 195–204.

Borbély, A.A. and Achermann, P. 1999. Sleep homeostasis and models of sleep regulation. *Journal of Biological Rhythms*, 14, 557–68.

Buijs, R.M. and Kalsbeek, A. 2001. Hypothalamic integration of central and peripheral clocks. *Nature Reviews Neuroscience*, 2, 521–6.

Campbell, S.S. and Murphy, P.J. 1998. Extraocular circadian phototransduction in humans. *Science*, 279, 396–9.

Christie, M.A., Bolortuya, Y., Chen, L.C., McKenna, J.T., McCarley, R.W. and Strecker, R.E. 2008. Microdialysis elevation of adenosine in the basal forebrain produces vigilance impairments in the rat psychomotor vigilance task. *Sleep*, 31, 1393–8.

Claustrat, B., Brun, J. and Chazot, G. 2005. The basic physiology and pathophysiology of melatonin. *Sleep Medicine Reviews*, 9, 11–24.

Cohen, R.A. and Albers, H.E. 1991. Disruption of human circadian and cognitive regulation following a discrete hypothalamic lesion: A case study. *Neurology*, 41, 726–9.

Czeisler, C.A., Shanahan, T.L., Klerman, E.B., Martens, H., Brotman, D.J., Emens, J.S. *et al.* 1995. Suppression of melatonin secretion in some blind patients by exposure to bright light. *New England Journal of Medicine*, 332, 6–11.

Dacey, D.M., Liao, H.W., Peterson, B.B., Robinson, F.R., Smith, V.C., Pokorny, J. *et al.* 2005. Melanopsin-expressing ganglion cells in primate retina signal colour and irradiance and project to the LGN. *Nature*, 433, 749–54.

Dijk, D.J., Duffy, D.J., Riel, E., Shanahan, T.L. and Czeisler, C.A. 1999. Ageing and the circadian and homeostatic regulation of human sleep during forced desynchrony of rest, melatonin and temperature rhythms. *Journal of Physiology*, 516, 611–27.

Dunlap, J.C., Loros, J.J. and DeCoursey, P.J. 2004. *Chronobiology: Biological Timekeeping*. Sunderland, MA: Sinauer.

Foster, R.G. 1998. Shedding light on the biological clock. *Neuron*, 20, 829–32.

Foster, R.G. and Helfrich-Forster, C. 2001. The regulation of circadian clocks by light in fruitflies and mice. *Philosophical Transactions of the Royal Society of London Series B – Biological Sciences*, 356, 1779–89.

Foster, R.G. and Kreitzman, L. 2004. *Rhythms of Life: The Biological Clocks that Control the Daily Lives of Every Living Thing*. London: Profile Books.

Foster, R.G. and Lucas, R.J. 1999. Clocks, criteria and critical genes. *Nature Genetics*, 22, 217–9.

Foster, R.G., Provencio, I., Hudson, D., Fiske, S., De Grip, W. and Menaker, M. 1991. Circadian photoreception in the retinally degenerate mouse (*rd/rd*). *Journal of Comparative Physiology*, 169, 39–50.

Freedman, M.S., Lucas, R.J., Soni, B., von Schantz, M., Munoz, M., David-Gray, Z.K. and Foster, R.G. 1999. Regulation of mammalian circadian behavior by non-rod, non-cone, ocular photoreceptors. *Science*, 284, 502–4.

Fuller, P.M., Gooley, J.J. and Saper, C.B. 2006. Neurobiology of the sleep-wake cycle: Sleep architecture, circadian regulation, and regulatory feedback. *Journal of Biological Rhythms*, 21, 482–93.

Hattar, S., Lucas, R.J., Mrosovsky, N., Thompson, S., Douglas, R.H., Hankins, M.W. *et al.* 2003. Melanopsin and rod-cone photoreceptive systems account for all major accessory visual functions in mice. *Nature*, 424, 76–81.

Herzog, E.D., Takahashi, J.S. and Block, G.D. 1998. Clock controls circadian period in isolated suprachiasmatic nucleus neurons. *Nature Neuroscience*, 1, 708–13.

Honma, S., Kawamoto, T., Takagi, Y., Fujimoto, K., Sato, F., Noshiro, M. *et al.* 2002. Dec1 and Dec2 are regulators of the mammalian molecular clock. *Nature*, 419, 841–4.

Keesler, G.A., Camacho, F., Guo, Y., Virshup, D., Mondadori, C. and Yao, Z. 2000. Phosphorylation and destabilization of human period I clock protein by human casein kinase I epsilon. *Neuroreport*, 11, 951–5.

Krueger, J.M., Rector, D.M., Roy, S., Van Dongen, H.P., Belenky, G. and Panksepp, J. 2008. Sleep as a fundamental property of neuronal assemblies. *Nature Reviews Neuroscience*, 9, 910–19.

Kume, K., Zylka, M.J., Sriram, S., Shearman, L.P., Weaver, D.R., Jin, X. *et al.* 1999. mCRY1 and mCRY2 are essential components of the negative limb of the circadian clock feedback loop. *Cell*, 98, 193–205.

Landolt, H.P. 2008. Sleep homeostasis: A role for adenosine in humans? *Biochemical Pharmacology*, 75, 2070–79.

Lockley, S.W., Skene, D.J., Arendt, J., Tabandeh, H., Bird, A.C. and Defrance, R. 1997. Relationship between melatonin rhythms and visual loss in the blind. *Journal of Clinical Endocrinology and Metabolism*, 82, 3763–70.

Lowrey, P.L. and Takahashi, J.S. 2000. Genetics of the mammalian circadian system: Photic entrainment, circadian pacemaker mechanisms, and posttranslational regulation. *Annual Review of Genetics*, 34, 533–62.

Lucas, R.J., Douglas, R.H. and Foster, R.G. 2001. Characterization of an ocular photopigment capable of driving pupillary constriction in mice. *Nature Neuroscience*, 4, 621–6.

Melyan, Z., Tarttelin, E.E., Bellingham, J., Lucas, R.J. and Hankins, M.W. 2005. Addition of human melanopsin renders mammalian cells photoresponsive. *Nature*, 433, 741–5.

Millar-Craig, M.W., Bishop, C.N. and Raftery, E.B. 1978. Circadian variation of blood-pressure. *Lancet*, 1, 795–7.

Moore, R.Y. and Eichler, V.B. 1972. Loss of a circadian adrenal corticosterone rhythm following suprachiasmatic lesions in the rat. *Brain Research*, 42, 201–6.

Moore, R.Y. and Lenn, N.J. 1972. A retino-hypothalamic projection in the rat. *Journal of Comparative Neurology*, 146, 1–14.

Mrosovsky, N. 1990. *Rheostasis: The Physiology of Change*. Oxford and New York, NY: Oxford University Press.

Okamura, H., Miyalke, S., Sumi, Y., Yamaguchi, S., Yasui, A., Muijtjens, M. *et al.* 1999. Photic induction of mPer1 and mPer2 in cry-deficient mice lacking a biological clock. *Science*, 286, 2531–4.

Panda, S., Nayak, S.K., Campo, B., Walker, J.R., Hogenesch, J.B. and Jegla, T. 2005. Illumination of the melanopsin signaling pathway. *Science*, 307, 600–604.

Pittendrigh, C.S. 1981. Circadian Systems: Entrainment. In: J. Aschoff (ed.) *Handbook of Behavioral Neurobiology: Biological Rhythms*. New York, NY, and London: Plenum Press, 95–124.

Pittendrigh, C.S. 1993. Temporal organization: Reflections of a Darwinian clock-watcher. *Annual Review of Physiology*, 55, 17–54.

Pittendrigh, C.S., Caldarola, P.C. and Cosbey, E.S. 1973. A differential effect of heavy water on temperature-dependent and temperature-compensated aspects of circadian system of *Drosophila pseudoobscura*. *Proceedings of the National Academy of Sciences of the United States of America – Biological Sciences*, 70, 2037–41.

Pittendrigh, C.S. and Daan, S. 1976. A functional analysis of circadian pacemakers in nocturnal rodents. IV Entrainment: Pacemaker as clock. *Journal of Comparative Physiology*, 106, 333–55.

Preitner, N., Damiola, F., Lopez-Molina, L., Zakany, J., Duboule, D., Albrecht, U. *et al.* 2002. The orphan nuclear receptor REV-ERBalpha controls circadian transcription within the positive limb of the mammalian circadian oscillator. *Cell*, 110, 251–60.

Provencio, I., Rodriguez, I.R., Jiang, G., Hayes, W.P., Moreira, E.F. and Rollag, M.D. 2000. A novel human opsin in the inner retina. *Journal of Neuroscience*, 20, 600–605.

Qiu, X., Kumbalasiri, T., Carlson, S.M., Wong, K.Y., Krishna, V., Provencio, I. *et al.* 2005. Induction of photosensitivity by heterologous expression of melanopsin. *Nature*, 433, 745–9.

Ralph, M.R., Foster, R.G., Davis, F.C. and Menaker, M. 1990. Transplanted suprachiasmatic nucleus determines circadian period. *Science*, 247, 975–8.

Ralph, M.R. and Menaker, M. 1988. A mutation of the circadian system in golden hamsters. *Science*, 241, 1225–7.

Reppert, S.M. and Weaver, D.R. 2002. Coordination of circadian timing in mammals. *Nature*, 418, 935–41.

Richter, C.P. 1967. Sleep and activity: Their relation to the 24-hour clock. *Research Publications – Association for Research in Nervous and Mental Disease*, 45, 8–29.

Richter, C.P. 1971. Inborn nature of the rat's 24-hour clock. *Journal of Comparative and Physiological Psychology*, 75, 1–4.

Roenneberg, T. and Foster, R.G. 1997. Twilight times: Light and the circadian system. *Photochemistry and Photobiology*, 66, 549–61.

Roenneberg, T. and Merrow, M. 2001. Circadian systems: Different levels of complexity. *Philosophical Transactions of the Royal Society of London Series B – Biological Sciences*, 356, 1687–96.

Schibler, U. 1998. Circadian rhythms: New cogwheels in the clockwork. *Nature*, 393, 620–21.

Schwartz, W.J. and Gainer, H. 1977. Suprachiasmatic nucleus: Use of 14C-labeled deoxyglucose uptake as a functional marker. *Science*, 117, 1090–91.

Sekaran, S., Foster, R.G., Lucas, R.J. and Hankins, M.W. 2003. Calcium imaging reveals a network of intrinsically light-sensitive inner-retinal neurons. *Current Biology*, 13, 1290–98.

Shearman, L.P., Sriram, S., Weaver, D.R., Maywood, E.S., Chaves, I., Zheng, B. *et al.* 2000. Interacting molecular loops in the mammalian circadian clock. *Science*, 288, 1013–9.

Shearman, L.P., Zylka, M.J., Reppert, S.M. and Weaver, D.R. 1999. Expression of basic helix-loop-helix/PAS genes in the mouse suprachiasmatic nucleus. *Neuroscience*, 89, 387–97.

Shearman, L.P., Zylka, M.J., Weaver, D.R., Kolakowski, L.F. and Reppert, S.M. 1997. Two period homologs: Circadian expression and photic regulation in the suprachiasmatic nuclei. *Neuron*, 19, 1261–9.

Shigeyoshi, Y., Taguchi, K., Yamamoto, S., Takekida, S., Yan, L., Tei, H. *et al.* 1997. Light-induced resetting of a mammalian circadian clock is associated with rapid induction of the mPer1 transcript. *Cell*, 91, 1043–53.

Stehle, J., Vanecek, J. and Vollrath, L. 1989. Effects of melatonin on spontaneous electrical activity of neurons in rat suprachiasmatic nuclei: An *in vitro* iontophoretic study. *Journal of Neural Transmission*, 78, 173–7.

Stephan, F.K. and Zucker, I. 1972a. Circadian rhythms in drinking behavior and locomotor activity of rats are eliminated by hypothalamic lesions. *Proceedings of the National Academy of Sciences of the United States of America – Biological Sciences*, 69, 1583–6.

Stephan, F.K. and Zucker, I. 1972b. Rat drinking rhythms: Central visual pathways and endocrine factors mediating responsiveness to environmental illumination. *Physiology and Behaviour*, 8, 315–26.

Stokkan, K.A., Yamazaki, S., Tei, H., Sakaki, Y. and Menaker, M. 2001. Entrainment of the circadian clock in the liver by feeding. *Science*, 291, 490–93.

Takumi, T., Taguchi, K., Miyake, S., Sakakida, Y., Takashima, N., Matsubara, C. *et al.* 1998. A light-independent oscillatory gene mPER3 in mouse SCN and OVLT. *Embo Journal*, 17, 4753–9.

Ueda, H.R., Chen, W., Adachi, A., Wakamatsu, H., Hayashi, S., Takasugi, T. *et al.* 2002. A transcription factor response element for gene expression during circadian night. *Nature*, 418, 534–9.

Vielhaber, E., Eide, E., Rivers, A., Gao, Z.H. and Virshup, D.M. 2000. Nuclear entry of the circadian regulator mPER1 is controlled by mammalian casein kinase I epsilon. *Molecular and Cellular Biology*, 20, 4888–99.

Vitaterna, M.H., King, D.P., Chang, A., Kornhauser, J.M., Lowrey, P.L., McDonald, J.D. *et al.* 1994. Mutagenesis and mapping of a mouse gene, clock, essential for circadian behavior. *Science*, 264, 719–25.

Welsh, D.K., Logothetis, D.E., Meister, M. and Reppert, S.M. 1995. Individual neurons dissociated from rat suprachiasmatic nucleus express independently phased circadian firing rhythms. *Neuron*, 14, 697–706.

Wigren, H.K., Schepens, M., Matto, V., Stenberg, D. and Porkka-Heiskanen, T. 2007. Glutamatergic stimulation of the basal forebrain elevates extracellular adenosine and increases the subsequent sleep. *Neuroscience*, 147, 811–23.

Wright, K.P. Jnr and Czeisler, C.A. 2002. Absence of circadian phase resetting in response to bright light behind the knees. *Science*, 297, 571.

Yu, W., Nomura, M. and Ikeda, M. 2002. Interactivating feedback loops within the mammalian clock: BMAL1 is negatively autoregulated and upregulated by CRY1, CRY2, and PER2. *Biochemical and Biophysical Research Communications*, 290, 933–41.

Zeitzer, J.M., Morales-Villagran, A., Maidment, N.T., Behnke, E.J., Ackerson, L.C., Lopez-Rodriguez, F. *et al.* 2006. Extracellular adenosine in the human brain during sleep and sleep deprivation: An *in vivo* microdialysis study. *Sleep*, 29, 455–61.

Zylka, M.J., Shearman, L.P., Weaver, D.R. and Reppert, S.M. 1998. Three period homologs in mammals: Differential light responses in the suprachiasmatic circadian clock and oscillating transcripts outside of brain. *Neuron*, 20, 1103–110.

Chapter 3

AIRCREW AND ALERTNESS

Anthony N. Nicholson and Michael B. Spencer

Duty periods of varying duration occurring at any time over the 24 hours and the disengagement of the circadian rhythm from the alternation of the day and night are potent causes of impaired alertness in aircrew. Indeed, the schedules operated by aircrew often have periods of rest and activity that predispose to disturbed sleep and/or prejudice alertness, and these difficulties have been appreciated since the advent of aircraft that could cross several time zones within a single duty period. However, although the importance of designing schedules that are compatible with acceptable levels of alertness has been generally recognized, there has been no consistent approach. These considerations apply both to the crew piloting the aircraft and to the flight attendants, subject to differences in the nature of their work.

Some authorities have implemented fairly detailed guidelines for flight-time limitations, based mainly on the experience of the aviation community rather than on empirical data. Others, with few guidelines in place, have relied on industrial agreements between the aircrew and the airlines. With the increasing complexity of worldwide operations, especially those involving transmeridian flights, and the advent of flights of extremely long duration,

together with the mounting commercial pressures on the airline industry, there is clearly a requirement for a scientifically based approach to the problem. In this chapter, laboratory and field studies related to the duty hours of aircrew are reviewed, and the emergence of models that attempt to predict the suitability or unsuitability of schedules examined. The implications for the formulation of flight-time limitations are then considered.

Rest and Activity

Early investigations of the sleep of aircrew were carried out during round-the-world flights with the Boeing 707 (Nicholson, 1970). They revealed that, during extended periods away from base, sleep patterns were disrupted by a combination of the timing of the duty periods, which often interfered with the normal sleep opportunity, and the desynchronization of circadian rhythms with the local environment. Almost a quarter of all sleep periods were naps of less than three hours, and a similar number were short sleeps of between three and five hours. In addition, some very long sleeps, extending beyond ten hours, were reported. Similar irregular patterns that appear to be typical of long-haul schedules involving several time-zone transitions have been observed on polar routes (Stone *et al.*, 1993) and during flights that involve inversion of the day–night cycle.

The first electroencephalographic recordings of the sleep of aircrew on arrival in a new time zone were carried out as part of an international collaborative venture in the mid-1980s (Graeber *et al.*, 1986). The routes studied were return flights between the United States, Europe and Japan, with time-zone transitions of eight or nine hours in both an eastward and a westward direction. They provided an indication of the large differences in the patterns and quality of sleep after eastward and westward flights. After westward flights, aircrew tended to go to bed in advance of their normal local bedtime, in the middle of their circadian night. More time than usual was spent in slow-wave sleep in the early part of the night, as a consequence of the sleep deficit associated with the extended daytime on the outward flight. However, because of the early bedtime and the rising circadian trend in alertness, sleep was generally terminated well before normal local wake-up time.

Sleep after a westward flight is normally consolidated into one sleep period per day. In contrast, sleep after a long eastward transition tends to be considerably fragmented, with individuals adopting different strategies. Sleep may, in some cases, be disrupted to the same extent as during the schedules involving several large time-zone transitions described above. Typically, after eastward flights across eight time zones, crews may sleep on three or four separate occasions during a two-day rest period and on four or five occasions in a three-day rest period, where the majority of the sleep periods would be less than five hours. Nevertheless, most aircrew achieve sufficient sleep overall,

averaging over seven hours of sleep in each 24-hour period. Many aircrew may deliberately split their daily sleep into two shorter periods, one during the local night and one during the night-time at home base. Thus, after a 12-hour transition the proportion of crews sleeping at different times during the 24-hour day was bimodal (Figure 3.1), with peaks corresponding to the home and the local nights. Other studies have shown that the sleep timing tends to be more closely related to the social rather than the biological night (Kandelaars *et al.*, 2006a).

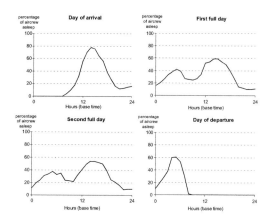

Figure 3.1   Percentage of aircrew sleeping at different times during the day after a 12-hour transition

Incidence is bimodal with peaks corresponding to home and local nights. Crews arrived at 07:15 base time on the first day and departed at 10:00 base time on the fourth day. Illustration derived from Spencer *et al.*, 2005. QinetiQ Limited: Report No D&TS/CHS/CR 50288/1.0.

Recovery of Sleep

The recovery of the sleep process after five time-zone transitions is quicker after westward than after eastward flights (Nicholson *et al.*, 1986). After a westward flight, subjects tend to fall asleep quickly and sleep more deeply as the rest period is delayed, but there is less sleep during the later part of the rest period (Figure 3.2). The normal pattern of sleep is re-established within a couple of days. After an eastward flight, sleep is delayed and disturbed for several days, with a delay also in the cyclical appearance of rapid eye movement sleep (Figure 3.3).

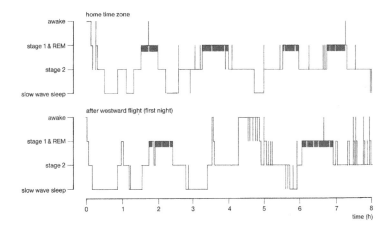

Figure 3.2   Sleep patterns (hypnogram) after a westward flight with a time-zone change of five hours (see colour section)

Source: A.N. Nicholson and I.B.Welbers (eds.) 1986. *Sleep and Wakefulness: Physiology, Pathology and Pharmacology*. Ingelheim, Boehringer (reprinted with permission).

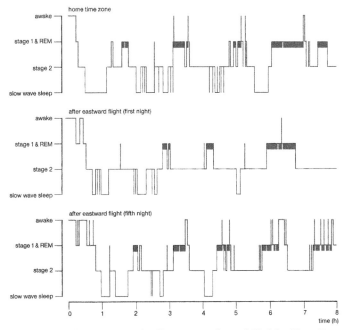

Figure 3.3   Sleep patterns (hypnogram) after an eastward flight with a time-zone change of five hours (see colour section)

Source: A.N. Nicholson and I.B.Welbers (eds.) 1986. *Sleep and Wakefulness: Physiology, Pathology and Pharmacology*. Ingelheim, Boehringer (reprinted with permission).

After ten-hour eastward transitions with rest at the normal bedtime, sleep times are reduced and sleep efficiency is degraded on the second and third nights, and some subjects experience sleep difficulties up to the fourth night. Furthermore, there is sometimes evidence of a rebound of rapid eye movement (REM) sleep, with reduced levels of REM sleep on the nights immediately after the flight, being followed, several nights later, by a large increase in REM sleep, amounting to as much as 40 per cent of the total sleep time. A rebound in REM sleep was observed on the fifth night in pilots on return from the polar route (Spencer *et al.*, 1991), and it may be that this event marks the completion of the recovery process, as subsequent sleep periods returned to normal.

With the exception of schedules involving multiple flights, such as those between Europe and Australasia, most long-haul operations now involve an outward and a return flight, separated by a rest period usually of two or three days (approximately 48 or 72 hours). In such cases, the length of the rest period does not allow sufficient time for adaptation to the new environment. However, the advantage of a short rest period is that the circadian disruption is limited in the new time zone, and crews are able to recover relatively quickly on return. Rest periods of only one day are generally not favoured unless it is clear that the timing and duration of the flights enable the crews to obtain sufficient rest. Such a short period of rest may not allow aircrew sufficient time to reverse the effect of any sleep loss generated by the outgoing flight (Lamond *et al.*, 2006). After a 72-hour rest following an inversion of the day–night cycle, sleep may return to normal after only three nights, though this does not necessarily

imply that the endogenous circadian rhythm has readjusted within that time.

Sleep disruption is not only a problem on long-haul operations across multiple time zones. A feature of many short-haul operations involving domestic and intracontinental flights is the requirement to provide a service to cover the early-morning rush-hour period. With a typical reporting time of one hour before the start of the flight, there are examples of operations in which almost half of all duty periods start before 07:00 (Powell *et al.*, 2007). Although aircrew tend to advance their bedtime to allow for the earlier wake-up times, they rarely achieve a normal amount of sleep. This is partly due to the problems of sleeping at an earlier time on the circadian clock (Folkard and Barton, 1993). As a consequence, the duration of sleep tends to be reduced by approximately 30 minutes for each hour that the report time is earlier than 09:00 (Figure 3.4). There is little evidence that aircrew adapt their sleep pattern to the earlier start times, even when the early report times continue over several consecutive days.

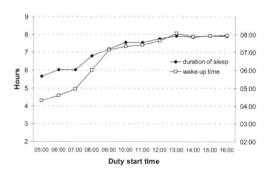

Figure 3.4   Duration of sleep in hours and wake-up time prior to the start of duty

Source: Illustration derived from Spencer & Robertson, 2000. Defence Evaluation and Research Agency: Report No CHS/PPD/CRO00394.

Other operations, particularly those involving charter flights for the leisure industry, contain a mixture of early starts, late finishes and duties that continue through the night. Sleep disruption is likely to be associated with these irregular patterns and particular problems are associated with night duties (Samel *et al.*, 1997a). The amount of sleep that is lost after a late finish depends on the time at which the duty ends. Sleep may average more than six hours when duties end between midnight and 02:00, but average around five hours when duty ends between 03:00 and 05:00, and around four hours when duty ends between 06:00 and 08:00 (Figure 3.5). The extent to which sleep patterns may adapt over consecutive nights is uncertain, but given the lack of evidence of a significant circadian adaptation, it is unlikely that any substantial recovery of sleep is achieved in the majority of cases.

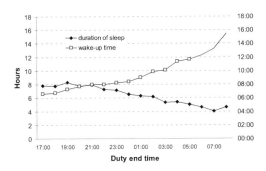

Figure 3.5   Duration of sleep in hours and wake-up time after the end of duty

Source: Illustration derived from Robertson & Spencer, 2003. QinetiQ Limited: Report No KI/CHS/CR021911/1.0.

In-Flight Sleep

Sometimes aircrew may be able to obtain some sleep in the form of a short nap during the flight itself. It has been proposed (Rosekind *et al.*, 1994) that a planned period of one hour could be set aside during the cruise, when one of the operating crew would be given the opportunity to sleep for up to 40 minutes. Such a procedure must be carefully managed to ensure that the other crew member remains awake and alert during that period, and that sufficient time is provided after waking to ensure that any subsequent sleep inertia has dissipated before the pilot returns to the controls. On longer flights additional aircrew may be carried, and this has been shown to lead to reduced levels of sleepiness (Eriksen *et al.*, 2006).

Often a sleep facility is provided in the form of a compartment in the cabin area with a bunk, separated from the passengers. Various studies using polysomnography have shown that pilots are able to obtain recuperative sleep in such a facility, and sleep of as much as six hours has been recorded in flight. Other studies have used subjective data from a large number of different flights to derive predictions for the quantity and quality of in-flight sleep, dependent on the time of day and the length of the rest period. Except at the most unfavourable times of day, crews are able to sleep during at least a quarter of the time allocated to them for rest, and this rises to over a half if the rest period is overnight (Figure 3.6). However, when crews are unacclimatized at the point of departure, their sleep is liable to be less restful.

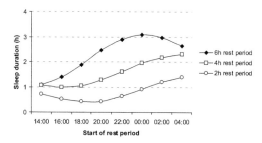

Figure 3.6   Trends in sleep duration (hours) in a bunk related to the start of the rest period

Source: Illustration derived from Spencer, 2002. QinetiQ Limited: Report No HS/PPD/CRO10406/1.0.

To overcome the problems of trying to sleep during a rest period at a difficult time of day when not yet sufficiently tired, it is sometimes preferable for a pilot to take two short rest periods rather than a single long rest period. The allocation of two rest periods per pilot has been shown to work well on the new generation of very long-range aircraft, where individual flights may last for 18 hours or even longer. On flights of over 18 hours most crews report achieving a total of between two and five hours of sleep, and on very few flights do they fail to sleep at all. However, to achieve reasonable sleep it is important that the rest facilities are well designed and that care is taken to limit sources of disturbance. Noise, including the background noise from the aircraft, is a major disturbing factor, together with poor temperature control and inadequate bedding. In well-designed facilities sleep disturbance can be eliminated or reduced considerably, but aircraft turbulence may still cause a problem.

Where in-flight sleep facilities are not available, crews are sometimes provided with a reclining seat, possibly screened from the other passengers. Few data are available on the quality of sleep of aircrew resting in such conditions, though crews report greater difficulty in getting to sleep and remaining asleep in a passenger seat and report that their sleep is reduced by approximately a quarter compared with sleeping in a bunk. They also report more frequent use of earplugs and eyeshades. However, much depends on the quality of the seat provided. In a laboratory study of sleep in a seat with various back angles to the vertical of less than 90 degrees, adequate sleep was obtained as long as the back angle to the vertical approached 40 degrees (Nicholson and Stone, 1987), though a fully reclining seat on the flight deck is unlikely to provide much good-quality sleep.

Circadian Adaptation

A critical issue for aircrew operating many different types of schedules is their ability to adapt to duties at a different time of day or in a new time zone. After a long transmeridian flight, their circadian rhythms do not adjust immediately to the new local time and a full adjustment may take several days. Various simple rules have been suggested for the rate of resynchronization, including a shift in the circadian phase of one hour per day or a halving of the phase difference every two days (Klein and Wegmann, 1980). However, the patterns of adaptation tend to be more complex and to differ between eastward and westward flights (Sasaki, 1964). Wegmann and Klein (1985) reported that adjustment of the temperature rhythm to a six-hour time-zone shift was not complete until ten days after a westward transition and 13 days after an eastward transition. However, after a nine-hour eastward shift, the same authors noted that, whereas some individuals readapted by a phase advance, others readapted by a phase delay (Klein and Wegmann, 1980). Thus, their circadian rhythm had delayed by a full 24 hours before resynchronizing with home time. A similar division between those advancing and those delaying their rhythm has also been reported after a simulated ten-hour eastward transition, and in all these studies there were uneven patterns of adaptation as well as large individual differences in the rates of adaptation.

The practical difficulties of monitoring physiological parameters in operating aircrew have meant that most studies of circadian rhythms have been carried out on volunteers rather than on the aircrew themselves. However, recordings of rectal temperature have been made in aircrew operating the polar route from the United Kingdom to Tokyo, throughout the trip itself and for nine days after the return (Spencer *et al.*, 1991). The eight-hour eastward transition was accomplished by two consecutive westward transitions of nine and seven hours, with individual rest periods of approximately 24, 72 and 24 hours in Anchorage, Tokyo and Anchorage respectively. From the pattern of adaptation on return (Figure 3.7), it was clear that the circadian rhythms of the crews had responded very differently to the various time-zone transitions. This emphasizes the extent of the variability in the patterns and speed of readaptation after schedules involving long transmeridian flights.

Estimation of rates of adaptation of physiological parameters is complicated by the presence of confounding factors that tend to conceal the underlying rhythm. These so-called 'masking effects' may themselves contain rhythmical elements related, for example, to the patterns of sleep and wakefulness, activity, or eating and drinking. These exogenous patterns are often difficult to distinguish from the endogenous rhythm, even in a laboratory environment. The problem becomes many times more

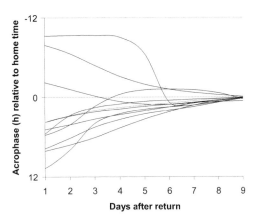

Figure 3.7   Circadian rhythms of aircrew on return from a polar flight

Source: Spencer et al., 1991. *Aviation Space and Environmental Medicine*, 62, 3–13: with permission.

complex in the uncontrolled or partially controlled setting of a field trial. Masking effects have ruled out the majority of biochemical and hormonal variables as markers for the endogenous rhythm. One exception is the timing of the normal nocturnal onset of urinary melatonin that has been found to be a reliable marker of circadian phase (Lushington *et al.*, 1996). However, the estimation of the onset is limited by the frequency of urinary collection, and precision may be considerably reduced when the onset occurs in the middle of a long period of sleep. Even rectal temperature, which has been used in many laboratory experiments and field trials as a marker of circadian phase, is subject to masking effects, particularly those related to the pattern of rest and activity. Attempts of varying mathematical complexity (Spencer, 1989; Folkard *et al.*, 1991) have been made to correct for masking, and in many cases these may provide the most reliable estimates of the underlying rhythm that can be achieved.

Mathematical Models

Mathematical models to predict the behaviour of circadian rhythms have been derived from experiments where time cues have either been completely removed (temporal isolation) or systematically controlled. Many of these models have been based on an extended van der Pol equation:

$$\frac{d^2y}{dt^2} + \varepsilon\left(y^2 - 1\right)\frac{dy}{dt} + y = z$$

where y represents the state of the system (the circadian oscillation) as a function of time, ε is the non-linear damping or 'stiffness' parameter, and z represents the external forces or time cues. In the absence of an external force, the solutions of the van der Pol equation are oscillations of constant period which, in the current area of application, may be taken to represent a free-running circadian rhythm. However, the oscillations can become entrained by a sufficiently strong periodic force within a given frequency range, thereby replicating the entrainment of the circadian rhythm by time cues with periodicities in the region of 24 hours.

The model was first adopted by Wever (1984) who simulated time-zone transitions of six and 12 hours by phase-shifting the external force z (Wever, 1966). Kronauer (1984) proposed a system of two coupled van der Pol oscillators, one representing the temperature rhythm, the other the pattern of rest and activity, and simulations based on this model were compared with the results of experimental time-zone shifts (Gander et al., 1985). Indeed, parameter values for a single oscillator representing the temperature rhythm have been derived from various laboratory and flight experiments (Gundel and Spencer, 1992; Spencer, 1992). Simulations using this model fit well with the results from a field trial involving a large eastward transition (Gundel and Spencer, 1999), in which individual differences in the pattern of adaptation were represented by a different choice of parameters. This model is able to reproduce the uncertainty in the direction of readaptation observed after long eastward transitions. Further, depending on the choice of the stiffness parameter, it predicts that the period of readaptation may be accompanied by a marked reduction in the amplitude of the rhythm, lasting for several days.

The question arises whether some form of circadian adaptation can occur when aircrew undertake irregular schedules that do not involve any flights across times zones. This possibility is most likely when crews undertake a series of night flights. Although there are, as yet, no studies of the circadian adaptation of aircrew to night operations, many studies have been carried out on night workers engaged in various other forms of activity. In a review of the literature on the adjustment to permanent night work of the endogenous melatonin rhythm (Folkard, 2008), it was concluded that less than a quarter of night workers adjust sufficiently to derive any significant benefit. Until suitable data from air operations are available, it would be difficult to argue that aircrew are a special case and that night operations generate a significant circadian disruption.

Alertness of Aircrew

Early studies on the alertness of aircrew were carried out during transatlantic flights (Samel et al., 1997b). The crews were assessed at set times throughout the flights using electroencephalography and the monitoring of microsleeps. Various questionnaires and subjective assessments were also completed at hourly intervals. One of the checklists reflected the momentary subjective feeling of the aircrew. During the flights there was a steady move away from the 'Very Alert' extreme of the list, and this was consistent with the physiological recordings (Figure 3.8).

Nowadays, for reasons of economy, the majority of in-flight investigations mainly use subjective assessments of levels of alertness either recorded into a diary format or entered into a portable computer. The most commonly used subjective measures are the modified version of the Samn–Perelli seven-point fatigue scale (SPS) and the nine-point Karolinska Sleepiness Scale (KSS). The SPS (Samn and Perelli, 1981) is a validated scale with ranges between 1 (fully alert, wide awake) and 7 (completely exhausted), and when it reaches a value of 5 or 6, it is considered that some performance impairment is probably occurring and that flying duty is permissible but not recommended.

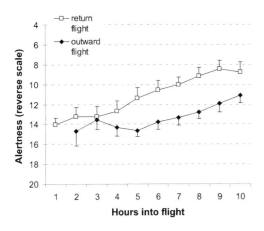

Figure 3.8   Alertness ratings during flights

Outward flights departed from Hamburg at 13:30 local time with the return flight departing from Los Angeles (nine time zones west of Hamburg) two days later at 18:00 local time. Ratings were obtained from the 20-point Samn-Perelli checklist (low scores correspond to low levels of alertness). The bars represent one standard error of the mean. Illustration derived from: Samel et al.,1997b. Aircrew fatigue in long-haul operations. *Accident Analysis and Prevention*, 29,439–452.

The nine-point Karolinska Sleepiness Scale (KSS) is a measure of sleepiness (Akerstedt and Gillberg, 1990) and has been validated with respect to decrements in performance and objective measures of sleepiness (Gillberg *et al.*, 1994). A rating of 7 has been equated with visual correlates of sleepiness such as drooping eyelids. In some studies, subjective information has been augmented by data from simple tests of vigilance and reaction time that aircrew carry out on the flight deck. However, the uninterrupted administration of these tests in the flight-deck environment can be difficult to achieve, and the results are not always easy to interpret.

Studies of aircrew operating from the United Kingdom (Civil Aviation Authority, 2005) and New Zealand (Powell *et al.*, 2007; Powell *et al.*, 2008) have substantially increased our understanding of the factors that contribute to impaired alertness in civil air operations, and have led to the development of models relating impaired alertness to the schedules operated by aircrew (Belyavin and Spencer, 2004). In particular, these studies have helped to clarify the impact of the start time of duty on long-haul two-crew operations. Flights have been carried out under similar conditions at different times of day, and ratings obtained at approximately equally spaced times during each duty period. The trends are illustrated in Figure 3.9 as a function of the time of day at the start of duty. The highest levels of impaired alertness on reporting for duty are between 02:00 and 04:00, at times when an unfavourable circadian phase is combined with short pre-duty sleep. However, the sharpest increase during the flights themselves occurs on duties starting in the late afternoon and early evening, when the duration of the flight corresponds with the ongoing reduction in circadian alertness.

Limited information is available on the effects of layovers of different duration on subsequent levels of alertness (Powell *et al.*, 2010). Crews require time to recover from the most severe effects of sleep disruption, and a 12-hour period is insufficient if the return flight is overnight (Samel *et al.*, 1997a). However, it appears that increasing the length of the layover from one to two days may confer limited benefit for alertness levels during an overnight return (Figure 3.10). Where large time-zone differences are involved, an important consideration is that a longer layover increases the exposure to time cues in the new location and hence promotes circadian adaptation. Crews are therefore likely to take longer to resynchronize their rhythms to home time on return.

Levels of alertness during flights that involve additional pilots (augmented crews) are strongly influenced by the timing of the rest periods. There is a steady decrease in levels of alertness throughout flights, except during the rest periods themselves where this is

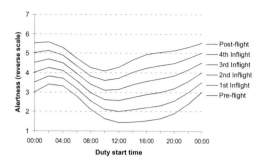

Figure 3.10 Alertness on outward and return flights after one- and two-day layovers

Alertness, on the seven-point Samn-Perelli scale (high values correspond to low levels of alertness), on flights between Dubai and Perth. The flights departed at approximately 02:00 (outward) and 22:00 (return) local time, and the durations were 10.5 and 11.5 hours respectively. Illustration derived from Spencer et al., 2004. QinetiQ Limited: Report No KI/CHS/CR03236/2.0.

temporarily either halted or reversed (Figure 3.11). Overall, the lowest levels are at the end of the flight when the departure time is in the morning, and at the start of the mid-flight rest period when the departure time is in the evening. Low levels of alertness can arise on very long flights involving continuous periods at the controls, and these are a cause for concern. For this reason, two rest periods may be appropriate on many ultra-long-range operations, and this has proved to be a successful strategy for maintaining alertness levels throughout the longest flights.

On operations over a shorter range, several factors have been shown to influence levels of alertness. Among the most important, as on long-haul operations, are the time of day and the duration of the duty period (Powell *et al.*, 2008). The lowest levels of alertness are observed during long duty periods that have continued through the night and where the final top of descent is in the late morning (Figure 3.12). Unlike many long-haul flights, where the level of activity during the cruise phase is often very low, the workload on short-

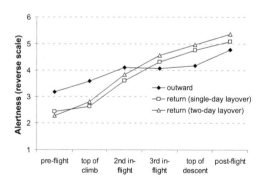

Figure 3.9   Trends fitted to alertness levels as a function of time of day at the start of duty

Alertness, on the seven-point Samn-Perelli scale (high values correspond to low levels of alertness), as reported by crews on the outward flight from Indonesia to Saudi Arabia. Duty periods were between 11 and 11.5 hours. Illustration derived from Spencer & Robertson, 1999. Defence Evaluation and Research Agency: Report No DERA/CHS/PPD/ CR980207.

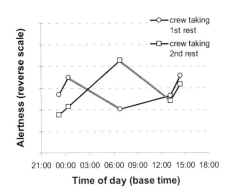

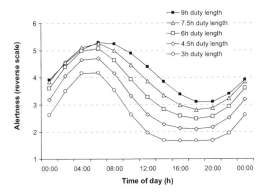

Figure 3.11 Alertness levels on flights with double crews

Alertness, on the seven-point Samn-Perelli scale (high values correspond to low levels of alertness), on flights from Singapore to London. The grey lines correspond to times when that particular crew has been allocated a rest period. Illustration derived from Spencer et al., 200. QinetiQ Limited: Report No &TS/CHS/CR50288/1.0. With acknowledgements to Civil Aviation Authority, Singapore (J. Singh).

Figure 3.12 Trends in alertness at top of descent related to time of day and time on duty

Alertness on the seven-point Samn-Perelli scale (high values correspond to low levels of alertness). Trends derived from a wide range of medium-haul flights leaving from or arriving in New Zealand. With acknowledgements to Air New Zealand.

A small decrease in levels of alertness is associated with consecutive duty periods even when the duty periods are during the day. This effect is more marked when the sleep loss associated with early start times is repeated over consecutive days. There are also indications that alertness may be impaired over the first two or three consecutive nights of duty (Samel *et al.*, 1997a), and this would be consistent with both the reduction in the duration of sleep during the day and the increase in the accident rates of shift workers observed with successive nights (Folkard, 2008).

Models of Alertness

Patterns and trends in aircrew alertness have led to the development of various alertness models, and many studies have been undertaken, at least in part, with the purpose of validating such models. By encapsulating current knowledge of the impact of different duty schedules, the most appropriate models are able to provide an expert assessment of

haul operations is a significant factor. Increased activity is associated with every additional take-off and landing, especially when these are delayed due to unforeseen circumstances. Pilots identify this as one of the major causes of increased levels of fatigue on this type of operation.

any proposed variation of the existing rosters, and hence to inform the regulatory authority of the implications of any proposed changes.

The first alertness models were derived from the results of laboratory experiments, and were used to predict the physiological impact of irregular patterns of work and rest, irrespective of the type of duty that was being undertaken (Folkard and Akerstedt, 1987; Spencer, 1987). Essentially, they included two components (Figure 3.13), one related to the time of day, the other the time that had elapsed since the end of the last sleep period (time since sleep). The time-of-day component was usually represented by a sinusoidal function, with peak alertness in the late afternoon, between 17:00 and 18:00, while the time-since-sleep component contained two separate elements. The first of these was the recovery in alertness immediately after waking (the 'sleep inertia' effect), and the second was an exponential reduction in alertness associated with increasing time since sleep. This second element is modelled

by the so-called 'S Process' (Daan *et al.*, 1984), which represents the requirement for sleep as a function of the pattern of sleep and wakefulness. It enables the model to generalize the time-since-sleep component to include sleep periods that are not sufficiently long to be fully restorative.

These two models have been identified as 'two-process models', the two processes being sleep, represented by S, and the circadian rhythm, or C process. There is now a proliferation of alertness models, almost all of which may be characterized, in one form or another, as two-process models. The performance of several of these models has been compared over a range of scenarios (Mallis *et al.*, 2004; Van Dongen, 2004). However, the results of the comparison are inconclusive, mainly because the individual models have been developed for different purposes and tend to include special features that are relevant to their particular area of application. As has been concluded in a recent review, individual models perform best when they are applied to the area in

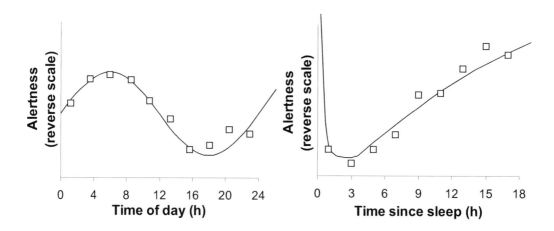

Figure 3.13 Alertness related to time of day and time since sleep

Source: Spencer, M.B. 1987. The influence of irregularity of rest and activity on performance: a model based on time since sleep and time of day. *Ergonomics*, 30, 1275–76 (With permission from Taylor and Francis Group http://www.informaworld.com.

which they were validated (Gundel *et al.*, 2007).

Aircrew Fatigue Evaluation

A typical configuration for a model with application to the aircrew environment is shown in Figure 3.14. This structure has been used as the basis for a computer program known as SAFE (System for Aircrew Fatigue Evaluation, © Civil Aviation Authority and QinetiQ Limited), which has been specifically designed for the prediction of the impact of duty schedules on aircrew fatigue (Belyavin and Spencer, 2004). The model includes both physiological and task-related elements. The core of the physiologically based part of the model is the sleep–wake cycle (S) and the circadian rhythm (C), whose combined influence on fatigue is represented by the two-process model as outlined above. The sleep–wake cycle itself is subject to the direct influence of the duty schedule, for example when sleep is displaced by early start times or night duties, and to the influence of both biological time,

through the circadian rhythm, and the local time of day. The modelling of the pattern of sleep and wakefulness during schedules which are subject to time-zone transitions is particularly difficult due to the complex interaction of competing influences and to the large individual differences. An initial approach has been suggested by Kandelaars *et al.* (2006b), based on an analysis of sleep patterns on return flights between Sydney and London. This involves splitting the longer (> 32 hours) layovers into three separate phases, a post-duty phase, an intermediate period and a pre-duty phase, to take account of the influence of duty time at the start and end of the layover period.

There is also a two-way interaction between the circadian rhythm and the sleep–wake cycle. As has been demonstrated both in laboratory simulations of irregular work–rest schedules (Akerstedt *et al.*, 1998), and in a statistical analysis of experiments carried out in isolation (Strogatz, 1986), the quantity, quality and the timing of sleep are strongly influenced by the phase of the circadian clock. Figure 3.15 shows the quantity of sleep reported by aircrew and by Japanese and German shift workers (Kogi, 1985) related to the time of sleep onset. There is a consistent pattern, with the amount of sleep reducing from midnight to the middle of the afternoon, when sleep averages approximately two hours. There is a window of considerable variability, between 18:00 and 21:00, when there are some very short sleeps, together with some sleeps of eight hours or more.

The influence of the sleep–wake cycle on the circadian rhythm is less direct. At

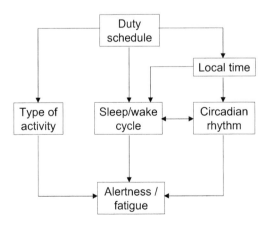

Figure 3.14 Schematic representation of a model with application to aircrew

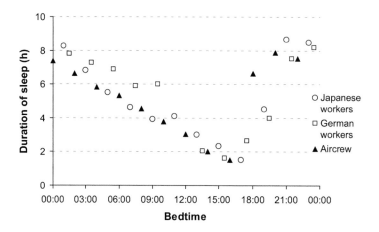

Figure 3.15 Duration of sleep (hours) related to the time of going to bed

Source: Shiftwork data derived from Kogi, K. 1985. Introduction to the problems of shiftwork. In: Folkard, S. and Monk, T.H. (eds.) *Hours of Work: Temporal Factors in Work-scheduling.* Chichester: John Wiley & Sons, pp. 165–84. Aircrew data derived from Robertson and Spencer, 2003. QinetiQ Limited: Report No Ki/CHS/CR021911/1.0.

one time it was thought that sleep, wake and activity exerted a strong influence on the circadian rhythm as a time cue, or *zeitgeber*. However, it is now recognized that by far the most powerful *zeitgeber* is bright light, and studies have been carried out to derive its phase response curve (Khalsa *et al.*, 2003). A phase delay is generated when light exposure is centred on a point in advance of the minimum of core body temperature (normally between 04:00 and 06:00), and a phase advance when exposure is after the minimum. The timing of sleep can, therefore, have an indirect effect on the body clock by providing a period free of exposure to bright light, for example when sleeping during the day after a time-zone transition. However, with one main exception (Jewett and Kronauer, 1999), current alertness models do not incorporate directly the phase-resetting properties of light.

Task-related elements include the effect of multiple sectors in short-haul operations and the timing of the rest periods and their impact on sleep in long-haul operations. An additional factor is the effect of the length of

duty or 'time-on-task'. In most aircrew studies, the results for length of duty include both a time-on-task and a time-since-sleep effect, although some attempts have been made to estimate the two effects separately. The workload or 'hassle' factor will contribute to the time-on-task effect which may, therefore, vary between different types of operation or indeed between different types of aircraft and different operators. However, little is known about the adverse effects of different types of work, though this is the subject of current investigations (Richter *et al.*, 2005).

A factor that is not well represented in current models is the accumulation of fatigue associated with high rates of working over several consecutive days, especially when the duties disrupt the normal pattern of sleep. Laboratory studies have demonstrated cumulative effects on alertness and performance of the reduction in sleep over consecutive nights (Van Dongen *et al.*, 2003), and it is likely that cumulative fatigue in aircrew has its origin in the various factors, social and environmental as well as physiological, that disrupt their sleep.

However, the realistic incorporation of cumulative effects into alertness models would require more information from real-life studies.

Flight-Time Limitations

Alertness models are likely to have an increasing role in the design and evaluation of aircrew rosters when it is considered that there is the ever-present need to maintain or even improve on current levels of safety. For the regulatory authorities, models provide guidance on the definition of flight-time limitations and assistance with the evaluation of variations requested by the operators. For the operators, they provide a means of assessing proposed rosters, as well as current schedules. It is likely that, in the near future, models will be integrated into the software used to create the rosters, so that alertness issues will be addressed at the early stages of roster generation. In addition, the increasing emphasis on fatigue risk management as an adjunct, or even as an alternative, to flight-time limitations, will place an even greater importance on the assessment of work patterns, and this is likely to result in the increasing use of modelling tools.

It is clear that there are many issues that have direct implications for the regulation of the rest and duty hours of aircrew. Evidence from studies of the work and rest of aircrew can be used as the basis for the definition of flight-time limitations, and any scheme should include considerations of duty periods, number of sectors, time zones crossed and provision of rest. The flight duty period (FDP) should be defined relative to the start of duty to take into account the different trends in aircrew alertness at different times of day. For example, the level of alertness that can be sustained for 14 hours in a duty starting in the late morning can only be sustained for at most ten hours when the duty starts close to midnight. Further, the FDP needs to be reduced for each take-off and landing after the first, to allow for the reduction in alertness associated with multi-sector operations.

When aircrew are not acclimatized to local time, it is not sensible to use local time to determine the maximum FDP, but it may be possible to use an estimated 'body clock' time based on an approximation to circadian adaptation. After large time-zone transitions, which can be associated with severe disruption to both sleep and circadian rhythms, the maximum FDP may need to be restricted even further. On the other hand, the FDP can be extended in flights with an augmented complement, where the increase in the duty period may reasonably be based on the amount of time that the crew members are able to rest. For example, with three pilots on a 14-hour flight, it would normally be possible for each to rest for approximately four hours, which would permit, on a conservative assumption, one hour of good-quality sleep for each pilot. It might be argued that one hour of sleep would permit the FDP to be extended by three hours. However, if the facilities for sleep were poor, or if such facilities were not provided, the extension would need to be reduced to account for the inevitable poorer quality of the sleep, and the advantage of an augmented crew would be eroded.

Ideally, the rest period between flights should provide sufficient time to enable an individual to be fully rested before the start of the next duty (minimum rest). In normal circumstances, after allowing for commuting and for personal activities, 12 hours might be considered sufficient, although this could be reduced if good-quality accommodation is provided close to the airport. However, as sleep tends to be much reduced during the day due to both physiological and environmental factors, it would be reasonable to extend the duration of minimum rest whenever the rest period falls during the day.

The requirement for sufficient time off for recovery after a duty period depends on the type of duty undertaken. When aircrew return home from a sequence of duties, it may take several days to reacclimatize, depending on both the time away and the number of time zones crossed. After a sequence of night duties, at least two days off, including two full local nights, would normally be required before they might be considered sufficiently recovered to undertake duties at other times of day. Where duties are less disruptive, extra days off may be necessary to protect against the accumulation of fatigue, but, to date, cumulative fatigue has received little attention except for the possibility that there is a gradual decrease in the number of duty hours per day that are compatible with acceptable alertness.

Approach to Aircrew

Despite the advances that have been made in understanding how aircrew cope with sleep disturbance and time-zone changes, an overarching evidence-based system that identifies schedules free of impaired alertness has not yet been achieved. Indeed, from time to time, schedules within currently used guidelines lead to difficulties. In such circumstances, consideration of the rest and activity patterns of all the aircrew involved in the schedule usually establishes where the problem resides. However, some aircrew, from time to time, may have a problem in coping with a route structure that presents little difficulty to other aircrew, and it may be appropriate to pursue the matter further. The question of the 'shift work disorder' may be raised, but intolerance to shift work is common and there is much uncertainty about the claim that such a pathological entity exists (Sack *et al.*, 2007). Nevertheless, it is important to ensure that the lifestyle of the individual is conducive to good sleep and to exclude a psychological illness (particularly depression) or a social problem. The practitioner should establish whether there is any possibility of a sleep disorder and whether there is excessive daytime sleepiness when the individual is not operational (see Chapter 11, Excessive Daytime Sleepiness: Clinical Considerations).

It is more than likely that an individual aircrew with a difficulty in coping with schedules will be free of any sleep pathology, and so the occasional use of an hypnotic at the appropriate time in a schedule (always after a flight) may be helpful. It is important to stress *occasional* use. The hypnotic must be free of residual effects on performance during the next duty period, and that is achieved by using low doses of hypnotics that are rapidly metabolized (Nicholson, 2006). However, at the time of writing, there continues to be much uncertainty concerning the appropriate use of hypnotics in aircrew. Indeed, there are differences between the recommendations of the various aeromedical authorities. There can be a firm recommendation concerning the use of a particular drug from one direction and reservations concerning the use of the same drug from another. The reason for these differences is that, though much work has been carried out on residual effects, insufficient attention is being given to mode of action, the determinants of duration of action, appropriate dose and clinical experience with respect to efficacy and adverse effects. The data required to ensure that the profile of a hypnotic is acceptable for transport aircrew is discussed in detail in a commentary in *Aviation, Space, and Environmental Medicine* (Nicholson, 2011).

Melatonin is also used to alleviate perceived difficulties that arise from transmeridian flights, and its adherents include aircrew. Melatonin induces a behavioural state resembling quiet wakefulness and that could lead to sleep in a suitable environment, though its effect is limited to parts of the day when endogenous plasma levels are low. Recommendations for its use are often based on the assumption that it accelerates the realignment of the sleep–wakefulness rhythm with the new day and night, but, at the time of writing, there is no convincing evidence of its potential to realign endogenous rhythms in humans (Agency for Healthcare Research and Quality, 2004). Many studies concerned with its potential chronobiotic activity have relied on subjective data and often lacked acceptable methodology (Auger and Morgenthaler, 2009; Nicholson, 2009). Further, the sedative nature of the compound prohibits its use if ingestion would be required during a duty period. The use of melatonin by aircrew is proscribed by most aeromedical authorities.

References

Agency for Healthcare Research and Quality. 2004. Melatonin for treatment of sleep disorders. *Evidence Report/Technology Assessment No. 108. Publication No. 05-E002-2*. Rockville, MD: United States Department of Health and Human Services.

Akerstedt, T. and Gillberg, M. 1990. Subjective and objective sleepiness in the active individual. *International Journal of Neuroscience*, 5, 29–37.

Akerstedt, T., Hume, K., Minors, D. and Waterhouse, J. 1998. Experimental separation of time of day and homeostatic influences on sleep. *American Journal of Physiology*, 43, R1162–8.

Auger, R.R. and Morgenthaler, T.I. 2009. Jet-lag and other sleep disorders relevant to the traveller. *Travel Medicine and Infectious Disease*, 7, 60–68.

Belyavin, A.J. and Spencer, M.B. 2004. Modelling performance and alertness: The QinetiQ approach. *Aviation, Space, and Environmental Medicine*, 75, 3 (Suppl.), A93–103.

Civil Aviation Authority. 2005. *Aircrew Fatigue: A Review of Research Undertaken on Behalf of the UK Civil Aviation Authority*. Available at: http://www.caa.co.uk/docs/33/CAAPaper2005_04.pdf

Daan, S., Beersma, D.G. and Borbély, A.A. 1984. Timing of human sleep: Recovery process gated by a circadian pacemaker. *American Journal of Physiology*, 246, R161–78.

Eriksen, C.A., Akerstedt, T. and Nilsson, J.P. 2006. Fatigue in trans-Atlantic airline operations: Diaries and actigraphy for two- vs. three-pilot crews. *Aviation, Space, and Environmental Medicine*, 77, 605–12.

Folkard, S. 2008. Do permanent night workers show circadian adjustment? A review based on the endogenous melatonin rhythm. *Chronobiology International*, 25, 215–24.

Folkard, S. and Akerstedt, T. 1987. Towards a Model for the Prediction of Alertness and/or Fatigue on Different Sleep/Wake Schedules. In: A. Oginski, J. Pokorski and J. Rutenfranz (eds) *Contemporary Advances in Shiftwork Research*. Krakow: Medical Academy, 231–40.

Folkard, S. and Barton, J. 1993. Does the 'forbidden zone' for sleep onset influence morning shift sleep duration? *Ergonomics*, 36, 85–91.

Folkard, S., Minors, D.S. and Waterhouse, J.M. 1991. 'Demasking' the temperature rhythm after simulated time zone transitions. *Journal of Biological Rhythms*, 6, 81–91.

Gander, P.H., Kronauer, R.E. and Graeber, R.C. 1985. Phase shifting two coupled circadian pacemakers: Implications for jet lag. *American Journal of Physiology*, 249, R704–19.

Gillberg, M., Kecklund, G. and Akerstedt, T. 1994. Relations between performance and subjective ratings of sleepiness during a night awake. *Sleep*, 17, 236–41.

Graeber, R.C., Dement, W.C., Nicholson, A.N., Sasaki, M. and Wegmann, H.M. 1986. International collaborative study of aircrew layover sleep: Operational summary. *Aviation, Space, and Environmental Medicine*, 57, 12 (Suppl.), B10–13.

Gundel, A. and Spencer, M.B. 1992. A mathematical model of the human circadian system and its application to jet-lag. *Chronobiology International*, 9, 148–59.

Gundel, A. and Spencer, M.B. 1999. A circadian oscillator model based on empirical data. *Journal of Biological Rhythms*, 14, 516–52.

Gundel, A., Marsalek, K. and ten Thoren, C. 2007. A critical review of existing mathematical models of alertness. *Somnologie*, 11, 148–56.

Jewett, M.E. and Kronauer, R. 1999. Interactive mathematical models of subjective alertness and cognitive throughput in humans. *Journal of Biological Rhythms*, 14, 588–97.

Kandelaars, K.J., Fletcher, A., Eitzen, G.E., Roach, G.D. and Dawson, D. 2006a. Layover sleep prediction for cockpit crews during transmeridian flight patterns. *Aviation, Space, and Environmental Medicine*, 77, 145–50.

Kandelaars, K.J., Fletcher, A., Dorrian, J., Baulk, S.D. and Dawson, D. 2006b. Predicting the timing and duration of sleep in an operational setting using social factors. *Chronobiology International*, 23, 1265–76.

Khalsa, S.B.S., Jewett, M.E., Cajochen, C. and Czeisler, C.A. 2003. A phase response curve to single bright light pulses in human subjects. *Journal of Physiology*, 549, 945–52.

Klein, K.E. and Wegmann, H.M. 1980. Significance of circadian rhythms in aerospace operations. *AGARDograph 24*. London: NATO Technical Editing and Reproduction.

Kogi, K. 1985. Introduction to the Problems of Shiftwork. In: S. Folkard, and T.H. Monk (eds) *Hours of Work: Temporal Factors in Work-Scheduling*. Chichester: John Wiley & Sons, 165–84.

Kronauer, R.E. 1984. Modeling Principles for Human Circadian Rhythms. In: M.C. Moore-Ede and C.A. Czeisler (eds) *Mathematical Models of the Circadian Sleep-Wake Cycle*. New York, NY: Raven Press, 105–28.

Lamond, N., Petrilli, R.M., Dawson, D. and Roach, G.D. 2006. Do short international layovers allow sufficient opportunity for pilots to recover? *Chronobiology International*, 23, 1285–94.

Lushington, K., Dawson, D., Encel, N. and Lack, L. 1996. Urinary 6-sulfatoxymelatonin cycle-to-cycle variability. *Chronobiology International*, 13, 411–21.

Mallis, M.M., Mejdal, S., Nguyen, T.T. and Dinges, D.F. 2004. Summary of the key features of seven biomathematical models of human fatigue and performance. *Aviation, Space, and Environmental Medicine*, 75, 3 (Suppl.), A107–18.

Moore-Ede, M.C. and Czeisler, C.A. (eds). 1984. *Mathematical Models of the Circadian Sleep-Wake Cycle*. New York, NY: Raven Press.

Nicholson, A.N. 1970. Sleep patterns of an airline pilot operating world-wide east-west routes. *Aerospace Medicine*, 41, 626–32.

Nicholson, A.N. 2006. Sleep and intercontinental flights. *Travel Medicine and Infectious Disease*, 4, 336–9.

Nicholson, A.N. 2009. Intercontinental air travel: The cabin environment and circadian realignment. *Travel Medicine and Infectious Disease*, 7, 57–9.

Nicholson, A.N. 2011. Prescription sleep medicine for aircrew. *Aviation, Space, and Environmental Medicine*, 82, 564–6.

Nicholson, A.N. and Stone, B.M. 1987. Influence of back angle on the quality of sleep in seats. *Ergonomics*, 30, 1033–41.

Nicholson, A.N., Pascoe, P.A., Spencer, M.B., Stone, B.M., Roehrs, T. and Roth, T. 1986. Sleep after transmeridian flights. *Lancet*, 2, 1205–8.

Powell, D.M.C., Spencer, M.B., Holland, D., Broadbent, E. and Petrie, K.J. 2007. Pilot fatigue in short-haul operations: Effects of number of sectors, duty length and time of day. *Aviation, Space, and Environmental Medicine*, 78, 698–701.

Powell, D., Spencer, M.B., Holland, D. and Petrie, K.J. 2008. Fatigue in two pilot operations: Implications for flight and duty time limitations. *Aviation, Space, and Environmental Medicine*, 79, 1047–50.

Powell, D.M.C., Spencer, M.B. and Petrie, K.J. 2010. Fatigue in airline pilots after an additional day's layover period. *Aviation, Space, and Environmental Medicine*, 81, 1013–7.

Richter, S., Marsalek, K., Glatz, C. and Gundel, A. 2005. Task-dependent differences in subjective fatigue scores. *Journal of Sleep Research*, 14, 393–400.

Rosekind, M.R., Graeber, R.C., Dinges, D.F., Connell, L.J., Rountree, M.S., Spinweber, C.L. and Gillen, K.A. 1994. Crew factors in flight operations IX: Effects of planned cockpit rest on crew performance and alertness in long-haul operations. *NASA Technical Memorandum*, 108839.

Sack, R.L., Auckley, D., Auger, R., Carskadon, M., Wright, K.P. Jr, Vitello, M.V. and Zhdanova, I.V. 2007. Circadian rhythm sleep disorders: Part 1, Basic principles, shift work and jet lag disorders. *Sleep*, 30, 1460–83.

Samel, A, Wegmann, H.-M., Veyvoda, M., Drescher, J., Gundel, A., Manzey, D. and Wenzel, J. 1997a. Two crew operations: Stress and fatigue during long-haul flights. *Aviation, Space, and Environmental Medicine*, 68, 679–87.

Samel, A., Wegmann, H.M. and Veyvoda, M. 1997b. Aircrew fatigue in long-haul operations. *Accident Analysis and Prevention*, 29, 439–52.

Samn, S.W. and Perelli, L.P. 1981. Estimating aircrew fatigue: A technique with application to airlift operations. *United States Air Force School of Aviation Medicine Report*, SAM-TR-82-21.

Sasaki, T. 1964. Effect of rapid transportation around the earth on diurnal variation in body temperature. *Proceedings of the Society for Experimental Biology and Medicine*, 11, 1129–31.

Spencer, M.B. 1987. The influence of irregularity of rest and activity on performance: A model based on time since sleep and time of day. *Ergonomics*, 30, 1275–6.

Spencer, M.B. 1989. Regression models for the estimation of circadian rhythms in the presence of effects due to masking. *Chronobiology International*, 6, 77–91.

Spencer, M.B. 1992. A mathematical model of the human circadian rhythm of temperature during irregular sleep-wake schedules. *Journal of Interdisciplinary Cycle Research*, 23, 178–9.

Spencer, M.B., Stone, B.M., Rogers, A.S. and Nicholson, A.N. 1991. Circadian rhythmicity and sleep of aircrew during polar schedules. *Aviation Space and Environmental Medicine*, 62, 3–13.

Stone, B.M., Spencer, M.B., Rogers, A.S., Nicholson, A.N., Barnes, R. and Green, R. 1993. Influence of polar route schedules on the duty and rest patterns of aircrew. *Ergonomics*, 36, 1465–77.

Strogatz, S.H. 1986. *The Mathematical Structure of the Human Sleep-Wake Cycle (Lecture Notes in Biomathematics)*. Berlin: Springer-Verlag.

Van Dongen, H.P.A. 2004. Comparison of model predictions to experimental data of fatigue and performance. *Aviation, Space, and Environmental Medicine*, 75, 3 (Suppl.), A15–36.

Van Dongen, H.P.A., Maislin, G., Mullington, J.M. and Dinges, D.F. 2003. The cumulative cost of additional wakefulness: Dose-response effects on neurobehavioral functions and sleep physiology from chronic sleep restriction and total sleep deprivation. *Sleep*, 26, 117–26.

Wegmann, H.M. and Klein, K.E. 1985. Jetlag and Aircrew Scheduling. In S. Folkard and T.H. Monk (eds). *Hours of Work: Temporal Factors in Work-Scheduling*. Chichester: John Wiley & Sons, 263–76.

Wever, R.A. 1966. The duration of re-entrainment of circadian rhythms after phase shifts of the zeitgeber. *Journal of Theoretical Biology*, 13, 187–201.

Wever, R.A. 1984. Toward a Mathematical Model of Circadian Rhythmicity. In: M.C. Moore-Ede and C.A. Czeisler (eds) *Mathematical Models of the Circadian Sleep-Wake Cycle*. New York, NY: Raven Press, 17–79.

Chapter 4

SPATIAL ORIENTATION

AND

DISORIENTATION

J. R. Rollin Stott

Orientation implies a sense of location, an awareness of position in relation to our immediate or more remote surroundings. When considering a sense of orientation in flight, a pilot certainly needs to be aware of the location of the aircraft on the map of the area, but there are many other aspects to orientation in flight. A pilot must be aware of the vertical dimension, the separation of the aircraft from the ground but also from other aircraft, and from obstacles such as hillsides or radio masts that may lie in the flight path of the aircraft. These aspects of orientation might properly be described as 'geographic orientation'. There is, however, another aspect of orientation that assumes particular significance in flight and which does not have an exact counterpart in pedestrian life. This is the need for a pilot to maintain a continued awareness of the attitude of the aircraft. Is it flying straight and level? Is it banked and turning? Is it pitched up or pitched down? Could it be upside down? On the ground we would have no difficulty in answering these questions in relation to our own body attitude. We would not even need to think about them.

Life on two feet, while freeing the hands for other purposes, brings with it a critical need for stability when standing, walking or running. Because of its importance, it is not surprising that several physiological mechanisms, visual, proprioceptive and vestibular, combine to achieve bipedal stability, and that it is an activity of which humans remain largely unaware. The ability to maintain balance on two feet is based on certain assumptions about the external world: in particular, that the visual environment is predominantly earth-fixed and that gravity remains constant in direction and intensity. What is it about the flight environment that does not allow a pilot, who is generally firmly strapped into the aircraft, to use similar mechanisms to achieve an accurate awareness of the aircraft attitude in flight? The answer to this question can be summarized in the following five statements, four of which relate to the flight environment and only one to human sensory deficiency:

○ In flight, the external visual world becomes remote and may be significantly degraded or totally obscured.

○ The aircraft generates forces through the aerodynamics of flight which, because of their sustained nature, are perceived as the effect of gravity, but may no longer indicate the true vertical.

○ In flight, manoeuvres that involve rotation in pitch or roll do not necessarily generate the sense of tilt with respect to gravity that would be expected.

○ Accelerative forces in flight can induce a sense of tilt without any accompanying rotation.

○ Sensors of angular motion in the inner ear become increasingly inaccurate in the presence of rotation that is sustained for more than a few seconds.

These statements will be considered further in the course of this chapter. However, in coming to a broad understanding of spatial disorientation in flight, it is important to view the subject from both perspectives – how, through its aerodynamics and the flight environment, the aircraft has the capacity to deceive the pilot and how, through misperceptions and sensory shortcomings, the pilot has the capacity to be deceived.

Part 1:
NEUROPHYSIOLOGY OF ORIENTATION

Any creature that is able to move about within its environment will have a need for some form of spatial orientation. In more complex organisms the capacity to orientate allows for purposeful activity in the search for food or a mate and

to return home to a secure refuge. The migration of birds and the homing abilities of pigeons have for long excited the fascination of naturalists. No less surprising, given the size of their brain, is the orientation capabilities of insects, notably bees and wasps. There have been many behavioural studies on a wide variety of species carried out over many years in an attempt to understand the mechanisms involved in orientation (Healy, 1998). On the basis of such studies, the notion of a cognitive map was proposed (Tolman, 1948). Such an idea might be regarded as self-evident. There must be a neural basis for the human capacity to recall many years later the layout of a once familiar environment, and also the ability rapidly to acquire a spatial awareness of a previously unfamiliar environment. The form of such a map, and indeed whether the term 'map' is the correct metaphor to use, remains the subject of debate and continued experimentation.

Cues to Orientation and Navigation

The sense of awareness of our surroundings that we call orientation is closely associated with an ability to navigate within that environment. For the purposes of navigation, a sense of place needs to be complemented by a sense of direction. A fundamental distinction can be drawn between information derived from the external environment, so-called allothetic cues, and information derived from sensors internal to the body, so-called idiothetic cues. Allothetic cues are predominantly visual landmarks, but may for some animals be tactile or olfactory cues. Idiothetic cues come from what is known as efference copy of the cortical motor outflow that brings about locomotion, and from the proprioceptive feedback from muscle stretch receptors and skin pressure receptors as a consequence of locomotor activity. Also included in the category of idiothetic cues is information derived from the vestibular system, though it could be argued that this organ is a sensor of the external inertial and gravitational force environment and in a sense therefore allothetic.

Allothetic cues, as conventionally defined, allow navigation by the use of landmarks. Idiothetic cues facilitate navigation by a process termed path integration, or what a sailor would know as dead reckoning – a knowledge of present position derived from a previously known position and the distance travelled in a known direction. In a visually rich environment it seems likely that allothetic cues predominate, but there is still a requirement for them to remain concordant with internally derived sensory information. Path integration on the basis of vestibular cues alone would be prone to accumulated errors and can only be relied on for relatively short periods of time.

Hippocampus and Entorhinal Cortex

An insight into the neurophysiological basis of orientation began with the discovery that the hippocampus of rats and the adjacent entorhinal cortex contained cells that showed activity only when the experimental animal was at a particular location within its environment (O'Keefe, 1976). Complementary to this finding was the observation that rats with lesions of the hippocampus were unable to find their way around a previously familiar environment (Morris *et al.*, 1982). The pattern of place cell activity is a neural representation of the environment, each cell having its own 'place field' that represents a particular region of that environment (Figure 4.1a). If the animal is moved to a different environment, the same place cell may take on a new place field. What determines the location in which a place cell will fire has been the subject of much experimentation (Best *et al.*, 2001). Visual landmarks exert a powerful influence on place cell firing,

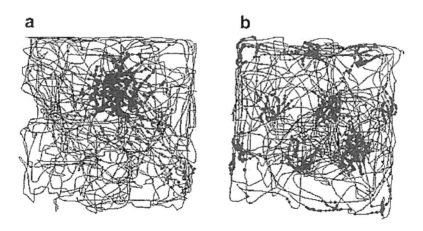

Figure 4.1   Pattern of activity in a) a place cell in the hippocampus and b) a grid cell in the entorhinal cortex (see colour section)

particularly those on the periphery of an animal's enclosure.

Experiments in which visual landmarks on the periphery of a circular enclosure were rotated to a new location showed a corresponding change in the location of firing of place cells. If, however, the animal was confined to an open maze within a larger environment whose fixed external landmarks it could see, place cell firing remained tied to the location of these external landmarks despite reorientation of the maze. Other experiments in which an animal was free to move between two identical visual environments connected by a corridor found that place cell firing changed between the two environments, suggesting that the locomotor or vestibular cues had played a part in the place cell representation of the environment as a whole.

Head Direction Cells

The next development was the discovery of head direction cells (Taube *et al.*, 1990). Whereas place cells are largely confined to the hippocampus and entorhinal cortex, head direction cells are more widely distributed, being found in the lateral mammillary nucleus, anterodorsal thalamus, posterior subiculum and entorhinal cortex. As their name implies, head direction cells show a peak of activity when the head is facing in a particular direction independent of the location (Figure 4.2). The preferred firing direction of these cells is determined, as with place cells, by the visual surroundings, particularly distant rather than nearby landmarks. It has been shown that the preferred firing direction is retained with reasonable accuracy if an animal is free to move through a passage containing two right-angle corners into a new visual

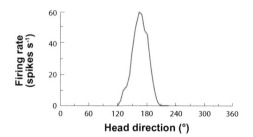

Figure 4.2   Firing rate of a typical head direction cell from the anterodorsal thalamic nucleus plotted against head orientation relative to the environment

Head direction cells vary in their peak firing rates from between 5 and 120 spikes per second and also in the angular range over which they show activity above their baseline from 60 to 150 degrees (from Taube, 2007).

environment. The accuracy of retention is somewhat less if the animal has to make the journey in the dark, and much less if it is passively transported to the new location. If the animal is free to move about its familiar environment and the light is switched off, the preferred firing direction of these cells, though initially maintained, tends to drift with time.

Groups of head direction cells appear to be networked in that all cells tend to drift by similar amounts in the same direction. When the light is switched on again, the initial preferred firing direction of the cell is restored within 80 milliseconds. This observation raises an interesting parallel with a phenomenon known to aircrew as 'the leans' which involves an erroneous sense of roll attitude after manoeuvring in cloud and which is rapidly dispelled once a view of the ground is regained. Thus head direction cells are behaving as a form of internal compass that is maintained not by the Earth's magnetic field but by visual, locomotor and vestibular cues. The afferent signal from the semicircular canals conveys information about head angular velocity. Cells similarly coded for head angular velocity can be found in brainstem nuclei, in particular the medial vestibular nucleus, the dorsal tegmental nucleus and the lateral mammillary nucleus. Angular velocity of the head derived from vestibular inputs has a significant influence on head direction cell activity. Neurotoxic lesions to the vestibular system abolish the head direction signal in the anterodorsal thalamic nucleus and the posterior subiculum and, in addition, disrupt location-specific firing of place cells in the hippocampus (Taube, 2007).

Grid Cells

A more recent discovery is the presence of grid cells located in the entorhinal cortex (Hafting *et al.*, 2005). These cells are so named because they show activity when an animal is at multiple locations within its environment. In addition, when the firing locations of an individual cell are mapped on to that environment, they form a regularly spaced hexagonal grid pattern (Figure 4.1b). This arrangement suggests the possibility that these cells act as some form of measurement system for spatial navigation. Grid cells within the entorhinal cortex are arranged in multiple layers, each with a different spatial resolution and orientation. It has been suggested that this arrangement might form the basis of a memory for location. There is now an extensive literature (reviewed in Moser *et al.*, 2008) exploring the determinants of cell activity and the interaction between these various types of cell. Cells of different types coexist in certain nuclei. For example, the lateral mammillary nucleus contains both head velocity cells and head direction cells, and the entorhinal cortex contains place, grid and head direction cells.

The importance of the hippocampus for memory is exemplified by the patient H.M., described by Scoville and Milner (1957). This 29-year-old man, who suffered from intractable epilepsy, underwent bilateral resection of the medial temporal lobes which included removal of the anterior two-thirds of the hippocampus. Post-operatively he suffered profound loss of recent memory which persisted for the rest of his life. He died in 2008 (Anon., 2008). He was unable to remember events that had occurred only minutes before. When the family subsequently moved to a new house on the same street, he was unable to find his way home and could not remember the location of familiar objects within it. It is likely that the hippocampal region of the brain, which has connections not only with the entorhinal cortex but also with other cortical areas, acts as an assembly point for contextual memory to link events to the location in which they occurred.

Part 2:
THE VESTIBULAR SYSTEM

Comparison of the mammalian vestibular system with an inertial navigation system, as currently installed in commercial aircraft, shows a strong resemblance. Both incorporate separate structures to detect linear and angular motion. Although, for aircraft navigation purposes, the technology of inertial navigation is being superseded by the high-precision position information that is continuously available from satellites through the global positioning system, it remains in use to supply reliable aircraft attitude information to the cockpit displays. An inertial navigation system incorporates two functional elements: a sensor of angular motion formed by three orthogonal laser ring gyros and a sensor of linear motion in the form of three orthogonal accelerometers. The system can measure aircraft motion in all three linear and all three rotational axes. This information is made available to the pilot through the attitude indicator and, by a process of integration over time, can be used to determine the current position of the aircraft. In the vestibular system, the analogous functional elements are the three semicircular canals sensitive to angular motion and the two otolith organs which between them have the capability to sense the intensity and direction of accelerative forces in any axis (Figure 4.3).

Similarly, therefore, the vestibular system functions as an inertial navigation system and there is increasing neurophysiological evidence of its role in navigation and in the related function of orientation. The information derived from the vestibular system is also used in the maintenance of postural stability and balance and, most significantly, through the vestibulo-ocular reflex, in the stabilization of the eyes to enable them to maintain visual acuity for an earth-fixed visual world in the presence of head movements resulting from locomotion and other externally generated forces. Though popularly known as the balance organ, the vestibular system shares the role of maintaining balance with visual and proprioceptive systems. An intact vestibular system on its own is unable to maintain balance in an individual with loss of joint position sense in the legs who is also deprived of vision. Classically, this occurred in the late manifestation of syphilis known as tabes dorsalis and was the condition for which Romberg's test was originally developed. The vestibular system plays a more exclusive role in maintaining stability of the retinal image.

The involvement of three separate sensory systems in the maintenance of balance has obvious advantages in circumstances in which the sensory information to one or other modality is lacking, since the redundancy will allow balance function to be maintained. However, such a system requires that there are rules of engagement between each of the constituent systems. For example, a sense of rotation has

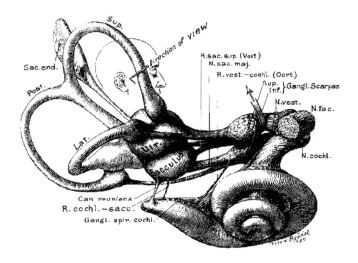

Figure 4.3   Human inner ear (an illustration by Max Brödel, 1934)

The vestibular component of the inner ear comprises the three semicircular canals whose neural output indicates the angular velocity of the head in any plane, and the utricle and saccule whose combined output indicates the direction and magnitude of linear acceleration, notably that of gravity.

implications for what is expected visually from an inertially stable visual world. Similarly, a vestibular sense of tilt should be accompanied by proprioceptive information, from the neck if only a head movement has been involved or from the feet and legs if such a tilt sensation represents an impending loss of balance. These rules of engagement have been built up on the basis of constant features of terrestrial life in which what is seen is predominantly inertially stable, and that what is experienced as gravity is vertical with respect to the surface of the Earth, and maintains a constant intensity. Part of the problem of disorientation in flight arises because in the flight environment these rules are broken. Reliance on innate terrestrial rules leads to erroneous conclusions about aircraft attitude, whether the aircraft is flying wings level, whether it is climbing or descending.

The Semicircular Canals

The orthogonal arrangement of the three semicircular canals of the vestibular system ensures that rotation of the head in any plane is detected by activation of one or more of the canals. Canals in the right and left inner ears that are co-planar operate in opposing pairs. Thus the two horizontal canals act as a pair. The orientation of the anterior and posterior vertical canals at roughly 45 degrees to the sagittal plane means that the anterior vertical canal of one side is in the same plane as, and forms a pair with, the posterior vertical canal of the opposite side and vice versa. With the head in the upright position, the vestibular labyrinth is tilted backwards such that the plane of the horizontal canals is deviated by about 20 degrees from the earth-referenced horizontal. Palaeontologists have used this anatomical information to suggest that humans evolved to walk and run with the head tilted forwards in order to scan the ground ahead, and also that determination of the orientation of the horizontal canals from fossilized remains can yield evidence of the head posture and mode of locomotion of extinct animals.

The neural signal from the semicircular canals represents the angular velocity of the head in the plane of each canal. At rest, a rate of firing of about 80 spikes per second can be measured in vestibular afferent nerves. A rotation in one direction results in an increase in the rate of firing proportional to the instantaneous angular velocity, and in the opposite direction, a decrease. Comparison of the signals from corresponding canals in each inner ear shows that, in the presence of a rotational stimulus, when one canal generates an increase in the rate of firing, the opposite canal will register a decrease. This so-called push–pull arrangement is familiar to electronic engineers and is used, for example, in the output of an amplifier to improve the linearity of the response and thereby reduce distortion. It appears that physiology is doing the same.

The semicircular canal does not sense rotational velocity directly but responds to the angular head accelerations that initiate and then retard head rotation (Figure 4.4). In deriving angular velocity from an angular acceleration stimulus, the canal is behaving as a mechanical integrator; it senses the accumulation of angular acceleration over time which is, by definition, angular velocity. The way this is achieved depends on three characteristics of the system. First, the cupula, the gelatinous membrane that separates the ampulla into two halves is an elastic structure that at rest maintains a central position within the ampulla. However, it is very compliant and readily displaced by movement of the endolymph. Second, the

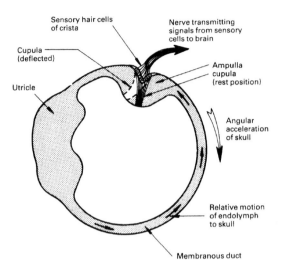

Figure 4.4   Diagram to illustrate the function of a semicircular canal

The endolymph in the fluid ring formed by the semicircular canal and the utricular cavity exerts an inertial force on the cupula within the ampulla when the whole structure is subjected to angular acceleration (clockwise in the diagram). The fluid drag exerted by the walls of the narrow canal means that, while angular acceleration continues, fluid will continue to accumulate in one half of the ampulla and drain form the other half increasing the deflection of the cupula. On account of this property of the system, cupular deflection, and hence the neural signal derived from the hair cells embedded in it, is related to the angular velocity of the head. This system shows a high degree of accuracy during natural head movements in which angular accelerations are short-lived and angular velocity is unsustained.

semicircular canal is narrow in cross section and exerts a significant drag on any movement of endolymph within it. By contrast, it communicates with a relatively capacious ampulla. Third, the endolymph, by virtue of its mass, exhibits inertia so that when the whole structure is rotated, the fluid within the canal tends to remain stationary. However, the drag exerted by the walls of the canal on the movement of endolymph ensures that, although the rate of endolymph flow is proportional to the applied acceleration, only a relatively small amount enters one half of the ampulla and drains out of the other half. The compliant cupula initially offers little resistance to the movement of endolymph and for small deflections acts as an almost passive indicator of fluid movement in and out of the ampulla. The result of this is that, for short-duration angular acceleration, cupular deflection is proportional to the accumulation over

time of the accelerative force on the endolymph and hence an indication of instantaneous angular velocity of the head.

This system operates very successfully for natural head movements in which an accelerative force is immediately followed by a decelerative force as the head adopts a new angular position. In this situation the cupula is constrained by inertial fluid movement, first in one direction, then immediately in the opposite direction, to return to its central position at the end of the head movement. However, the semicircular canal is not a perfect integrator (Figure 4.5). If an initial angular acceleration is followed by a period of constant angular velocity, there will no longer be an inertial force from the endolymph to maintain the cupula in its deflected position, and the inherent elasticity of the cupula will gradually return it to its central position, pushing fluid back around the canal against the

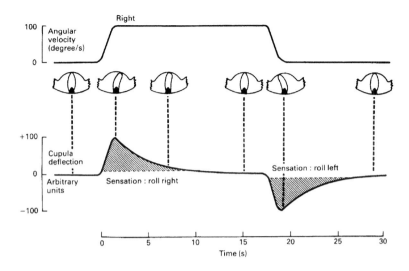

Figure 4.5   Response of the semicircular canal to sustained angular velocity
Once a constant velocity is attained, the absence of any further angular acceleration stimulus allows the cupula by virtue of its elasticity gradually to return to its rest position and thus no longer to indicate any rotation. Once this state has been reached, a deceleration stimulus is sensed as the onset of rotation in the opposite direction.

retarding force of viscous drag from the walls. Because the restoring force of the cupula becomes less the closer it comes to its central position, the pattern of the neural firing rate as it returns to its resting level will have the form of a decaying exponential which can be characterized by its time constant – a measure of the rate of return to the resting level. The consequence of a return to the resting level of neural discharge under conditions of sustained angular velocity is that the sense of rotation gradually decays to zero and, with it, any vestibular signal to maintain visual stability. When a period of sustained rotation is eventually stopped, the decelerative force involved results in a cupular deflection which, if the cupula has already returned to its central position, now deviates it in the opposite direction and signals to the brain an illusory rotation in this direction and, with it, inappropriate and destabilizing eye movements. This sequence of events is familiar to children who, after turning on the spot for a while, when they stop,

enjoy seeing the world spinning round and having difficulty in keeping their balance.

When measured using electrodes inserted into the vestibular nerve to record the firing rate in the afferent neurons, the time constant of decay following a stopping stimulus from a period of constant velocity rotation is of the order of 5 seconds (Goldberg and Fernandez, 1971; Fernandez and Goldberg, 1971). An alternative indication of semicircular canal activity is provided by the recording of eye movements induced by a vestibular stimulus – a technique that is used as the basis of clinical tests of vestibular function. However, the time constant derived from the measurement of eye movements following a stopping stimulus is found to be in the region of 15 seconds. This prolongation of the time constant beyond that of the vestibular end organ is brought about by the vestibular nuclei and other midbrain structures and is known as velocity storage.

The apparent shortcoming of semicircular canal function in failing to sense prolonged rotation at constant velocity can be viewed in a different light. As already discussed, the semicircular canal behaves as an integrator. An integrator generates its output by a process of accumulation over time of a given input. However, any spurious offset in the input signal, however small, will accumulate over time and lead to a progressive drift of the output. An aircraft inertial navigation system, though prone to drift by only 0.01 degrees per hour, has periodically to be reset by reference to a fixed location either by satellite or by radio beacons on the ground. The potential problem of drift in the physiological integrator formed by the semicircular canal is more severe, and is overcome by the tendency of the canal to return gradually towards its resting state when no further accelerative input is present. This means that any errors that would otherwise accumulate and lead to persistent dizziness are rapidly eliminated, but, as a consequence, the semicircular canal system is only accurate as a transducer of angular velocity for time periods of a few seconds. A more abrupt resetting can be achieved by central mechanisms. The velocity storage mechanism can be 'dumped', for example, by a change of head position that takes the head out of the plane of sensed rotation. Also visual fixation can largely suppress vestibular-induced eye movements. It appears that evolution has optimized the response of the vestibular system to provide an accurate measure of angular velocity at the frequencies encountered in normal head movements during pedestrian life.

The Otolith Organs

The otolith organs, the utricle and saccule lying in two chambers below the semicircular canals, are sensitive to linear accelerations. On two feet, such accelerations are generated by locomotor activities as well as by the force of gravity. The forces of locomotion and that of gravity are physically equivalent and when both are present they act as a single force. However, it is unlikely that the brain should have difficulty in distinguishing between the transient or oscillatory nature of locomotor forces and the invariant nature of gravity. Travel in moving vehicles complicates this simple distinction since accelerations and decelerations may be of comparatively long duration and consequently may alter the intensity and direction of what the brain perceives as gravity. This effect, the somatogravic effect, is particularly evident in aircraft and is an important cause of orientation errors and accidents.

Each otolith organ contains a sensory epithelium, the macula, consisting of a carpet of hair cells, the hairs of which project into the base of the overlying statoconial membrane (Figure 4.6). This membrane is rendered more dense than the surrounding endolymphatic fluid by the incorporation within it of crystals of calcium carbonate, giving the membrane a stony appearance, from which the name otolith is derived. The hair cells of the sensory epithelium have a directional sensitivity and will change their rate of firing if there is relative movement in the appropriate direction between the sensory epithelium and the statoconial membrane. Such movement comes about if, as a result of tilt, there is a change in the component of gravity acting on the statoconial membrane in the plane of the macula, or if, as a result of a dynamic acceleration, it is

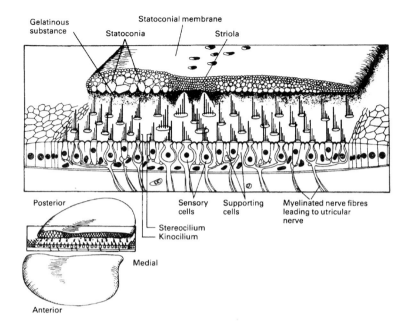

Figure 4.6   Structure of the otolith organ

The macula of the utricle or saccule consists of a carpet of hair cells, the hairs of which project upwards into gelatinous material beneath the statoconial membrane. This membrane is rendered more dense than the endolymph that surrounds it by the incorporation within it of crystals of calcium carbonate. Bending of the hairs and the consequent change in the rate of depolarisation of the cell is brought about by movement of the statoconial membrane through the effect of gravity if the structure is tilted or by the inertial effect of linear accelerations associated with locomotion.

subject to an inertial force. The direction of maximum sensitivity of the hair cells changes progressively across the surface of the macula in such a way that, whatever the direction of acceleration acting in the plane of the macula, there will always be a group of hair cells that are maximally stimulated. Since the macula of the utricle lies approximately in the horizontal plane and that of the saccule in the sagittal plane, the anatomical arrangement of these two structures allows sensation of the direction and intensity of any acceleration acting on the head. The only force in terrestrial life that acts continuously on the inner ear is that associated with gravity. As a result, though sensitive to the transient accelerations associated with locomotion, the predominant function of the otolith organs is to act as sensors of tilt of the head with respect to the direction of gravity.

Just as there is a rule of engagement that links angular head motion and its effect on vision of the static visual world, so there is a link between angular motion of the head and its effect on the otolith organs. Specifically, because the force of gravity is invariant in direction, angular head movements in pitch or roll must be associated with a corresponding angular change in tilt as sensed by the otoliths. While this rule is transiently broken in everyday life, for example when changing direction while running, infringements become far more evident when manoeuvring in an aircraft that may be travelling 100 times faster. Changes in roll attitude of an aircraft are seldom associated with any change in the direction of what is perceived as gravity. As a result, it is likely that the ability of a pilot to detect an inadvertent roll of the aircraft is much reduced for lack of any confirmatory tilt sensation.

Vestibulo-ocular Reflexes

Individuals with a total lack of vestibular function are likely to have difficulty with maintaining balance in the dark, but their gait is little affected in daylight. However, there will be a persistent effect on vision which consists of apparent motion of the stable visual scene during any physical activity, a symptom known as oscillopsia.

> Imagine the results of a sequence taken by pointing the camera straight ahead, holding it against the chest and walking at a normal pace down a city street. In a sequence thus taken and viewed on the screen, the street seems to career crazily in all directions, faces of approaching persons become blurred and unrecognizable. (J.C., 1952)

This problem is the consequence of the loss of the vestibulo-ocular reflex which serves to stabilize the retinal image against the effects of head movement, either voluntary or induced by activities such as walking, running and jumping.

The angular velocity signal generated by the semicircular canals in response to angular head movement in any plane is relayed through a three-neuron reflex arc to the appropriate eye muscles to produce a contrary rotation of the eyeball in that plane. The activity of this reflex can be explored in the laboratory by the measurement of eye movements in a subject undergoing angular motion on a turntable. The system can be characterized by its frequency response which gives a measure of the gain and phase of the eye movement in response to sinusoidal oscillation over a range of frequencies (Figure 4.7). For perfect compensatory function, it would be expected that the gain of the response would be unity at all frequencies – that is, the angular amplitude of eye

movement would be the same as the angular amplitude of the turntable stimulus – and that the phase would be 180 degrees, indicating accurate timing of the response but in the opposite direction. This is indeed what is found if the experiment is carried out in the light. However, in darkness, although the phase is compensatory over a wide range of frequencies from 0.1 to 10.0 Hertz, the gain is below unity at the lower frequencies (typically 0.6 at 0.1 Hertz) and increases with increasing frequency of oscillation to approach unity gain at a frequency of 2 to 3 Hertz. It is evident that in the light the gain at low frequency is being enhanced by visual mechanisms.

It is also possible to detect an eye movement response to linear motion mediated through the otolithic component of the vestibular system, the

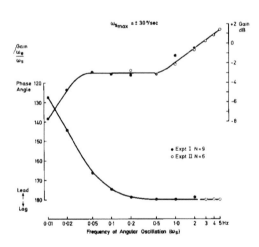

Figure 4.7   Frequency response of the vestibular system to angular oscillation about a vertical axis in the dark as measured by the induced angular eye movements

Gain is defined as the angular motion of the eye, we, as a ratio of the angular motion of the subject, ws, here expressed in dB (20 $\log_{10}(w_e/w_s)$). Full gain compensation (0dB) is only achieved at 2 Hz, ideal phase compensation (phase angle 180 degrees) is achieved at frequencies above about 0.2 Hz. In visual conditions the deficit in gain of the vestibulo-ocular response at lower frequencies is augmented by visual pursuit mechanisms to achieve ideal gain compensation over the full range of frequencies.

so-called otolith-ocular reflex. However, attempts to measure this reflex have yielded variable results. Unlike the expected one-to-one relationship between stimulus and response for angular motion, the ideal angular eye movement response to linear motion depends on the distance from the eye to the visual target. If the visual target is at infinity, no eye movement is required. The nearer the target, the greater is the angular eye movement required to stabilize the retinal image.

In summary, the vestibulo-ocular reflex is responsible for the capacity to perceive a stable visual world. This reflex can also be viewed as an essential neurological link that maintains concordance between the visual frame of reference represented by the stable external world and the inertial frame of reference that relates to forces and accelerations.

Part 3:
SITUATIONAL AWARENESS AND ORIENTATION

It is a primary requirement of flight that a pilot maintains the aircraft on the desired flight path. This task involves awareness of aircraft attitude, heading, airspeed and altitude – in other words, maintaining spatial orientation. The amount of attention that a pilot needs to devote to this task varies considerably in different phases of flight. In level flight, given a clear horizon and a ground separation of a few thousand feet, the task of maintaining an appropriate aircraft attitude is, to a trained pilot, an almost automatic activity that only requires an occasional, though regular, cross-check against the aircraft instruments. In these circumstances the pilot will have spare mental capacity to deal with other aspects of the flight. At

low level, however, particularly when manoeuvring, small errors in aircraft attitude can have fatal consequences and the scope for attending to anything other than flying the aircraft is severely limited.

Although the aphorism 'First, fly the aircraft' emphasizes the prime importance of remaining in control of the aircraft, there are, of course, other aspects of the flying task that also demand the attention of the pilot, and about which the pilot must remain aware. These include knowledge of aircraft position with respect to location on the ground (geographic orientation), weather conditions, fuel status and, for a military pilot, the location of supporting aircraft and of potential threats. This wider aspect of what a pilot needs to keep in mind has come to be known as situational awareness. The concept of situational awareness has gained currency since the early 1980s though uncertainty remains about what should be included within its definition. For some it has become synonymous with spatial orientation, and therefore of little additional value. To be of use, its scope is generally widened to include an awareness by the pilot of all aspects of the current state of the aircraft and of the external environment, at the time that it is necessary to be aware of this information. It also incorporates an element of anticipation of future events. The inclusion of a time dimension in this definition recognizes the limit on the number of pieces of information of which a pilot can simultaneously be aware. It has to be recognized that in dealing with these other aspects of the flight there is a temporary loss of awareness of aircraft orientation. In most circumstances this is of no consequence to flight safety, but in other circumstances it is crucial. It is often termed 'distraction' on the accident report rather than disorientation, but it represents a failure, for whatever reason, to 'First, fly the aircraft'.

Spatial Disorientation and Illusions

Spatial disorientation is concerned with the way in which the flight environment can deceive a pilot, either because the visual environment is degraded or obscured, or because the force environment is altered by the dynamics of the aircraft. When a pilot makes an error in the attitude or spatial position of the aircraft, the pilot is said to be disorientated and to have suffered an illusion. The nature of the illusion forms a basis on which to classify the type of disorientation. However, a pilot can be aware of an illusion without being disorientated. The two terms are not synonymous. Illusions are universal; the loss of awareness of speed with increasing altitude, the nose-up sensation during forward acceleration, the feeling of wings level during a banked turn are present every time an aircraft flies whether or not a pilot reports the experience of them. By contrast, disorientation incidents are relatively rare. When pilots describe such incidents, they seldom speak of illusions; to them the incident was reality. A further problem associated with an illusion-based approach to disorientation is that it gives no indication of the likelihood that a given illusion will lead to a disorientation incident or accident. The illusion that an aircraft feels straight and level when it is not is probably the most frequent underlying cause of disorientation episodes, yet this illusion hardly merits inclusion in any list of illusions of flight; it is just too commonplace.

To a pilot, disorientation presents itself in just one of two ways. Either there is a sense of confusion about the attitude of the aircraft on account of deteriorating visual information or the presence of conflicting sensations (termed recognized, or Type 2, disorientation), or else all feels well until there is a sudden realization that the aircraft is not in the attitude or position that it was expected to be (termed unrecognized, or Type 1, disorientation).

Illusions in flight can be classified according to their physiological origin. Some illusions are visual in origin; others can be linked to the function of the vestibular system, either the angular motion sensing capacity of the semicircular canals or the linear motion or tilt sensing capacity of the otolith organs. Because of the link between the vestibular and visual systems through the vestibulo-ocular and otolith-ocular reflexes, there are also visual illusions that have a vestibular basis. Vestibular-based illusions can be separated into those that are seen and those that are felt, that is, those that would be evident with eyes closed. They can also be separated into those that are based on the semicircular canal sensation of rotation and those based on the otolithic sensation of tilt. This leads to four categories:

- ❍ Illusions that are felt have the prefix 'somato-'.
- ❍ Illusions that are seen have the prefix 'oculo-'.
- ❍ Illusions that involve rotation have the suffix '-gyral'.
- ❍ Illusions that involve tilt have the suffix '-gravic'.

Thus, the terminology of vestibular-based illusions involves somatogravic, oculogravic, somatogyral and oculogyral illusions.

Vision and Spatial Disorientation

Flying an aircraft is an inherently visual activity. It is estimated that at least 80 per cent of the information acquired by a pilot in flight is through the visual system, either from the external visual scene or from the aircraft instruments. To an earthbound individual, the visual scene is generally earth-stable and detailed. Within this detail are multiple visual cues to self-orientation in the form of verticals and horizontals. Much of this visual detail is retained in low-level flight, together with the added pleasure of gaining a new perspective on the world. However, even at 500 feet the visual sense of speed over the ground is much reduced and this perception continues to diminish with increasing altitude. Pilots who are used to flying at low level in fast jet aircraft, on transferring to a lower-performance aircraft, may find themselves flying too low in an attempt to achieve their accustomed sense of speed over the ground.

As the height above the ground increases, ground features lose visual detail and appear increasingly two-dimensional. Eventually, the one remaining visual cue to aircraft attitude is the line of the horizon. Because of the lack of redundancy in visual information, an excessive reliance on this one orientation cue can give rise to error. The horizon may be rendered indistinct by haze. A distant bank of cloud may suggest a horizon that is significantly below the true horizon.

During a rapid descent to low level over the sea I was aware that the cloud was not 'coming up to meet me' as expected. The 'cumulus' cloud was in fact a bank of sea fog sitting at around 200 feet. Thankfully meticulous height checks from both cockpits prevented an embarrassing/fatal outcome.

Other false horizons are generated by sloping cloud tops, by mountain ridges and, at night, by lines formed by cultural lighting, for example along a coastline.

Although low-level flight generally offers good visual orientation cues, there is little margin for attitude errors that may arise when a pilot is distracted either by something within the cockpit or by searching the sky for the presence of another aircraft. The problem is particularly acute when executing turns at low level, when the need for good lookout conflicts with the requirement for accuracy in flying the aircraft.

I was leading a pair of aircraft with a third aircraft acting as a bounce. I was solo and the sortie was flown at low level. Conditions were perfect with little or no cloud and good visibility. I gained tally on the bounce aircraft attempting to attack my pair of aircraft and countered towards it. I was sharing the lookout between the bounce over my left shoulder and the terrain ahead of my aircraft. Approximately 20 seconds into the counter whilst looking over my shoulder I became aware of ground-rush in my peripheral vision. Looking forward I was about 10 to 15 degrees nose-down in a hard left turn. I aggressively recovered the aircraft to straight and level flight at 250 feet (using approximately 7 to 8 G) and then continued fighting. Only afterwards did I realize how lucky I had been. Neither of the other aircraft had noticed the proximity of my aircraft to the undulating terrain. I suggest that I had become target (bounce) fixated.

There are, however, circumstances in which the visual cues at low level, though clearly visible, are impoverished or deceiving. It may be difficult to judge height over the ground when flying over featureless terrain such as snow or sand or over open water where the apparent size of waves is a poor indicator of separation. The pilot of a float-plane attempting to land on the glassy surface of a lake may be obliged to set up a descent rate of no more than 150 feet per minute and wait until the aircraft touches down on the water rather than risk rounding out too soon or impacting the water at too high a descent rate. A similar technique may be required by a pilot when landing on featureless snow.

Other problems arise from the scale of ground features. A pilot who mistakes conifer saplings for fully grown trees may find himself to be closer to the ground than he intended. A helicopter pilot described the following incident:

> We had been flying at low level down a lake in Wales and then over a forest. Beyond the forest we crested a ridge and came upon what appeared to be a very large sheep! Only then did we realize how close we were to the ground. On re-flying the route, we discovered the pine trees, that we had assumed were 60 feet, were only 8 to 10 feet high.

On the approach to land, a pilot needs to maintain an accurate glide slope that brings the aircraft to the runway threshold at the correct airspeed. At major airfields, the pilot is assisted by Precision Approach Path Indicators (PAPIs) adjacent to the runway threshold, but in their absence the pilot uses the gradually changing appearance of the runway to judge the approach. If an unfamiliar runway is unusually long or narrow, a pilot may feel he is making too high an approach and tends to land short. The opposite tendency is induced by a runway that is abnormally wide or short.

There can also be problems in certain sunlight conditions when the distant terrain masks the contour of more imminent high ground that is lying in the flight path of the aircraft.

> While flying a navigational turn during an evasion sortie the pilot and navigator failed to spot a hill in the foreground that blended into a larger hill beyond. The low height warning sounded and the aircraft was levelled and climbed away. The lowest radar altimeter height seen was 170 feet. (Minimum Separation Distance 250 feet, radar altimeter bug set at 225 feet.) Causes of this incident were insufficient contrast between foreground and mid-distance objects due to sparse tree cover and snow. Both aircrew were concentrating on lookout for the bounce aircraft.

Similarly, a snow-covered ridge may become invisible against a background of uniform brightly lit cloud. This last scenario was a contributory factor in the accident in 1979 when a commercial aircraft crashed on the slopes of Mount Erebus in Antarctica.

In search and rescue operations, helicopter pilots may be required to maintain hover over a visual background of moving waves. In a similar fashion, the rotor downdraught can create a moving wave-like appearance when hovering over crops or grassland. Such conditions call for close coordination between the pilot and the rear-end crew to maintain accurate aircraft position. There is an added risk to helicopters when landing on snow or dusty terrain that the pilot may become unsighted at a critical phase by snow or dust blown into the air by the rotor downwash – so-called 'whiteout' or 'brownout'.

Night Vision

A pilot has to be particularly alert to the possibility of confusion when visual conditions are deteriorating, either from increasing haze or at dusk or, more abruptly, with inadvertent cloud penetration. With abrupt loss of external vision, there may be a delay before an inexperienced pilot transfers attention to attitude instruments, during which time the aircraft may have departed significantly from its intended flight path and the attitude indicator may be difficult to interpret or believe. At night, what remains visible to the pilot outside the aircraft depends on many factors such as the presence of moonlight or ground lights from towns and cities and the prevailing weather conditions. However, even in apparently clear conditions there may be no distinct horizon and, in consequence, starlight and points of light on the ground may become confused.

> I was descending from medium level to low level to conduct a detail at a bombing range. It was twilight with good visibility and there was a thin broken cloud layer at about 2,000 feet. After a safe level-off at 500 feet and while entering a positioning turn for the range, I became immediately disorientated, unable to determine visually which way was up. The aircraft descended approximately 200 feet before I locked on to head-down instruments and climbed away. On the subsequent pass we determined that we had over-flown a number of fishing vessels and had almost certainly become confused between stars and their lights. I believe the good weather had caught me between VFR (Visual Flight Rules) and IFR (Instrument Flight Rules) flying. Spatial disorientation training was useful. It reinforced the need to get on to instruments if in any doubt.

In the absence of a visual context, stationary isolated lights may appear to be in motion, and this can lead to misinterpretation of their true nature. This phenomenon, known as autokinesis, is particularly evident from isolated flashing lights. The effect is probably the result of ocular drift occurring in the dark intervals between flashes, so that the next flash falls on an adjacent portion of the retina which the brain interprets as movement of the light source.

In military operations, there are important tactical advantages to be gained from the use of night vision devices. However, the potential increase in safety that such devices might afford may be outweighed by the increased hazard associated with the night-time operations that they enable. Night vision goggles amplify the residual light to create a monochromatic image of the view ahead. However, they restrict the field of view to about 40 degrees and so deprive the pilot of important peripheral visual orientation cues. The image presented to the pilot is of lower resolution and its single green colour leads to problems with depth perception. In helicopter operations, the spatial disorientation accidents associated with the use of night vision goggles have most frequently involved undetected drift or descent from the hover or controlled flight into terrain or water. Other night vision devices generate a visible image using the thermal radiation from ground features. Contrast within the image is determined by the amount of infrared radiation from different objects in the field of view. This does not remain constant over time since it is dependent on the amount of previously absorbed solar radiation and the rate at which it is re-radiated during the night. More so than with daytime flying, the pilot has to exercise particular care during flight over featureless terrain when using these devices.

Instrument Flying

In daylight with clear external visual conditions, pilots gain the information they need about the aircraft attitude from looking outside the aircraft. In these circumstances they are said to be flying in visual meteorological conditions. In cloud, at night or when visual conditions deteriorate to the extent that they cease to give an unambiguous attitude reference to pilots, they are obliged to transfer to the aircraft instruments and are said to be flying in instrument meteorological conditions. The most important of these instruments is the attitude indicator, which is generally placed centrally on the instrument panel in front of the pilot, though it may be less prominent in aircraft in which the head-up display has become the primary attitude reference. In older aircraft, in which there is a separate instrument for each function, the flight control instruments are typically laid out in the form of a T, with the airspeed indicator to the left of the attitude indicator, the barometric altitude to the right and the gyro compass below. For this configuration, the pilot has to set up a radial scan pattern centred around the attitude indicator to check in turn the aircraft attitude, heading, attitude, airspeed, attitude, altitude and so on.

The transition from visual to instrument meteorological conditions can give rise to problems in inexperienced pilots. If the external conditions undergo a gradual deterioration, it becomes a matter of judgement as to when to make the transition. If, on the other hand, the transition is abrupt but unexpected, it may take many seconds to establish a working instrument scan. By this time the aircraft may have taken on an unusual attitude that no longer corresponds to the attitude the pilot last remembers or to the sensation of straight and level flight that is likely still to be felt. This may make it difficult for the pilot to interpret and to believe the attitude indicator. With the advent of cathode ray tube displays, it became possible to group multiple functions on to a single screen. The primary flight display screen typically incorporates a central attitude display with airspeed shown on a vertical scale to the left, pressure altitude and vertical speed on a similar scale to the right, and heading on a horizontal scale below it. While this arrangement reduces the need to make large visual scanning eye movements, it is still necessary to assimilate the multiple pieces of information in a systematic manner.

The way in which aircraft attitude is displayed has long been the subject of debate (Johnson and Roscoe, 1972). There are two principal alternatives known as the 'inside-out' and the 'outside-in' displays. The inside-out display, also known as a moving horizon display, is the standard attitude display in all Western-built aircraft. It shows an aircraft symbol that remains fixed with respect to the aircraft. Behind it is a line, blue above and brown below, which represents the horizon and is free to move so that it remains aligned with the true horizon when the aircraft rolls and pitches. This type of display behaves as if it were a forward-facing hole in the aircraft through which the pilot could see the true horizon. While this might seem a logically correct way in which to convey attitude information to the pilot, to the untrained it tends to be perceptually incorrect. Its very name, a moving horizon display, betrays the dilemma. The pilot tends to perceive the aircraft to be the stable environment against which the representation of the outside world is seen to move. This is probably because, when flying on instruments, the cockpit environment occupies much of the peripheral vision, whereas the horizon is represented only in the central vision, and also because, whatever its attitude, the aircraft continues to feel level. A pilot who responds to an unexpected roll attitude error by attempting to move the horizon back to its level position will do the reverse of what is required. This so-called roll reversal error has been held responsible for a number of accidents (Roscoe, 1997).

The alternative configuration for the attitude display, the outside-in or moving aircraft display, has been widely fitted to Russian commercial and military aircraft. Here a representation of the aircraft moves with respect to a horizon line that remains transverse with respect to the aircraft cockpit. Experiments have indicated that while pilots can be trained to use either type of display, naive individuals can assimilate and respond to aircraft attitude information more rapidly and reliably from the moving aircraft display (Ponomarenko, 2000). However, only roll information is displayed in this way. Pitch is represented within the same instrument by a moving pitch ladder that remains vertical with respect to the aircraft.

A commercial aircraft crashed into the sea about three minutes after take-off in the dark. To attain the desired outbound heading and avoid high ground, the captain, who was the handling pilot, was instructed to make a 270 degree climbing turn to the left over the sea. He duly established the aircraft in a 30 degree banked turn to the left. However, he must have become distracted as, over the next 30 seconds, the bank angle slowly decreased and the aircraft continued to roll past wings-level until it was banked 30 degrees to the right. At this point the co-pilot alerted the captain that the aircraft was now turning to the right. The captain evidently had some difficulty in understanding the situation as his next action was to bank the aircraft a further

30 degrees to the right, as a consequence of which it became impossible to recover the aircraft in the available height and it crashed into the sea. It is probably of significance that the captain was an ex-military pilot who had accumulated many hours flying Soviet-built aircraft fitted with a moving aircraft attitude display.

Part 4:
THE FORCE ENVIRONMENT OF FLIGHT

All pilots should be made aware at an early stage in their training, even before they take to the air, of the precept 'You cannot fly an aircraft by the seat of the pants'. This means that if external vision is lost, it is not possible to maintain aircraft attitude simply by the feel of the aircraft. Why this should be so involves an understanding of the other major cue to orientation, the force environment, and how in flight this is affected by the aerodynamics of the aircraft. Many of the accidents and incidents involving spatial disorientation are the result of a transient neglect of this precept.

To remain in straight and level flight, an aircraft has to exert, through the aerodynamics of the wings, a force of 1 G to counteract the effect of gravity, an upward force that for a terrestrial object is ultimately provided by the surface of the Earth. An important difference between the aircraft and the terrestrial environment is that the pilot is in control of this force through the aerodynamic lift of the wings. Lift is determined by a combination of airspeed and the angle of attack of the wings. This latter is controlled by the pilot through fore-aft movement of the control column. In other words, the pilot can determine within certain limits the intensity of gravity that is perceived by the aircraft occupants. If the pilot pulls back on the control column to increase the angle of attack, the occupants will feel heavier than usual; if the control column is pushed forward, the angle of attack will decrease and they will feel lighter. If the control column is pushed still further, they will feel weightless; further still and they will need to be strapped into the seat and may feel upside down as the aerodynamic 'gravity' now acts upwards through the roof of the aircraft. These changes in the perceived intensity of gravity occur because the pilot's control action puts the aircraft into a curved flight path.

The radial acceleration (metres. second $^{-2}$) is dependent on the radius of curvature (metres) and the airspeed (metres per second) according to the formula $- A = V^2 / R$ (alternatively, A = ω. V) where A is the radial acceleration, R is the radius of curvature, V is the airspeed and ω is the rate of turn in radians per second. These formulae are often of use when determining from flight data records the forces that a pilot may have experienced, for example in the moments leading up to an accident. In practice, the alternative formula is more useful since the rate of turn can be estimated from the sequence of values of aircraft heading whereas the radius of the turn is not immediately available from the flight data.

Not only can the pilot vary the intensity of the aerodynamic lift force on the aircraft, but also its direction with respect to the true vertical. The most familiar example of this occurs when an aircraft is in a coordinated turn and leads to the sensation familiar to airline passengers that the aircraft is flying wings level when it is, in fact, banked (Figure 4.8). This is an example of the somatogravic illusion, a false sense of the gravitational vertical produced by the presence of an additional inertial force,

in this case the radial force engendered by the change of heading.

In a coordinated turn, the lift force continues to act at right angles to the main wing in a vertical direction with respect to the aircraft, but it now serves two purposes. As with any force, the lift force can be resolved into two components at right angles. If the aircraft is to maintain height, the earth-vertical component must continue to be sufficient to oppose the effect of gravity. At the same time, the horizontal component is required to produce the desired change in aircraft heading. The overall aerodynamic force must therefore be increased. However, for small angles of bank this increase is small and hardly perceptible. At a bank angle of 20 degrees typical of a commercial aircraft in a level turn, this force is only 1.06 G, but what the passengers perceive as gravity is now at an angle of 20 degrees to the true vertical. In cloud, the pilot has only the attitude instrument to indicate the true situation.

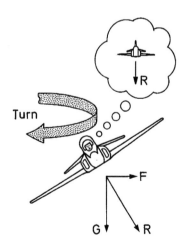

Figure 4.8   The coordinated turn

The aerodynamic force, R, generated by the wings serves two purposes: the vertical component, G, opposes the effect of gravity; the horizontal component, F, results in a change of heading in the earth-horizontal plane. Without a view of the outside world, force R is readily perceived as indicating the true vertical.

The Graveyard Spiral

Because any sensation of gravity in an aircraft is determined by the position of the control column, the pilot could maintain a reassuring sensation of 1 G downwards through the floor of the aircraft while inadvertently allowing the bank angle of the aircraft to increase. At 60 degrees of bank, the component of the lift force is only half what is required to maintain level flight so the aircraft will begin to lose height. At 90 degrees of bank all of the 1 G of lift is acting to change the aircraft heading and none of it to maintain height. The aircraft will now, at least initially, be in free-fall, though it may still feel wings level. Any increase in the bank angle beyond this point will cause the lift force to augment the effect of gravity in pulling the aircraft towards the ground and lead to a rapid descent. The loss of life from this inadvertent manoeuvre has earned it the name of 'graveyard spiral'.

I was undertaking a solo night navigation exercise in training for my Commercial Pilot Licence. After take-off I found the cloud base to be lower than my safety altitude but hoped to be able to climb through the cloud into clear skies. After about ten minutes I was still in cloud so I decided that I would abandon the exercise and turn back. I put the aircraft into a 20 degree banked turn and set about establishing a reciprocal heading on my navigation equipment. Fortunately for me the aircraft had windows in the cockpit roof, as, on glancing up, I suddenly became aware of what I realized was a row of street lights – the aircraft had now descended below the cloud base. A glance at the altimeter and airspeed indicator showed that I was in a spiral dive. I recovered the aircraft as best I could using the visual horizon, but with very little height to spare. I remember going into mild shock when two years later I first told a colleague of what had happened. A few seconds later and I might have been too low to recover.

The effect of the gravitational attraction of the Earth imposes one physical constraint on the pilot of an agile aircraft. Though the pilot has the facility aerodynamically to control the force acting in the vertical direction with respect to the aircraft, the component of the aerodynamic force acting in the vertical direction with respect to the Earth must average over time to 1 G. Any period for which this component of force is decreased below 1 G must be paid for by a corresponding period of increased vertical force. However, for short periods, given sufficient height above ground, an aerobatic pilot can enjoy a degree of freedom from the effect of gravity that is denied to mere earthbound mortals.

Longitudinal Forces

A further force on a fixed-wing aircraft that acts in the long axis of the aircraft approximately at right angles to the lift force comes from the thrust of the engines and the retarding effect of the airbrakes. Though this force contributes to problems with spatial orientation during changes in airspeed, its intensity in all aircraft is substantially less than the lift force that can be generated by the wings. In a helicopter there is no similar longitudinal force. The force that both lifts the aircraft off the ground and drives it forwards (or backwards or sideways) is generated by the main rotor and this force is always vertically upwards with respect to the fuselage of the helicopter, again, whatever the aircraft attitude with respect to the surface of the Earth.

These examples form part of a group of disorientating problems known as somatogravic effects or illusions. (The distinction between 'effect' and 'illusion' depends on whether you are the pilot experiencing the problem in flight or thinking about it afterwards. In flight, significant illusions tend to present to the pilot as reality.) Specifically, they describe situations in which the combination of forces acting on the aircraft are perceived as gravity and are erroneously assumed by the pilot to indicate the true earth vertical. They comprise situations in which the aircraft feels level, both in the pitch and roll axes, when it is not, and also situations in which the aircraft is felt to be pitched up or down to a greater extent than it actually is.

The Somatogravic Effect

The somatogravic effect is important for two reasons. First, it is involved in almost every aircraft manoeuvre and provides an explanation of why, in the absence of external vision, a pilot can readily be deceived by what is felt to be the attitude of the aircraft. Second, it is an underlying factor in many aircraft accidents. It is therefore important to understand how this effect comes about and in what circumstances in flight it can lead to problems.

The sensation of level flight when the aircraft is in a banked attitude during a coordinated turn is one example of the somatogravic effect that has already been described. A similar effect can be experienced in the pitch axis by longitudinal acceleration or deceleration of the aircraft. With take-off power applied to the engines, a commercial aircraft will accelerate typically at 0.25 G as it gains speed along the runway. A high-performance military aircraft can do much better than this with its ability

to generate levels of forward thrust approaching, or even exceeding, 1 G. After take-off, the thrust of the engines has to achieve two things: to cause the aircraft to climb against the force of gravity and to increase airspeed towards that required in the cruise. The pilot of a commercial aircraft, for reasons of noise abatement, will use the engine thrust to gain altitude as soon as possible, and only later will reduce the rate of climb and gain further airspeed. With greater power, the military pilot is able to climb and increase airspeed simultaneously. For a given power setting, the rate of climb and the rate of increase in airspeed are inversely related and the balance between them is determined by the aircraft pitch attitude that the pilot maintains. A reduction in pitch angle favours forward acceleration of the aircraft at the expense of climb, and vice versa.

In clear external visual conditions, a pilot should have no difficulty in maintaining an appropriate climb angle. If, however, the aircraft enters cloud, the pilot will have to transfer to instruments. Any attempt to continue the climb simply by the feel of the aircraft is likely to lead to an error in pitch attitude. The reason for this is that forward acceleration of the aircraft produces an equal inertial acceleration acting backwards on the pilot and increasing the sense of pressure from the back of the seat. This sensation is exactly the same as would occur if the seat were actually tilted backwards when some of the support against the force of gravity provided by the seat base when in the upright position would now be taken by the back of the seat. The sensory information provided by the otolithic system is exactly similar to the cutaneous sensation of backward tilt. Forward acceleration exerts an inertial force on the otolith and produces a displacement on the hair cells that is the same as would occur had the head been tilted backwards (Figure 4.9). Thus, from non-visual sensations a pilot is unable to distinguish between an actual backward tilt associated with the climb and an illusory sense of tilt associated with forward acceleration (Figure 4.10).

Furthermore, any adjustment the pilot makes to the pitch attitude of the aircraft in the climb is unlikely to make much difference to the perceived sense of pitch-up. This is because a reduction in climb angle allows a greater proportion of the engine thrust to accelerate the aircraft in the line of flight and hence to add to the illusory component of the sensation of pitch-up. Equally, if a pilot were inadvertently to increase the climb angle of the aircraft, there would be a reduced forward acceleration since more of the thrust would be required for the climb. As a result, any sensation associated with actual pitch change would be offset by a reduction in the illusory sensation of pitch-up and thus little change in perceived pitch attitude.

Low-level climb-out at night, scattered cloud at 2,000 to 4,000 feet, limited moonlight, night vision goggles worn. Whilst climbing out VMC approximately 15 degrees nose-up, I was distracted by a cockpit minor emergency. When I looked back at the head-up display the attitude was 40 degrees nose-up. I felt I was still in a shallow climb. However, instruments were trusted and having bunted back to 20 degrees nose-up, the body readjusted to this attitude.

An almost identical situation led to the opposite outcome in the following incident:

Low-level abort, reducing cloud base. Low-level abort carried out, however flew incorrect technique (flew head-up not head-down). Experienced severe pitch-up resulting in a bunt to 20 degrees nose-down. Second more severe abort then carried out head-down. Navigator was totally unaware of risk at any time.

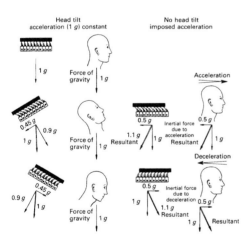

Figure 4.9   Equivalent effect of tilt and linear acceleration on the otolith organ

In the presence of gravity the same effect on the otolith is produced by backward tilt of the head as occurs as a consequence of acceleration in the forward direction. Likewise forward tilt of the head produces the same effect as forward deceleration. In consequence, a sustained forward acceleration can produce an illusory sensation of backward tilt and deceleration a sensation of forward tilt.

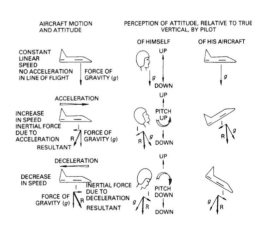

Figure 4.10 Somatogravic effect during acceleration and deceleration in the line of flight

Forward acceleration is associated with a false sensation that the aircraft is pitched up and deceleration with a false sensation of pitch down. These sensations can lead to errors of pitch attitude in conditions where there are limited or absent external visual cues such as in cloud or at night.

There is one difference between the sensation of tilt produced by changes in pitch attitude and that produced by forward acceleration. With change in pitch attitude, there is a corresponding semicircular canal signal to indicate a rotation in the pitch plane, whereas in forward acceleration this is absent. This difference may explain why experiments carried out in the laboratory and in flight suggest that the perceived tilt produced by linear acceleration is generally an underestimate of what would be predicted by a trigonometric analysis of the forces involved.

The consequences of the somatogravic effect produced by forces in the line of flight are that an aircraft that is accelerating will tend to feel more nose-up than it actually is, and, correspondingly, a decelerating aircraft will tend to feel more nose-down. It does not matter how these accelerations and decelerations come about. The example cited above has considered the forward acceleration of the aircraft that results from the level of engine thrust required for take-off and climb-out. However, if a pilot flying straight and level at constant speed inadvertently allows the nose to drop, the aircraft will begin to accelerate under the influence of gravity – it will be going downhill. As a result it will feel more nose-up than it actually is. Until the aerodynamic drag increases and establishes a new constant airspeed, the aircraft will continue to feel level. Similarly, if the pilot allows the nose to rise, the aircraft will decelerate and will therefore tend to feel more nose-down than it actually is, again will continue to feel level. This sequence of events could be termed the 'accidental somatogravic effect' in that it does not come about as a result of a deliberate control action by the pilot. It can occur in all aircraft types, even gliders. An increased nose-down attitude in a glider causes it to accelerate

and its low aerodynamic drag may allow the aircraft to build up excessive airspeed before the pilot becomes aware from the feel of the aircraft of any change in pitch attitude.

There are particular circumstances in flight when pilots have to remain very aware of possible errors of aircraft attitude arising from the somatogravic effect. Mention has already been made of take-off into low cloud where the transition from external vision to instruments must be anticipated and an appropriate rate of climb maintained. A similar situation occurs when a pilot intending to land the aircraft has for some reason to overshoot the runway and go around for a second approach. Poor weather conditions may often underlie the need to overshoot and a pilot may be distracted by the other tasks involved in the manoeuvre and fail to establish a positive rate of climb. Low-level flight in a military aircraft may have to be aborted on account of deteriorating visual conditions, low cloud or failing light. This manoeuvre involves a rapid climb to a safe altitude with full thrust applied to the engines. The desire to correct what feels like an excessive pitch angle has to be resisted in favour of what the aircraft instruments are saying. A further disconcerting sensation for the pilot arises from the curved flight path (bunt) as the aircraft, possibly still at full thrust, levels off at a safe altitude. The increased forward acceleration of the aircraft as the rate of climb is reduced coupled with the reduced and possibly negative lift force associated with the bunt manoeuvre can leave the pilot with the sensation that the aircraft has become inverted.

The Leans

After a series of turning manoeuvres when flying in cloud, and therefore on instruments, a pilot may find that on returning the aircraft to straight and level flight as indicated by the attitude indicator he is aware of a sensation that the aircraft is flying with one wing low. This effect is known as 'the leans' and takes its name from the fact that the sensation may be sufficiently compelling to cause the pilot to lean sideways in the seat in order to align his head with the perceived vertical. Its intensity can vary from a mild distraction to one that is powerful enough to cause the pilot to mistrust the instruments. Although the phenomenon could be considered another example of a somatogravic effect in that it involves an erroneous sensation of the gravitational vertical, it is atypical in that it affects a pilot who is flying straight and level at constant

airspeed and thus in circumstances where no additional force other than the earth-vertical lift required to oppose gravity is acting on the aircraft. In consequence, the leans require a physiological rather than an aerodynamic explanation.

A sequence of events that may lead to the leans is illustrated in Figure 4.11. A pilot is flying without any external visual reference. An unperceived rightward bank causes the aircraft to enter a coordinated turn to the right. Having recognized this unintended aircraft attitude, the pilot rolls the aircraft to the left at a supra-threshold rate to restore level flight. Because the pilot considered the aircraft to be straight and level when in fact it was banked to the right, he has reason, following an abrupt roll to the left, to feel that the aircraft is now banked to the left. The sensation provoked by the leans is not, however, the same as would be felt if one wing were actually low, for then the aircraft would tend

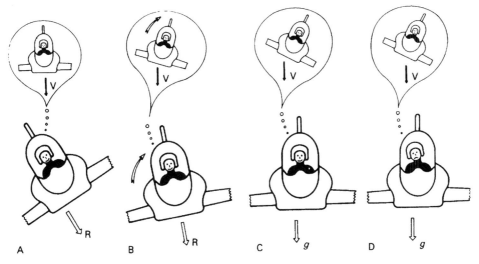

A	B	C	D
Aircraft in co-ordinated turn to right. Pilot feels that wings are level	Pilot rolls out of turn, feels that aircraft is banking to left	Aircraft in straight and level flight. Pilot feels left wing low	Pilot aligns head and trunk to perceived vertical and leans to right

Figure 4.11 The leans

The diagram shows a possible sequence of events that, in the absence of an external visual scene, may lead to the false perception that the aircraft is flying one wing low.

to enter a coordinated turn and, in consequence, continue to feel level. The false sensation of tilt is therefore perhaps surprising. Though instructors fly this sequence of manoeuvres in an attempt to demonstrate the leans to their student, they do not always succeed. Similarly, when pilots do develop the leans, they are often unable to say what sequence of manoeuvres brought it about.

When flying in close formation, the pilot of the number two aircraft in the formation takes his orientation cues from the leader and in so doing tends to lose awareness of his spatial orientation with respect to the outside world. The pilot of the lead aircraft has the major responsibility to maintain spatial orientation on behalf of the formation and to ensure that his manoeuvres are sufficiently gentle to allow his number two to respond to them. Formation flying often continues despite cloud penetration; the only difference may be that the aircraft fly closer to each other in order to maintain visual contact. In these circumstances, even greater concentration is required to maintain separation from the lead aircraft. Should visual contact be lost and the number two is obliged to break away, he may have great difficulty reorientating himself relative to the real world, as best he can perceive it through his aircraft instruments. Aircrew reports indicate that formation flying in cloud is particularly conducive to producing the leans in the number two aircraft. The sensation can be very disconcerting and the task of staying with the lead aircraft becomes increasingly demanding. The alternative of breaking away from the formation means losing the orientation cue provided by the leader and having to use instruments, without necessarily alleviating the leans.

I was solo on the wing of an aircraft that was being flown by a student pilot with his instructor in the rear. Whilst in cloud the attitude of my aircraft did not correspond to my physiological perception of it. Indeed, a look at the instruments at one point, when I felt we had about 90 degrees of bank on, revealed that the aircraft was straight and level. Flying my aircraft in this condition was very difficult and very disorientating, and many times I thought of breaking out of the formation, but I wasn't sure of which way was up. In the subsequent debrief, it transpired that the student in the lead aircraft had been rolling quite swiftly into turns and using more bank than is recommended when in cloud in formation – a lesson for me in formation leading!

The leans can be experienced by any instrument-rated pilot, though it is most frequently reported in military flying in which frequent manoeuvres may be called for when flying on instruments. In surveys of military pilots, over 90 per cent have experienced the leans. For many this is their only reported experience of disorientation. If in these circumstances the pilot is aware of the need to fly the aircraft according to the instruments and continues to do so, it could be argued that he is not disorientated in that he remains aware of the true attitude of the aircraft. However, when the leans occur at critical times in flight, such as on an instrument approach or when flying in formation, the experience can be very alarming. It is all the more memorable for its tendency to persist for as long as the flight continues without external visual reference. However, once an unambiguous view of the external world becomes visible, the sensation of the leans is instantly dispelled.

Although there is an understanding of the sequence of flight manoeuvres in cloud that may give rise to the leans, the underlying neurophysiology of the condition is difficult to understand. It seems that the pilot's perception of the roll attitude of the aircraft is derived from what might be described as 'path integration' of the preceding roll attitude changes as sensed by the relevant semicircular canals. This involves a double integration of the angular accelerative forces in roll that are the stimulus to the canals. This process is prone to the accumulation of errors. In sensing angular motion, the semicircular canals behave as a high-pass filter. As a result, lower-frequency components of the angular acceleration input signal are under-represented in the brainstem nuclei compared with the higher-frequency components. It might be theorized that there is a population of roll-axis head direction cells that, in the absence of an earth-orientated visual input, have modified their preferred firing direction in response to roll canal inputs. It has also to be assumed that these putative head direction cells are uninfluenced by an otolithic input which in straight and level flight could be expected to indicate the true vertical. Animal studies of head direction cells have hitherto only explored head direction cells that are responsive to direction changes in the horizontal plane as the animal navigates within its surroundings.

The Somatogyral Effect

As already outlined when dealing with the vestibular system, if a rotation, once established, is maintained at constant velocity, there will be a gradual return of the neural signal to resting levels over the next 10 to 15 seconds accompanied by a diminishing sense of rotation. If at this stage rotation is stopped, the deceleration involved will be falsely sensed as the start of a rotation in the opposite direction. This illusory post-rotational sensation is known as the somatogyral effect. It comes into the category of felt, non-visual, illusions – hence the prefix 'somato-'. In flight, prolonged rotations occur during changes of heading and also in aerobatic and spinning manoeuvres. In this latter situation, the illusory post-rotation sensation can contribute to difficulties in re-establishing straight and level flight following spin recovery. Even the comparatively benign manoeuvre of a roll attitude change from 45 degrees of left bank to 45 degrees of right bank can lead to a post-rotational sensation of rolling back towards wings level, which, if not countermanded by the visual evidence of bank angle, can lead to a compensatory over-bank to the right.

The Cross-Coupled (Coriolis) Effect

A subject who undergoes a sustained period rotation at constant velocity, for example about a vertical axis on a turntable, will experience a diminishing sensation of rotation. If at this stage the subject makes a head movement out of the plane of rotation, for example in roll (left ear to left shoulder), there will be an illusory sensation of rotation forwards or backwards in pitch. Likewise, if the head movement were made in pitch, an illusory sensation would be felt in roll. This is known as the cross-coupled or Coriolis effect. As originally defined, a Coriolis force arises when a mass mounted on a radial arm rotating at constant angular velocity moves inward or outward along the arm. The initial motion of the mass on the arm describes a circle. If the mass were to move outwards along the radial arm, it would have to travel around the circumference of a bigger circle and would therefore have to move at an increased circumferential velocity. The tangential force required to accelerate the mass to this increased velocity is known as the Coriolis force.

It might be thought from this physical definition that the origin of the Coriolis effect was based on physical principles with no regard to the behaviour of the semicircular canal under conditions of prolonged rotation. This, however, is not so. The illusory sensation is more evident the longer has been the preceding period of constant velocity rotation. The illusory component of the sensation provoked by a head movement in a rotating environment can be explained by the physiological behaviour of one semicircular canal (Figure 4.12).

For simplicity, assume that the canals are anatomically orientated within the head in the transverse, sagittal and coronal planes and are correspondingly named. Assume also that a head movement in roll can be made through 90 degrees. If this idealized subject is rotated about a vertical axis on a turntable, the acceleration associated with the onset of rotation will stimulate the transverse canal. However, once a constant velocity of rotation is established, the cupula of this canal will gradually revert to its rest position and cease to signal any rotation to the brain. A head movement at this point through 90 degrees in roll will carry the transverse canal into the sagittal plane, and will bring the canal that was previously in the sagittal plane into the transverse plane. The canal newly arrived in the plane of rotation will experience the onset of rotation and will correctly signal the ongoing yaw rotation to the brain. Correspondingly, the canal

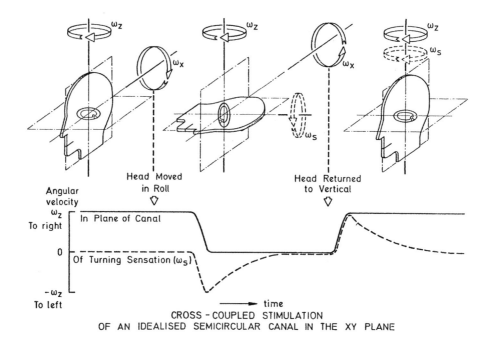

CROSS - COUPLED   STIMULATION
OF AN IDEALISED SEMICIRCULAR CANAL IN THE XY PLANE

Figure 4.12 The cross-coupled (Coriolis) stimulus: Response of an idealized canal in the transverse plane of the head

The subject with head upright has been rotated at constant velocity about a vertical axis for sufficient time (>30 seconds) for the sensation of turning to have decayed away. A head movement through 90 degrees in roll produces an illusory sensation of rotation in pitch. When this sensation decays, a return to the head upright position gives a renewed, but decaying, sensation of the original rotation.

that has been taken out of the plane of rotation and is now in the sagittal plane will register a stopping stimulus.

However, because this canal was previously signalling no rotation, the stopping stimulus will be registered as a rotation in the opposite direction. The perceptual process within the brain takes account of the altered position of the head on the trunk and refers any sense of rotation to the orientation of the body, so that this post-rotational sensation will be perceived as a rotation of the body in the sagittal plane, in pitch. The illusory sense of pitch is explained by the response of the one canal taken out of the plane of rotation. The canal brought into the plane of rotation by the head movement is responsible for a renewed sense of yaw-axis rotation. The overall sensation provoked by a head movement is therefore somewhat more complex than originally described – a combination of the underlying rotation and of rotation in the plane at right angles to that of the head movement.

The cross-coupled illusion is easily provoked in the laboratory or even in a rotating office chair, and it is regularly demonstrated to aircrew in rotating spatial disorientation trainer devices. However, the circumstances in which it is provoked in flight are probably not very frequent. The rate of yaw rotation in turns at low angle of bank in the aircraft may be sustained but are of low angular velocity. The standard rate-one turn involves a yaw rate of 3 degrees per second, significantly less than the 40 to 60 degrees per second of yaw rotation that might be used in a disorientation simulator to impress aircrew with the effects of head movement. Roll manoeuvres in aircraft can involve high rates of rotation but are not usually sustained for many seconds. Spinning manoeuvres involve high rotation rates for more prolonged periods,

but, though regularly practised, are otherwise manoeuvres that are avoided. Nonetheless, there have been sufficient reports from pilots flying in poor visual conditions who have experienced powerful but illusory sensations following an abrupt head movement to advise aircrew that they should not make unnecessary head movements when manoeuvring in cloud or at night. It is likely that even low-intensity spurious rotational sensations can be difficult to ignore in conditions where they cannot be countermanded by a clear view of the stable external world.

The weather at our destination was amber with a 200 feet cloudbase. We were positioned for a radar approach but, having arrived at the bottom of the descent a little late and fast in instrument meteorological conditions we were instructed to carry out a 270 degree turn to the right. I elected to complete the checks while in the turn but had to move my head down and to the left in order to check the hydraulic and brake pressures. On returning to a normal head position and recommencing my instrument scan, I experienced an incredibly strong case of disorientation. I have experienced the leans many times and handled it without difficulty, but this was something else. The feeling of being in a descending right-hand turn was incredibly strong. I was staring at the attitude indicator which showed straight and level flight, but was absolutely convinced it was wrong. By instinct, I cross-checked with the stand-by attitude indicator, which also showed straight and level flight. However, so strong was the disorientation that I began to doubt the accuracy of both attitude indicators; all my instincts told me I was continuing a descending turn and would shortly impact the sea. Luckily, I managed to maintain a straight and level picture on the attitude indicator, but was having to stare at it intently to do so. This was followed by a call of 'Airspeed!' from the front cockpit. In concentrating on the aircraft attitude, I had allowed the airspeed to drop below the 150 knots required at this stage of the approach. I applied power and handed control to the front cockpit. After about a minute I took control again, asking the front seat pilot to keep an eye on me. We broke cloud at decision height and made a successful landing. However, I had to fight the feeling of disorientation all the way down the approach and only when visual with the runway did I begin to feel a little (but not a lot) more comfortable.

Oculogravic and Oculogyral Effects

The force environment of aviation leads to illusory sensations of either tilt or rotation, the former termed somatogravic, the latter somatogyral. The prefix 'somato-' is designed to indicate that these sensations are bodily sensations that are non-visual; they are felt rather than seen. However, for every somatic illusion there is often a visual counterpart which, when evident, acts in such a direction as to confirm the somatic sensation.

As already described, a change of airspeed in level flight is associated with an illusory sensation of a change of pitch attitude, pitch-up during sustained acceleration and pitch-down during deceleration. The visual counterpart of this sensation is a visual perception of upward slope of the forward visual scene on acceleration and downward slope on deceleration. This illusion is little evident when viewing in daylight a highly structured terrestrial visual scene. In fact, the external view tends to countermand any sensation of tilt so that forward acceleration in the horizontal

direction is perceived for what it is. The high-performance sports car accelerating away from traffic lights on a level road neither feels nor appears to be going uphill. However, the same cannot be said for a catapult launch of an aircraft from the deck of an aircraft carrier. In this situation, the forward acceleration on the aircraft, which until it leaves the deck of the ship is about 4 G, generates a strong pitch-up sensation (Cohen *et al.*, 1973). To avoid the possibility of an inappropriate control action, the pilot is required to keep his hands clear of the control column during the launch.

The perception of tilt of the external scene is likely to be more evident when the visual information is limited, as when viewing isolated lights at night. In these circumstances, there is the possibility of misinterpretation of what is seen on account of the apparent change of position. Possibly of more significance is that the illusory appearance of tilt affects not just the external scene, but also the visual perception of the aircraft. This effect is perhaps best noticed by passengers in the rear aisle seats of a commercial aircraft who may observe that while the aircraft is accelerating along the runway, and well before the pilot lifts the nose wheel off the ground prior to becoming airborne, the floor of the cabin appears to slope upwards. A corresponding appearance of downward slope of the floor occurs when the brakes are applied after touch-down. The absence of any sensation of tilt when an aircraft is in a coordinated level turn is associated with the visual impression that the external horizon is tilted. This effect is particularly marked when external vision is lost and the horizon is now represented by the blue/brown boundary on the attitude indicator. The pilot may perceive the horizon to be tilted with respect to the aircraft rather than the reverse, even though it is the aircraft that moves, not the horizon. These are examples of what is termed the oculogravic illusion, a situation in which a false perception of the gravitational vertical induces a corresponding perception of tilt of the visual world.

A further example of this illusion is known as the elevator illusion. Passengers in a lift may observe during upward acceleration that the wall of the lift appears to move upwards even though there is in fact no relative movement between the wall of the lift and the observer. The effect is only observed during acceleration and deceleration and is therefore more readily observed in high-speed lifts when these phases of travel are more prolonged.

Angular motion is also associated with visual illusions that are the counterpart to the non-visual somatogyral illusions. The perceptual consequences of sustained rotation in the aviation environment are well illustrated by the effect of spinning manoeuvres. An aircraft when put into a spin may undergo several turns of a somewhat complex rotation, involving a combination of pitch, roll and yaw, from which the pilot has to recover the aircraft to straight and level flight.

The somatogyral (non-visual) effect of this manoeuvre consists of an accurate sensation of rotation in the early seconds of the spin, followed by a diminishing sense of rotation and finally an illusory sense of rotation in the opposite direction once straight and level flight is re-established. The visual counterpart of this sequence of sensations consists of an initial accurate perception of a static external visual world sweeping away in the opposite direction of the spin. There follows an increased perception of movement of the visual world in this direction as the somatic perception of self-rotation dies away, during which time it may only

be possible to determine the number of turns that the aircraft has made by counting the number of times the sun comes round. Finally, immediately after spin recovery the illusory sense of turning in the opposite direction of the spin is accompanied by a perception of the visual world moving in the same direction as the original spin. If the reader is confused by this description, it is perhaps some indication of the sensory confusion that a pilot may experience, made worse if the spin was inadvertent and happened in poor visual conditions.

The oculogyral effect can be defined as an illusory appearance of turning of the visual scene which does not accord with the angular motion of the observer. Aisle-seated airline passengers can also observe a manifestation of this illusion, most convincingly seen at night when there are no external visual cues through the aircraft windows. When the aircraft is taxiing, each turn that the aircraft makes between the runway and the terminal can be detected by the apparent left or right movement of what is visible looking along the length of the aircraft, even though the view is entirely confined to the interior of the aircraft. A similar observation can be made looking along the carriage of a tube train. A laboratory-based study of this effect required a subject seated in the dark on a turntable to view a solitary light, itself attached to the turntable a metre or so in front of the subject. The onset of rotation of the turntable was associated with an apparent movement of the light in the direction of rotation even though there had been no relative movement between the subject and the light. Studies that have compared the detection threshold of rotation with and without the light have shown that the presence of the light reduces the threshold of detection by a factor of 2.5 (Benson and Brown,

1989). The most likely explanation for this phenomenon is that the vestibular stimulus that accompanies the rotation elicits an eye movement that tends to keep the eye directed to a point fixed in space. This results in a displacement of the retinal image of the light, which the brain interprets as a movement of the light.

Also in the category of oculogyral effects is the visual counterpart to the cross-coupled illusion. A subject rotating in the dark at constant velocity on a turntable while viewing a fixed light mounted on the turntable will be aware of apparent upward and downward movement of the light as a result of making small angular head movements from side to side in roll. The direction of the apparent up and down movement of the light is in the same direction as the illusory sensation of pitch motion that would accompany more generous roll-axis head movements. As with the other manifestations of the oculogyral illusion, vestibular-induced eye movements are the most likely basis of the perceived motion of the visual target.

Alternobaric Vertigo

The change in atmospheric pressure with altitude can in certain circumstances lead to a disturbance of vestibular function. This takes the form of an abrupt onset of vertigo during rapid ascent in an aircraft. The vertigo is usually short-lived and decays over 15 to 20 seconds, a time period typical of the decay of rotation sensation following a transient angular velocity change on a laboratory turntable. This problem may, however, occur at a critical time in the flight and, if there is no sight of the ground, it may be very difficult to dispel the perception that the sensed rotation is affecting the whole aircraft. The phenomenon of

alternobaric, or pressure, vertigo is more familiar to divers on ascent from depth on account of the much greater changes in pressure associated with diving. Here too, it is associated with the hazard of disorientation. The affected individual usually reports that the onset of vertigo is triggered by clearing of the ears when, on ascent, air is vented from the middle ear via the eustachian tube, and particularly when one ear clears and the other does not. The problem can also occur on descent if an over-energetic Valsalva manoeuvre leads to excess pressure in the middle ear.

The precise mechanism for the vertigo is not well understood. Overpressure of the middle ear will result in outward bulging of the tympanic membrane which in turn pulls the stapes outward from the oval window. An abrupt relief of excess pressure in the middle ear will result in a sudden inward movement of the stapes and a corresponding movement of perilymph and endolymph. For this to result in vertigo implies that there has been a displacement of one or more of the cupulae of the semicircular canals. The plane of the sensed vertigo varies between affected individuals which suggests that more than one semicircular canal may be affected by the inner ear pressure disturbance. Problems with pressure vertigo are more likely to occur if there is congestion around the nasopharyngeal openings of the eustachian tubes as a consequence of an upper respiratory infection, since a higher pressure difference is required between the middle ear and the pharynx before venting occurs. This is a further reason, in addition to the risk of barotrauma, why aircrew should not fly with sticky ears.

It was an early morning take-off. I had not eaten before departure as I expected a good breakfast on arrival. I had had a cold two weeks before and appeared to have fully recovered. As the aircraft was levelling at 3,000 feet with the sea in sight below but the only horizon being the top of the haze layer at about 2,000 feet, my ears cleared and I suddenly had the most powerful impression that the aircraft was yawing very fast to the left. Fortunately the autopilot was flying the aircraft and all the instruments were showing normal straight and level flight. I realized very quickly that I was disorientated but found myself fighting the autopilot on the controls. The only way I stopped myself from doing this was by placing my feet on the floor and sitting on my hands. I am sure that the only reason I had the impression of yaw alone was because of the definite but featureless horizon. I felt airsick while all this was going on and was only able to relieve the sensation when I stared for some time at a small cloud that I found above the horizon at about 4 o'clock.

Alcohol

The loss of inhibitions and the impairment of cognitive function are well-recognized central effects of alcohol. Giddiness and unsteadiness of gait are also typical of excessive alcohol consumption. While this effect on balance may have a central component, the effect on the labyrinth is thought to arise as a consequence of a density disparity within the semicircular canal system. To function correctly as a rotation sensor, it is essential that the cupula within the ampulla of each semicircular canal remains insensitive to gravity. This is achieved by the cupula having exactly the same density as the endolymphatic fluid that surrounds it. Provided this is so, whatever the position of the head, the cupula tends neither to float nor to sink. Were it to do either, it would send

a spurious signal to the brain to indicate rotation. It appears that alcohol in the circulation diffuses into the cupula before it reaches the endolymphatic fluid, and because alcohol is less dense than water sets up a density difference between the cupula and the endolymph. As a result, when a head movement brings the cupula into a more horizontal position, the subject becomes aware of a sense of vertigo.

This effect can be demonstrated clinically by the positional test in which the subject from a sitting position adopts a lying posture with the head turned to one side and tilted below the horizontal. A sustained horizontal nystagmus can be seen either by recording eye movements with the eyes closed by means of the electro-oculogram, or else by direct inspection of the eyes through Frenzel lenses, strong magnifying lenses worn by the subject which prevent visual fixation by defocusing any image of the surroundings. This explanation of the origin of alcohol-induced vertigo receives support from experiments using deuterium oxide (heavy water) in place of alcohol (Money and Myles, 1974). This substance, which has a density that is greater than that of water, also induces vertigo and a positive positional test, but the induced nystagmus is in the opposite direction to that produced by alcohol. If alcohol intake is continued over several hours, it penetrates into the endolymphatic fluid, the density disparity becomes less and the positional nystagmus is reduced or abolished. However, once alcohol ingestion is stopped, it clears from the circulation and from the cupulae more rapidly than from the endolymph and a density disparity is re-established that can remain for 48 hours or more.

The implication for flying is that a prolonged generous alcohol ingestion may require longer than the rule that specifies the 12-hour alcohol-free 'bottle-to-throttle' interval before flying. Though alcohol may be cleared from the blood and cognition unimpaired after this time, it is sequestered in the endolymph for a longer period and may cause positional vertigo after a much longer interval. If flying involves high G manoeuvres, the increased G amplifies the effect of any density disparity and thus any related vertigo.

Part 5:
SPATIAL DISORIENTATION – ACCIDENTS AND INCIDENTS

In the process of acquiring any physical skill, there is a gradual transfer of a student's attention away from the individual components of the activity and towards an integrated approach to the task. With continued practice, it becomes possible to achieve the individual components without evident thought and this liberates the student's mental capacity to concentrate on the overall purpose of the activity. In the early stages of training, a student military pilot is learning to fly various aircraft manoeuvres accurately. As training progresses, other skills are added, for example instrument flying, navigation, airmanship, weapons delivery and combat tactics. By the time these new skills are achieved, the basic skill of handling an aircraft is largely taken for granted. The trained pilot is no longer thinking about the manoeuvre that he is flying but rather about what he is trying to achieve by the manoeuvre.

A common theme in spatial disorientation incidents, and, by extension, accidents, is a preoccupation with one aspect of the flying task to the exclusion of accurately flying the aircraft. Many pilots have commented on how quickly a flight trajectory can go from safe to unsafe when attention is diverted away from the flying task. This is particularly true when the aircraft is manoeuvring at low level.

> I was the lead of a pair conducting low-level close air support. I was repositioning for another talk-on. I entered a right-hand turn whilst typing in coordinates in our navigational kit located on the left quarter light. About 4 seconds after I started inputting the data, the low height warning sounded. I immediately recovered. The nose had sliced to 10 degrees nose-down and my turn took me towards rising ground. My number two, an experienced pilot, had not been aware of the danger to the aircraft. If we had not been flying with a minimum separation distance of 500 feet, I believe the aircraft would have become more nose-down and I would have missed the ground very narrowly. The weather was excellent throughout. I have chalked this up to experience. Spatial disorientation happens very insidiously, especially as I was effectively 'heads-up' while typing in the navigational information. The real learning point is how quickly my flight path went from safe to unsafe.

It is unsurprising that a pilot's loss of awareness of aircraft attitude at a critical phase of flight can lead to an accident. Analysis of accidents often reveals multiple causal factors leading up to the final event. An assessment of the role played by disorientation in any accident may have to rely on circumstantial evidence, such as a knowledge of weather conditions at the time and the manoeuvre being attempted, in order to arrive at a conclusion. Any conclusion is always open to investigator bias. For these reasons, accident surveys, almost all of them dealing with military accidents, vary quite widely in the reported percentage of accidents attributable to spatial disorientation.

A recent survey of military accidents (Bushby, 2004) covering the years 1983–1992 and 1993–2002 showed a reduction in the rate of all accidents, particularly in rotary wing aircraft, between the two time periods, but little change in the rate of spatial disorientation-related accidents. Several factors were identified that increased the relative risk of a disorientation-related accident. Risk was increased by a factor of two when night-flying and by a factor of about three when flying in cloud or in degraded visual conditions. Failure of communication within the cockpit led to an almost fourfold increase in risk. Of particular significance in this survey were the findings that 50 per cent of disorientation-related accidents involved distraction and that, at the point at which the accident became inevitable, disorientation remained unrecognized in 85 per cent of accidents. The accident rates per 100,000 flying hours are given below. For comparison, the accident rate for commercial aircraft belonging to major airlines recorded between 1995 and 1998 was 0.29 per 100,000 flying hours.

	1983–1992	1993–2002
Fast jet aircraft		
All accidents	7.0	5.8
Disorientation-related accidents	1.7	1.6
Rotary wing aircraft		
All accidents	4.1	2.4
Disorientation-related accidents	1.0	1.0

Questionnaire surveys of pilots to determine their experience of spatial disorientation have tended to concentrate on the incidence of known in-flight illusions. There are several difficulties with this approach. One problem was highlighted by an unpublished survey of 100 pilots who were asked to report their most recent experience of disorientation and its impact on flight safety. In four of the five reported incidents in which flight safety was considered at risk, the pilot was unable to say what illusion he had suffered. It could be argued that a pilot is only disorientated when he does *not* experience an illusion in flight, in that to be aware of an illusion requires a simultaneous appreciation of the reality of the situation and the discrepancy between the misperception and reality. It is only when the illusion is reality to the pilot that he is truly disorientated. It has to be acknowledged, however, that there are circumstances in flight in which, despite knowing from flight instruments the reality of aircraft attitude, the illusory sensation can be very powerful and difficult to countermand.

An alternative approach to assess the incidence of spatial disorientation is to obtain from pilots a description of occasions in flight when either they became confused about the attitude or spatial position of the aircraft or they suddenly became aware that the aircraft was not in the attitude or position that it was expected to be. The first of these two categories describes a situation that is almost a daily occurrence in flying, in that all pilots have to recognize that the potential to become confused is an essential feature of flight. The second potentially more dangerous category describes the moment of recognition of a previously overlooked deviation from the intended flight path. In a survey of this type, it then becomes the task of the investigator to identify from the description of the incident the precipitating factors and the underlying illusions that may have been involved. It is likely that this approach gives a truer picture of the functional significance of the spatially disorientating aspects of flying.

Aircrew Spatial Disorientation Training

Many scientific disciplines contribute to the avoidance of accidents attributable to spatial disorientation. Aircraft design engineers are developing new forms of display to maintain pilot awareness of the attitude and flight path of the aircraft. Other engineering developments have involved pilot-activated automatic attitude recovery systems, the so-called 'panic button', and also ground collision avoidance systems that intervene without the pilot's request if the predicted aircraft trajectory would lead to a crash. Of perpetual importance is the specialist aeromedical training of aircrew to understand the deceptiveness of the flight environment and human physiological limitations and also the training, both in flight and in the simulator, to develop in aircrew safe flying practices in potentially disorientating situations.

In addition to lectures and video presentations, aircrew are given the opportunity to experience spatial disorientation in a dedicated simulator. These devices have evolved from relatively simple rotating chairs to enclosed rotating cabins with visual presentations of an aircraft instrument panel and a computer-generated external visual scene. While the aim of the earlier devices was to demonstrate the fallibility of vestibular sensors of motion, later devices with additional motion capabilities have attempted to demonstrate, with variable degrees of fidelity, the disorientating illusions of flight. Some air forces have supplemented ground-based training with dedicated flights designed to demonstrate manoeuvres that can deceive the pilot.

The problem of unrecognized disorientation, the situation in which everything feels normal despite a worsening deviation from the intended flight path, is not well addressed by ground-based disorientation simulators. The confusing sensations that they demonstrate, if experienced in flight, act as the trigger to alert the pilot to rely on the aircraft instruments to determine the true situation. However, the great majority of disorientation-related accidents occur without the alerting benefit of confusing sensations. For these it is necessary to familiarize pilots in the circumstances, such as go-around, take-off into cloud or low-level abort manoeuvres, in which the risk of unrecognized disorientation is high. An equally important aspect of disorientation training is prioritization of tasks and the apportionment of time devoted to them in relation to the demands of maintaining an accurate flight path. These considerations are well suited to the use of modern training simulators, in which the motion environment is far less important than the ability to create a large range of scenarios that tax the pilot's airmanship and create the potential for unrecognized disorientation. This use of conventional simulators is being introduced for disorientation training in both fixed and rotary-wing aircraft at multiple stages throughout a pilot's career. Whether this development will have a beneficial impact on the accident statistics only time will tell.

References

Anon. 2008. Obituary. H.M. *The Economist*, 20th December, 146.

Benson, A.J. and Brown, S.F. 1989. Visual display lowers detection threshold of angular, but not linear, whole body motion stimuli. *Aviation Space and Environmental Medicine*, 60, 629–33.

Best, P.J., White, A.M. and Minai, A. 2001. Spatial processing in the brain: The activity of hippocampal place cells. *Annual Review of Neuroscience*, 24, 459–86.

Bushby, A.J.R. 2004. An assessment of the influence of spatial disorientation upon military aircraft accidents from 1983 to 2002. Thesis: Membership of the Faculty of Occupational Medicine, Royal College of Physicians, London.

Cohen, M.M., Crosbie, R.J. and Blackburn, L.H. 1973. Disorienting effects of aircraft catapult launchings. *Aerospace Medicine*, 47, 39–41.

Fernandez, C. and Goldberg, J.M. 1971. Physiology of peripheral neurons innervating semicircular canals of the squirrel monkey. II. Response to sinusoidal stimulation and dynamics of peripheral vestibular system. *Journal of Neurophysiology*, 34, 661–84.

Goldberg, J.M. and Fernandez, C. 1971. Physiology of peripheral neurons innervating semicircular canals of the squirrel monkey. I. Resting discharge and response to constant angular accelerations. *Journal of Neurophysiology*, 34, 635–60.

J.C. 1952. Living without a balancing mechanism. *New England Journal of Medicine*, 246, 458–60.

Johnson, S.L. and Roscoe, S.N. 1972. What moves, the airplane or the world? *Human Factors*, 14, 107–29.

Hafting, T., Fyhn, M., Molden, S., Moser, M.B. and Moser, E.I. 2005. Microstructure of a spatial map in the entorhinal cortex. *Nature*, 436, 801–6.

Healy, S. 1998. *Spatial Representation in Animals*. Oxford: Oxford University Press.

Money, K.E. and Myles, W.S. 1974. Heavy water nystagmus and effects of alcohol. *Nature*, 247, 404–5.

Morris, R.G.M., Garrud, P., Rawlins, J.N.P. and O'Keefe, J. 1982. Place navigation impaired in rats with hippocampal lesions. *Nature*, 297, 681–3.

Moser, E.I., Kropff, E. and Moser, M.B. 2008. Place cells, grid cells, and the brain's spatial representation system. *Annual Review of Neuroscience*, 31, 69–89.

O'Keefe, J. 1976. Place units in the hippocampus of the freely moving rat. *Experimental Neurology*, 51, 78–109.

Ponomarenko, V.A. 2000. *Kingdom in the Sky – Earthly Fetters and Heavenly Freedoms. The Pilot's Approach to the Military Flight Environment*. Neuilly-sur-Seine: NATO Research and Technology Organization AGARDograph 338.

Scoville, W.B. and Milner, B. 1957. Loss of recent memory after bilateral hippocampal lesions. *Journal of Neurology, Neurosurgery and Psychiatry*, 20, 11–21.

Roscoe, S.N. 1997. Horizon control reversals and the graveyard spiral. *Gateway: United States Department of Defense Crew System Ergonomics Information Analysis Centre*, 7, 1–4.

Taube, J.S. 2007. The head direction signal: Origins and sensory-motor integration. *Annual Review of Neuroscience*, 30, 181–207.

Taube, J.S., Muller, R.U. and Ranck, J.B. Jnr 1990. Head direction cells recorded from the postsubiculum in freely moving rats. I. Description and quantitative analysis. *Journal of Neuroscience*, 10, 420–35.

Tolman, E.C. 1948. Cognitive maps in rats and men. *Psychology Review*, 55, 189–208.

Chapter 5

CEREBRAL CIRCULATION AND GRAVITATIONAL STRESS

Anthony N. Nicholson

Observations on the effect of accelerations experienced by aircrew in high-performance aircraft suggest that intracranial fluid dynamics play an important part in mitigating, though to a limited extent, the influence of hypotension on cerebral blood flow. However, as with the cerebral circulation of the giraffe (Goetz *et al.*, 1960), the literature is not overwhelmed by experimental data on the cerebral circulation when the gravitational vector is orientated along the long axis of the body, particularly when, as in the case of aircrew, the stress can exceed that experienced on the surface of the Earth. Indeed, the means to investigate the immediate effects of increased gravity on the cerebral circulation of humans is not currently within the methodological inventory of physiological research. Studies related to cerebral blood flow have been limited to the supine, near supine and upright postures and to techniques that induce hypotension, while invasive measurement of intracranial pressure is normally restricted to neurosurgical procedures.

Nevertheless, this chapter is concerned with the cerebral circulation during gravitational stress when the individual is subject to significant falls in arterial pressures (positive acceleration). In an attempt to predict the changes in intracranial dynamics during positive accelerations, experimental data related to changes in posture and during hypotension have been used. It is appreciated that such extrapolations may have limitations, but the approach has the advantage of using data derived from observed effects on intracranial fluid dynamics, and so is based on physiological evidence. In that context the initial part of this chapter is concerned with the cerebral circulation during change in posture and during hypotension. The latter part attempts to apply these findings to observations during positive accelerations, and raises the question of an active participation of the nervous system in the preservation of consciousness[1] during increased gravitational stress.

Cerebral Blood Flow

Various techniques have been used to study cerebral blood flow. Since the

---

1   In this chapter, considerations of impaired consciousness are limited to its physical manifestations. See Chapter 1 (Wakefulness, Awareness and Consciousness).

1980s changes have been estimated from velocity measurements in the middle cerebral artery using the transcranial Doppler technique (Aaslid *et al.*, 1989). Flow within the artery is proportional to its cross-sectional area as well as to the velocity, but, as changes in the diameter of the middle cerebral artery are minimal in healthy conscious humans, flow is considered to be directly proportional to velocity (Schondorf *et al.*, 1997; Serrador *et al.*, 2000). It is also considered that flow in the middle cerebral artery is an indication of blood flow through all regions of the brain (Levine *et al.*, 1994). Simultaneous measurements of total cerebral blood flow, intracranial compliance and intracranial pressure have been provided by imaging techniques (Alperin *et al.*, 2005, 2006), while the venous drainage system has also been studied by angiography (Epstein *et al.*, 1970, Dilemge and Perry, 1973) and by sonography (Valdueza *et al.*, 2000; Suarez *et al.*, 2002; Cirovic *et al.*, 2003; Gisolf *et al.*, 2004; Doepp *et al.*, 2004).

Adequate cerebral blood flow is essential if consciousness is to be preserved in the upright posture and during increased gravitational stress. Arterial pressures are determined by the cardiac output and by reflex baroreceptor activity: the outflow venous pressures depend on the patency of the internal jugular vein and/or the vertebral venous plexus, as well as being a passive reflection of the gravitational environment. The arterial and venous pressures also create a siphon across the cerebral circulation, and these pressures, as well as the resistance exerted by the blood and cerebrospinal fluid contained within the cranium, are also determinants of cerebral blood flow.

In the supine position, venous outflow is predominantly through the internal jugular vein, but in the upright posture there is a partial or complete collapse of the internal jugular vein with outflow shifted to secondary veins such as the epidural, vertebral and deep cervical that comprise the vertebral venous plexus (Valdueza *et al.*, 2000; Alperin *et al.*, 2005). However, it would appear that any fall in cerebral blood flow on assuming the upright position related to the closure or partial closure of the internal jugular vein is not completely compensated by any increased drainage through the venous plexus. On the other hand, in the upright position there is a considerably smaller volume of cerebrospinal fluid (Alperin *et al.*, 2005, 2006) than when supine, and that would assist cerebral blood flow even though overall it may be slightly reduced.

Autoregulation and Hypotension

In addition to the pressures that influence perfusion, the cerebral vasculature has an inherent ability to preserve blood flow within a limited range of arterial pressure (possibly from 50 to 170 mm Hg). The autoregulatory response to hypotension is located in small vessels in the brain parenchyma (Stromberg and Fox, 1972; Kontos *et al.*, 1978; Baumach and Heistad, 1983), and its response to hypotension has been investigated during fluid shifts and during changes in posture. A variety of manoeuvres have been used. Fluid shifts have involved reductions in central blood volume induced by lower body negative pressure and by deflation of thigh cuffs that encouraged a sudden flow of blood into the lower limbs. The effect of posture has been explored by using head-up tilt which exposes the individual to the near upright posture in the absence of muscular activity in the lower limbs, and by assuming the upright posture from the squat position which involves compensatory vasodilatation in the lower limbs on standing. In some studies, these manoeuvres have been combined.

Studies during fluid shifts and changes in posture have demonstrated the resilience of cerebral autoregulation during hypotensive states. During head-up tilt (80 degrees up to ten minutes) in normal subjects aged between 29 and 77 years, Novak *et al.* (1998) observed that there were no correlations between brain flow velocity and arterial pressures, suggesting that autoregulation had been preserved. Carey *et al.* (2001) also concluded from studies in normal subjects aged between 19 and 90 years that there was no deterioration in cerebral autoregulation during head-up tilt (70 degrees for 30 minutes). Similar conclusions were drawn by Leftheriotis *et al.* (1998) from studies in normal subjects using thigh-cuff deflation during head-up tilt (40 degrees for five minutes), and by Guo *et al.* (2006) who observed that autoregulation was preserved during systemic hypotension induced by thigh-cuff deflation during lower body negative pressure.

However, reduced cerebral blood flow has been observed during lower body negative pressure (Levine *et al.*, 1994; Zhang *et al.*, 1998, 2002), though not of sufficient magnitude to lead to impaired responsiveness. It was ascribed to sympathetic activation rather than to any intrinsic change in autoregulation. A similar vasoconstrictor effect could also be induced during reductions in central blood volume due to falling arterial tensions of carbon dioxide arising from hyperventilation (Cencetti *et al.*, 1997; Novak *et al.*, 1998). It would be important to bear in mind that a tendency to even a modest degree of reduced cerebral blood flow could be significant in the presence of a severe systemic hypotension.

Lower body negative pressure or head-up tilt, even when combined with deflation of thigh cuffs, may be stresses of insufficient severity to investigate autoregulation at the bottom of the regulatory range (around and below 70 mm Hg). In that context Rickards *et al.* (2007) have used the squat–stand test, paying particular attention to the initial 10 to 15 seconds of standing. On standing (from the squat position) mean arterial pressures fell to below 70 mm Hg with concomitant falls in cerebral blood flow velocity. However, the delays to the nadir and to the recovery of cerebral blood flow velocity were less than those of the mean arterial pressures. It was concluded that, though transient falls in cerebral blood flow occurred during precipitous falls in arterial pressures, the dynamic component of autoregulation remained intact, even with arterial pressures around the lower limit of the autoregulatory range.

Positive Acceleration

Positive acceleration is a term used in aviation physiology that refers to an acceleration in the headwards direction with the resultant inertial force in the head to foot direction (+ Gz) leading to hypotension. Essentially, the pressure gradients that normally exist due to gravity in the upright position are accentuated. Positive accelerations exceeding +4 Gz are likely to lead to total loss of vision with loss of consciousness when they exceed +5 to +6 Gz. Above +6 Gz loss of consciousness is likely to be the initial event. Arterial pressures fall rapidly during the first 10 seconds or so of an exposure due to reduced cardiac output and falls in peripheral resistance. At head level the mean arterial pressure falls to around zero at accelerations exceeding +4 Gz, and there are negative transmural pressures across the jugular veins with increased resistance to flow. These cardiovascular effects are counteracted by reflex baroreceptor activity with arteriolar vasoconstriction and tachycardia and by increased venous return. They tend to restore the arterial pressure toward that which exists in the upright posture, but the degree of recovery depends on the magnitude of the continuing acceleration (Glaister and Prior, 1999).

Accelerations around and in excess of +3 Gz reduce arterial pressures at head level to values that under normal gravity would be far below those needed to maintain an adequate cerebral blood flow. However, during positive accelerations of such magnitude, consciousness may be preserved. During increased gravitational stress, cerebral blood flow is likely to be favoured by the reduced volume of intracranial blood due to the preferential distribution of blood to the lower part of the body in excess of that experienced in the upright state, and by reductions in the volume of the cerebrospinal fluid within the cranium. Further, though the partial or even complete closure of the jugular vein as observed in the upright posture could be of significance during the positive accelerations encountered in flight, it is possible that the increased gravitational environment may encourage venous flow either through the jugular veins or through the venous complex.

Changes in the compliance of the cerebral vasculature during orthostatic stress, particularly when enhanced by systemic hypotension, would also play their part in mitigating the immediate effects of positive accelerations. Though precipitous falls in arterial pressure may be associated with an acute, though transient, fall in cerebral blood flow (Aaslid et al., 1989; Levine et al., 1994; Immink et al., 2006; Guo et al., 2006; Rickards et al., 2007), recovery of blood flow may take place while the arterial pressure is still depressed. With the onset of positive acceleration, even of limited magnitude, there is an immediate fall in arterial pressure. The dynamic component of cerebral autoregulation has a more rapid influence on cerebral blood flow than the baroreceptor effect on arterial pressures, and so may assist in the maintenance of consciousness before the partial recovery of arterial pressures. However, ultimately, with accelerations of significant magnitude, the fall in arterial pressures becomes the overriding risk to cerebral function.

Consciousness and Gravitational Stress

Understanding the tendency for consciousness to be preserved during positive accelerations of limited magnitude has been a long-standing puzzle in aviation medicine. Assumed changes in fluid dynamics during hypotension have been invoked to interpret the sequence of events. Impaired vision precedes impaired consciousness, and that has been explained, at least partially, by the resistance to flow in the retina due to the intraocular pressure (20 mm Hg). The explanation assumes that the normal intraocular pressure is maintained during accelerations, but the system that supports the intraocular pressure is not a closed one. Indeed, there is evidence that intraocular pressure is elevated during microgravity (Mader, 1991; Mader et al., 1993; Draeger et al., 1995) and by head-down rest (Xu et al., 2010) and altitude (Ersanli et al., 2006). Further, studies in animals have shown that intraocular pressure falls, pari passu, with an induced fall in arterial blood pressure (Nicholson et al., 1968). There is no evidence to support the contention that the intraocular pressure is maintained during acute hypotension.

Nevertheless, impaired vision does precede the impairment of consciousness during increased gravitational stress, and the sequence of events is clearly related to the maintenance of cerebral blood flow due to autoregulation and to the changes in intracranial dynamics rather than to any undue resistance to retinal blood flow. Even so, it is difficult to accept that autoregulatory and haemodynamic factors alone account for the tendency for consciousness to be preserved beyond the loss of vision. That would imply that the neural systems that support consciousness are entirely passive, and that the nervous system does not possess any coping mechanisms in response to an acute stress that could impair consciousness. It is beyond discussion that the brain

possesses systems that, when activated, modulate responsiveness, and so it is possible that these ascending systems may be activated during hypotension.

In that context studies in animals on conduction in the retino-optic tract and in the thalamocortical circuit during acute hypotension induced by a reduction in circulating blood volume suggest that activity within these pathways is differentially modulated (Nicholson et al., 1968). The electroretinogram and potentials along the optic tract evoked by flashes of light are markedly reduced and almost disappear during hypotension, while conduction in the thalamocortical pathway and the activity of cortical neurons evoked by stimulation of the optic tract are enhanced (Figures 5.1 and 5.2). During

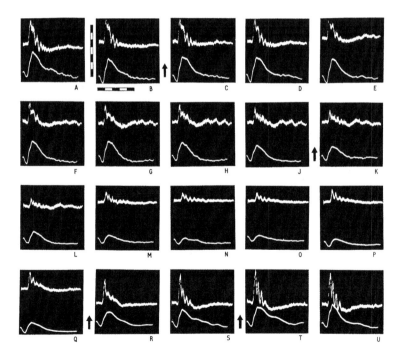

Figure 5.1   Optic tract discharges (upper traces) and electroretinograms (lower traces) of the cat induced by flashes of light during hypotension

Recordings A and B are the control potentials. Recordings C to Q are the potentials during a 90 second period of hypotension and recordings R to U are the potentials during the recovery phase. (Calibrations: vertical divisions – 200 microvolts; horizontal divisions – 20 milliseconds)

Source: Nicholson, A.N., Macnamara, W.D. and Borland, R.G. 1968. Responsiveness of the cortex and visual pathway during transient hypotension. *Electroencephalography and Clinical Neurophysiology*, 25, 330–337. (Reprinted with permission from Elsevier)

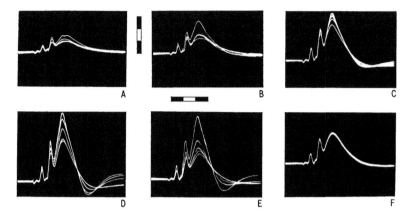

Figure 5.2   Cortical responses of the cat elicited by stimulation of the optic tract during hypotension

Recording A is the control response. Recordings B to F are superimposed potentials at 10 second intervals during hypotension. (Calibrations: vertical divisions – 200 microvolts; horizontal divisions – 20 milliseconds)

Source: Nicholson, A.N., Macnamara, W.D. and Borland, R.G. 1968. Responsiveness of the cortex and visual pathway during transient hypotension. *Electroencephalography and Clinical Neurophysiology*, 25, 330–337. (Reprinted with permission from Elsevier)

hypotension there is no evidence of enhanced activity within the retino-optic tract level, and so the enhancement observed in cortical potentials, even though afferent sensory signals are depressed, arises in the thalamocortical system. The enhancement of the cortical responses suggests that forebrain activity during hypotension may be preserved by a neurally mediated activation of thalamocortical transmission.

Similar changes are observed in the same cortical potentials during positive accelerations (Nicholson, 1966), as well as in cortical potentials evoked by flashes of light (Nicholson, 1964). There is marked enhancement of post-synaptic cortical activity (Figure 5.3). As with the studies on hypotension induced by a rapid reduction in the central blood volume, the enhancement of cortical responses suggests that forebrain activity during hypotension may be preserved by a neurally mediated activation of thalamocortical transmission. The relevance of these findings to the preservation of consciousness is uncertain, though the thalamocortical

system could well be related to the neural substrate of consciousness (Llinás, 1990; Llinás and Ribary, 2001; Llinás and Steriade, 2006; Llinás *et al.*, 1998; Steriade, 2001; Steriade and Deschenes, 1984) – an issue discussed more fully in Chapter 1 (Wakefulness, Awareness and Consciousness). Adaptations within the system could suggest that activity within the thalamocortical system is preserved preferentially, at least for a while, during a hypotensive stress that leads to unconsciousness. In that way impaired consciousness may be delayed.

Summary

Both cerebrovascular and neurological adaptations must be sought in understanding the preservation of consciousness during increased gravitational stress. Cerebral blood flow may be assisted by reduced intracranial volumes of blood and cerebrospinal fluid and, possibly, by a boost to the siphon effect. It is also reasonable to assume that autoregulation will be preserved

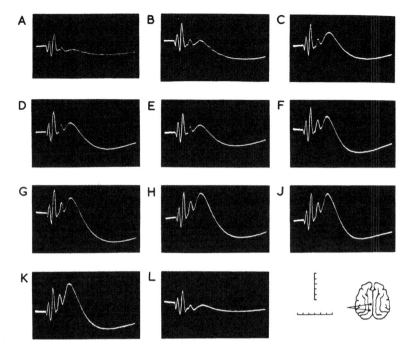

Figure 5.3   Cortical responses of the cat evoked by stimulation of the optic tract during a positive acceleration (+3 Gz)

Source: Nicholson, A.N. 1968. Thalamo-cortical activity during increased gravitational stress. Electroencephalography and Clinical Neurophysiology. 21,168-167. Reprinted with permission from Elsevier.

during positive accelerations of limited magnitude, up to +3 Gz and possibly beyond, and that the influence of its dynamic component (dynamic cerebral autoregulation) may be crucial during the rapid fall in arterial pressure that occurs with the onset of acceleration. As far as the central nervous system is concerned, there is some evidence to suggest that there is increased synchrony of neuronal activity in the thalamocortical system during hypotension, and that could also be concerned with the preservation of consciousness. There is much interest in the role of the thalamocortical system in the process of consciousness, and this is discussed earlier in this volume (Chapter 1: Wakefulness, Awareness and Consciousness).

References

Aaslid. R., Lindegaard, K.F., Sorteberg, W. and Nornes, H. 1989. Cerebral autoregulation dynamics in humans. *Stroke*, 20, 45–52.

Alperin, N., Lee, S.H., Sivaramakrishnan, A. and Hushek, S.G. 2005. Quantifying the effect of posture in intracranial physiology in humans by MRI flow studies. *Journal of Magnetic Resonance Imaging*, 22, 591–6.

Alperin, N., Mazda, M., Lichtor, T. and Lee, S.H. 2006. From cerebrospinal fluid pulsation to noninvasive intracranial compliance and pressure measured by MRI flow studies. *Current Medical Imaging Reviews*, 2, 117–29.

Baumach, G.L. and Heistad, D.D. 1983. Effects of sympathetic stimulation and changes in arterial pressures on segmental resistance of cerebral vessels in rabbits and cats. *Circulation Research*, 52, 527–33.

Carey, B.J., Manktelow, B.N., Panerai, R.B. and Potter, J.F. 2001. Cerebral autoregulatory responses to head-up tilt in normal subjects and patients with recurrent vasovagal syndrome. *Circulation*, 104, 898–902.

Cencetti. S., Bandinelli, G. and Lagi, A. 1997. Effect of PCO_2 changes induced by head-upright tilt on transcranial Doppler recordings. *Stroke*, 28, 1195–7.

Cirovic, S., Walsh, C., Fraser, W.D. and Gulino, A. 2003. The effect of posture and positive pressure breathing on the hemodynamics of the internal jugular vein. *Aviation, Space, and Environmental Medicine*, 74, 125–31.

Dilemge, D. and Perry. B. 1973. An angiographic study of the meningorachidian venous system. *Radiology*, 108, 333–7.

Doepp, F., Schreiber, S.J., von Munster, T., Klingebiel, R. and Valdueza, J.N. 2004. How does the blood leave the brain? A systematic ultrasound analysis of cerebral venous drainage patterns. *Neuroradiology*, 46, 565–70.

Draeger, J., Schwarftz, R., Groenhoff, S. and Stern, C. 1995. Self-tonometry under microgravity conditions. *Aviation, Space, and Environmental Medicine*, 66, 568–70.

Epstein, M.H., Linde, H.W. and Crampton, A.R. 1970. The vertebral venous plexus as a major cerebral outflow tract. *Anesthesiology*, 32, 332–7.

Ersanli, D., Yildiz, S., Sonmez, M., Akin, A., Sen, A. and Uzun, G. 2006. Intraocular pressure at a simulated altitude of 9000 m with and without 100% oxygen. *Aviation, Space, and Environmental Medicine*, 77, 704–6.

Gisolf, J., van Lieshout, J.J., van Heusden, K., Pott, F., Stock, W.J. and Maremaker, M. 2004. Human cerebral venous outflow pathway depends on posture and central

venous pressure. *Journal of Physiology*, 560, 317–27.

Glaister, D.H. and Prior, A.R.J. 1999. The Effects of Long Duration Acceleration. In: J. Ernsting, A.N. Nicholson and D.J. Rainford (eds) *Aviation Medicine*. Oxford: Butterworth-Heinemann, Ch. 9.

Goetz, R.H., Warren, J.V., Gauer, O.H., Patterson, J.L., Doyle, J.T., Keen, E.N. *et al.* 1960. Circulation of the giraffe. *Circulation Research*, VIII, 1049–58.

Guo, H., Tierney, N., Schaller, F., Raven, P.B., Smith, S.A. and Xiangrong, S. 2006. Cerebral autoregulation is preserved during orthostatic stress superimposed with systemic hypotension. *Journal of Applied Physiology*, 100, 1785–92.

Immink, R.V., Secher, N.H., Roos, C.M., Pott, F., Madsen, P.L. and van Lieshout, J.J. 2006. The postural reduction in middle cerebral artery velocity is not explained by $PaCO_2$. *European Journal of Applied Physiology*, 96, 609–14.

Kontos, H.A., Wei, E.P., Navari, R.M., Levasseur, J.E., Rosenblum, W.I. and Patterson, J.L. 1978. Responses of cerebral arteries and arterioles to acute hypotension and hypertension. *American Journal of Physiology*, 234, H371–83.

Leftheriotis, G., Preckel, M.P., Fizanne, L., Victor, J., Dupuis, J.M. and Saumet, J.L. 1998. Effect of head-upright tilt on the dynamic of cerebral autoregulation. *Clinical Physiology*, 18, 41–7.

Levine, B.D., Giller, C.A., Lane, L.D., Buckley, J.C. and Blomqvist, C.G. 1994. Cerebral versus systemic hemodynamics during graded orthostatic stress in humans. *Circulation*, 90, 298–306.

Llinás, R.R. 1990. Intrinsic Electrical Properties of Mammalian Neurons and CNS Function. In: *Fidia Research Foundation Neuroscience Award Lectures*. New York, NY: Raven Press, 40, 1–10.

Llinás, R. and Ribary, U. 2001. Consciousness and the brain: The thalamocortical dialogue in health and disease. *Annals of the New York Academy of Sciences*, 929, 166–75.

Llinás, R., Ribary, U., Contreras, D. and Pedroarena, C. 1998. The neuronal basis for consciousness. *Philosophical Transactions of the Royal Society of London Series B – Biological Sciences*, 353, 1841–9.

Llinás, R. and Steriade, M. 2006. Bursting of thalamic neurons and states of vigilance. *Journal of Neurophysiology*, 95, 3297–308.

Mader, T.H. 1991. Intraocular pressure in microgravity. *Journal of Clinical Pharmacology*, 31, 947–50.

Mader, T.H., Gibson, C.R., Caputo, M., Hunter, N., Taylor, G., Charles, J. and Meehan, R.T. 1993. Intraocular pressure and retinal vascular changes during transient exposure to microgravity. *American Journal of Ophthalmology*, 115, 347–50.

Nicholson, A.N. 1964. Gravitational stress: Changes in cortical excitability. *Science*, 145, 1458–9.

Nicholson, A.N. 1966. Thalamo-cortical activity during increased gravitational stress. *Electroencephalography and Clinical Neurophysiology*, 21, 168–79.

Nicholson, A.N., Macnamara, W.D. and Borland, R.G. 1968. Responsiveness of the cortex and visual pathway during transient hypotension. *Electroencephalography and Clinical Neurophysiology*, 25, 330–37.

Novak, V., Novak, P., Spies, J.M. and Low, P.A. 1998. Autoregulation of cerebral blood flow in orthostatic hypotension. *Stroke*, 29, 104–11.

Novak, V., Spies, J.M., Novak, P., McPhee, B.R., Rummans, T.A. and Low, P.A. 1998. Hypnocapnia and cerebral hypoperfusion in orthostatic intolerance. *Stroke*, 29, 1876–81.

Rickards, C.A., Cohen, K.D., Lindsey, L., Bergeron, B., Burton. L., Khatri, P.J. *et al.* 2007. Cerebral blood flow response and its association with symptoms during orthostatic hypotension. *Aviation, Space, and Environmental Medicine*, 78, 653–8.

Schondorf, R., Benoit, J. and Wein, T. 1997. Cerebrovascular and cardiovascular measurements during neurally mediated syncope induced by head-up tilt. *Stroke*, 28, 1564–8.

Serrador, J.M., Picot, P.A., Rutt, B.K., Shoemaker, J.K. and Bondar, R.L. 2000. MRI measures of middle cerebral artery diameter in conscious humans during simulated orthostasis. *Stroke*, 31, 1672–8.

Steriade, M. 2001. Impact of network activities on neuronal properties in corticothalamic systems. *Journal of Neurophysiology*, 86, 1–39.

Steriade, M. and Deschenes, M. 1984. The thalamus as a neuronal oscillator. *Brain Research Reviews*, 8, 1–63.

Stromberg, D.D. and Fox, J.R. 1972. Pressures in the pial arterial microcirculation of the cat during changes in systemic arterial blood pressure. *Circulation Research*, 31, 229–39.

Suarez. T., Baerwald, J.P. and Kraus, C. 2002. Central venous access: The effects of approach, position, and head rotation on internal jugular vein cross-sectional area. *Anesthesia & Analgesia*, 95, 1519–24.

Valdueza, J.M., von Munster, T., Hoffman, O., Schreiber, S. and Einhaupl, K.M. 2000. Postural dependency of the cerebral venous outflow. *Lancet*, 355, 200–201.

Xu, X., Li, L., Cao, R., Tao, Y., Guo, Q., Geng, J. *et al.* 2010. Intraocular pressure and ocular perfusion pressure in myopes during 21 min head-down rest. *Aviation, Space, and Environmental Medicine*, 81, 418–22.

Zhang, R., Zuckerman, J.H., Iwasaki, K., Wilson, T.E., Crandall, C.G. and Levine, B.D. 2002. Autonomic neural control of dynamic cerebral autoregulation in humans. *American Journal of Physiology – Heart and Circulatory Physiology*, 106, 1814–20.

Zhang, R., Zuckerman, J.H. and Levine, B.D. 1998. Deterioration of cerebral autoregulation during orthostatic stress. *Journal of Applied Physiology*, 85, 1113–22.

Chapter 6

OXYGEN DELIVERY AND ACUTE HYPOXIA: PHYSIOLOGICAL AND CLINICAL CONSIDERATIONS

Jane Ward

One of the most important potential problems in aviation is the acute hypoxia that is associated with exposure to altitude, and this chapter is concerned with the physiology of oxygen transport and discusses acute hypoxia in relation to the aviation environment using relevant experimental studies in animals and humans, as well as clinical observations. Subsequent chapters deal with adaptation and acclimatization to hypobaric hypoxia (Chapter 7) and exposure to the profound hypoxia of extreme altitude and space (Chapter 8). They are concerned with the cabin environment of transport aircraft, the means of, and the limitations of, adaptation and acclimatization to high altitudes and the sequelae of acute exposure to extreme altitudes[1] as with decompression in supersonic transports and space operations.

Part 1: OXYGEN DELIVERY AND ACUTE HYPOXIA

Inspired and Alveolar Gases

Dry air contains 20.95 per cent oxygen (O_2), 78.08 per cent nitrogen (N_2), 0.93 per cent argon, traces of other inert gases and just under 0.04 per cent carbon dioxide (CO_2). In physiology and medicine it is usual to put all the physiologically inert gases together under the heading 'nitrogen' and to view the carbon dioxide present as too low to be of functional significance. Consequently, for physiological and medical purposes the fractional (F_I) composition (= percentage/100) of dry inspired air is often simplified to:

Concentration of oxygen (F_IO_2) = 0.21
Concentration of nitrogen (F_IN_2) = 0.79
Concentration of carbon dioxide (F_ICO_2) = 0.00

The total pressure of the atmosphere (barometric pressure) at any point is

---

1   In this text extreme altitudes refer to altitudes that would be experienced in the event of a decompression in a transport aircraft, an ejection from a high-performance aircraft, or loss of pressurization of a space capsule or of a space suit during extravehicular activity.

affected by altitude (Figure 6.1), and it also varies with the seasons and weather conditions. The partial pressure of each component gas in a mixture is equal to the fractional concentration of the gas × total pressure (Dalton's Law). At sea level, barometric pressure (P_B) averages around 101.3 kPa (760 mm Hg) and the partial pressure of oxygen (PO_2) of dry inspired air (= $F_IO_2 \times P_B$) is about 21 kPa (159 mm Hg). At altitude, F_IO_2 remains 0.2095, but barometric pressure, and therefore dry P_IO_2, is reduced.

Atmospheric air normally contains some water vapour which dilutes the other gases so that the actual fraction of inspired oxygen is lower than the dry value by a variable amount. The partial pressure of water vapour (PH_2O) in a gas mixture is determined by the temperature of the gas and the relative humidity. The temperature determines the maximum water vapour pressure that is possible, and this is known as the saturated water vapour pressure at that temperature. Saturated water vapour pressure is higher for a warm gas than for a cool gas. The relative humidity is the percentage saturation of the gas with water vapour (= (actual PH_2O / saturated water vapour pressure) × 100 per cent). Air that has been exposed to water as it crosses a large ocean will tend to have a higher relative humidity than air that has crossed a large land mass.

As the inspired air passes through the conducting airways of the respiratory system, it is warmed to around 37°C, and the contact with moist epithelial surfaces saturates it with water vapour. Consequently, in the lungs water vapour pressure is constant at 6.3 kPa (47 mm Hg), the saturated water vapour pressure at 37°C. This addition of water vapour dilutes the other inspired gases and effectively reduces the dry pressure that the other gases share. The partial pressure of oxygen in inspired air is indicated as P_IO_2.

P_IO_2 (dry) = 0.2095 × PB
PO_2 of the moistened inspired air,
P_IO_2 (moist) = 0.2095 × (PB − 6.3).
At sea level (PB=101.3 kPa, 760 mm Hg) P_IO_2 (dry) = 159 mm Hg;
P_IO_2 (moist) = 19.9 kPa (149 mm Hg)

This unavoidable addition of water vapour is important at high altitude because it lowers the P_IO_2 by the same absolute amount (about 10 mm Hg) whatever the altitude. Moistening the inspired air causes a 6 per cent fall in P_IO_2 at sea level, but a 19 per cent fall on the summit of Everest ($P_B \approx 250$ mm Hg, dry $P_IO_2 \approx 52$ mm Hg, moist $P_IO_2 \approx 42$ mm Hg).

In the remaining sections of this chapter, if P_IO_2 is unqualified, it refers to the partial pressure of oxygen in moistened inspired air.

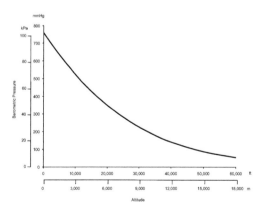

Figure 6.1   Effect of altitude on barometric pressure

The values used here are based on the International Civil Aviation Organization (ICAO) international standard atmospheric pressure. Actual values will vary, especially with season and latitude. It closely predicts average barometric pressure at latitude of 45° North.

Oxygen Consumption and Carbon Dioxide Production

In the alveolar region, oxygen moves into the pulmonary capillary blood to replenish the oxygen that has been removed in the tissues, and the carbon dioxide produced in the tissues moves into the alveolar gas; alveolar PO_2 falls and alveolar PCO_2 rises. At rest, tissue oxygen consumption in a normal adult male (about 3.4 mL/kg/min or 250 mL/min) is usually slightly more than tissue carbon dioxide production (about 2.7 mL/kg/min or 200 mL/min). Oxygen consumption and carbon dioxide production rise by five to 20 times in heavy exercise depending on the fitness of the person, their weight, age and gender (Hossack and Bruce, 1982). In the steady state, the tissue oxygen consumption and carbon dioxide production are the same as the oxygen uptake ($\dot{V}O_2$) and carbon dioxide output ($\dot{V}CO_2$) measured at the mouth from inspired and expired gas analysis.

The respiratory gas exchange ratio (R) = $\dot{V}CO_2/\dot{V}O_2$, and in the steady state its precise value depends on what substances are being metabolized. If carbohydrate alone is being metabolized, one molecule of carbon dioxide is produced for every molecule of oxygen consumed and R = 1. Fat metabolism uses more oxygen, and if it was the sole fuel being metabolized, R would be about 0.7. Using the resting values given above, the typical value of around 0.8 (= 200/250 mL/min) reflects the mixture of fuels normally being metabolized.

There are times when the body is not in a steady state. For example, for some time after the onset of hyperventilation more carbon dioxide is expelled than is being produced in the tissues, and as oxygen uptake is less affected by hyperventilation, R increases, often to values > 1. If hyperventilation continued at the same rate, after about 20 minutes a new steady state would be reached and R would again reflect tissue metabolism (Nunn and Matthews, 1959; Lumb, 2000a).

Alveolar oxygen

When R = 1, each molecule of oxygen taken up by the pulmonary capillary blood is replaced by a carbon dioxide molecule. In this case, P_AO_2 (alveolar PO_2) = moist inspired PO_2 (P_IO_2) – alveolar PCO_2. The simple equation above also applies when the subject is breathing pure oxygen, whatever the value of R. When oxygen and carbon dioxide are not exchanged on a one-for-one basis (R ≠ 1), then P_AO_2 ≈ moist inspired PO_2 – alveolar PCO_2/R. This is a simplified, but useful version of the alveolar air equation.[2] The approximately equal sign in this version of the equation arises from the fact that the volume of expired air is not quite the same as the volume of inspired air when R ≠ 1, but for most medical and aviation purposes this version is adequate for estimating the effect on alveolar PO_2 of changes in barometric pressure and/or alveolar PCO_2. At sea level, moist P_IO_2 = 19.9 kPa (149 mm Hg) and P_ACO_2 is 5.3 kPa (40 mm Hg), giving the normal sea-level P_AO_2 (with a typical R of 0.8) of 13.3 kPa (100 mm Hg).

Alveolar-Capillary Membrane

Diffusion of oxygen across the alveolar-capillary membrane is a passive process, driven by the partial pressure gradient between the alveolar gas and pulmonary capillary blood. The partial pressure of

---

2   The full version of the alveolar air equation is: $P_AO_2 = P_IO_2 - P_ACO_2 (F_IO_2 + (1 - F_IO_2)/R)$. Even this assumes a steady state so that the inert gases are in equilibrium after any change in inspired gas composition or barometric pressure (Lumb, 2000b).

X in the gas mixture is the product of the fractional concentration of X and the total gas pressure as discussed above. The partial pressure of a gas, X, in a liquid (or 'tension') is defined as equal to the partial pressure of gas X in a gas mixture with which it is in equilibrium (no net movement of the gas between gas and liquid). For example, if blood is exposed to a gas mixture containing oxygen, oxygen will diffuse into or out of the blood until the blood and gas mixture has come into equilibrium, at which point the gas mixture PO_2 will be neither falling nor rising. If at that point the gas $PO_2 = 5$ kPa, then the liquid PO_2 will also be 5 kPa.

The concentration of gas in simple solution in a liquid (mL gas/L liquid) is proportional to the partial pressure of the gas in the liquid, with the constant of proportionality being the solubility of the gas in the liquid (Henry's Law). The concentration of gas in liquid (mL/L) = solubility (mL/kPa/L) × Pgas (kPa). The solubility depends on both the gas and the liquid. If two different liquids, L1 and L2, are equilibrated with the same gas mixture containing gas X at partial pressure P_X, the partial pressure of gas X in both liquids will be P_X, but the concentrations C_{X1} and C_{X2} will be different. The liquid with the higher solubility for gas X will contain more molecules of X per litre at the same partial pressure than the liquid with the lower solubility. Partial pressure determines the direction and rate of diffusion of gases, and concentration (mL/L) gradients do not reliably predict gas movement between different fluids such as blood and lipid or blood and alveolar gas.

In the lung, oxygen diffuses from the alveolus, where PO_2 is normally about 13.3 kPa (100 mm Hg) at sea level, into the pulmonary capillary, where mixed venous blood in a resting subject normally enters the capillary with a PO_2 of about 5.3 kPa (40 mm Hg). So, at sea level in a resting subject, there is normally a partial pressure gradient of 8.0 kPa (60 mm Hg) driving oxygen diffusion from alveolus to blood at the start of the pulmonary capillary. This partial pressure gradient diminishes along the pulmonary capillary as oxygen is added to the blood until equilibration with alveolar PO_2 is achieved. At sea level, with a normal alveolar-capillary membrane, pulmonary capillary blood PO_2 equals alveolar PO_2 by one third of the way along the pulmonary capillary at rest (Figure 6.2a). For the remaining time in the pulmonary capillary the blood takes up no more oxygen. Improving the ease with which oxygen diffuses through the alveolar-capillary membrane would mean equilibration occurred a little earlier in the journey through the pulmonary capillary, but would not improve oxygen uptake per minute. Oxygen uptake (L/min) can be raised by increasing pulmonary blood flow as happens in exercise, and consequently oxygen uptake is said to be 'perfusion limited' in health at sea level.

In exercise, as cardiac output and pulmonary blood flow increase, the time taken for blood to traverse the pulmonary capillary is reduced and equilibration is reached further along the capillary. In heavy exercise, the time taken for blood to traverse the pulmonary capillary may be reduced to a third of the time at rest, but, in normal subjects at sea level, this is still just enough time to ensure equilibration of the blood with alveolar gas. In some highly trained elite athletes, arterial hypoxaemia does occur during heavy exercise. One possible cause of this 'exercise-induced hypoxaemia' is failure of equilibration of the pulmonary capillary blood with alveolar PO_2, as the time in the pulmonary capillary is severely reduced. However, other mechanisms such as increased ventilation–perfusion mismatching now seem more likely (Prefaut *et al.*, 2000; Zavorsky *et al.*, 2003).

If diffusion through the alveolar-capillary membrane is impaired, alveolar and pulmonary capillary PO_2 may not reach equilibrium by the end of the pulmonary capillary, and under these circumstances oxygen uptake will be 'diffusion limited' (Figure 6.2a – dashed line). This may occur in disease if the diffusion pathway is lengthened, for example by the fluid of pulmonary oedema or in lung fibrosis. Diffusion will also be slowed if alveolar PO_2 is reduced (Figure 6.2b), for example because inspired PO_2 is reduced at altitude. Even though both alveolar and mixed venous PO_2 will both be lowered in this situation, alveolar PO_2 will be

more affected than mixed venous PO_2, causing a reduction in the pressure difference driving diffusion.

In addition, if the final oxygen saturation in the pulmonary capillary oxygen is below the normal sea level value of > 97 per cent, as the equilibrium PO_2 is approached, the haemoglobin is still being loaded with oxygen. This will slow the final rise in dissolved oxygen concentration and consequently pulmonary capillary PO_2. With exercise at high altitude, the two stresses of reduced partial pressure gradient and reduced time in the pulmonary capillary are combined, and, even in healthy subjects, oxygen uptake may then be diffusion-limited with failure of equilibration of the pulmonary capillary blood with alveolar gas (West *et al.*, 1962; Torre-Bueno *et al.*, 1985).

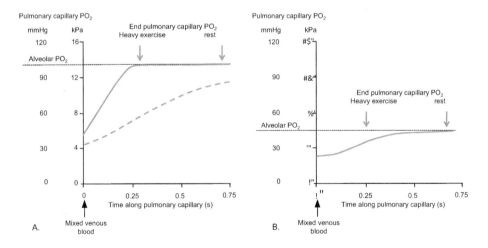

Figure 6.2   a) Time course of the rise in PO_2 along the pulmonary capillary in a healthy person at sea level (solid line) and b) Time course of the rise in PO_2 along the pulmonary capillary in a healthy person at high altitude

a)   The pressure gradient driving diffusion at the start of the pulmonary capillary is about 8 kPa (60 mm Hg) and equilibrium is reached by about a third of the way along the pulmonary capillary at rest and by the end of the pulmonary capillary in heavy exercise when the time along the capillary is reduced. In a person with a very abnormal diffusion pathway (dashed line, for example caused by pulmonary oedema or thickening of the alveolar wall in pulmonary fibrosis) diffusion is slowed and equilibrium with alveolar gas may not have been reached by end of the pulmonary capillary even at rest.

b)   At 15,000 feet alveolar PO_2 is about 6 kPa (45 mm Hg) and the pressure gradient driving diffusion is less than half the sea level value. This slows diffusion of oxygen across the alveolar-capillary membrane. At this altitude equilibrium with alveolar PO_2 may still be reached by the end of the pulmonary capillary at rest but in heavy exercise end-pulmonary capillary PO_2 may not reach alveolar PO_2, leading to a further reduction in arterial PO_2.

Carriage of Oxygen

Oxygen solubility in blood (0.000225 mL oxygen per mL of blood per kPa; 0.00003 mL/mL/mmHg) is low and with the normal arterial PO_2 (PaO_2) of about 13 kPa (100 mmHg), dissolved oxygen is just 3 mL/L. Most of the 200 mL of oxygen normally present in each litre of arterial blood is combined to haemoglobin. Haemoglobin has a molecular weight of 64,500 and consists of four haem groups, each attached to a protein chain. In normal adult haemoglobin (HbA) there are two alpha chains and two beta chains. The haem group contains an iron atom in the ferrous form and this is where oxygen binds. When oxidized to the ferric form (methaemoglobin), the haem group can no longer bind oxygen.

The binding of oxygen to haemoglobin is described by the oxyhaemoglobin dissociation curve (Figure 6.3). As blood is equilibrated with gas of progressively higher PO_2, the oxygen saturation (per cent of available binding sites filled) increases. The sigmoidal relationship is produced by two features of oxygen carriage by haemoglobin. One is 'cooperative binding', by which the binding of the first and subsequent oxygen molecules increases the affinity of the remaining binding sites to oxygen as the molecule changes from its 'tense' to its 'relaxed' form. The other factor is the limited number of oxygen binding sites. The dissociation curve becomes steeper above about 2 kPa (15 mm Hg) as the affinity of the remaining binding sites increases, and then after about 8 kPa (60 mm Hg) it flattens again as the number of free binding sites runs out. Each gram of haemoglobin (Hb) can combine with a maximum of about 1.34 mL oxygen, and the oxygen content of the blood (mL/L) is the sum of the bound oxygen

and the small amount of dissolved oxygen. Oxygen content (mL/L) = 1.34 × [Hb] x oxygen saturation + PO_2 × oxygen solubility.

The oxygen content axis of the dissociation curve in Figure 6.3 gives values for blood when the haemoglobin concentration is 150 g/L. When fully saturated, this normal blood has an oxygen content of just under 200 mL/L. In anaemia, with a normal arterial PO_2, the arterial oxygen saturation will be normal, but arterial oxygen content will be reduced in proportion to the reduction in haemoglobin concentration.

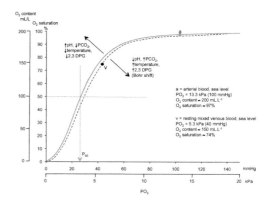

Figure 6.3   Oxygen–haemoglobin dissociation curve

The affinity of haemoglobin for oxygen is affected by pH, PCO_2, temperature and the concentration of the red cell metabolite 2,3-diphosphoglycerate, causing right or left shifts of the dissociation curve as shown. The position of the curve can be described by the P_{50} which is the PO_2 at which the haemoglobin is 50 per cent saturated. P_{50} is normally about 27 mm Hg when pH = 7.4, PCO_2 = 5.3 kPa (40 mm Hg), temperature = 37°C and with a normal sea level 2,3-DPG concentration. Increased affinity of haemoglobin for oxygen is associated with a reduced P_{50} and decreased affinity with an increased P_{50}. The normal sea level values of PO_2, O_2 content and saturation are shown for arterial (a) and mixed venous blood (v) in a resting subject. The mixed venous point (v) lies on a dissociation curve to the right of the curve for arterial blood. The increased P_{50} is because of the increased PCO_2 and reduced pH of venous blood.

Oxyhaemoglobin Dissociation Curve

In a healthy person at sea level, the PO_2 at the arterial end of all systemic tissue capillaries is about 13 kPa or 100 mm Hg (that is, arterial PO_2), and it falls along the capillaries as oxygen diffuses to the tissues. The size of the PO_2 fall from the arterial to the venous end of the capillary varies from tissue to tissue, depending on both the local oxygen consumption and the local tissue blood flow. The kidneys and cardiac muscle both have a high oxygen consumption per kilogram of tissue, but the kidney has a much more generous blood supply per kilogram than the myocardium. As a result, PO_2 is high in the venous blood emerging from the renal capillaries and low in that emerging from the myocardial capillaries.

In a normal resting sea level subject, PO_2 at the venous end of an average systemic capillary is about 5.3 kPa (40 mm Hg). This is the resting mixed venous PO_2, which can be sampled from the pulmonary artery where venous blood from the different systemic circulations are fully mixed together. This average venous PO_2 is on the steep part of the oxyhaemoglobin dissociation curve: a small further fall in tissue capillary PO_2, for example caused by an increased metabolism, will cause a large further release of oxygen from the haemoglobin. This ready release of oxygen where it is needed is an important feature of normal haemoglobin that is enhanced by the Bohr effect, which is discussed in the next section. Within any organ, PO_2 will not be uniform. Tissue PO_2 will be lower in the regions furthest from a capillary, and at any given distance from a capillary, tissue PO_2 will be lower on the venous side than on the arterial side of the capillary. The regions that normally have the lowest PO_2 are often known as 'lethal corners' as they are the most vulnerable if anything, such as falling arterial PO_2 or ischaemia, impairs the tissues oxygen supply.

The sea-level alveolar and arterial PO_2 of around 13 kPa (100 mm Hg) is on the plateau of the dissociation curve

('a' on Figure 6.3) close to full saturation (> 97 per cent). As there are few empty binding sites, if alveolar PO_2 rises above this value (either by hyperventilation or breathing oxygen-enriched air), the oxygen saturation and content of the arterial blood will be little affected. This explains why mental and physical performance is not greatly enhanced when a healthy person breathes oxygen at sea level. A modest fall in alveolar ventilation or inspired PO_2 will also have little effect on oxygen delivery to the tissues in a normal person; the oxygen saturation is still 95 per cent when PO_2 is 10 kPa (75 mm Hg) (Severinghaus, 1966, 1979).

When arterial PO_2 falls below about 8 kPa (60 mm Hg), as occurs in a healthy person at altitudes above 10,000 feet (3,000 metres) or in hypoxic respiratory disease, there is a significant reduction in arterial oxygen saturation, arterial oxygen content, tissue oxygen delivery and exercise tolerance. Even if oxygen saturation and tissue oxygen delivery are adequate for current needs, once the arterial PO_2 is in the steep region of the dissociation curve, the individual is vulnerable. A small worsening of the situation, resulting in a small further fall in arterial PO_2, will cause a significant fall in oxygen saturation and possibly a fatal reduction in tissue oxygen delivery. On the other hand, when PO_2 is on the steep part of the curve, a small rise in arterial PO_2, produced by a small increase in the inspired oxygen concentration from the 21 per cent in air to 24 or 28 per cent, can produce worthwhile improvements in oxygen saturation.

Pulse oximeters measure arterial oxygen saturation indirectly by measuring the pulse-related absorption of different wavelengths of light passed though the finger or earlobe. Oximeters are non-invasive, convenient and relatively cheap, and, as well as their use for monitoring patients, they have been used by pilots flying in unpressurized aircraft to warn them of impending hypoxic deterioration. In either situation it is important that the physiology and the limitations of oxygen saturation as an early warning system are understood. If a normal person at sea level (oxygen saturation 97 per cent) holds their breath, there may be little or no change in the pulse oximeter reading for 30 seconds or more. Alveolar and arterial PO_2 will have been falling progressively during the breath-hold, but oxygen saturation will be little affected until PaO_2 falls below about 8–9 kPa (60–70 mm Hg). Averaging due to electronic processing within the oximeter often further increases the response time.

Oxygen Affinity of Haemoglobin

At any given PO_2, the affinity of the oxygen binding sites is influenced by the environment to which the haemoglobin is exposed. Increased hydrogen ion concentration (reduced pH), increased temperature and increased PCO_2 all reduce the affinity of haemoglobin for oxygen, and this is reflected by a rightward shift of the dissociation curve (Figure 6.3 – dashed line). The shifts in the position of the oxyhaemoglobin dissociation curve caused by these factors are often referred to as 'Bohr shifts' after the Danish physiologist Christian Bohr (1885–1962) who first described the rightward shift in the presence of increased PCO_2. An increase in the red cell metabolite, 2,3-diphosphoglycerate (2,3-DPG), also causes a rightward shift in the dissociation curve. This may occur in anaemia or when arterial PO_2 is reduced at high altitude or in chronic hypoxic lung disease.

A convenient way of quantifying the affinity of haemoglobin for oxygen and the position of the oxyhaemoglobin dissociation curve is the P_{50}. This is the PO_2 at which the haemoglobin is 50 per cent saturated and the normal value at sea level is 26.8 mm Hg. A reduced affinity and rightward shift of the dissociation curve, for example caused by increased PCO_2, will raise the P_{50}, while increased affinity and a leftward shift causes a fall in P_{50}. The 'standard P_{50}' is the PO_2 at which the haemoglobin is 50 per cent saturated when the blood is corrected to standard conditions of temperature, PCO_2 and pH (37°C, 5.3 kPa (40 mm Hg) and 7.4 respectively). Standard P_{50} will reflect any change in affinity due to altered 2,3-DPG or the presence of a variant haemoglobin. The physiological significance of these changes in oxygen affinity is discussed below.

Haemoglobin Variants

In both health and disease many different variants of haemoglobin are synthesized. They often differ from normal adult haemoglobin in the shape and/or position of their oxyhaemoglobin dissociation curve. Normal foetal haemoglobin differs from normal adult haemoglobin in that the two beta globin chains are replaced by two gamma globin chains. This difference results in a much higher affinity for oxygen than normal adult haemoglobin, so that its dissociation curve is shifted to the left (low P_{50}). Most of the abnormal haemoglobin variants involve simple inherited gene mutations resulting in substitution of a single amino acid in one of the globin chains.

The most well-known haemoglobin variants are important because of problems not caused primarily by any effect on oxygen affinity. In the case of sickle cell anaemia, the polymerization of deoxygenated haemoglobin, leading to sickling, causes the clinical symptoms. Sickle cell trait itself does not present a problem to passengers at cruising altitudes, but those with sickle cell anaemia are advised to travel with supplemental oxygen and to delay travel following a sickling crisis (United Kingdom Civil Aviation Authority, 2010). The affinity of sickle cell haemoglobin is also reduced, and this may have both positive and negative effects. As in other forms of anaemia, the reduced oxygen affinity aids oxygen unloading in the tissues, which helps the individual to tolerate the reduced oxygen delivery, but it also increases the concentration of deoxyhaemoglobin in the tissues, increasing the risk of red cell sickling (Hsia, 1998). More than 90 different abnormal haemoglobin variants have been described that increase the affinity of haemoglobin for oxygen, leading to a low P_{50} (Rumi et al., 2009), and there are at least 65 variants described that lower the affinity, raising the P_{50} (Deyell et al., 2006). The inheritance of most of these variants is autosomal dominant and most are rare.

Affinity of Haemoglobin

A reduction in affinity and a rightward shift of the oxyhaemoglobin dissociation curve (increased P_{50}) happens to the haemoglobin in normal people every time blood passes through a tissue microcirculation. In exercising skeletal muscle, the effect of the increased PCO_2, acidity and temperature can be large and greatly increase the release of oxygen. As the blood returns to the lungs, these changes are largely or completely reversed and the affinity of haemoglobin for oxygen increases. This aids oxygen uptake in the lungs and is reflected by a left shift in the dissociation curve and decreased P_{50}.

In many abnormal situations PCO_2 and pH mediated changes in oxygen affinity occur that help optimize the balance between uptake and unloading, maximizing oxygen transport between lungs and tissues in that situation (Hsia, 1998). For example, if oxygen loading is impaired (perhaps because of exposure to reduced inspired PO_2 at high altitude), hypoxic stimulation of ventilation reduces arterial PCO_2, which then increases oxygen affinity, helping to improve oxygen loading. On the other hand, impaired unloading of oxygen in the tissues (for example because of anaemia or inadequate blood flow), leads to tissue acidosis, which reduces oxygen affinity, improving release of oxygen in the tissues.

2,3-DPG and Haemoglobin Variants

When changes of affinity and P_{50} occur because of increased 2,3-DPG or the presence of a haemoglobin variant, the altered affinity is present in both lungs and tissues. Raising affinity (lowering P_{50}) will increase uptake in the lungs, but reduce release of oxygen from the haemoglobin in the tissues. Lowering affinity (raising P_{50}) will aid release in the tissues, but impair oxygen uptake in the lungs. Consequently, with these permanent or semi-permanent changes in oxygen affinity, it is less obvious whether they confer an overall benefit or hindrance to oxygen transport from ambient gas to tissue mitochondria. The answer to this depends on the nature of the primary problem with oxygen transport and the situation in which the altered affinity occurs.

In the foetus, the increased affinity of haemoglobin confers a net benefit because, here, the major challenge is oxygen uptake from the respiratory organ, the placenta, where PO_2 is much lower (28 mm Hg, 3.7 kPa) than in the adult lung (100 mm Hg, 13.3 kPa). The net benefit has been demonstrated in experiments on lambs, where exchange transfusion of foetal blood with blood containing adult haemoglobin leads to a fall in uterine vein saturation, a fall in foetal oxygen consumption and the development of metabolic acidosis. Fortunately, in the human the effects of exchange transfusion (for example, as used for treating rhesus incompatibility) are less severe because the difference between foetal and maternal P_{50} is less in humans than in sheep.

In anaemia at sea level, the reduction in affinity caused by the increase in red blood cell 2,3-DPG levels also confers a net benefit to oxygen transport. Arterial PO_2 is normal in anaemia and the shift in the oxyhaemoglobin curve is smaller in the plateau region ($PO_2 > 8$ kPa, 60 mm Hg) than in the steep region ($PO_2 < 8$ kPa, 60 mm Hg). Consequently, the rightward shift has only a small detrimental effect on oxygen uptake in the lungs and this is more than outweighed in terms of overall oxygen transport, by the improvement in oxygen release in the tissues.

Oxygen Affinity at High Altitude

Attempts to measure the position of the oxyhaemoglobin dissociation curve and P_{50} at high altitude initially produced variable results (Barcroft, 1923; Aste-Salazar and Hurtado, 1944; Hurtado, 1964; for review, see Winslow, 2007), as well as different opinions as to whether a right or left shift would be adaptive. It is now generally agreed that when measured under standard conditions of PCO_2, pH and temperature, living at high altitude or indeed any form of chronic hypoxia, leads to a rightward shift of the oxyhaemoglobin dissociation curve. This reduced affinity of haemoglobin

for oxygen is now known to be due to an increased concentration of 2,3-DPG in the red cell (Brewer, 1974). However, at high altitude ventilation increases and arterial PCO_2 falls, leading to respiratory alkalosis. This will lead to the opposite effect on oxygen affinity, opposing and potentially reversing the reduction of affinity caused by the increased 2,3-DPG.

The American Medical Research Expedition to Everest (AMREE) in 1981 (Winslow et al., 1984) found that the in vivo P_{50} at 6,300 metres (c. 20,000 feet) was very similar to the sea-level value, but it became progressively lower at higher altitudes as the effect of increasing alkalosis overwhelmed the effects of the increased 2,3-DPG. In the one subject whose alveolar PCO_2 was measured on the summit of Everest, it was found to be only 7.5 mm Hg (1 kPa). In contrast, during a simulated ascent of Mount Everest (Operation Everest II) in which arterial and venous blood samples were collected from five subjects decompressed in stages in a chamber over 42 days, it was found that the in vivo P_{50} changed little, even at a simulated altitude equivalent to that on the summit of Mount Everest (Wagner et al., 2007). At all altitudes the leftward shift caused by hyperventilation almost exactly balanced the rightward shift caused by the increased 2,3-DPG. It is difficult to be sure what the typical P_{50} at extreme altitude is because so few subjects have been studied. The degree of hyperventilation and alkalosis is likely to be variable between subjects and may be very different in a real mountain environment to that found in the less threatening environment of a hypobaric chamber.

Observations on patients with haemoglobin variants that either raise or lower the affinity of haemoglobin for oxygen shed some interesting light on the effects of altered affinity and on the problem of what might be useful at high altitude. In most cases these haemoglobin variants are surprisingly well tolerated and generally discovered by chance. People with high-affinity haemoglobins often have polycythaemia with high haemoglobin concentration due to an erythropoietin-mediated compensatory response to chronic tissue hypoxia at sea level. Low-affinity haemoglobins are often associated with a mild anaemia, presumably resulting from the higher than normal tissue PO_2 causing a compensatory suppression of erythropoietin levels.

Both high- and low-affinity haemoglobin variants cause few if any symptoms and may be discovered during routine screening because of the unexplained polycythaemia, anaemia or cyanosis or because of surprisingly low pulse oximetry oxygen saturation readings in the presence of a normal arterial PO_2. The reduced pulse oximetry value and cyanosis are not simply related to the rightward shift of the dissociation curve in low-affinity haemoglobinopathies. Cyanosis can also be a feature of some high-affinity variants and is probably mostly due to the abnormal light absorbance by many variant haemoglobins.

Many animals and birds resident at high altitude such as yaks, llamas, alpacas, pikas and bar-headed geese have high-affinity haemoglobin, with values of P_{50} that are typically about 10 mm Hg lower than in similar lowland animals and birds. In humans, a small but interesting study was carried out on four young (12–18 years) members of a family with a high-affinity haemoglobin variant (Hebbel et al., 1977). Two had normal haemoglobin (P_{50} 26.9 and 27) and two (matched for age, size and gender) had high-affinity haemoglobin Andrew-Minneapolis (P_{50} 17.0 and 17.2). Maximum oxygen consumption was lower at sea level in the two affected individuals (average 34.9 + 4.3 mL/min/kg) compared with the two normal individuals (43.0 + 4.6 mL/min/ kg). When the $\dot{V}O_2max$ measurements were repeated at an altitude of 3,100 metres (c. 10,000 feet), as expected, the normal subjects showed a fall in their $\dot{V}O_2max$ (by about 26 per cent to 32.6+3.3 mL/min/kg). In contrast, the two affected individuals with high-affinity haemoglobin showed a small rise in their $\dot{V}O_2max$ (13 per cent to 39.5+3.2 mL/min/kg).

This was a very small study, but, taken together with observations in other species, it suggests that high oxygen binding affinity may be a small disadvantage for exercise at sea level, but an advantage at high altitude. In line with these observations, it has been suggested that the increase in 2,3-DPG that occurs on ascent to altitude is not an adaptive mechanism, but rather a potentially unhelpful consequence of a mechanism that has evolved to respond to sea-level oxygen transport problems such as anaemia (Hsia, 1998; Wagner et al., 2007).

It might be expected that low-affinity variants would be a disadvantage at high altitude, but, if so, this seems to be mild. A 16-year-old boy was found to have haemoglobin Chico (P_{50} = 40 mm Hg) following the chance observation of a low pulse oximetry reading at a sports medical. He had lived at 5,395 feet (1,644 metres) and, following exercise testing, was cleared to participate in sports, which he carried out without complication. It seems, in humans at least, that a wide range of oxygen affinities and P_{50} values can be tolerated, both at sea level and high altitude, with little detrimental affect on oxygen delivery and consumption. There is plenty of redundancy in the oxygen delivery system, so impaired uptake or release can be compensated for by increased ventilation and increased cardiac output (Hsia, 1998; Winslow, 2007).

Anaemia and Carbon Monoxide Poisoning

In a person with a normal haemoglobin concentration (150 g/L), to supply a normal resting oxygen consumption of 250 mL/min with a normal resting cardiac output of about 5,000 mL/min, about 0.05 mL oxygen needs to be removed from each mL of blood passing through the systemic capillaries (50 mL/L), leaving a mixed venous oxygen saturation of 75 per cent (Figure 6.4 – thick unbroken line). In an anaemic person at rest with a similar cardiac output, a similar amount of oxygen would have to be removed from each litre of blood passing through the tissues. Figure 6.4 (thin unbroken line) shows the dissociation curve for anaemic blood when haemoglobin concentration is half normal (75 g/L). Arterial PO_2 is normal since the inspired air and respiratory system are normal. Arterial oxygen saturation is also nearly normal at sea level.

With arterial oxygen saturation near normal, but with only half the normal number of oxygen binding sites, the arterial oxygen content at sea level is half normal at about 100 mL/L. To release the required 50 mL from each litre of blood, venous oxygen saturation will have to fall to 50 per cent and venous PO_2 will need to fall lower (point B) than in the normal person (point A). The reduced partial pressure gradient for diffusion to the tissues will be adequate at rest, but will quickly become inadequate as oxygen consumption increases, leading to fatigue and exercise intolerance. In chronic anaemia, an

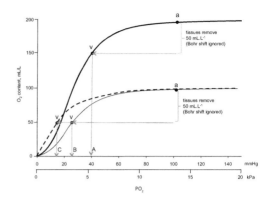

Figure 6.4   Oxygen–haemoglobin dissociation curve

Oxygen – haemoglobin curves are shown for blood with a normal haemoglobin concentration of 150 g/L (thick line), anaemic blood with a haemoglobin concentration of 75 g/L (thin line) and for 50% carboxyhaemoglobin blood (broken line; normal haemoglobin concentration, 150 g/L, with 50 per cent of the oxygen binding sites combined to carbon monoxide). If cardiac output is the same in these three situations approximately 50 mL O_2 will need to be unloaded from each L of blood passing through the tissues to supply the resting O_2 consumption of about 250 mL/min. In the normal subject this unloading is associated with a fall in the PO_2 at the end of the 'average' capillary (= mixed venous PO_2) to about 5.3 kPa (40 mmHg) (point A). In anaemia the fall is greater (B) but with this degree of anaemia capillary PO_2 is still adequate to drive adequate diffusion of O_2 at rest and in light exercise. With 50 per cent carboxyhaemoglobin the fall in PO_2 by the venous end of the capillary is greater still (C) because in addition to the reduced arterial O_2 content, the affinity of the remaining O_2 binding sites for oxygen is increased, as reflected by the leftward shift of the dissociation curve. The severely reduced capillary PO_2 will impair diffusion, leading to tissue hypoxia even at rest.

increase in red blood cell 2,3-DPG raises P_{50} and has a net beneficial effect on tissue PO_2 and oxygen delivery by aiding oxygen unloading in the tissues without significantly impairing oxygen loading in the lungs.

In carbon monoxide poisoning, the adverse effect on oxygen transport is due to the combination of reduced arterial oxygen content and impaired oxygen unloading in the tissues. The affinity of the haem group for carbon monoxide (CO) is 250 times higher than its affinity for oxygen. Consequently, prolonged breathing of even a very low concentration of CO can lead to a progressive replacement of a significant proportion of the oxygen with CO. In addition, with CO attached to some binding sites, the affinity of the remaining sites for oxygen is increased; the dissociation curve for carboxyhaemoglobin is hyperbolic and left-shifted.

Figure 6.4 (dashed line) shows the curve for a person with a normal haemoglobin concentration, but with half the oxygen binding sites occupied by CO. Oxygen release in the tissues is impaired, and to remove the required 50 mL O_2/L the mixed venous PO_2 must fall to a value (point C) which is inadequate to drive the required diffusion from capillary to cell. In contrast with the anaemic person with the same arterial oxygen content, this person will be symptomatic at rest. The main effects are due to poor cerebral oxygen delivery and include headache, nausea, confusion and possibly seizures, coma or death.

Oxygen Transport System

Alveolar PO_2 is determined by the inspired PO_2, alveolar ventilation ($\dot{V}_A$) and oxygen consumption ($\dot{V}O_2$): $P_AO_2 = P_IO_2 - \dot{V}O_2/\dot{V}_A$. The greater the alveolar ventilation, the closer the alveolar PO_2 approaches moist inspired PO_2. By the end of the pulmonary capillary, the blood has normally fully equilibrated with alveolar gas so that its PO_2 equals alveolar PO_2 (P_AO_2). This blood returns to the left heart, but the arterial blood that emerges into the aorta has a PO_2 that is lower than P_AO_2. The reason is that even with normal people there is some 'right to left shunting' or 'venous admixture' because of some anomalies of the normal human circulation. Some of the bronchial circulation venous blood (from the 'right' side of the systemic circulation) with reduced oxygen content drains into the pulmonary veins, contaminating the oxygenated blood

returning from the lungs to the left heart ('left' sided blood). In addition, although the bulk of the coronary venous blood is directed appropriately to the right side of the heart, a small quantity of this blood empties directly into left atrium or left ventricle, adding to venous admixture.

The amount by which arterial PO_2 (P_aO_2) is lower than alveolar PO_2 (P_AO_2) (the 'A–a PO_2 gradient') increases with age, being about 1–2 kPa (7.5–15 mm Hg) at 20 years but 3–5 kPa (22.5–37.5 mm Hg) at 80 years. Conditions that increase the A–a PO_2 gradient include abnormal sources of right-to-left shunting of blood and ventilation–perfusion mismatching. Abnormal right to left shunts occur when there is a region of lung which fails to gas exchange (for example, lobar pneumonia, atelectasis) or in some types of congenital heart disease (for example, Fallot's tetralogy). Ventilation–perfusion ($\dot{V}_A/\dot{Q}$) mismatching occurs when there is uneven distribution of alveolar ventilation ($\dot{V}_A$) in relation to blood flow (perfusion, $\dot{Q}$) within the lung. Regions that are overventilated in relation to perfusion have a dead-space effect (high $\dot{V}_A/\dot{Q}$) and represent wasted ventilation. Regions that are underventilated in relation to perfusion (low $\dot{V}_A/\dot{Q}$) have a right-to-left shunt effect, with the incompletely saturated blood from these regions depressing arterial oxygen content and PO_2.

Ventilation–perfusion mismatching is an important cause of arterial hypoxia in many respiratory diseases including asthma and chronic obstructive pulmonary disease (COPD). Increased ventilation–perfusion mismatching is also the main reason for the increased A–a PO_2 gradient with increased age. Arterial oxygen saturation is determined by the arterial PO_2 and the oxyhaemoglobin dissociation curve (Figure 6.3). Arterial oxygen content is determined by the oxygen saturation and the haemoglobin concentration. Each gram of haemoglobin can combine with about 1.34 mL oxygen when fully saturated. Arterial oxygen content (mL/L) = haemoglobin concentration (g/L) × oxygen saturation × 1.34.

Haemoglobin acts as a reservoir for oxygen, replenishing the dissolved oxygen as it diffuses to the tissues. In anaemia this reservoir is reduced and so tissue capillary PO_2 falls faster than normal and mean tissue capillary PO_2 and mixed venous PO_2 will be reduced at rest. Chronic hypoxia due to lung disease or a prolonged stay at high altitude often leads to polycythaemia mediated by increased erythropoietin production by the kidney. Polycythaemia increases arterial oxygen content and tissue PO_2, which partly compensates for the reduced oxygen saturation in chronic hypoxia. However, polycythaemia increases blood viscosity and the workload of the heart and, when excessive, the disadvantages outweigh the benefits. Oxygen delivery to a tissue = blood flow x arterial oxygen content, so, as well as the factors discussed above, tissue hypoxia can result from poor perfusion.

Oxygen Delivery to Tissues

In the paper 'On Anoxaemia' by Barcroft (1920) three mechanisms of tissue hypoxia were described: reduced arterial PO_2 ('anoxic anoxaemia'), reduced oxygen-carrying capacity, usually due to a reduced haemoglobin concentration ('anaemic anoxaemia') and reduced tissue blood flow ('ischaemic anoxaemia'). The classification remains useful today although the terminology has evolved. 'Hypoxia' and 'hypoxaemia' have replaced the terms 'anoxia' and 'anoxaemia' and the terms in brackets, as well as their more modern equivalents ('hypoxic hypoxia', 'anaemic hypoxia' and

'ischaemic hypoxia'), are probably best avoided. 'Hypoxia' and 'hypoxic', when unqualified, are now used to refer to a low arterial PO_2. The statement 'This patient is hypoxic' means 'This patient has a low arterial PO_2' and would not be used to describe a patient with anaemia or low cardiac output. The expression 'anaemic hypoxia' is potentially confusing, as anaemia does not lead to a low arterial PO_2. The term 'anaemic tissue hypoxia' would avoid this problem.

Oxygen is required in the tissues for the production of adenosine triphosphate (ATP), the main energy source of cells. When ATP production fails, many aspects of tissue function will be affected, ultimately leading to cell death. In addition to impairment of oxygen delivery by the three mechanisms cited above, ATP production can be impaired by inadequate utilization of the delivered oxygen. This 'histotoxic' form of tissue hypoxia can be caused by poisoning of the electron transport chain in the mitochondria, for example by cyanide or sepsis.

Part 2:
CLINICAL CONSIDERATIONS: SIGNS AND SYMPTOMS

Tissues vary in their tolerance to hypoxia. Without its oxygen supply, loss of function occurs in the heart within about four minutes, but in skeletal muscle it may take more than an hour. The most vulnerable tissue is the brain. Loss of cerebral blood flow caused by sudden onset of high positive acceleration (+Gz) or occlusion of the arteries to the head using a pressurized sphygmomanometer cuff around the neck causes loss of consciousness within 5 to 8 seconds (Ernsting, Personal Communication).

Below is a list of the most common signs and symptoms of acute hypobaric hypoxia, and, as expected, many reflect cerebral dysfunction. Although the list is long, it is important to realize that in many cases of acute hypoxic exposure only a few of them occur and a key feature is their subtlety (Cable, 2003). Many factors affect the occurrence of these symptoms, especially the severity and the rate of onset of the hypoxia. With rapid exposure to hypobaric environments, the first sign of hypoxia may be loss of consciousness. The common patterns of effects of acute exposure at different altitudes are discussed further under 'Hypoxia in Aviation'.

- lightheadedness and dizziness[*]
- sensory loss and paraesthesia (numbness and tingling)[*]
- personality change
- lack of insight and judgement
- loss of self-criticism
- euphoria
- loss of memory
- cognitive impairment
- disorientation
- muscular incoordination
- impaired speech
- cyanosis
- increased ventilation and breathlessness
- hot and cold flushes
- decreased visual acuity and tunnel vision[*]
- clouding of consciousness
- headache
- non-specific malaise
- shaking of limbs
- lethargy
- loss of consciousness
- death

[*] These are common symptoms of hyperventilation and hypocapnia that occur in the absence of arterial hypoxia.

Acute Hyperoxia

Whilst tissue hypoxia is a major threat to performance and survival in the presence of disease or a reduced inspired PO_2, it is important to recognize that hyperoxia can also be harmful. Awareness of the possibility of oxygen toxicity is important in aviation, since the prevention and treatment of hypobaric hypoxia and decompression illness often involve the administration of oxygen-enriched gases, sometimes at increased pressure. Although the mechanisms of toxicity are not fully understood, many of them are thought to relate to increased production of reactive oxygen species. The occurrence and severity of symptoms depend on the inspired P_IO_2 (= oxygen fraction × (barometric pressure – 47) mm Hg) and the duration of exposure to the raised P_IO_2. At sea level, normal adults do not usually show symptoms of oxygen toxicity if oxygen concentration is below 50 per cent.

The main targets of oxygen toxicity are the lung, the central nervous system (CNS) and the eye (Altemeier and Sinclair, 2007; Bitterman, 2004, 2009). The earliest symptoms are those of tracheobronchitis, including tickling, substernal distress and inspiratory pain, and occur within 4 to 24 hours of breathing 100 per cent oxygen at one atmosphere. Longer exposures (> 48 hours) can lead to reduced vital capacity, diffuse alveolar damage and the acute respiratory distress syndrome. CNS toxicity includes nausea, dizziness, headache, visual disturbance, and seizures. Such effects do not occur at normal atmospheric pressures and are a feature of diving, or exposure to oxygen in a hyperbaric chamber.

Oxygen administration may also lead to absorption collapse. Alveolar gas normally contains about 80 per cent nitrogen, and when this is replaced by oxygen, alveolar gas may be absorbed into the blood faster than it is replaced in regions of the lung with low ventilation–perfusion ratios. In aviation, a similar problem occurs in pilots when they are subjected to +Gz acceleration forces, as airways in dependent areas of the lung close. This 'acceleration atelectasis' is much more likely to occur when high inspired oxygen concentrations (> 70 per cent) are used and it may lead to chest pain, dyspnoea and coughing (Tacker *et al.*, 1987). Other problems associated with oxygen administration are specific to particular patient groups. In premature babies, complications associated with oxygen therapy include retinopathy (retrolental fibroplasia) and bronchopulmonary dysplasia. Retinopathy of prematurity can follow even quite brief periods (a few hours) of hyperoxia (Sola, 2008).

Individuals with severe hypercapnic ('type 2') respiratory failure sometimes experience a further, potentially dangerous, rise in their arterial PCO_2 if given air enriched with too high a concentration of oxygen. One possible reason is that chronically hypercapnic patients have reduced sensitivity to changes in P_ACO_2 and rely on their hypoxia to maintain their respiratory drive. A large rise in arterial PO_2 can then lead to respiratory depression and increased P_ACO_2. However, increased ventilation–perfusion mismatching following loss of hypoxic vasoconstriction in poorly ventilated areas is probably also important.

Fortunately, in patients with type 2 respiratory failure, the problem can usually be avoided by restricting oxygen enrichment to 24 or 28 per cent, which leads to a small rise in arterial PO_2. Hypoxic pulmonary vasoconstriction and respiratory drive (P_AO_2 dependent) will be maintained, but oxygen delivery (arterial oxygen content dependent)

should be significantly improved. The initially low PaO_2 of these patients is on the steep part of the oxygen dissociation curve where a small increase in PO_2 can give a worthwhile increase in arterial oxygen content. Another important problem associated with the use of high-concentration oxygen is the increased fire risk.

Cyanosis

Cyanosis refers to a blue-grey tinge of a tissue, usually due to poor oxygenation of that tissue. When present in the tongue, buccal mucosa, conjunctivae and lips, it is termed 'central cyanosis' and indicates arterial hypoxaemia (low arterial PO_2). When cyanosis is seen in other tissues, most commonly finger and toe nails, it is known as 'peripheral cyanosis'. In the absence of central cyanosis, peripheral cyanosis is caused by low blood flow, leading to greater oxygen extraction from the tissue capillary blood. When present in both hands and feet in the absence of central cyanosis, it indicates a low cardiac output and/or widespread peripheral vasoconstriction as occurs in cardiovascular shock. More localized cyanosis indicates a local reduction in blood flow to that area, for example because of an arterial embolus.

Studies by Lundsgaard and Van Slyke (1923) showed that cyanosis was caused by an increased concentration of the darker red/purple deoxygenated form of haemoglobin and was not related to the blood CO_2 concentration. They found that it occurred when the concentration of deoxyhaemoglobin in the tissue microcirculation reached about 5 ± 1 g/dl (50 ± 10 g/L) and the blue colour became more intense as the concentration rose above this threshold. Subsequently, they have been repeatedly misquoted in both papers and textbooks as saying that cyanosis only appears when arterial deoxygenated haemoglobin reaches 5 g/dl (50 ± 10 g/L), which, in a human with a normal haemoglobin concentration of 15 g/dl (150 g/L), would mean an arterial saturation of only 66 per cent. In clinical practice, in patients with normal haemoglobin concentration, cyanosis can usually be detected when oxygen saturation has fallen to about 80 to 90 per cent, with the exact value varying with skin colour, lighting, the observer, etc. A saturation of 80 to 90 per cent corresponds to about 10 to 20 per cent or 1.5–3.0 g/dl (15–30 g/L) deoxygenated haemoglobin in the arterial blood, which would be expected to give a tissue capillary deoxygenated haemoglobin in the 4–6 g/dl (40–60 g/L) range quoted in the original papers (Martin and Khalil, 1990; Martin, 2009).

Whilst the presence of central cyanosis is a useful warning of arterial hypoxia, its absence cannot be taken to indicate the absence of hypoxia. It is not a very sensitive sign and, even in the best of conditions in a patient with a normal haemoglobin concentration, arterial PO_2 will have to fall from a normal sea-level value of about 13 kPa (100 mm Hg) to below 8 kPa (60 mm Hg) before cyanosis will be detected. As it is the absolute concentration of deoxygenated haemoglobin that determines whether cyanosis will be seen (not the percentage of deoxygenated blood), the arterial oxygen saturation will have to be lower before cyanosis is visible in an anaemic person. Once haemoglobin concentration is below about 9 g/dl (90 g/L), arterial hypoxia will usually cause death before cyanosis appears. In contrast, in the presence of polycythaemia, cyanosis appears more readily and may be present with oxygen saturations above 90 per cent.

Less common causes of cyanosis include the alteration of haemoglobin by drugs or other chemicals to give high concentrations of methaemoglobin (sulphonamides, dapsone, nitrates, nitrites, aniline dyes) or sulphaemoglobin (suphonamides, sulphasalasine, sumatriptan) where sulphur has become attached to the haemoglobin. Finally, as discussed above, some rare haemoglobinopathies may be associated with cyanosis. Methaemoglobinaemia, sulphaemoglobinaemia and haemoglobinopathies can all cause cyanosis with a normal arterial PO_2.

Carriage of Carbon Dioxide

Carbon dioxide (CO_2) is 20 times more soluble than oxygen and about 10 per cent of the expired CO_2 comes from CO_2 that was carried in the blood in simple solution. Of the rest, about 30 per cent originates from carbamino compounds, mostly in combination with haemoglobin, and about 60 per cent from bicarbonate. Bicarbonate is formed when CO_2 reacts with water to form carbonic acid, which then dissociates:

$$CO_2 + H_2O \underset{i}{\Leftrightarrow} H_2CO_3 \underset{ii}{\Leftrightarrow} H^+ + HCO_3^-$$

Reaction i is slow in plasma, but in the red blood cell it is catalyzed by carbonic anhydrase. Consequently, most of the bicarbonate is formed inside red blood cells, after which it diffuses into the plasma down its concentration gradient. The H^+ formed at the same time is buffered by haemoglobin, helping the above reaction to continue to the right.

Carbamino compounds are formed when CO_2 reacts with proteins at the terminal amino (NH_2) groups or the amino groups on the side chains of amino acids like lysine and arginine ($RNH_2 + CO_2 \Leftrightarrow RNHCOOH$). Most carbamino compounds in the blood are formed by combination of CO_2 with the amino groups on the globin chains of haemoglobin; haemoglobin has a lot of available NH_2 groups and there is a high concentration of haemoglobin in the blood. The amount of carbaminohaemoglobin formed is little affected by PCO_2 but very affected by the state of oxygenation of the haemoglobin. Deoxygenated haemoglobin forms carbamino compounds more readily than oxyhaemoglobin and it is also a better buffer, which enhances bicarbonate formation. Both these changes contribute to the Haldane effect – at any given PCO_2, the quantity of carbon dioxide carried is greater in deoxygenated than oxygenated blood. Figure 6.5 gives the CO_2 dissociation curve for blood with high and low oxygen content. It can be seen that there is no plateau and the relationship is fairly linear and steep over the range of values for PCO_2 seen in health and disease.

At any one moment there is about 1.5 litres of oxygen in the body, of which about 850 mL is combined with haemoglobin in the blood, about 450 mL is in the alveolar gas, about 200 mL is combined with myoglobin in muscle and less than 50 mL is dissolved in the plasma and tissues. This is a very small store considering that resting oxygen consumption is 250 mL per minute and following a change in alveolar ventilation arterial PO_2 will rapidly reach its new steady-state value. In contrast, there are about 120 litres of carbon dioxide in various forms (dissolved, carbamino compounds, bicarbonate and carbonates) and at various sites in the body (plasma, fat and bone) (Cherniack and Longobardo, 1970). When alveolar ventilation changes, CO_2 will diffuse to or from these stores until a new equilibrium is reached with the plasma. It takes 10 to 20 minutes for arterial PCO_2 to fall to its steady-state value following an increase

in alveolar ventilation and even longer to rise to its final value following a fall in alveolar ventilation (Lumb, 2000b).

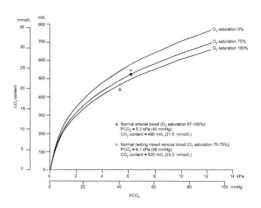

Figure 6.5   Carbon dioxide dissociation curves for whole blood

Three carbon dioxide dissociation curves are shown for blood with 0 per cent, 75 per cent and 100 per cent O_2 saturation. At any given PCO_2 the blood has a higher CO_2 content the lower the oxygen saturation (the Haldane effect). Over the range of values usually found in health and disease the curve is fairly linear. Normal arterial (a) and resting mixed venous points (v) are shown.

Ventilation and Alveolar Gases

Figure 6.6 gives the final steady-state values for alveolar PCO_2 and PO_2 when alveolar ventilation is altered at constant metabolic rate. Alveolar O_2 and CO_2 concentrations are determined by the balance of O_2 and CO_2 entering and leaving the alveolar region – that is, into or out of the pulmonary capillary blood and to and from the inspired and expired air. Alveolar O_2 concentration expressed as a fraction (F_AO_2 e.g. 0.13) is determined by the O_2 fraction of the gas entering the alveolar region in the inspired air (F_IO_2) and the rate of oxygen entering the pulmonary capillary blood ($\dot{V}O_2$) relative to alveolar ventilation ($\dot{V}_A$).

Alveolar oxygen fraction (F_AO_2) =
    Moist inspired FO_2 – Oxygen
    consumption $(\dot{V}O_2)$/Alveolar
    ventilation $(\dot{V}_A)$.

With a constant metabolic rate, as alveolar ventilation $(\dot{V}_A)$ increases, the difference between moist inspired fraction and alveolar oxygen fraction decreases. Theoretically, with an infinitely large alveolar ventilation, alveolar oxygen fraction would equal that of moistened inspired air. The important practical consequence is that F_AO_2 and, therefore, P_AO_2 (= $F_ACO_2 \times P_B$) are limited by inspired PO_2. At an altitude of 10,500 feet (3,200 metres) barometric pressure is 524 mm Hg (70 kPa), and

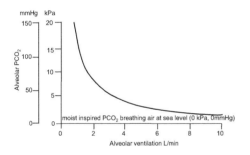

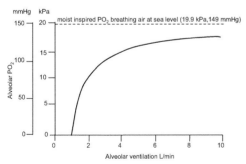

Figure 6.6   Effect on PCO_2 (top) and PO_2 (lower) of changing ventilation with metabolic rate constant

These relationships are hyperbolic; the higher the alveolar ventilation the closer the alveolar gas approaches the composition of moist inspired air. As inspired air is usually CO_2-free the relationship is simpler for CO_2 than for O_2.

Alveolar PCO_2 = P_B (Alveolar fraction CO_2) = P_B (CO_2 production/Alveolar Ventilation).

Alveolar PO_2 = P_B (Alveolar fraction O_2) = P_B (Inspired O_2 concentration – O_2 uptake/Alveolar ventilation)

when saturated with water at 37°C, the moistened inspired PO_2 is 100 mm Hg (13.3 kPa), so only with an infinitely high ventilation could the normal sea-level value of alveolar PO_2 be reached when breathing air.

At higher altitudes when breathing air, normal sea-level PO_2 is not achievable even with this imaginary ventilatory feat. In real life, acute ascent to altitudes up to 10,000 feet (c. 3,000 metres) is associated with very little increase in alveolar ventilation (see 'Chemical Control of Breathing' below), and although this increases over the next few days as part of the acclimatization process, it remains modest. This means that, in real life, ascent to any altitude above sea level whilst breathing ambient air results in an alveolar PO_2 below that at sea level. Any reflex increase in ventilation that occurs in response to the hypoxaemia improves the arterial PO_2 but never restores it to the normal sea-level value in a subject breathing air.

Alveolar CO_2 fraction is similarly determined by the balance of CO_2 entering and leaving the alveolus, but the equation is simpler because inspired CO_2 fraction (0.0004) is low enough to be considered to be zero.

Alveolar carbon dioxide fraction (F_ACO_2)
    = carbon dioxide production
    $(\dot{V}CO_2)$/alveolar ventilation
    $(\dot{V}_A)$.

Since alveolar PCO_2 (P_ACO_2) = F_ACO_2 $\times$ P_B and arterial PCO_2 is equal or close to alveolar PCO_2 in both health and disease, alveolar and arterial PCO_2 are also determined by the ratio of carbon dioxide production and alveolar ventilation. At constant metabolic rate, the alveolar FCO_2 and PCO_2 are inversely proportional to alveolar ventilation, producing the so-called metabolic hyperbola of Figure 6.6.

Hypoventilation and Hyperventilation

The relationship $P_ACO_2 \propto \dot{V}CO_2/\dot{V}_A$ is used to define the terms hypoventilation and hyperventilation. Hyperventilation is present when alveolar ventilation is high relative to CO_2 production. Hypoventilation is present when alveolar ventilation has fallen proportionally more than CO_2 production. Hyperventilation leads to a reduced P_ACO_2 (< 4.7 kPa: 35 mm Hg) and hypoventilation to an increased P_ACO_2 (> 6.1 kPa: 46 mm Hg). It is important to note that hypoventilation and hyperventilation are only present if P_ACO_2 is abnormal; they do not simply mean low and high minute ventilation, the correct terms for which are 'hypopnoea' and 'hyperpnoea'.

Hypoventilation leading to hypercapnia (high P_ACO_2) occurs when ventilatory drive is decreased, for example as a result of head injury or the respiratory depressant effects of drugs (opioids, barbiturates, anaesthetics) or when something prevents the drive being effective at maintaining ventilation (respiratory muscle weakness). Although ventilation–perfusion mismatching and right-to-left shunting do impair CO_2 excretion, a rise in arterial PCO_2 is not inevitable or even usual. A reflex increase in ventilation usually occurs and is sufficient to normalize or lower the arterial PCO_2, even though the hypoxia persists. The hypercapnia found in some patients with severe hypoxic chronic obstructive pulmonary disease (COPD) indicates hypoventilation, the cause of which remains uncertain, as are the reasons why it occurs in some patients with COPD and not others.

The effects of hypercapnia (high arterial PCO_2) are the result of multiple mechanisms, some of which act via the increased [H^+] that is generated by the increased CO_2 ($CO_2 + H_2O \Leftrightarrow H_2CO_3 \Leftrightarrow H^+ + HCO_3^-$). Hypercapnia has direct depressant effects on the central nervous system, cardiac muscle and is vasodilator in all systemic vascular beds. It also activates peripheral and central chemoreceptors causing reflex effects, both directly (bradycardia and vasoconstriction) and also secondary to the ventilatory reflex responses it initiates (tachycardia and vasodilatation). The strength of the various components differs between subjects and species, and symptoms and signs are also dependent on the cause of the hypercapnia.

Rebreathing exhaled gas or breathing CO_2 containing gas mixtures in a normal person produces a strong reflex increase in ventilation and marked breathlessness (dyspnoea), but when hypercapnia is caused by respiratory depression, dyspnoea and any effects secondary to increased ventilation will be absent. In humans, the typical effects of a moderately raised PCO_2 are flushed skin, full pulse, muscle twitching, hand flap, cardiac extrasystoles, headache and usually a raised blood pressure. Very high $PaCO_2$ (> 10 kPa) causes confusion, depressed ventilation and eventually convulsions, coma and death. These symptoms and their severity are also influenced by whether the hypercapnia is acute or chronic. Chronic hypercapnia is better tolerated because of compensatory mechanisms such as a metabolic alkalosis mediated by the kidneys, which can return arterial pH to within or close to the normal range.

Hyperventilation arises whenever there is some additional stimulus to breathing over and above the normal respiratory drive. The increased alveolar ventilation that accompanies mild to moderate exercise is not hyperventilation because it is in proportion to the increased $\dot{V}CO_2$ and arterial PCO_2 is unchanged. In heavy exercise, the extra stimulus to breathing caused by the lactic acidosis produced by anaerobic respiration does lead to an alveolar ventilation disproportionally high compared with the CO_2 production, and this can be correctly described as hyperventilation. There are many other sources of additional respiratory drive. In the aviation environment, anxiety-driven hyperventilation may be seen in a passenger with a flying phobia or in any crew member or passenger during an in-flight emergency. Pain is another important respiratory stimulus. An injured person, who is anxious and in pain, may have the signs and symptoms of their injuries complicated by those arising from hyperventilation. Hypoxia, when severe (below about 7.5–8.0 kPa: 56–60 mm Hg), is a potent respiratory stimulus that will increase ventilation out of proportion to CO_2 production.

Hypoxia is an especially important cause of hyperventilation in the aviation environment, as here it may warn of a problem with cabin pressurization or the oxygen system and with it imminent loss of function or consciousness. It follows from this that if symptoms or signs of hyperventilation occur at an altitude above 12,000 feet (3,660 metres), it is necessary to assume and act as if the cause is hypoxia until proven otherwise. Positive-pressure breathing, as used by military pilots for hypoxia protection at altitude or for G-protection in high-performance aircraft, almost invariably produces some degree of hyperventilation. High skin and core body temperature as well as whole-body immersion in cold water are potent causes of hyperventilation. Whole body vibration especially at low frequency (4–8 Hz), as produced by clear-air turbulence when flying at low altitudes, can also produce hyperventilation (Ernsting, 1961). In disease, hyperventilation may arise from the added respiratory stimulus from lung receptors (for example, with pulmonary embolus or lung fibrosis),

hypoxia or metabolic acidosis (diabetic ketoacidosis).

The effects of hypocapnia vary with the severity of the fall in arterial PCO_2 (P_ACO_2). Symptoms usually start when P_ACO_2 falls from its normal value of 5.3 kPa (40 mm Hg) to about 2.7–3.3 kPa (20–25 mm Hg) with lightheadedness, dizziness, visual disturbance, anxiety and tingling of various regions especially the face, lips, and fingers (Macefield and Burke, 1991; Rafferty et al., 1992). The visual disturbance takes various forms, but scotoma and eventually complete blackout of vision are common. At this level of hypocapnia, it is also possible to measure a significant fall in psychomotor performance (Rahn et al., 1946; Balke and Lillehei, 1956), although this seems to be much more to do with a decrement in motor performance than to intellectual performance (Gibson, 1978). Below 2.7 kPa (20 mm Hg), muscle spasms or tetany in hands and feet (carpopedal spasm) and face are likely to occur (Macefield and Burke, 1991; Rafferty et al., 1992). At a P_ACO_2 of 1.3–2.0 kPa (10–15 mm Hg), clouding of consciousness, whole body muscle spasms and unconsciousness occur (Perkin and Joseph, 1986; Burden et al., 1994).

The dizziness, lightheadedness, cognitive and visual disturbances are caused by the cerebral vasoconstriction that occurs in the presence of hypocapnia. The cerebral circulation has long been known to be very sensitive to arterial PCO_2 (for review, see Ainslie and Duffin, 2009) and cerebral blood flow falls by about 2 per cent for each 1 mm Hg fall in arterial PCO_2 until P_ACO_2 reaches about 22 mm Hg, when the fall levels off (Reivich, 1964; Raichle and Plum, 1972). The fall in cerebral blood flow is severe enough to lead to cerebral hypoxia despite arterial oxygen content being maintained or slightly increased. The mechanism of the paraesthesia and muscle spasms is still not completely certain. There is an increased excitability of cutaneous and motor axons, which begins before the paraesthesia and tetany start (Macefield and Burke, 1991). The usual explanation is that the alkalosis causes increased binding of calcium to plasma proteins, leading to a reduction of free ionized calcium, which in turn increases neuronal excitability. However, other mechanisms such as hypophosphataemia have been proposed (Gardner, 1996).

It is important to note that many of the symptoms of hypocapnia described here, with the exception of tetany, are indistinguishable from those caused by hypoxia. Moreover, as severe hypoxia causes a reflex stimulation of ventilation and therefore can lead to hypocapnia, it is not always easy to determine whether the signs and symptoms experienced are due to hypoxia, hypocapnia or a combination of the two.

Part 3:
CONTROL OF VENTILATION

Rhythmic output to the respiratory muscles originates in the brainstem where it is controlled in response to a wide variety of inputs. The most important of these, especially in relation to the challenge of high altitude, is the afferent input from the central and the peripheral respiratory chemoreceptors. Many other reflexes also affect breathing, including those from lung and airway receptors, arterial baroreceptors, facial and laryngeal receptors, muscle and joint receptors, temperature and pain receptors. These other receptors, which will not be discussed in detail here, can be of great importance to breathing regulation in specific situations, for example breath-hold diving and exercise.

Chemical control of breathing

It has been known for more than 100 years that changes in both alveolar PCO_2 and alveolar PO_2 can affect ventilation and that changes in alveolar PCO_2 have the largest effect. The first quantitative descriptions were by Haldane and Priestley (1905). Their main findings have been confirmed and extended by many authors since (for reviews, see Cunningham *et al.*, 1986; Lahiri and Forster, 2003). The typical ventilatory response to raising alveolar PCO_2 by progressively raising inspired PCO_2 is shown schematically in Figure 6.7 (solid lines). The key features are:

1. The CO_2 response curve is linear as P_ACO_2 is raised above normal up to a P_ACO_2 of about 10.7 kPa (80 mm Hg). In conscious subjects, the intense breathlessness (dyspnoea) induced makes it hard to study the responses at very high P_ACO_2. The slope of the response curve is reduced after this and eventually (PCO_2 > 13 kPa) ventilation declines below control values as the respiratory centre is depressed. In anaesthetized subjects, the P_ACO_2 at which respiratory depression occurs is lower.

2. The equation for linear part of the CO_2 response curve is: $\dot{V}_E = S(P_ACO_2 - B)$ where S is the CO_2 sensitivity (L/min rise in ventilation for each kPa or mm Hg rise in PCO_2). B is the intercept on the P_ACO_2 axis produced by extrapolation (light dashed lines), which predicts the PCO_2 value at which ventilation will fall to zero. The sensitivity to CO_2 is high; a 1 kPa (7.5 mm Hg) rise usually causes an increase in ventilation of about 20 L/min. However, CO_2 responsiveness is very variable (see below).

3. Ventilation values at P_ACO_2 below the normal value are obtained by prior hyperventilation of the subject to lower the P_ACO_2. Anaesthetized subjects, who are often hyperventilated during surgery, are often apnoeic when the anaesthetic is reversed and artificial ventilation terminated. They start breathing again when P_ACO_2 rises to a value (B) similar to that predicted by extrapolation of the CO_2 response curve. For this reason, anaesthetists commonly add CO_2 to the inspired gas shortly before the end of the operation to raise P_ACO_2 above the apnoeic threshold, thereby avoiding a period of hypoxia. In conscious subjects, the relationship between ventilation and P_ACO_2 in this region is variable and probably depends on the subjects and the precise experimental protocol. The early physiologists frequently used themselves as subjects and they experienced apnoea when P_ACO_2 was reduced below the intercept, B (Haldane and Priestley, 1905). With ventilation so influenced by higher cortical control, it is possible that their findings were influenced by their expectations. At low P_ACO_2 (25 mm Hg) following a period of hyperventilation, Fink (1961) found that naive subjects continued to breath, and this produces a 'dog leg' on the CO_2 response curve (dotted line on Figure 6.7). In conscious humans, ventilation post-hyperventilation may also depend on the time after the end of the hyperventilation (Meah and Gardner, 1994: Gardner, 1996). They found that when most subjects were asked to stop hyperventilation, ventilation initially remained above the pre-hyperventilation control

level, with apnoeic pauses occurring later, starting 0.8 to 5.6 minutes after the end of the hyperventilation.

4. The ventilatory response to $PaCO_2$ is affected by the arterial PO_2 (see below).

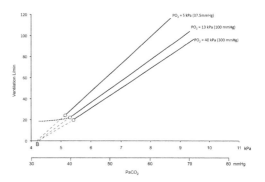

Figure 6.7   Carbon dioxide response curve
CO_2 response curves are shown for blood with normal P_AO_2 (13 kPa, 100 mm Hg), low PO_2 (5 kPa, 37.5 mm Hg) and high PO_2 (40 kPa, 300 mm Hg). The open circles represent the resting P_ACO_2 and expired ventilation values whilst breathing CO_2-free gas. Hypoxia increases and hyperoxia decreases the sensitivity to PCO_2 with little change of the intercept (B) of the ventilation / P_ACO_2 line. Responses to changing P_ACO_2 at values below the normal PCO_2 are obtained by prior hyperventilation and are variable. Conscious, naïve subjects often continue to breath with a ventilation similar to or a little below the pre-hyperventilation rate to give a 'dog leg' as shown by the dotted black line. Some conscious and most anaesthetized subjects show the ventilation predicted by extrapolation of the CO_2 response curves at low values of P_ACO_2 (grey dashed lines). In these subjects when P_ACO_2 falls below the intercept on the $PaCO_2$ axis (about 4.3 kPa, 32 mm Hg), apnoea occurs and breathing is resumed when P_ACO_2 rises above it.

Hypoxic ventilatory response

The typical ventilatory response to reducing alveolar PO_2 by lowering inspired PO_2 is shown schematically in Figure 6.8 (solid line). The important features are:

1. Lowering alveolar PO_2 from its normal sea-level value of 13.3 kPa (100 mm Hg) causes very little increase in ventilation until PO_2 falls below about 8 kPa (60 mm Hg).

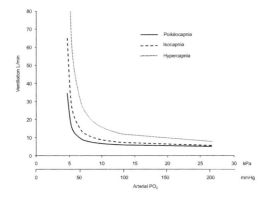

Figure 6.8   Ventilatory response to changing arterial PO_2

The solid line shows the ventilatory response to progressive hypoxia when arterial PCO_2 is allowed to fall naturally as ventilation increases (poikilocapnia). The dashed line shows the ventilatory response to progressive hypoxia with arterial CO_2 held constant by adding CO_2 to the inspired gas to compensate for the increased ventilation (isocapnia). The dotted line shows the ventilatory response to progressive hypoxia in the presence of an increased arterial PCO_2 (hypercapnia). There is little ventilatory response to hypoxia until P_AO_2 falls below about 8 ka (60 mmHg). Increase PCO_2 increases the ventilatory response to hypoxia.

2. Raising PO_2 from its normal sea-level value causes only a very slight depression of ventilation.
3. Below about 8 kPa (60 mm Hg), ventilation begins to increase more steeply and below about 6.7 kPa (50mm Hg) there is usually marked hyperventilation.
4. The main part of the hypoxic response curve can be described by a hyperbola with its equation $V_E = Vo + A/(P_AO_2 - C)$ (Weil and Zwillich, 1976; Hirshman *et al.*, 1975). V o is the ventilation asymptote (the ventilation at infinitely high PO_2 when there is no hypoxic drive), and the constant C is the PO_2 asymptote (the PO_2 value that the extrapolated data predicts will lead to infinitely high ventilation). In conscious humans, this value is usually around 32 mmHg (Weil and Zwillich, 1976; Hirshman *et al.*, 1975). In reality, experiments are terminated at a higher PO_2 such as 40 mm Hg and

with very severe degrees of hypoxic ventilation falls (not shown in Figure 6.7) as the hypoxic brainstem respiratory centres fail. The value A is a constant that is a measure of the subject's hypoxic drive; the higher the value, the higher the ventilatory response to hypoxia.

5. It is clear from Figures 6.7 and 6.8 that, for a normal person at sea level, changes in P_ACO_2 have much larger effects on ventilation than changes in P_AO_2. One of the factors limiting the ventilatory response to a fall in P_AO_2 is that any increase in alveolar ventilation inevitably leads to a fall in alveolar PCO_2, and this acts as a potent brake on the hypoxic ventilatory response. If CO_2 is added to the inspired gas in quantities just sufficient to hold the alveolar PCO_2 constant, the hypoxic ventilatory response is increased (Figure 6.8 – dashed line), although it still modest in comparison with the CO_2 response. There is synergy between the hypoxic and hypercapnic ventilatory responses. In the presence of hypoxia, the sensitivity to CO_2 increases (Nielsen and Smith, 1952) as shown by the increased slope of the CO_2 response curve (Figure 6.7 – PO_2 = 5 kPa line). In the presence of increased PCO_2, the sensitivity to hypoxia increases (Cormack *et al.*, 1957) (Figure 6.8 – dotted line).

Variability of CO_2 and O_2 Responses

The size of the ventilatory response to both hypoxia and hypercapnia is very variable. Haldane and Priestley (1905) noted that although subjects usually experienced hyperpnoea when the inspired oxygen concentration was reduced to 15 per cent (which would give an alveolar PO_2 of about 57 mm Hg), one of their subjects had continued to breathe air with diminishing oxygen concentration until unconsciousness occurred without the subject having experienced any hyperpnoea or discomfort. A variety of steady-state and rebreathing methods have been used to measure CO_2 responsiveness, and the actual values of S and B in an individual depend on the technique used (Read and Leigh, 1967; Rebuck et al., 1974; Avery et al., 1963; Berkenbosch et al., 1989).

Using a rebreathing method in 44 healthy subjects between the ages of 21 and 51, Hirshman et al. (1975) found the mean CO_2 response slope (S) was 2.69 ± 1.23 l/min/mmHg (20.7 ± 9.2 l/min/kPa) with individual values of between 1 and 5.95 l/min/mmHg (7.5 and 44.6 l/min/kPa). In the same subjects, the measure of hypoxic sensitivity, A, varied between 59 and 400, with a mean value of 185.8 ± 84.85 (SD) (ventilation in L/min and P_AO_2 in mmHg). There was a correlation between hypoxic and CO_2 sensitivity, subjects, with high CO_2 sensitivity tending to have high O_2 sensitivity. For a given subject, the values of both oxygen and CO_2 sensitivity are fairly constant when the measurements are repeated over periods of a few hours, but tend to be more variable when repeated on different days. The between-day variability in hypoxic ventilatory response may partly be explained by daily variations in arterial PCO_2 and pH (Sahn et al., 1977).

Response to Changes in Arterial (H+)

A rise in arterial PCO_2 leads to increased acidity via the increased production of carbonic acid, which then dissociates to form hydrogen and bicarbonate ions. An increase in hydrogen ions (decreased pH) produced in this way is a 'respiratory acidosis'. If an increase in hydrogen ion is produced in any other way, by convention the condition is known as a 'metabolic acidosis'. The terminology is not completely logical as CO_2 is a metabolite and many drugs and chemicals, which are not metabolites, are capable of producing a 'metabolic' acidosis. Experimentally, increased hydrogen ion stimulates increased ventilation independent of changes in PCO_2 and PO_2.

For example, if normal subjects are given oral ammonium chloride over several days, a metabolic acidosis is produced which increases resting ventilation, lowering arterial PCO_2 (Cunningham et al., 1961). Production of a chronic metabolic alkalosis by ingestion of bicarbonate produces a fall in ventilation, but the magnitude of the response is small. Most studies have shown little effect of increased hydrogen ion on the sensitivity to PCO_2 or PO_2. If CO_2 response curves are obtained from subjects with chronic metabolic acidosis and or chronic metabolic alkalosis, they are usually parallel to those obtained when starting at normal arterial pH (Cunningham et al., 1961; Mitchell and Singer 1965; Fencl et al., 1969).

Common causes of metabolic acidosis include the excess production of lactic acid in heavy exercise or circulatory shock and ketoacids in starvation or uncontrolled diabetes. In renal failure, metabolic acidosis usually results from the failure to excrete the acid anions, such as sulphate and phosphate, produced by normal metabolic pathways. Patients with metabolic acidosis often show deep, gasping respiration at rest, the breathing described by Kussmaul (1822–1902). Lactic acidosis is the extra stimulus responsible for increased rate of rise of ventilation as exercise work rate rises above moderately severe. The work rate at which this happens is known as the anaerobic threshold (Wasserman *et al.*, 1973).

Chemoreceptors

The respiratory chemoreceptors responsible for the reflex responses to changes in arterial PCO_2, PO_2 and pH are the central chemoreceptors located in the brainstem and the peripheral chemoreceptors in the carotid and aortic bodies. In anaesthetized animal experiments, the central chemoreceptors were originally found to be located near the surface of the ventrolateral medulla (Mitchell *et al.*, 1963; Loeschcke, 1982). More recently, using approaches such as recording the phrenic nerve response to focal acidosis produced by microinjection, central respiratory chemosensitivity has been found in other regions of the brainstem and cerebellum (Richerson *et al.*, 2005; Nattie, 2000). It is not yet clear whether all these regions contribute equally to central chemoreception or whether one group is dominant (Guyenet, 2008).

The exact mechanism of chemoreception at the central chemoreceptor is still uncertain, but it almost certainly involves a change in the intracellular pH of the chemoreceptors (Putnam *et al.*, 2004; Lahiri and Forster, 2003). In the intact animal, changes in intracellular pH are usually caused by changes in arterial blood PCO_2. The CO_2 diffuses readily across the blood brain barrier where its reaction with water generates hydrogen ion (H^+) at the chemoreceptor ($CO_2 + H_2O \Leftrightarrow H_2CO_3 \Leftrightarrow H^+ + HCO_3^-$). The buffering power of brain extracellular fluid is low, so small changes in PCO_2 can cause large

changes in hydrogen ion concentration, $[H^+]$, at the chemoreceptor.

Changes in bicarbonate concentration will also affect brain tissue $[H^+]$ and this may be important following a long-term change in arterial PCO_2. In chronic hypercapnia, an increase in cerebrospinal fluid (CSF) bicarbonate concentration occurs and this moves the above reaction to the left, restoring CSF pH to a more normal value than occurs in acute hypercapnia. This helps explain why patients with severe hypoxic COPD may tolerate a very high arterial PCO_2 without breathlessness at rest. A similar level of hypercapnia produced acutely in a normal person would lead to a much higher CSF $[H^+]$, a strong reflex stimulation of ventilation and severe breathlessness.

A gradual reduction in CSF bicarbonate concentration has long been thought to contribute to the ventilatory acclimatization that happens over the first few days after ascent to high altitude (Severinghaus *et al.*, 1963). It was thought that transport of bicarbonate out of the CSF helped correct the initial alkalosis to permit the ventilatory response to hypoxia to be more fully expressed. However, the CSF pH compensation is incomplete and develops too slowly to explain the ventilatory acclimatization (Forster *et al.*, 1975; Robbins, 2007). In recent years it has been recognized that this is probably not the main mechanism of respiratory acclimatization to altitude; changes in carotid body sensitivity to PO_2 are likely to play an important role in the increased ventilation that develops in the hours and days following ascent to high altitude (Robbins, 2007).

Subjects who have had their carotid bodies surgically removed (to treat bilateral carotid body tumours, or in the 1960s and 1970s as an experimental treatment for asthma and COPD) fail to show the increased slope of the ventilation versus oxygen consumption curve that normally occurs above the anaerobic threshold (Wasserman *et al.*, 1975). This suggests that carotid bodies, rather than central chemoreceptors, mediate the ventilatory response to metabolic acidosis in humans. However, this may depend on the severity and duration of the acid-base disturbance. The charged hydrogen ions present in the arterial blood do not readily cross the blood–brain barrier, but with severe or prolonged acidaemia the CSF [H$^+$] is likely to rise and lead to stimulation of ventilation via the central chemoreceptors.

Humans without carotid bodies show no significant increase in ventilation when breathing hypoxic gas mixtures (Lugliani *et al.*, 1971; Swanson *et al.*, 1978), which suggests that, in humans, the hypoxic ventilatory response is mediated almost entirely by the carotid bodies. A response can be demonstrated if these subjects are exposed to hypoxia when their arterial PCO$_2$ is also experimentally raised by about 10 mm Hg, but even then the response is very small (Swanson *et al.*, 1978). These patients would be particular vulnerable at high altitude, especially above about 10,000 feet (c. 3,000 metres), as their lack of ventilatory response (see Figure 6.9 and below) would result in more severe hypoxia than in normal subjects.

These observations suggest that the central chemoreceptors are not stimulated by hypoxia, and indeed in carotid body-denervated animals severe hypoxia may depress ventilation, as the hypoxia impairs respiratory centre function. However, even this apparently straightforward conclusion has been challenged recently. It is increasingly recognized that complete loss of sensory input to the central nervous system (CNS), as happens when carotid bodies are removed or denervated, may alter the

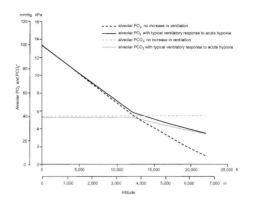

Figure 6.9   Effects of acute exposure to high altitude on alveolar PO$_2$ and PCO$_2$

If ventilation remained constant as altitude increased, the alveolar PCO$_2$ (grey broken line) would be unchanged (assuming constant CO$_2$ production) and alveolar PO$_2$ would fall progressively (black broken line). The actual ventilatory response to the acute hypoxia is variable. The solid lines show alveolar PO$_2$ (black line) and PCO$_2$ (grey line) with a typical observed ventilatory response to acute altitude exposure (for example, Rahn & Otis, 1949). There is little increase in ventilation below 10,000 feet (3,000 m) but at altitudes above this there is a progressive increase in ventilation which slows the decline in PO$_2$ and reduces alveolar PCO$_2$.

sensitivity of the CNS to other inputs, and in the long term there may also be remodelling within the CNS (Forster, 2003). In unanaesthetized sleeping dogs, a modest ventilatory response to cerebral hypoxia has been demonstrated using a preparation in which the carotid bodies are intact and perfused with blood with normal PO$_2$, PCO$_2$ and pH (Curran *et al.*, 2000). The mechanism and importance of this modest CNS hypoxic response in dogs is currently difficult to assess, but there is little doubt that in all mammals studied the carotid body is by far the most important source of the hypoxic ventilatory response.

Peripheral Chemoreceptors

Peripheral chemoreceptors are located in the carotid bodies at the bifurcation of the common carotid artery. The carotid body contains neuron-like glomus or type 2 cells that are believed to act as the chemoreceptor, surrounded by glial-like type 1 cells. Each carotid body is normally just a few grams in weight, and the afferents join the carotid sinus nerve, which also carries afferents from the arterial baroreceptors in the nearby carotid sinus. The carotid sinus nerve is a branch of the glossopharyngeal nerve via which the afferent information from both chemoreceptors and baroreceptors passes to the nucleus of the tractus solitarius (NTS) in the brainstem. Similar chemoreceptors are found in the aortic bodies scattered around the aortic arch. Afferents from the aortic bodies pass to the NTS via the vagus nerve. Carotid bodies are stimulated by increased arterial PCO_2, increased arterial hydrogen ion (reduced pH) and reduced arterial PO_2. As discussed above, in humans the reflex ventilatory response to arterial hypoxia and also to acute metabolic acidosis is largely, if not solely, due to the stimulation of the carotid body chemoreceptors.

Hypoxia is believed to increase the firing of the type 2 glomus cells of the carotid body by inhibition of potassium channels leading to depolarization and Ca^{2+} entry leading to transmitter release and activation of afferent nerve fibres. The exact mechanism(s) involved are still uncertain and the various theories are beyond the scope of this chapter, but discussed in many excellent reviews (Peers, 2002; Peers and Wyatt, 2007; Kumar and Bin-Jaliah, 2007; Lopez-Barneo et al., 2008). The carotid body has an extremely high total blood flow per gram of tissue and the blood in the veins emerging from it often looks as bright red as the arterial blood entering it. These observations led to the idea that it 'tasted arterial blood' (De Castro, 1927). It was thought that the carotid body's oxygen needs could be met from the dissolved oxygen in

the blood and that carotid body tissue PO_2 was close to arterial PO_2. As often happens, the picture that has emerged is more complicated. Not all the carotid body blood flow passes through the carotid body tissue capillaries; much of it passes through arteriovenous shunts (De Castro, 1940). Direct measurements of the microcirculation and tissue PO_2 deep in the carotid body have revealed values considerably below arterial PO_2 (Acker, 1980; Acker and O'Regan, 1981; Delpiano and Acker, 1980; Lahiri et al., 1993).

The similarity between the shape of the hypoxic ventilatory response curve (ventilation versus arterial PO_2) and the oxyhaemoglobin dissociation curve (oxygen saturation versus PO_2) has been noted on many occasions (Comroe et al., 1962; Weil et al., 1970). Ventilation shows little increase until arterial PO_2 falls below about 7–8 kPa (50–60 mm Hg) (Figure 6.8), which is the also the PO_2 region at which oxygen saturation begins to decline more steeply (Figure 6.3). Indeed, plotting ventilation against O_2 saturation reveals a linear relationship suggesting the possibility that it is oxygen saturation, or the directly related oxygen content, that is the stimulus causing the reflex increase in ventilation. However, anaemic patients (low oxygen content, normal PO_2 and normal O_2 saturation) do not usually have increased ventilation or breathlessness at rest, and experimentally moderate anaemia causes neither increased carotid body discharge nor increased ventilation (Hatcher et al., 1978; Matsuoka et al., 1994).

Similarly, moderately severe carbon monoxide poisoning (low oxygen content, low O_2 saturation with normal arterial PO_2) causes little increase in ventilation or breathlessness, and in animal experiments moderately high concentrations of carboxyhaemoglobin fail to cause carotid body chemoreceptor stimulation (Duke *et al.*, 1952). Moreover, in the cat carotid body, chemoreceptor activity in the carotid sinus nerve has been shown to increase progressively when arterial PO_2 is lowered from hyperoxic to normoxic values, a range over which oxygen saturation changes little (Lahiri and DeLaney, 1975). For example, in one cat, lowering PO_2 from 495 mm Hg to 97 mm Hg, with PCO_2 and pH constant, had little effect on oxygen saturation but caused chemoreceptor discharge, in a single fibre recording, to increase from 1.9 to 4.4 impulses/second. Taken together, these findings indicate that the arterial hypoxic stimulus to the carotid body is PO_2 and not arterial oxygen content or saturation. Part of the synergistic interaction between PCO_2 and hypoxia on ventilation occurs at the level of the carotid body; carotid body firing in response to high PCO_2 is increased by hypoxia and the increased firing in response to hypoxia is increased by high PCO_2 (Lahiri and DeLaney, 1975).

Increased Arterial PCO_2: Reflex Contributions

The central and peripheral chemoreceptors both contribute significantly to the reflex ventilatory response to increased arterial PCO_2. Most physiology textbooks state that the central chemoreceptors contribute 80 per cent of the response to raised CO_2 and the peripheral chemoreceptors 20 per cent. This statement is based on studies of the ventilatory responses to breathing CO_2 containing gas mixtures in animals before and after carotid body denervation. In humans, bilateral carotid body resection causes CO_2 responsiveness to fall by 20–30 per cent (Lugliani *et al.*, 1971; Bellville *et al.*,

1979; Honda *et al.*, 1979; Whipp, 1994; Timmers *et al.*, 2003).

With newer, more sophisticated experimental approaches, a wide range of different values for the relative importance of the carotid body chemoreceptors and the central chemoreceptors has been found. Important factors that affect the conclusions include the species studied, whether anaesthesia was used, the technique used to separate central from peripheral chemoreceptor responses and, in the case of carotid body denervation studies, the time that has elapsed since the denervation. As discussed above in relation to hypoxia sensitivity, carotid sinus and carotid body denervation leads to loss of the normal tonic input to the brainstem, which can lead to remodelling of the central reflex pathways and their responses (Curran *et al.*, 2000; Brooks and Sved, 2005; Smith *et al.*, 2006; Dahan *et al.*, 2007). Loss of tonic input from the carotid body may impair central chemoreceptor responsiveness initially but, with time, this brainstem plasticity may allow recovery of CO_2 responsiveness (Pan *et al.*, 1998).

Even if it is not possible, or even sensible, to assign a percentage to their role in CO_2 sensitivity, it is clear that peripheral chemoreceptors contribute to the steady-state responses to PCO_2, both by their direct reflex effects and also because their tonic input to the brainstem increases the chemoreceptor responsiveness of the system as a whole. In addition, the reflex responses initiated by the carotid body in response to a change in arterial PCO_2 are much faster than those initiated by central chemoreceptors (Smith *et al.*, 2006), and in many situations this further increases the importance of the carotid body. Following a sudden rise in PCO_2, the rapid carotid body-mediated ventilatory response may correct the P_ACO_2 before the central chemoreceptors are activated. There also seems to be large individual variability in the apparent contribution of the peripheral and central chemoreceptors, even when the same species is studied under the same experimental approach (Smith *et al.*, 2006).

Part 4: Cardiovascular Responses To Acute Hypoxia

Acute hypoxia has multiple effects on the systemic circulation (Marshall, 1999) and this gives rise to considerable variability in the net response between and within individuals, depending on such things as the intensity and duration of the hypoxia. Hypoxia has a direct vasodilator effect on systemic vessels and causes reflex effects mediated by peripheral chemoreceptors both directly (bradycardia and vasoconstriction) and secondary to the reflex increase in ventilation. Increased ventilation stimulates pulmonary stretch receptors and these in turn have reflex cardiovascular effects (tachycardia and vasodilatation). In addition, in animal experiments, hypoxic stimulation of the peripheral carotid body chemoreceptors has been shown to activate the defence or alerting areas of the brain, which initiate a complex pattern of respiratory, cardiovascular and other responses including increased arousal (Hilton and Marshall, 1982). The cardiovascular effects include tachycardia, increased blood pressure, and vasoconstriction in many vascular beds with vasodilatation in skeletal muscle.

In humans, too, the carotid bodies almost certainly activate the defence areas, and this mediates the arousal from life-threatening hypoxia that occurs during sleep in patients with obstructive sleep apnoea, leading to repeated awakening and daytime sleepiness. Activation of the

defence response and some of the reflex responses to hypoxia leads to increased sympathetic activity and also increased circulating adrenaline (norepinephrine). The following is a description of the net effects of all the mechanisms discussed above in humans during acute hypoxic exposure. Prolonged exposure to high altitude modifies these responses and this is discussed in Chapter 7 (Hypobaric Hypoxia: Adaptation and Acclimatization).

Cardiac Output and Heart Rate

In humans, acute hypoxia sufficient to lower saturation to about 85 per cent (altitude approximately 12,000 feet (c. 3,600 metres)) increases both heart rate and cardiac output at rest, usually with little effect on mean arterial blood pressure (Korner, 1959; Richardson *et al.*, 1966, 1967; Wagner *et al.*, 1986; Wagner, 2000). During exercise at any submaximal level of oxygen consumption, the cardiac output and heart rate are also higher than at the same level of oxygen uptake at sea level. The maximum exercise cardiac output during acute altitude exposure is unchanged, but the maximum oxygen uptake and the work rate associated with it are reduced. For example, during a hypobaric chamber exposure at 15,000 feet (4,600 metres: P_B = 430 mm Hg) in eight normal subjects at rest, mean arterial PO_2 was 48 $\pm$ 3 mm Hg (Wagner *et al.*, 1986). During exercise carried out within an hour of the start of exposure to this altitude, the maximum heart rate and maximum cardiac output (172 $\pm$ 7 beats/minute and 24.8 $\pm$ 2.6 litres/minute), were very similar to the maximum sea level values (176 $\pm$ 8 beats/minute and 23.9 $\pm$ 1.2 litres/minute). However, the maximum oxygen consumption was only 2.27 $\pm$ 0.12 litres/minute at 15,000 feet (4,600 metres) compared with 3.72 ± 0.56 litres/minute at sea level.

Coronary blood flow increases as cardiac output increases with ascent to high altitude. Electrocardiographic changes, such T wave flattening, ST depression, lengthening of QT interval and an increased incidence of supraventricular and ventricular extrasystoles, do occur, but they are mostly mild, at least at altitudes up to about 23,000 feet (7,000 meters) (Laciga and Koller, 1976; Boutellier and Koller, 1981; Saurenmann and Koller, 1984; Koller et al., 1988; Kujanik et al., 2000). Some of these changes are due to the increased sympathetic and reduced parasympathetic drive to the heart that occurs with acute hypoxic exposure, but some changes, especially at the higher altitudes, are probably the direct result of cardiac hypoxia.

Cerebrovascular System

It has been known for a long time that a fall in arterial PO_2 or a rise in arterial PCO_2 dilates cerebral blood vessels, increasing cerebral blood flow (Kety and Schmidt, 1948). The cerebral circulation is very sensitive to changes in alveolar PCO_2. Cerebral blood flow is linearly related to PCO_2 over the 20–50 mm Hg range usually encountered in normal people. It decreases by 2–3 per cent for every mm Hg fall in PCO_2, so that halving PCO_2 from 40 to 20 mm Hg (5.3 to 2.7 kPa) will cause a 40–60 per cent reduction in cerebral blood flow (Brugniaux et al., 2007). In contrast, if P_ACO_2 is held constant, changes in arterial PO_2 in the range 60–150 mm Hg (8–20 kPa) have only a small effect on cerebral blood flow ($\pm$ 5–10 per cent) (Ainslie and Poulin, 2004; Brugniaux et al., 2007). As PO_2 falls below about 40 mm Hg, larger (> 30 per cent) increases

in blood flow are seen, even if PCO_2 is not prevented from falling (Kety and Schmidt, 1948; Shapiro et al., 1970).

When humans are exposed to high altitude, arterial PO_2 falls, but any increase in ventilation lowers arterial PCO_2, which opposes the vasodilator effects of the hypoxia. The net effect on cerebral blood flow is variable, depending on the degree of hypoxia and also on the hypoxic ventilatory response (Brugniaux et al., 2007). Some studies show relatively little effect on cerebral blood flow as PO_2 falls progressively to 45 mm Hg, as the hypoxic vasodilatatory effects seem to be balanced by the vasoconstrictor effects of the reduced P_ACO_2 (Ainslie and Poulin, 2004). If the fall in P_ACO_2 is prevented by adding CO_2 to the inspired gas (eucapnia), hypoxia consistently increases cerebral blood flow (Ainslie and Poulin, 2004; Shapiro et al., 1970), and the magnitude of any increase is larger than when P_ACO_2 is permitted to fall. The duration of the hypoxic exposure may also be important. When ventilation and P_ACO_2 were permitted to change spontaneously during 20 minutes of hypoxia with PaO_2 held at 45 mm Hg, Steinback and Poulin (2008) found there was a transient fall in cerebral blood flow followed by an increase. The transient fall was abolished when the experiments were repeated under eucapnic conditions.

In summary, in humans exposed to altitude, with a typically hypoxic ventilatory response, an increased cerebral blood flow can be expected when $PO_2 \leq 45$ mm Hg, as occurs with acute exposure to an altitude of above approximately 15,000 feet (4,600 metres). Below this altitude, the cerebral blood flow response is more variable with some subjects showing an increase and others a decrease, as the effects of hypocapnia reduce or override the effects of hypoxia.

Pulmonary Circulation

The pulmonary blood vessels respond to hypoxia by constricting, a response that is opposite to that of systemic blood vessels. The exact mechanism of hypoxic pulmonary vasoconstriction (HPV) is still unknown, but it involves an increase in intracellular calcium in the pulmonary artery smooth muscle cells (Aaronson *et al.*, 2006; Ward and McMurtry, 2009). The effect is quite large in humans. In anaesthetized subjects with separate intubation of the right and left main bronchi, suddenly changing the gas mixture from 100 per cent oxygen in both lungs to 5 per cent oxygen in one lung caused a rapid (within minutes) decrease in the blood flow to the hypoxic lung, an increase in flow to the other lung, a 54 per cent increase in pulmonary artery pressure and a threefold increase in vascular resistance of the hypoxic lung (Bindslev *et al.*, 1985).

At sea level, this mechanism helps to improve ventilation–perfusion matching in the lungs. Regions of the lungs that are poorly ventilated, perhaps because of airway constriction, inflammation or secretions, will have a low local alveolar PO_2, causing the vessels in such regions to constrict. This constriction reduces the blood flow to the hypoxic regions and diverts more of the pulmonary blood flow to regions that remain well ventilated, improving overall gas exchange (West, 1990). At high altitude, alveolar PO_2 is low throughout the lung and the widespread pulmonary vasoconstriction that occurs is less useful. It raises pulmonary artery pressure and the right heart workload and in time may lead to right heart failure.

Although HPV occurs with both acute and chronic high-altitude exposure, it is probably a more important phenomenon in subacute and chronic hypoxia. A high HPV response has been associated with increased susceptibility to high-altitude pulmonary (o)edema (often referred to as HAPE) that affects climbers (Dehnert *et al.*, 2005; Bärtsch and Gibbs, 2007). The maladaptive nature of HPV with chronic hypoxia is seen in the development of chronic mountain sickness (Chapter 7 – Hypobaric Hypoxia: Adaptation and Acclimatization) and also in the right heart failure of chronic hypoxic lung disease. Interestingly, high-altitude-dwelling Ladakhi yaks and llamas (Anand *et al.*, 1986) have considerably reduced pulmonary vascular smooth muscle and reduced HPV, which has been shown to be an inherited trait. Well-adapted mountain-dwelling human populations such as Tibetans also seem to show a similar loss of HPV (Groves *et al.*, 1993).

Part 5:
THE AVIATION DOMAIN

Flying entails rapid ascent to high altitude and, with it, the potential for several problems related to the fall in barometric pressure that are predictable from the gas laws. The first and most important potential problem is the fall in inspired PO_2 (Dalton's law; see 'Inspired and Alveolar Gases') leading to alveolar and arterial hypoxia. Boyle's law (Volume α 1/pressure) predicts the expansion of pockets of gas in the body, and Henry's law (concentration of a gas dissolved in a liquid α partial pressure of the gas) predicts the fall in the amount of gas that can be held in solution at high altitude. These three consequences of the fall in barometric pressure can give rise to problems for the aircrew and passengers, both in normal flight and especially during emergency situations. The effects of exposure to low barometric pressure will be considered under several headings.

Body Cavities

Air trapped in body cavities will expand on ascent (by about 30 per cent between sea level and 8,000 feet (c. 2,400 metres)) and contract on descent as predicted by Boyle's law, which states that for a given mass of gas, volume α 1/pressure. In some sites, such in the gastrointestinal tract or in a pneumothorax, this will cause problems on ascent as the gas expands. In the middle ear, a feeling of fullness, reduced auditory acuity and earache may develop if a pressure difference develops across the eardrum, causing it to distort. On ascent, the eustachian tube is usually forced open by the increased pressure inside the middle ear, allowing equalization of pressure across the tympanic membrane. On descent, when pressure in the middle ear is lower than in the ear canal, it may remain closed. Thus earache is more likely on descent and especially in the presence of eustachian tube oedema associated with an upper respiratory tract infection. Pain due to expansion and contraction of air in a blocked sinus (barosinusitis) may occur on both ascent and descent. Pain from air in a tooth abscess or cavity tends to be worse on ascent.

Most of these problems can be reduced or alleviated by simple measures such as avoiding gas-producing foods before flight, decongestants for ear or sinus problems, and simple analgesics such as paracetamol (acetaminophen). Various manoeuvres such as swallowing, yawning, jaw movements, the Freznel (contracting floor of mouth and pharynx with the nose pinched) or Valsalva (forced expiration with closed mouth and nostrils) manoeuvre can help open the eustachian tube and relieve ear pain. However, an expanding pneumothorax would lead to increased pain and breathlessness, further lung collapse, worsening gas exchange and possibly a tension pneumothorax. Flying should be avoided until the pneumothorax is resolved, or when air evacuation is essential, a chest drain must be inserted to allow the expanding pneumothorax air to escape (Teichman et al., 2007; Beninati et al., 2008).

In very rapid decompressions to high altitude, as may happen with major structural failure of the aircraft, air within the lungs may expand more rapidly than it can be exhaled, leading to pulmonary barotrauma, which can give rise to subcutaneous or mediastinal emphysema or systemic air embolism. Very occasionally, fatal air embolism has been reported following ascent in commercial aircraft in passengers with large pulmonary cysts (Zaugg et al., 1998).

Decompression

The term decompression illness (DCI) is an umbrella term referring to both arterial gas embolism, as discussed in the previous section, and decompression sickness (DCS), in which the problem is gas evolved from blood and tissues which have become supersaturated with nitrogen on decompression. The quantity of a gas that dissolves in a liquid is dependent on the solubility of the gas in the liquid and the partial pressure of the gas to which the liquid is exposed, as described by Henry's law (concentration of gas X in liquid Y = solubility of gas X in liquid Y × partial pressure of gas X). Sudden exposure to the reduced pressure at high altitude can cause gases, especially nitrogen, to come out of solution in the blood and tissues, forming bubbles. These bubbles may expand tissues and cause blockage of blood vessels leading to subatmospheric decompression sickness. Once formed, the bubbles gradually increase in size and the peak onset of decompression sickness is about 20 to 60 minutes after the start of exposure to high altitude. It is rare for symptoms to appear in the first five minutes, and if they do, it is likely that they are caused not by 'evolved gas' but by arterial air embolism, for example following pulmonary barotrauma.

The symptoms of DCS and their origin are similar to those that occur when a deep-sea diver returns to sea level too quickly, but there are some important differences. The main symptoms are joint and limb pains ('the bends'), respiratory symptoms such as a sense of chest constriction, difficulty in taking a deep breath and coughing ('the chokes'), itching, tingling and mottling of the skin ('the creeps'), visual or neurological symptoms ('the staggers') and cardiovascular collapse (syncope). Venous gas emboli can be detected in the right heart using precordial Doppler ultrasound and they may be found in asymptomatic subjects exposed to high altitude. Fortunately, the symptoms of subatmospheric DCS usually improve rapidly on descent to low altitude, and treatment in a hyperbaric chamber is only rarely required (Harding, 2002; Macmillan, 2006; Risdale, 2006).

Decompression sickness is extremely rare with exposures to altitudes below 18,000 feet (c. 5,500 metres) and so decompression sickness is not usually a problem associated with normal passenger transport aircraft where the maximum cabin altitude is 8,000 feet (c. 2,500 metres), and even in the event of sudden decompression, the time spent at altitudes above 18,000 feet (c. 5,500 metres) would usually be short, making serious DCS unlikely. In contrast, for operational reasons, many military aircraft spend long periods in cabins pressurized at higher altitudes; the maximum cockpit altitude of current high-performance aircraft is around 22,500 feet (6,860 metres). The risk of DCS becomes greater with increasing altitude, although it is still quite rare with exposures up 22,500 feet. The incidence and severity of DCS increase with increased duration of exposure to high altitude, exercise and also with prior exposure to altitudes above one atmosphere (scuba diving in the 24 hours before flying). The risk of DCS is also greater with repeated exposure to high altitude because any bubbles remaining from the first exposure may then rapidly expand (Allan, 2003).

Hypoxia

The most important challenge of high-altitude exposure is the reduced inspired PO_2 that occurs as barometric pressure falls. It follows from the discussion above on the control of ventilation that the reflex responses to hypoxia are unable to maintain sea-level alveolar and arterial PO_2 at any altitude above sea level. The reflex increase in ventilation in response to hypoxia is negligible until PO_2 falls to about 60 mm Hg (Figure 6.8) at an altitude of about 8,000–10,000 feet (c. 2,400–3,000 metres), and so P_AO_2 falls steadily in line with the progressive fall in barometric pressure and inspired PO_2 (Figure 6.9). Above about 8,000–10,000 feet, the reflex increase in ventilation leads to a higher PO_2 (Figure 6.9, solid line) than would have occurred without an increase in ventilation (Figure 6.9, dashed line), but this only serves to slow the decline in alveolar PO_2. The P_AO_2 and P_ACO_2 values used to generate Figure 6.9 are 'typical' values for a subject exposed acutely (< 1 hour) to high altitude (Rahn and Otis, 1947, 1949; Ernsting, 1973; Gradwell, 2006). The exact values vary depending on such issues as the hypoxic ventilatory responses of the individuals studied and the exact duration of the acute exposure. Immediate values (< 5 minutes) of P_AO_2 tend to be higher and P_ACO_2 lower than later values (20–30 minutes) reflecting 'hypoxic ventilatory decline' from an early peak value (Weil and Zwillich, 1976; Powell et al., 1998).

There are several approaches to avoiding or at least reducing the severity of the problems associated with flying at high altitudes. The simplest, taken by small recreational aircraft, is to restrict flying to altitudes below about 8,000 to 10,000 feet (2,400–3,000 metres). Many commercial and military aircraft fly much higher than 10,000 feet, often above 40,000 feet (12,000 metres). The operating altitude of Concorde was around 55,000 feet (16,750 metres). The reasons include fuel efficiency, reduction of turbulence, air corridor management and tactical considerations. For these aircraft, cabin pressurization is used to reduce the equivalent altitude to which the occupants are exposed. For aircrew and passengers, it would be ideal to keep the pressure in the cabin at sea level, but a compromise has to be reached between human physiology, aircraft design and operational considerations (Ernsting, 1978; Macmillan, 2006).

The lower the cabin altitude, the greater the pressure difference across the fuselage when the aircraft is at high altitude and the stronger and heavier it will need to be. In addition, if the aircraft integrity is lost, the consequences of the sudden decompression are more severe with a high differential pressure. Commercial passenger transport aircraft are usually pressurized to an equivalent of about 5,000 to 6,000 feet (1,500 to 1,800 metres), with a maximum cabin altitude in normal flight of 8,000 feet (2,400 metres). With this degree of pressurization, aircrew can work without significant deficit and the majority of passengers will have no problems because oxygen saturation will have

fallen only a little with the fall in arterial PO_2 (from about 11–13 kPa (80–100 mm Hg) at sea level to about 8 kPa (60 mm Hg) at 8,000 feet).

Problems can arise at normal cabin altitudes in passengers with respiratory and/or cardiovascular disease. Those with severe respiratory disease may have an arterial PO_2 at sea level on the steep part of the oxyhaemoglobin dissociation curve (< 8–9 kPa), and in this region a further fall in arterial PO_2 will cause a large, potentially dangerous, fall in arterial oxygen saturation. Various indices (based on sea-level oxygen saturation and/or arterial PO_2, spirometry, walk test) have been proposed for screening such patients, in particular to determine which patients require supplemental oxygen during the flight (Mortazavi, 2003). The British Thoracic Society Guidelines (2004) recommend that oxygen supplementation is required if arterial oxygen saturation is less than 92 per cent at sea level, but not if it is greater than 95 per cent or greater than 92 per cent with no additional risk factors. If the saturation is 92 to 95 per cent with additional risk factors present (FEV_1 < 50 per cent predicted), a hypoxia challenge test is recommended to determine whether oxygen supplementation is needed.

In high-performance aircraft, a combination of cockpit pressurization and oxygen supplementation is used to prevent hypoxia in normal operations. For aircraft design and operational reasons, military aircraft cabins are usually pressurized rather less than civilian transport aircraft, with a cabin pressure that varies with altitude. Current high-performance aircraft may operate around or even above 60,000 feet (18,000 metres), at which altitude the maximum cockpit altitude is likely to be around 22,500 feet (6,800 metres). At these cockpit altitudes, breathing oxygen-enriched air is necessary both for protection against hypoxia and decompression illness. To prevent hypoxia as the altitude increases, the percentage of oxygen in the inspired gas is progressively increased. Normal sea-level alveolar PO_2 can be maintained by increasing the inspired oxygen fraction up to an altitude of 33,700 feet (c. 10,000 metres) where 100 per cent oxygen is required. With exposure to progressively higher altitudes above 33,700 feet, while breathing 100 per cent oxygen at ambient pressure, alveolar PO_2 will fall progressively until, at around 40,000 feet (12,200 metres), it is equivalent to that when breathing air at 10,000 feet (around 55 mm Hg). This is the minimum alveolar PO_2 that will ensure acceptable physical and psychometric performance.

In the event of a sudden decompression above 40,000 feet, oxygen needs to be supplied under pressure (30 to 70 mm Hg depending on the altitude) if unacceptable hypoxia is to be avoided and the aircrew enabled to respond appropriately. Positive pressure breathing has several disadvantages; it is tiring and the raised intrapleural pressure distends the lungs and reduces venous return. These problems require countermeasures, such as counter-pressure garments, which are beyond the scope of this chapter. They are discussed elsewhere (Gradwell, 2006). When there is a planned or possible exposure above 18,000 feet (5,500 metres), the risk of decompression illness can be reduced by breathing 100 per cent oxygen for 30 minutes to 3 hours beforehand to wash out the nitrogen stored in the blood and tissues (Macmillan, 2006). The exact time recommended depends on the expected altitude and duration of exposure to altitudes above 25,000 feet (7,600 metres). Finally, an alternative approach to cockpit pressurization is pressurization of the immediate environment around the person in the form of a pressure suit. These are used at very high altitudes or in space.

Physiological Hazards at Altitude

Although some problems related to exposure to reduced barometric pressure may occur when aircraft are operating normally, more serious problems can be expected when the normal protective measures fail. They fall into three broad categories: failure of pressurization, loss of pressure and loss of oxygen delivery to the occupants. Accidental failure to engage the pressurization system was the primary problem in the 2005 Helios Boeing 737 crash at Grammatiko. One issue that was addressed by the enquiry that followed was why the crew failed to respond in an appropriate and timely manner to the situation (Aircraft Accident Report, Helios Airways Flight HCY522, November 2006). It was concluded that a major contributor to the fatal outcome was likely to be that an insidious onset of cognitive impairment due to hypoxia was not recognized by the crew in time to take appropriate action. In high-performance aircraft where the crew often rely on oxygen breathing in normal flight, loss of the oxygen supply, poor mask seal or malfunction of oxygen regulators are common causes of aircrew hypoxia at high altitude (Cable 2003; Gradwell, 2006).

Sudden decompression of an aircraft occurs when the integrity of the fuselage of a pressurized aircraft flying at high altitude is prejudiced. The time taken for the cabin pressure to fall to the ambient pressure outside the aircraft is inversely proportional to the size of the hole, directly proportional to the volume of the cabin and directly proportional to the ratio of cabin to ambient pressure (Macmillan, 2006). Other factors that can affect the cabin pressure are air inflow from the engines and any aerodynamic suction, which may cause a subatmospheric pressure immediately outside the defect. The actual profile to which the occupants are exposed will determine the severity of the effects, and this will normally be influenced by the emergency descent action taken by the pilot. Following sudden fuselage damage, the cabin altitude usually rises and then falls as the aircraft descends. In many passenger aircraft the large cabin volume gives enough time to allow descent to occur before the initial ambient altitude is reached.

Explosive or rapid decompression is usually obvious to both aircrew and passengers, and provided the structural damage is not too great, rapid descent to a safe altitude (10,000 feet) followed by emergency landing is often possible. In the Qantas Flight 30 Boeing 747 accident in 2008, all passengers and aircrew survived uninjured, when at 29,000 feet (c. 8,800 metres) an oxygen cylinder in the cargo hold exploded causing a 2×1.5 metre hole in the fuselage (Australian Transport Safety Bureau, 2009).

The speed of onset of arterial hypoxia will vary with these different types of accidental exposure to high altitude. Generally, it will be slowest and the signs and symptoms insidious if an aircraft ascends from the ground to high altitude without cabin pressurization. In high-performance aircraft, a fault in the oxygen supply or a leaking mask in an aircraft that is either unpressurized or pressurized to a high cockpit altitude will usually give a fairly rapid fall in alveolar PO_2 as the initially normoxic alveolar gas is replaced by the hypoxic inspirate. The rate of fall of PO_2 will depend on the subject's ventilation.

The most rapid onset of hypoxia usually occurs with a rapid decompression because the total alveolar pressure and alveolar PO_2 fall instantly following the falling pressure. For example, a rapid decompression causing the cabin altitude to rise rapidly to 40,000 feet (12,000 metres) would lead to a similarly very rapid fall in alveolar PO_2 to about 14 mm Hg. Whatever the speed of development of alveolar hypoxia, whenever alveolar PO_2 reaches a value below mixed venous PO_2, oxygen will be lost from the blood to the alveolus until a new equilibrium is reached.

Any reflex increase in ventilation is inevitably accompanied by a fall in alveolar PCO_2 (solid line. lower panel, Figure 6.9), which has a cerebral vasoconstrictor effect that can partly offset the benefits of improved PO_2 and arterial oxygen content. The effects of acute exposure to high altitude are very variable both because of the variability of the ventilatory response to hypoxia, and hence the resultant P_AO_2 and P_ACO_2 at any given altitude, and also because the effects of hypoxia vary between individuals. Nevertheless, an attempt to describe typical effects in a healthy subject at different altitudes is given below. In this context, 'altitude' refers to the equivalent altitude, in terms of the barometric pressure to which the subject is exposed, rather than the height above sea level; a passenger flying at 35,000 feet (10,650 metres) in a commercial jet pressurized to 565 mm Hg is said to be at 8,000 feet.

Arterial PO_2 falls progressively on ascent to altitude from about 13.3 kPa (100 mm Hg) at sea level to about 7.3 kPa (55 mm Hg) at 10,000 feet with little change in P_ACO_2 (Figure 6.9). Fortunately, as can be seen from the oxyhaemoglobin dissociation curve, this 45 per cent fall in P_AO_2 causes a much smaller fall in oxygen saturation from about 97 per cent at sea level to about 87 per cent at 10,000 feet (Figure 6.3).

At rest or with mild/moderate exercise, increased cardiac output and a modest increase in oxygen extraction will compensate for the fall in oxygen content, and tissue oxygen consumption will be well maintained. Maximum oxygen consumption and work rate are reduced with acute exposure to altitudes from about 3,000 feet (1,000 metres) (Squires and Buskirk, 1982; Lawler *et al.*, 1988; Woorons *et al.*, 2005). During submaximal exercise, ventilation, heart rate and cardiac output are all higher than when the same work rate is performed at sea level. In practice, at the exercise levels required in the aviation environment, physical performance is usually acceptable when breathing air up to about 10,000 feet.

The exact altitude at which cognitive deficits can be detected has varied in different studies and is partly dependent on the psychomotor or cognitive test used. Most of these studies have been performed on resting subjects in a hypobaric chamber, but in some studies the subjects have exercised to mimic the energy expenditure of a working pilot (Denison *et al.*, 1966). Performance on simple or well-learned psychomotor tests is well maintained on acute exposure to altitudes up to about 10,000 feet (Kelman *et al.*, 1969; Crow and Kelman, 1971, 1973; Figarola and Billings, 1966; Pavlicek *et al.*, 2005). The results of studies looking at performance on complex tests and learning tasks have been more variable, with some studies finding (Denison *et al.*, 1966; Kelman and Crow, 1969; Ledwith, 1970; Billings, 1974) and others failing to find an effect at altitudes between 5,000 and 10,000 feet (Kelman *et al.*, 1969).

Denison *et al.* (1966) decompressed subjects to 5,000 and 8,000 feet and presented a spatial transformation test while they performed light cycling exercise (27 watts) to match the typical work rate of pilots. Compared with control subjects, the subjects at both 5,000 and 8,000 feet were significantly slower in these tests initially, but with practice their performance improved and with repetition the difference between controls and hypoxic subjects disappeared. Kelman and Crow (1969) confirmed these conclusions in resting subjects performing a novel complex task at 8,000 feet. Fowler *et al.* (1985) confirmed the finding of a reduced performance at 8,000 feet in subjects performing 27-watt exercise, but when oxygen saturation was held constant at the pre-exercise 8,000 feet level, performance was unaffected.

It can be concluded that the mild hypoxia associated with ascent to altitudes up to 10,000 feet has produced variable results, probably mainly depending on the complexity and novelty of the task, but also other factors such as whether the subjects were resting or exercising. In general, there seems to be little or no effect on simple well-learned tasks. In some studies, performance on more complex tasks has been shown to be affected at altitudes from about 8,000 feet, especially in the task-learning phase. In the aviation environment most healthy aircrew would be able to perform well-learned tasks at altitudes up to 10,000 feet, but probably from about 8,000 feet their ability to learn new skills would be slowed and their ability to cope with novel situations (such as in-flight emergencies) would possibly be slightly impaired.

Vision and Hearing

It has been known for a long time that adaptation of both rods and cones to the dark is affected by exposure to high altitude. McFarland and Evans (1939) studied subjects previously adapted to bright light and found that their dark adaptation curves (light threshold against time) were shifted up by breathing hypoxic gas mixtures, indicating reduced sensitivity. The part of the adaptation curve due to the responses of the rods (responsible for scotopic or low-light-level vision) was affected more than the initial part of the curve due to the responses of the cones (responsible for photopic or high-light-level vision). This reduced sensitivity occurred in most subjects exposed to hypoxia equivalent to 7,400 feet (2,250 metres) and in all subjects at 15,000 feet (4,600 metres), and the effect could be reversed by a few minutes of oxygen breathing. Pretorius (1970) found that night vision was impaired at altitudes starting from 4,000 to 5,000 feet (P_AO_2 about 75 mm Hg, 10 kPa).

In more recent studies of dark adaptation, it has been found that hypoxia delays the development of early scotopic (rods) sensitivity, as well as reducing it (Connolly and Hosking, 2006). Interestingly, moderate hypocapnia ($P_ACO_2 \approx 25$ mm Hg) enhances visual sensitivity, and hyperventilation partly protects against the reduced sensitivity and delay in development of early scotopic sensitivity produced by hypoxia (Wald et al., 1942; Connolly and Hosking, 2006). This effect of mild hyperventilation is probably related to the alkalosis, rather than the beneficial effects of increased ventilation on arterial PO_2 and oxygen saturation. More severe hypocapnia ($PaCO_2 <$ 20–25 mm Hg) is associated with visual disturbance including flashing lights, blurring and scotomata. These effects coincide with the onset of dizziness and lightheadedness and are related to the cerebral vasoconstrictor effect of hypoxia reducing both cerebral and retinal blood flow.

Colour sensitivity is also impaired by hypoxia, with the size of the effect varying with the level of light adaptation. For example, Connolly et al. (2008) found that in mesopic (twilight) lighting conditions colour sensitivity is impaired by mild hypoxia produced by breathing 14.1 per cent oxygen ($P_AO_2 \approx 60$ mm Hg, 8 kPa; arterial oxygen saturation $\approx$ 90 per cent) which is roughly equivalent to that produced by exposure to 10,000 feet. Colour sensitivity was not impaired by this level of hypoxia when there was higher (low photopic) background lighting.

In the aviation domain, darkening of the visual fields is a common subjective experience with hypoxic exposure at high altitude, with the effect being more noticeable in low-light conditions when the eyes are dark-adapted. As the onset of darkening caused by hypoxia is often gradual, the subject may appreciate the effect only when the hypoxia is relieved and vision suddenly brightens. Tunnel vision may occur as the function of the rods that are the main receptors in the periphery of the retina fails completely with severe hypoxia. The effect on scotopic vision is considered functionally significant when P_AO_2 falls to about 50 mm Hg and on photopic vision when PO_2 falls to about 40 mm Hg (Gradwell, 2006).

Fowler and Prlic (1995) found that reaction times to both visual and auditory stimuli were reduced by hypoxia once arterial oxygen saturation fell below about 81 per cent (as found with acute exposure to about 13,500 feet (4,100 metres). Beach and Fowler (1998) confirmed that reaction times to auditory stimuli were slowed in contrast with reaction times to kinesthetic stimuli which were unaffected by the degree of hypoxia used in these experiments (arterial oxygen saturation 65 per cent). These and other approaches suggest that the slowing of reaction times to visual or auditory stimuli occurs mostly early in the preprocessing stage of vision and audition and may not involve later, more central, stages of processing (Fowler and Kelso, 1992; Fowler and Nathoo, 1997; Beach and Fowler, 1998).

Cognition and Behaviour

10,000 (3,000 metres) to 15,000 feet (4,600 metres)

At 10,000 feet, alveolar PO_2 in a healthy resting subject is typically 55 to 60 mm Hg (7.3–8 kPa) and arterial oxygen saturation about 87–90 per cent, falling to about 45 mm Hg (6 kPa) and 80 per cent respectively at 15,000 feet. From the oxyhaemoglobin dissociation curve (Figure 6.3), it can be seen that below 60 mm Hg (8 kPa), arterial oxygen saturation falls more steeply. Tissue capillary PO_2 is the driving force for oxygen diffusion to the tissues, and when it becomes too low, oxygen diffusion fails to keep up with the oxygen requirements of the tissues, especially when these are increased by exercise or stress. In addition, when alveolar PO_2 is very low, diffusion across the alveolar-pulmonary capillary membrane is slowed, and during exercise pulmonary capillary blood may have inadequate time to equilibrate with alveolar PO_2 (Figure 6.2b). If this happens, arterial PO_2 falls below the already very low alveolar PO_2.

Despite the increasingly large effect on arterial oxygen content at altitudes above 10,000 feet, the psychomotor effects are subtle, and many studies have found no significant effect on the performance of simple psychometric tests when subjects are exposed to acute hypoxia equivalent to that at 10,000 and 15,000 feet (Crow and Kelman, 1973; Courts and Pierson, 1965; Pearson

and Neal, 1970; Pavlicek *et al.*, 2005). In contrast, other studies have found reduced performance at these altitudes (Barach *et al.*, 1938; Kida and Imai, 1993; Bartholomew *et al.*, 1999; Li *et al.*, 2000; Van der Post, 2002), and it is likely that the type of task the subjects are asked to perform is the main factor affecting whether a significant impairment is found. Bartholomew *et al.* (1999) found no effect of exposure to either 12,000 or 15,000 feet on the performance of either a simple vigilance task or a simultaneous low memory load read-back task. However, when the material the subjects were asked to recall and read back contained greater amounts of information, performance was reduced significantly at both altitudes.

There is also considerable individual variability in the susceptibility to hypoxia. Kida and Imai (1993) used an auditory reaction time test on a group of 38 subjects exposed to several different altitudes in a hypobaric chamber. The threshold for reduction of reaction time was 4,000 metres (13,120 feet) in six subjects and 5,000 meters (16,400 feet) in 20 subjects. In the remaining 12 subjects, reaction time was unaffected at all altitudes including the highest used, 6,000 metres (19,680 feet). Part of the individual variability may be due to some positive effects on psychomotor function of mild to moderate hypoxia that have been found in humans (Shepherd, 1956; Van der Post *et al.*, 2002) and monkeys (Nicholson and Wright, 1975) and which may offset to a variable degree the negative effects.

Van der Post *et al.* (2002) found that whilst hypoxia sufficient to lower arterial oxygen saturation to 80 per cent caused the expected fall in cognitive performance (using a binary choice task and a serial word recognition task), milder hypoxia (oxygen saturation of 90 per cent) actually significantly increased performance compared with when O$_2$ saturation was normal (97 per cent). The authors suggest several possible mechanisms including that the subjects may have noticed mild symptoms and over-compensated. In addition, hypoxia is known to activate the defence areas of the brain via carotid body stimulation and this has many effects including raising the alertness level of the subject, which could also be a possible mechanism that opposes the depressant effects of hypoxia.

In summary, the effects of acute exposure to altitudes from 10,000 to 15,000 feet are variable, and in many people psychomotor performance with simple or well-learned tasks is little affected by altitudes as high as 15,000 feet. As psychometric tasks become more complex and demanding (choice reaction time, high memory load tasks), deficits are more easily demonstrated and by 15,000 feet, as hypoxia worsens, simpler tasks (pursuit-meter tasks, simple reaction times) are affected in most subjects. In the aviation environment the effects of acute hypoxia at these altitudes may not be obvious to either the exposed person or to observers. However, the ability of a pilot to judge airspeed, heading and orientation (Denison *et al.*, 1966; Ledwith, 1970) is likely to be progressively impaired with increasing altitude, as is their ability to deal with novel and emergency situations. In addition, prolonged exposure to 15,000 feet usually results in a severe headache and muscle incoordination, which is likely to further impair performance.

Above 15,000 feet (4,600 metres)

Above 15,000 feet, symptoms and signs become increasingly obvious. Despite the length of the list of possible signs and symptoms of hypoxia (see section 'Clinical Considerations: Signs and Symptoms'), it is not uncommon to move from no, or only very subtle, signs and symptoms to unconsciousness in a very short period of time. The accounts of the early balloonists (Glaisher, 1862; De Fonvielle, 1875; Tissandier, 1985) are still worth reading today for their detailed accounts of the signs and symptoms of acute exposure to very high altitudes. In 1862, Glaisher and Coxwell just survived their intentional ascent to very high altitude (at least 29,000 feet) in a hot air balloon without the protection of pressurization or oxygen. In contrast, in 1875, two of the three occupants of the French balloon, the Zenith, died of hypoxia despite recognizing the danger and carrying oxygen bottles with them. As they ascended above 28,000 feet (8,500 metres), the surviving balloonists recorded visual disturbances, euphoria, lack of judgement, and inability to respond appropriately to the situation (De Fonvielle, 1875).

In 298 incidents between 1970 and 1980 in which United States Air Force crews reported experiencing in-flight hypoxia, most of them had more than one symptom. In order of frequency, the most common symptoms (number of occurrences) were paraesthesia (95), lightheadedness (41), dizziness (41), decreased mentation such as confusion, impaired concentration and judgement (38), hot and cold flashes (27), tunnel vision (26), numbness (23), loss of consciousness (16), impaired speech (14), fatigue/drowsiness (13), blurred vision (13), euphoria (12), decreased visual acuity (12), decreased coordination (10), headache (7) and disorientation (6) (Rayman and McNaughton, 1983). Cable (2003) reviewed 29 incidents of hypoxia in aircrew that occurred from 1990 to 2001. The symptoms they experienced (number affected) were cognitive impairment (9), dizziness/

lightheadedness (7), tingling/numbness (5), feeling non-specifically unwell (5), hot/cold flushing (3), shaking of limbs (3), numbness (2), visual changes (2), loss of consciousness (2), headache (1), lethargy (1) and death (1).

However, in both these studies (Rayman and McNaughton, 1983; Cable, 2003) there was a relatively high incidence where the cause of the presumed hypoxia was unknown (33 and 18.5 per cent respectively). It was assumed this was because a mask leak or other malfunction was transient, but it is likely that in some of these incidents the real cause of the symptoms was anxiety-provoked hyperventilation unaccompanied by significant hypoxia. This would mean that certain symptoms such as pins and needles were overrepresented and would probably be less common in cases of confirmed acute hypobaric hypoxic exposure. Many of the symptoms of hypoxia and hyperventilation are the same. Moreover, hypoxia, when PO_2 < 60 mm Hg, is an important cause of hyperventilation and so hypoxia and hypocapnia frequently coexist. It may be hard for an affected individual or an observer to distinguish the signs and symptoms of hypoxia accompanied by reflex hyperventilation from those caused by stress or anxiety-driven hyperventilation. In the aviation situation, and especially when a plane is flying at an actual altitude above 12,000 feet (c. 3,600 metres), it is essential that it is assumed that the cause of hyperventilation is hypoxia until proven otherwise. Action (such as descent, donning of oxygen masks) to correct the possible hypoxia must be immediate because loss of consciousness can quickly follow the first symptoms and signs.

Hypoxia Training

The subtlety of the early symptoms and the effects of progressive hypoxia on cognitive function described by the early balloonists remain important today. Military pilots are usually given hypoxia training so that they are familiar with their own personal symptoms of hypoxia, they can recognize the signs of hypoxia in others and they understand the importance of responding immediately to these warning signs. There is evidence that prior hypoxic training affords protection against loss of consciousness in emergency situations (Chisholm et al., 1974; Cable, 2003). Untrained subjects are more likely to lose consciousness, and many aircrew who have experienced accidental in-flight hypoxia report that they recognized that they were becoming hypoxic because of their altitude chamber training (Rayman and McNaughton, 1983).

In recent years there has been considerable debate over the optimum form of hypoxic training experience, as well as whether it should available to civilian as well as military aircrew. Traditionally, military pilots have received hypobaric hypoxic training in a decompression chamber. They breathe oxygen from a mask while the chamber is rapidly decompressed and when at the appropriate altitude, often 25,000 feet (c.7,600 metres), they remove their mask and breathe air. This form of hypoxic training exposes subjects to a small but significant risk of decompression illness. The safety observers who accompany them in the chamber may be at even greater risk because of such factors as their increased age, percentage body fat and because they experience repeated exposures (Bason et al., 1976, 1991). For this reason, systems and protocols for hypoxic training using normobaric breathing of reduced oxygen fraction gas mixtures have been developed (Artino et al., 2006; Westerman and Bassovitch, 2010).

Cable (2003) has proposed a mixed method involving breathing reduced oxygen fraction during hypobaric exposure to 10,000 feet. This method has the advantage of allowing aircrew to experience some effects of the hypobaric environment whilst using an altitude at which decompression illness does not occur. It also removes the need to have a hyperbaric facility available at the training site to treat possible cases. In a study comparing these different methods there were small differences in ventilation, oxygen saturation and heart rate, but these were considered to be physiologically and operationally insignificant and, importantly, symptoms and psychomotor performance were similar with the different methods (Evetts et al., 2005).

Hypoxia and the Oxygen Paradox

Administering oxygen to a subject suffering from hypobaric hypoxia usually results in rapid recovery, but in some subjects improvement is preceded by a period of worsening symptoms and signs of hypoxia lasting up to a minute. This unexpected effect of oxygen is known as the oxygen paradox. Westerman (2004) found it in 'at least 6' of 452 subjects undergoing hypoxia training using a reduced oxygen breathing method, and Izraeli et al. (1988) in one out of 35 times oxygen was administered to subjects exposed to 25,000 feet.

The cause of the oxygen paradox is uncertain, but it seems to be more likely in subjects who have been hyperventilating when hypoxic (Gradwell, 2006) and in subjects who are undergoing exercise during the hypoxia

and oxygen administration (Busby et al., 1976). Possible mechanisms that have been suggested are the sudden reversal of hypoxic vasoconstriction in the lung, loss of the cerebral vasodilator effect of hypoxia in the presence of continuing hypocapnic vasoconstriction, and reversal of the cardiovascular and/or respiratory reflex effects of carotid body chemoreceptor stimulation leading to systemic vasodilatation. In affected subjects, administration of oxygen often causes a fall in blood pressure and this will contribute to worsening cerebral hypoxia (Grandpierre and Franck, 1952; Gradwell, 2006). The practical importance of the oxygen paradox in aviation is that the subject or those looking after the subject must not be discouraged from continuing oxygen therapy. The worsening symptoms are transient and oxygen is essential in this situation.

Impaired Consciousness

Severe hypoxia eventually leads to loss of consciousness. When consciousness is lost, in most subjects this occurs in the presence of a normal or high blood pressure, and cerebral hypoxia caused by arterial hypoxia is the mechanism of the loss of consciousness. From the earliest studies of the effects of hypoxia, it was recognized that in some subjects hypoxia triggers vasovagal syncope. Loss of consciousness often occurs with milder degrees of hypoxia than expected, and it is preceded by a fall in blood pressure and heart rate and other typical vasovagal symptoms such as nausea and sweating. In these subjects, reduced cerebral PO_2 is caused by a combination of arterial hypoxia and reduced cerebral perfusion pressure secondary to hypotension.

The early studies on the effects of progressive arterial hypoxia used either rebreathing of a fixed volume of gas with CO_2 removal or breathing of hypoxic gas mixtures. The proportion of subjects showing vasovagal reactions was quite variable (at least 33 per cent in Schneider, 1918; 47 per cent in Schneider and Truesdell, 1921; 37 per cent in Ershler et al., 1943; and 23 per cent in Anderson et al., 1946). In most of these studies the proportion of subjects showing vasovagal reactions are higher than the 20 per cent usually quoted today based on hypobaric chamber experience (Gradwell, 2006). The proportions of subjects affected by vasovagal syncope are likely to depend on several experimental details, including the severity and speed of onset of the hypoxia.

'Time of Useful Consciousness'

Before consciousness is lost there is a period when the subject, though conscious, is unable to perform tasks in a purposeful way, including those needed to remedy the situation such as putting on and securing an oxygen mask, initiating descent or other emergency procedures. This has given rise to the concept of 'time of useful consciousness (TUC)' or 'effective performance time'. TUC is the time from the onset of an event such as sudden decompression or loss of oxygen supply to the time when the subject is unable to perform purposeful activity.

Time of useful consciousness is not a very precise term, and in experiments on subjects exposed to decompression, the end-point used to determine it has varied. Donaldson et al. (1960) required subjects to write numbers down while counting backwards from 100, with the end-point being when writing faltered or mistakes were made. In other studies subjects had to cancel light signals by pressing a button (Bryan and Leach, 1960), perform a complex light-cancelling task involving recent memory, choice reaction time and some manual dexterity – 'the Gedye task' (Billings, 1974; Billings and Ernsting, 1974) – or repeatedly recall a sequence of eight digital operations (Ernsting, 1978). These different tasks require different levels of mental functioning and so the time of useful consciousness determined by them is likely to vary with the choice of task. It is not certain which, if any, best represents the time in which aircrew are likely to be able to respond appropriately to an emergency situation, which itself will depend on what is required of the individual in the emergency situation.

In a sudden decompression, time of useful consciousness is affected by the initial cabin altitude, the pressure profile following the decompression including the maximum altitude reached, the gas being breathed at the time of the decompression and the time that elapses before pure oxygen is breathed following the decompression. As commercial jet aircraft began to fly at altitudes above 30,000 feet (9,150 metres), there was concern about the effects on crew and passengers of a sudden decompression at these altitudes.

Later, the development of supersonic civilian passenger aircraft (Concorde) and high-performance aircraft capable of operating at around or even above 60,000 feet (18,300 metres) meant that in the event of a sudden decompression the occupants risked exposure to low pressures combined with a long descent time to a safe altitude. It was important to understand the effects this would have on both aircrew and passengers and the speed at which oxygen needed to be delivered to enable the pilot to maintain control of the aircraft and take appropriate emergency action. In addition, there was a need to understand the effects on any passengers or aircrew who failed to don oxygen masks and were therefore exposed to significant hypoxia until the aircraft reached a safe altitude of around 10,000 feet.

Donaldson *et al.* (1960) used a hypobaric chamber to simulate the expected cabin pressure profile that would occur if a Boeing 707 flying at 42,000 feet (12,800 metres), with an initial cabin altitude of 8,500 feet (2,600 metres), lost a window and began to descend once the cabin altitude reached 14,000 feet (4,250 metres). In this model the maximum cabin altitude, 36,000 feet (11,000 metres), was reached in 25 to 30 seconds. When four subjects (on seven occasions) were exposed to this pressure profile with no oxygen given, the average time of useful consciousness (assessed from when their writing faltered or they produced errors) was 32 seconds. Three of the four subjects remained unconscious for an average of 83 seconds, recovering spontaneously with no ill effects during the descent. The fourth subject was given oxygen to breathe, as it was felt his oxygen saturation was too low to allow him to remain unconscious and untreated.

In further experiments with the same cabin altitude profile, oxygen was given either immediately 14,000 feet was reached (when oxygen masks would normally automatically deploy), or with a delay of 15 or 30 seconds. From the psychometric tests and oxygen saturations, Donaldson *et al.* (1960) concluded that the oxygen mask had to be donned within 15 seconds if impaired performance was to be avoided. Bryan and Leach (1960) simulated a faster decompression from 8,000 feet (2,450 metres) to 40,000 feet (12,200 metres) in 2.5 seconds and found the average time of useful consciousness in eight subjects to be 18 seconds. In this study, unconsciousness was noted to occur very suddenly, preceded by few symptoms. Using a decompression from 6,500 feet (2,000 metres) to 34,000 feet (10,350 metres) in 26 seconds followed by descent at the rate of 5,000 feet per minute, Busby *et al.* (1976) found a mean TUC (judged from a visual reaction time test) of 54 seconds and it was the same in men and women. A variety of different hypobaric chamber pressure profiles has been used to model sudden decompression at high altitude relevant to both passenger transport and military aircraft (Hall, 1949; Luft *et al.*, 1951; Billings and Ernsting, 1974; Busby *et al.*, 1976; Bryan and Leach, 1960; Yoneda and Watanabe, 1997; Gradwell, 2006). Many of these studies, including those in which subjects were allowed to remain unconscious for several minutes in a hypoxic environment, would be difficult to repeat today. However, this body of work has led to a good understanding of the approximate time of useful consciousness when sudden decompression occurs at different altitudes and also the key physiological changes that make unconsciousness likely.

Below are typical times of useful consciousness in a healthy resting subject, based on this body of work. The values are much more variable at the lower altitudes (Hall, 1949; Gradwell, 2006) and, as discussed below, these times are very much reduced by even light exercise.

Altitude		Progressive hypoxia: As when inspired oxygen is changed to air	Rapid decompression
Feet	Metres		
25,000	7,620	3–6 minutes	2–3 minutes
30,000	9,140	1.5–3 minutes	0.5–1.5 minutes
35,000	10, 670	45–75 seconds	25–35 seconds
40,000	12,190	25 seconds	18 seconds

The most important factor that will affect the time of useful consciousness is the oxygen consumption of the individual at the time of the sudden decompression or loss of oxygen supply. In the aviation environment, aircrew are unlikely to be at rest, as they usually are in experiments reproducing sudden decompression. Even mild exercise has been shown to cause large reductions in time of useful consciousness. In a study of ten men and ten women decompressed from 6,500 feet (2,000 metres) to 34,000 feet (9,900 metres) in 26 seconds followed by descent at 5,000 feet per second, when the subjects were at rest, mean time of useful consciousness was 54 seconds in both the men and the women (Busby *et al.*, 1976). When the experiments were repeated with subjects exercising at light work rates similar to those found in working flight attendants (50 watts for men, 40 watts for women), time of useful consciousness was reduced considerably and by a similar amount in the men and women (to 34 and 32 seconds respectively). Other factors that affect psychomotor performance, such as illness, cold exposure, fatigue, drugs and alcohol, can also be expected to reduce tolerance to hypoxia and reduce the TUC.

Binding of carbon monoxide to haemoglobin reduces oxygen content and impairs release of oxygen in the tissues, as discussed previously. Consequently, it might reasonably be expected that smokers (HbCO up to 8 per cent) would have increased susceptibility to hypobaric hypoxia and reduced TUC following rapid decompression. Indeed, it has often been stated that being a smoker at sea level is functionally equivalent to being a non-smoker at altitude and that this would add on to the effect of actual altitude. Dille and Mohler (1968) considered that a smoker at 10,000 feet is effectively at 14,000 feet, but experimental justification for this statement is difficult to find. Studies using acute CO administration show variable effects on vision and psychomotor performance, but with mild/moderate carboxyhaemoglobinaemia (5–10 per cent) any effects are mostly small or there is no significant change (Laties and Merigan, 1979).

Christensen *et al.* (1977) used a prolonged visual vigilance task to investigate whether breathing CO sufficient to produce 5 per cent carboxyhaemoglobin after two hours increased susceptibility to mild hypoxia produced by breathing 17 per cent O_2, equivalent to 5,060 feet (1,542 metres). The subjects performed worse when breathing 17 per cent O_2 than air (21 per cent O_2), but adding CO to the hypoxia appeared to improve rather than worsen performance on the vigilance test. In a large study of pilots and aircrew undergoing hypoxia training decompression to 25,000 feet (6,850 metres), there was no significant difference in TUC between smokers (n = 589, TUC = 213.5 ± 75.3 seconds) and non-smokers (n= 582, TUC = 214.5 + 75.1 seconds) (Yoneda and Watanabe, 1997).

The oxygen transport system has enough reserve that, with acute mild CO inhalation, oxygen delivery to the brain and other tissues can remain adequate and performance unaffected. In addition, in smokers, the carboxyhaemoglobinaemia is chronic and it is likely that there is well-developed adaptation to the altered oxygen delivery situation (Otis, 1970). The study by Yoneda and Watanabe (1997) did show a reduction in some of the symptoms of hypoxia in smokers, possibly because nicotine counters the effects of acute hypoxia symptoms such as reduced alertness. Even if, experimentally, TUC is not reduced, it is possible that smokers would be slower to recognize the onset of hypoxia in an emergency situation.

Rapid Decompression

Acute exposure to altitudes above 20,000 feet (c. 6,000 metres) will eventually lead to unconsciousness or other life-threatening acute altitude events. However, in aviation following sudden decompression the altitude profile is typically an initial increase in cabin altitude followed by descent to a safe altitude, assuming the correct emergency procedures are initiated. In the event of a decompression occurring below 25,000 feet (7,600 metres), there should be time to recognize the situation and descend to a safe altitude. The higher the altitude at which a rapid decompression occurs, the more difficult it is to avoid a significant performance deficit that could interfere with the safe recovery of the situation. Studies in humans simulating rapid decompression at high altitude have helped to understand the factors during a rapid decompression that are likely to lead to important performance deficit and/or unconsciousness.

Ernsting (1963) produced a rapid profound hypoxia in subjects using hyperventilation with 100 per cent nitrogen to permit measurements (including sampling of arterial blood and venous blood from the internal jugular vein, pulmonary artery and femoral vein) that would have not been possible inside a hypobaric chamber. When nitrogen hyperventilation was continued for 17 to 20 seconds, unconsciousness supervened and 'was accompanied on most occasions by a generalized convulsion'. With 15 seconds of nitrogen hyperventilation, slightly shorter than the time needed to producing unconsciousness, end-tidal (alveolar) PO_2 fell below 10 mm Hg, arterial PO_2 fell to a minimum of about 16 mm Hg, arterial saturation to about 35 per cent, mixed venous PO_2 to 35 mm Hg, and internal jugular PO_2 to about 20 mm Hg. In other studies, where subjects were decompressed from 8,000 feet (2,400 metres) to 41,000 feet (12,500 metres) in 2 seconds, giving an alveolar PO_2 less than 15 mm Hg, a severe performance decrement was found in all subjects even if oxygen was administered within 10 seconds of the onset of decompression (Billings and Ernsting, 1974; Ernsting, 1978). In both, nitrogen hyperventilation and rapid decompression to 40,000 feet (12,200 metres), alveolar PO_2 falls rapidly below mixed venous PO_2, causing oxygen to move from blood to alveoli.

No significant decrements in psychomotor performance using a learned sequence of eight operations were reported by Ernsting et al. (1973) if alveolar PO_2 remained above 30 mm Hg. However, Denison et al. (1974) reported a small effect on performance (spatial orientation task) when alveolar PO_2 fell below 35 mm Hg, though reaction times were not markedly prolonged until PO_2 had been below 32.5 mm Hg for 30 to 50 seconds. What seems to be important for maintaining consciousness is the time during which alveolar PO_2 is below 30 mm Hg and the severity of the fall below 30 mm Hg. If alveolar PO_2 is plotted against time, the area of the curve below $P_AO_2 = 30$ mm Hg, known as the P_{30} area, correlates with electroencephalographic recordings and psychometric performance (Ernsting *et al.*, 1973; Ernsting, 1978).

In 72 experiments in which subjects were rapidly decompressed from 8,000 feet (2,400 metres) to 37,000 feet (11,300 metres), 39,000 feet (11,900 metres) or 41,000 feet (12,500 metres) with oxygen delivered to the mask at 5, 10 or 15 seconds after the start of the decompression, there were 16 experiments in which the subject lost consciousness (Billings and Ernsting, 1974). In separate accounts of these experiments, Ernsting (1973, 1978) reported that in 15 of 16 of experiments where consciousness was lost, the P_{30} exceeded 140 mm Hg.seconds. A P_{30} greater than 140 mm Hg.seconds occurred in only four of the 56 occasions where the subject remained conscious. It seems likely that any profile of altitude exposure that causes an alveolar-time profile with a $P_{30} > 140$ mm Hg/seconds will lead to unconsciousness.

The importance of keeping P_AO_2 above 30 mm Hg if consciousness is to be preserved is supported by other quite different studies. In a study of cerebral blood flow and metabolism in humans, Cohen *et al.* (1967) produced a steady-state hypoxia by inhalation of 6.9–7.5 per cent for more than 15 minutes whilst keeping P_ACO_2 constant (39.12 + 0.82 mm Hg). With 6.9 per cent oxygen, they reported that the subjects were unable to complete the experiment 'due to restlessness, incipient loss of consciousness and nausea and vomiting'. In nine subjects with slightly less severe hypoxia, arterial PO_2 was 34.57 + 1.61 mm Hg and mean jugular venous PO_2

was 26.88 ± 1.10 mm Hg. These subjects all experienced dimming of vision and some also experienced lightheadedness, nausea and restlessness.

Long-term sequelae

If aircrew recognize and respond in a timely manner to an emergency such as rapid decompression, there is a good chance that the aircraft will be landed safely. Some passengers and aircrew may fail to don oxygen masks and lose consciousness. If the descent to 10,000 feet is rapid enough, they should recover consciousness with no ill effects, as did the subjects in some of the hypobaric chamber simulation studies discussed above. With aircraft capable of flying at extreme high altitudes (60,000 feet), the exposure is potentially more severe and prolonged, giving rise to the concern that survivors who failed to don oxygen masks might suffer permanent brain damage.

Using a decompression chamber, Nicholson and Ernsting (1967) exposed four baboons to three different altitude profiles, simulating sudden decompressions due to three different-sized holes in an aircraft flying at 60,000 feet. When the maximum altitude was 30,000 feet (9,150 metres) and the animals spent 3 minutes above 25,000 feet (7,600 metres) the baboons became unconscious, but recovered on recompression without any obvious signs of permanent damage. When the maximum altitude was 52,000 feet (15,850 metres) and the animals spent 6 minutes 40 seconds above 25,000 feet and 1 minute 30 seconds above 40,000 feet, three of the four animals survived the decompression, but had gross behavioural and neurological disturbance, with two of the three dying within five days.

In a subsequent study (Nicholson *et al.*, 1970), 12 monkeys previously trained to perform visual discrimination tests were exposed to an altitude of 37,500 feet for 10 to 16 minutes, the end-point being imminent respiratory arrest (respiratory frequency < 4 breaths/min). Eight animals (mean exposure time 13.5 minutes; range 10–16 minutes) showed neither impairment of performance on the visual discrimination tests nor locomotor abnormalities. Four of the animals (mean exposure time 13 minutes; range 10–15.5 minutes) showed impairment in the visual discrimination task and/or locomotor abnormalities. Seven showed post-mortem histological neuropathology, especially in the cortex in the boundary zone between cerebral arteries and also the basal ganglia. None of the animals without histological abnormalities had shown visual discrimination test abnormalities or locomotor problems after the hypobaric exposure, but two of the animals that appeared to recover without deficit showed some histological changes.

These experiments demonstrated that in primates hypobaric exposure of the sort that could occur following decompression at extreme altitude can lead to neurological damage in survivors. However, the majority of survivors showed no signs of permanent damage. These findings were extended in subsequent studies on primates exposed to prolonged hypobaric hypoxia (Nicholson *et al.*, 1970; Blagbrough *et al.*, 1973; Blagbrough and Nicholson, 1975). Permanent brain damage was more likely to occur with prolonged exposure to altitudes between 30,000 and 37,500 feet. Below 30,000 feet (c. 9,000 metres) or above 37,500 feet (11,400 metres), an uneventful recovery or death was likely. The behavioural and neuropathological aspects of these studies are described in more detail in Chapter 8 (Profound Hypoxia: Extreme Altitude and Space).

There is a considerable amount of evidence, both clinical and experimental, that suggests that a prolonged period of pure hypoxic hypoxia does not usually lead to permanent brain damage in survivors, in contrast to the high likelihood of brain damage when cerebral tissue hypoxia is caused by ischemia (Gray and Horner, 1970; Brierley, 1977; Pearigen *et al.*, 1996; Simon, 1999; Miyamoto, 2000). It seems likely that the animals that sustained permanent brain damage following the hypobaric exposures in the experiments described above suffered a prolonged period of reduced cerebral perfusion and/or hypotension which fits with the ischemic pattern of brain damaged seen histologically in these animals.

References

Aaronson, P.I., Robertson, T.P., Knock, G.A., Becker S., Lewis, T.H., Snetkov, V. and Ward, J.P.T. 2006. Hypoxic pulmonary vasoconstriction: Mechanisms and controversies. *Journal of Physiology*, 570, 53–8.

Acker, H. 1980. The meaning of tissue PO_2 and local blood flow for the chemoreceptive process of the carotid body. *Federation Proceedings*, 39, 2641–7.

Acker, H. and O'Regan, R.G. 1981. The effects of stimulation of autonomic nerves on carotid body blood flow in the cat. *Journal of Physiology*, 315, 99–110.

Ainslie, P.N. and Duffin, J. 2009. Integration of cerebrovascular CO_2 reactivity and chemoreflex control of breathing: Mechanisms of regulation, measurement, and interpretation. *American Journal of Physiology: Regulator, Integrative and Comparative Physiology*, 296, R1473–95.

Ainslie, P.N. and Poulin, M.J. 2004. Ventilatory, cerebrovascular, and cardiovascular interactions in acute hypoxia: Regulation by carbon dioxide. *Journal of Applied Physiology*, 97, 149–59.

Allan, G.M. and Kenny, D. 2003. High-altitude decompression illness: Case report and discussion. *Canadian Medical Association Journal*, 169, 803–7.

Altemeier, W.A. and Sinclair, S.E. 2007. Hyperoxia in the intensive care unit: Why more is not always better. *Current Opinion in Critical Care*, 13, 73–8.

Anand, I.S., Harris, E., Ferrari, R., Pearce, P. and Harris, P. 1986. Pulmonary haemodynamics of the yak, cattle and cross breeds at high altitude. *Thorax*, 41, 696–700.

Anderson, D.P., Allen, W.J., Barcroft, H., Edholm, O.G. and Manning, G.W. 1946. Circulatory changes during fainting and coma caused by oxygen lack. *Journal of Physiology*, I04, 426–34.

Artino, A.R., Jr, Folga, R.V. and Swan, B.D. 2006. Mask-on hypoxia training for tactical jet aviators: Evaluation of an alternate instructional paradigm. *Aviation, Space, and Environmental Medicine*, 77, 857–63.

Aste-Salazar, H. and Hurtado, A. 1944. Affinity of hemoglobin for oxygen at sea level and at high altitudes. *American Journal of Physiology*, 142, 733–43.

Australian Transport Safety Bureau. Transport Safety Report: Aviation Occurrence Investigation AO-2008-053, Interim Factual No. 2. Available at: http://www.atsb.gov.au/media/748064/ao2008053_2.pdf

Avery, M.E., Chernick, V., Dutton, R.E. and Permutt, S. 1963. Ventilatory response to inspired carbon dioxide in infants and adults. *Journal of Applied Physiology*, 18, 895–903.

Balke, B. and Lillehei, J.P. 1956. Effects of hyperventilation on performance. *Journal of Applied Physiology*, 9, 371–4.

Barach, L., McFarland, R.A. and Seitz, C.P. 1938. The effects of oxygen deprivation on complex mental functions. *Journal of Aviation Medicine*, 8, 197–207.

Barcroft, J. 1920. On anoxaemia. *Lancet*, 5062, 485–9.

Barcroft, J.A., Binger, C.A., Bock, A.V., Doggart, J.H., Forbes, H.S., Harrop, G. et al. 1923. Observations upon the effect of high altitude on the physiological processes of the human body, carried out in the Peruvian Andes, chiefly at Cerro de Pasco. *Philosophical Transactions of the Royal Society of London*, Series B, 211, 351–480.

Bärtsch, P. and Gibbs, J.S.R. 2007. Effect of altitude on the heart and the lungs. *Circulation*, 116, 2191–202.

Bartholomew, C.J., Jensen, W., Petros, T.V., Ferraro, F.R., Fire, K.M., Biberdorf, D. et al. 1999. The effect of moderate levels of simulated altitude on sustained cognitive performance. *The International Journal of Aviation Psychology*, 9, 351–9.

Bason, R., Pheeny, H. and Dully, F.E. 1976. Incidence of decompression sickness in Navy low-pressure chambers. *Aviation, Space, and Environmental Medicine*, 47, 995–7.

Bason, R., Yacavone, D. and Bellenkes, A.H. 1991. Decompression sickness: USN operational experience 1969–1989. *Aviation, Space, and Environmental Medicine*, 62, 994–6.

Beach, C. and Fowler, B. 1998. Evidence that the slowing caused by acute hypoxia is modality dependent. *Aviation, Space, and Environmental Medicine*, 69, 887–91.

Bellville, J.E., Whipp, B.J., Kaufman, R.D., Swanson, G.D., Aqleh, K.A. and Wiberg, D.M. 1979. Central and peripheral chemoreflex loop gain in normal and carotid body-resected subjects. *Journal of Applied Physiology*, 46, 843–53.

Beninati, W., Meyer, M.T. and Carter, T.E. 2008. The critical care air transport program. *Critical Care Medicine*, 36 (Suppl.), S370–76.

Berkenbosch, A., Bovill, J.G., Dahan, A., Degoede, J. and Olievier, I.C.W. 1989. The ventilatory CO_2 sensitivities from Read's rebreathing method and the steady-state method are not equal in man. *Journal of Physiology*, 411, 367–77.

Billings, C.E. 1974. Evaluation of performance using the Gedye task. *Aerospace Medicine*, 45, 128–31.

Billings, C.E. and Ernsting, J. 1974. Protection afforded by phased dilution oxygen equipment following rapid decompression: Performance aspects. *Aerospace Medicine*, 45, 132–4.

Bindslev, L., Jolin, A., Hedenstierna, G., Baehrendtz, S. and Santesson, J. 1985. Hypoxic pulmonary vasoconstriction in the human lung: Effect of repeated hypoxic challenges during anesthesia. *Anesthesiology*, 62, 621–5.

Bitterman, H. 2009. Oxygen as a drug. *Critical Care*, 13, 205–12.

Bitterman, N. 2004. CNS oxygen toxicity. *Undersea and Hyperbaric Medicine*, 31, 63–72.

Blagbrough, A.E., Brierley, J.B. and Nicholson, A.N. 1973. Behavioural and neurological disturbances associated with hypoxic brain damage. *Journal of the Neurological Sciences*, 18, 475–88.

Blagbrough, A.E. and Nicholson, A.N. 1975. Subatmospheric decompression: Neurological and behavioural studies. *Acta Astronautica*, 2, 197–206.

Boutellier, U. and Koller, E.A. 1981. Propranolol and the respiratory, circulatory, and ECG responses to high altitude. *European Journal of Applied Physiology*, 46, 105–19.

Brewer, G.Y. 1974. 2,3-DPG and erythrocyte oxygen affinity. *Annual Review of Medicine*, 25, 29–38.

Brierley, J.B. 1977. Experimental hypoxic brain damage. *Journal of Clinical Pathology*, 30 (Suppl.), 11, 181–7.

British Thoracic Society Guidelines. 2004. Managing Passengers with Respiratory Disease Planning Air Travel, Revised Recommendations. Available at: http://www.brit-thoracic.org.uk/clinical-information/air-travel/air-travel-guideline.aspx

Brooks, V.L. and Sved, A.F. 2005. Pressure to change? Re-evaluating the role of baroreceptors in the long-term control of arterial pressure. *American Journal of Physiology: Regulator, Integrative and Comparative Physiology*, 288, R815–8.

Brugniaux, J.V., Hodges, A.N.H., Patrick, J., Hanly, P.J. and Poulin, M.J. 2007. Cerebrovascular responses to altitude. *Respiratory Physiology & Neurobiology*, 158, 212–23.

Bryan, C.A. and Leach, W.G. 1960. Physiologic effects of cabin pressure failure in high altitude passenger aircraft. *Aerospace Medicine*, 31, 267–75.

Burden, R.J., Janke, E.L. and Brighouse, D. 1994. Hyperventilation-induced unconsciousness during labour. *British Journal of Anaesthesia*, 73, 838–9.

Busby, D.E., Higgins, E.A. and Funkhouser, G.E. 1976. Effect of physical activity of airline flight attendants on their time of useful consciousness in a rapid decompression. *Aviation, Space, and Environmental Medicine*, 47, 117–20.

Cable, G.G. 2003. In-flight hypoxia incidents in military aircraft: Causes and implications for training. *Aviation, Space, and Environmental Medicine*, 74, 169–72.

Cherniack, N.S. and Longobardo, G.S. 1970. Oxygen and carbon dioxide gas stores of the body. *Physiological Reviews*, 50, 196–243.

Chisholm, D.M., Billings, C.E. and Bason, R. 1974. Behavior of naive subjects during decompression: An evaluation of automatically presented passenger oxygen equipment. *Aerospace Medicine*, 45, 123–7.

Christensen, C.L., Gliner, J.A., Horvath, S.M. and Wagner, J.A. 1977. Effects of three kinds of hypoxias on vigilance performance. *Aviation, Space, and Environmental Medicine*, 48, 491–6.

Cohen, P.J., Alexander, S.C., Smith, T.C., Reivich, M. and Wollman, H. 1967. Effects of hypoxia and normocarbia on cerebral blood flow and metabolism in conscious man. *Journal of Applied Physiology*, 23, 183–9.

Comroe, J.H., Forster, R.E., Dubois, A.B., Briscoe, W.A. and Carlsen, E. 1962. *The Lung – Second Edition*. Chicago, IL: Year Book Medical Publishers.

Connolly, D.M., Barbur, J.L., Hosking, S.L. and Moorhead, I.R. 2008. Mild hypoxia impairs chromatic sensitivity in the mesopic range. *Investigative Ophthalmology & Visual Science*, 49, 820–27.

Connolly, D.M. and Hosking, S.L. 2006. Aviation-related respiratory gas disturbances affect dark adaptation: A reappraisal. *Vision Research*, 46, 1784–93.

Cormack, R.S., Cunningham, D.J.C. and Gee, J.B.L. 1957. The effect of carbon dioxide on the respiratory response to want of oxygen in man. *Experimental Physiology*, 42, 303–19.

Courts, D.E. and Pierson, W.R. 1965. Sport parachuting and hypoxia. *Aerospace Medicine*, 36, 372–4.

Cunningham, D.J.C., Shaw, D.G., Lahiri, S. and Lloyd, B.B. 1961. The effect of maintained ammonium chloride acidosis on the relation between pulmonary ventilation and alveolar oxygen and carbon dioxide in man. *Quarterly Journal of Experimental Physiology and Cognate Medical Sciences*, 46, 323–4.

Cunningham, D.J.C., Robbins, P.A. and Wolff, C.B. 1986. Integration of Respiratory Responses to Changes in Alveolar Partial Pressures of CO_2 and O_2 and in Arterial pH. In: A.P.F. Fishman (ed.) *Handbook of Physiology, Volume II, Part 2*. Bethesda, MD: American Physiological Society, Ch. 15.

Crow, T.J. and Kelman, G.R. 1971. Effect of mild acute hypoxia on human short-term memory. *British Journal of Anaesthesia*, 43, 548–52.

Crow, T.J. and Kelman, G.R. 1973. Psychological effects of mild acute hypoxia. *British Journal of Anaesthesia*, 45, 335–7.

Curran, A.K., Rodman, J.R., Eastwood, P.R., Henderson, K.S., Dempsey, J.A. and Smith, C.A. 2000. Ventilatory responses to specific CNS hypoxia in sleeping dogs. *Journal of Applied Physiology*, 88, 1840–52.

Dahan, A., Nieuwenhuijs, D. and Teppema, L. 2007. Plasticity of central chemoreceptors: Effect of bilateral carotid body resection on central CO_2 sensitivity. *Public Library of Science Medicine*, 4, 1195–203.

De Castro, F. 1927. Sur la structure et l'innervation du sinus carotidien de l'homine et des mammifères. Nouveaux faits sur l'innervation et la fonction du glomus caroticum. Études anatomiques et physiologiques. *Trabajos del Laboratorio de Investigaciones Biológicas de la Universidad de Madrid*, 25, 331–80.

De Castro, F. 1940. Nuevas observaciones sobra la inervación de la región carotídea. Los quimio-y pressoreceptores. *Trabajos del Instituto Cajal de Investigaciones Biológicas*, 32, 297–384.

De Fonvielle, W. 1875. The 'Zenith' balloon ascent. *Nature*, 11, 287, 513.

Dehnert, C., Grünig, E., Mereles, D., von Lennep, N. and Bärtsch, P. 2005. Identification of individuals susceptible to high-altitude pulmonary oedema at low altitude. *European Respiratory Journal*, 25, 545–51.

Delpiano, M. and Acker, H. 1980. Relationship between tissue PO_2 and chemoreceptor activity. *Brain Research*, 195, 85–93.

Denison, D.M., Byford, G.H., Allnutt, M.F. and Reader, D.C. 1974. Times of useful consciousness following rapid decompression from 8,000 feet to 25,000 feet or 27,000 feet. *Proceedings of the 45th Annual Meeting of Aerospace Medical Association*.

Denison, D.M., Ledwith, F. and Poulton, E.C. 1966. Complex reaction times at simulated cabin altitudes of 5,000 and 8,000 feet. *Aerospace Medicine*, 37, 1010–13.

Deyell, R., Jackson, S., Spier, S., Doan, L. and Poon, M.-C. 2006. Low oxygen saturation by pulse oximetry may be associated with a low oxygen affinity hemoglobin variant, hemoglobin Titusville. *Journal of Pediatric Hematology/Oncology*, 28, 100–102.

Dille, J.R. and Mohler, S.R. 1968. Drugs and toxic hazards in general aviation. *Aerospace Medicine Report AM-68/16*. Washington, DC: Federal Aviation Administration.

Donaldson, R.T., Carter, E.T., Billings, C.E. and Hitchcock, F.A. 1960. Acute hypoxia during rapid decompression and emergency descent in a commercial jet aircraft. *Aerospace Medicine*, 31, 842–51.

Duke, H.N., Green, J.H. and Neil, E. 1952. Carotid chemoreceptor impulse activity during inhalation of carbon monoxide. *Journal of Physiology*, 8, 520–27.

Ernsting, J. 1961. Respiratory effects of whole body vibration. *Flying Personnel Research Committee Report* 1164. London: Ministry of Defence.

Ernsting, J. 1963. The ideal relationship between inspired oxygen concentration and cabin altitude. *Aerospace Medicine*, 34, 911–7.

Ernsting, J. 1973. Hypoxia in the aviation environment. *Proceedings of the Royal Society of Medicine*, 66, 523–7.

Ernsting, J. 1978. The 10th Annual Harry G. Armstrong Lecture: Prevention of hypoxia-acceptable compromises. *Aviation, Space, and Environmental Medicine*, 49, 495–502.

Ernsting, J., Denison, D.M., Byford, G.H. and Fryer, D.I. 1973. Hypoxia induced by rapid decompression from 8,000 ft to 40,000 ft: The influence of rate of decompression. *Flying Personnel Research Committee Report 1324*. London: Ministry of Defence.

Ershler, I., Kossman, C.E. and White, M.S. 1943. Venous pressure and circulation time during acute progressive anoxia in man. *American Journal of Physiology*, 138, 593–8.

Evetts, G., Hartley, A., Keane, S., Keegan, J., Simpson, A., Taylor, A. et al. 2005. A comparison of acute hypoxia induced by low concentrations of oxygen at ground level, 10,000 feet and by air at 25,000 feet: Implications for military aircrew training. *Proceedings of the Survival and Flight Equipment Association*. Available at: http://www.safeeurope.co.uk/media/3570/george_evetts.pdf

Fencl, V., Vale, J.R. and Broch, J.A. 1969. Respiration and cerebral blood flow in metabolic acidosis and alkalosis in humans. *Journal of Applied Physiology*, 27, 67–76.

Figarola, T.R. and Billings C.E. 1966. Effects of meprobamate and hypoxia on psychomotor performance. *Aerospace Medicine*, 37, 951–4.

Fink, R.B. 1961. Influence of cerebral activity in wakefulness on regulation of breathing. *Journal of Applied Physiology*, 16, 15–20.

Forster, H.V. 2003. Plasticity in the control of breathing following sensory denervation. *Journal of Applied Physiology*, 94, 784–94.

Forster, H.V., Dempsey, J.A. and Chosy, L.W. 1975. Incomplete compensation of CSF [H$^+$] in man during acclimatization to high altitude (4,300 m). *Journal of Applied Physiology*, 38, 1067–72.

Fowler, B. and Kelso, B. 1992. The effects of hypoxia on components of the human event-related potential and relationship to reaction time. *Aviation, Space, and Environmental Medicine*, 63, 510–16.

Fowler, B. and Nathoo, A. 1997. Slowing due to acute hypoxia originates early in the visual system. *Aviation, Space, and Environmental Medicine*, 68, 886–9.

Fowler, B., Paul, M., Porlier, G., Elcombe, D.D. 1985. A re-evaluation of the minimum altitude at which hypoxic effects can be detected. *Ergonomics*, 28, 781–91.

Fowler, B. and Prlic, H. 1995. A comparison of visual and auditory reaction time and P300 latency thresholds to acute hypoxia.

Aviation, Space, and Environmental Medicine, 66, 645–50.

Gardner, W.N. 1996. The pathophysiology of hyperventilation disorders. *Chest*, 109, 516–34.

Gibson, T.M. 1978. The effects of hypocapnia on psychomotor and intellectual performance. *Aviation, Space, and Environmental Medicine*, 49, 943–6.

Glaisher, J. 1862. Notes of effects experienced during recent balloon ascents. *Lancet*, 2, 559–60.

Gradwell, D.P. 2006. Hypoxia and Hyperventilation; Prevention of Hypoxia. In: D.J. Rainford and D.P. Gradwell (eds) *Aviation Medicine – Fourth Edition*. London: Arnold. Ch. 3 and 4 respectively.

Grandpierre, R. and Franck, C. 1952. The paradoxical action of oxygen. *Aviation Medicine*, 23, 181–5.

Gray, F.D. and Horner, G.J. 1970. Survival following extreme hypoxemia. *Journal of the American Medical Association*, 211, 1815–7.

Groves, B.M., Droma T., Sutton, J.R., McCullough, R.G., McCullough, R.E., Zhuang, J. et al. 1993. Minimal hypoxic pulmonary hypertension in normal Tibetans at 3,658 m. *Journal of Applied Physiology*, 74, 312–8.

Guyenet, P.G. 2008. The 2008 Carl Ludwig Lecture: Retrotrapezoid nucleus, CO_2 homeostasis, and breathing automaticity. *Journal of Applied Physiology*, 105, 404–16.

Haldane, J.S. and Priestley, J.G. 1905. The regulation of the lung-ventilation. *Journal of Physiology*, 32, 225–66.

Hall, F.G. 1949. Interval of useful consciousness at various altitudes. *Journal of Applied Physiology*, 1, 490–95

Harding, R.M. 2002. Pressure changes and hypoxia in aviation. *The Textbook of Military Medicine: Medical Aspects of Harsh Environments*, 2, 984–1012.

Hatcher, J.D., Chiu, L.K. and Jennings, D.B. 1978. Anaemia as a stimulus to aortic

and carotid chemoreceptors in the cat. *Journal of Applied Physiology*, 44, 696–702.

Hebbel, R.P., Kronenberg, R.S. and Eaton, J.W. 1977. Hypoxic ventilatory response in subjects with normal and high oxygen affinity hemoglobins. *The Journal of Clinical Investigation*, 60, 1211–5.

Hellenic Republic Ministry of Transport and Communications: Air Accident Investigation and Aviation Safety Board. 2006. Aircraft Accident Report: Helios Airways Flight HCY522 Boeing 737-31S at Grammatiko, Hellas on 14 August 2005. Available at: http://www.moi. gov.cy/moi/pio/pio.nsf/All/F15FBD 7320037284C2257204002B6243/$file/ FINAL%20REPORT%205B-DBY.pdf

Hilton, S.M. and Marshall, J.M. 1982. The pattern of cardiovascular response to carotid chemoreceptor stimulation in the cat. *Journal of Physiology*, 326, 495–513.

Hirshman, C.A., McCullough, R.E. and Neil, J.V. 1975. Normal values for hypoxic and hypercapnic ventilatory drives in man. *Journal of Applied Physiology*, 38, 1095–8.

Honda, Y., Watanabe, S., Hashizume, I., Satomura, Y., Hata, N., Sakakibara, Y. and Severinghaus, J.W. 1979. Hypoxic chemosensitivity in asthmatic patients two decades after carotid body resection. *Journal of Applied Physiology*, 46, 632–8.

Hossack, K.F. and Bruce, R.A. 1982. Maximal cardiac function in sedentary normal men and women: Comparison of age-related changes. *Journal of Applied Physiology*, 53, 799–804.

Hsia, C.C.W. 1998. Respiratory functions of hemoglobin. *The New England Journal of Medicine*, 338, 239–47.

Hurtado, A. 1964. Animals in High Altitudes: Resident Man. In: D.B. Dill, E.F. Adolph and C.G. Wilber (eds) *Handbook of Physiology: Adaptation to the Environment*. Washington, DC: American Physiological Society, 843–60.

Izraeli, S., Avgar, D., Glikson, M., Shochat, I., Glovinsky, Y. and Ribak, J. 1988. Determination of the 'time of useful consciousness' (TUC) in repeated exposures to simulated altitude of 25,000 ft (7,620 m). *Aviation, Space, and Environmental Medicine*, 1103–5.

Kelman, G.R., Crow, T.J. and Bursill, A.E. 1969. Effect of mild hypoxia on mental performance assessed by a test of selective attention. *Aerospace Medicine*, 40, 301–3.

Kelman, G.R. and Crow, T.J. 1969. Impairment of mental performance at a simulated altitude of 8,000 feet. *Aerospace Medicine*, 40, 981–2.

Kety, S.S. and Schmidt, C.F. 1948. The effects of altered arterial tensions of carbon dioxide and oxygen on cerebral blood flow and cerebral oxygen consumption of normal young men. *Journal of Clinical Investigation*, 27, 484–92.

Kida, M. and Imai, A. 1993 Cognitive performance and event-related brain potentials under simulated high altitudes. *Journal of Applied Physiology*, 74, 1735–41.

Koller, E.A., Drechsel, S., Hess, T., Macherel, P. and Boutellier, U. 1988. Effects of atropine and propranolol on the respiratory, circulatory, and ECG responses to high altitude in man. *European Journal of Applied Physiology*, 57, 163–72.

Korner, P.I. 1959. Circulatory adaptations in hypoxia. *Physiological Reviews*, 39, 687–730.

Kujanik, S., Snincak, M., Vokal, J., Podracky, J. and Koval, J. 2000. Periodicity of arrhythmias in healthy elderly men at moderate altitude. *Physiological Research*, 49, 285–7.

Kumar, P. and Bin-Jaliah, I. 2007. Adequate stimuli of the carotid body: More than an oxygen sensor? *Respiratory Physiology & Neurobiology*, 157, 12–21.

Laciga, P. and Koller, E.A. 1976. Respiratory, circulatory, and ECG changes during acute exposure to high altitude. *Journal of Applied Physiology*, 41, 159–67.

Lahiri, S. and DeLaney, R.G. 1975. Stimulus interactions in the responses of carotid body chemoreceptor single afferent. *Respiratory Physiology*, 24, 299–366.

Lahiri, S. and Forster, R.E. 2003. Review: CO_2/H^+ sensing: Peripheral and central chemoreception. *The International Journal of Biochemistry & Cell Biology*, 35, 1413–35.

Lahiri, S., Rumsey, W.L., Wilson, D.F. and Iturriaga, R. 1993. Contribution of *in vivo* microvascular PO_2 in the cat carotid body chemotransduction. *Journal of Applied Physiology*, 75, 1035–43.

Laties, V.G. and Merigan, W.H. 1979. Behavioral effects of carbon monoxide on animals and man. *Annual Review of Pharmacology and Toxicology*, 19, 357–92.

Lawler, J., Powers, S.K. and Thompson, D. 1988. Linear relationship between VO_2max and VO_2max decrement during exposure to acute hypoxia. *Journal of Applied Physiology*, 64, 1486–92.

Ledwith, F. 1970. The effects of hypoxia on choice reaction time and movement time. *Ergonomics*, 13, 465–82.

Li, X.Y., Wu, X.Y., Yang, C.B., Wu, Y.H., Fu, C. and Shen, X.F. 2000. Effects of acute exposure to mild or moderate hypoxia on human psychomotor performance and visual-reaction time. *Space Medicine & Medical Engineering*, 13, 235–9.

Loeschcke, H.H. 1982. Central chemosensitivity and the reaction theory. *Journal of Physiology*, 332, 1–24.

Lopez-Barneo, J., Ortega-Sáenz, P., Pardal, P., Pascual, A. and Piruat, J.I. 2008. Carotid body oxygen sensing. *European Respiratory Journal*, 32, 1386–98.

Luft, U.C., Clamann, H.G. and Opitz, E. 1951. The latency of hypoxia on exposure to altitude above 50,000 feet. *Journal of Aviation Medicine*, 22, 117–22.

Lugliani, R., Whipp, B.J., Seard, C. and Wasserman, K. 1971. Effect of bilateral carotid-body resection on ventilatory control at rest and during exercise in man. *New England Journal of Medicine*, 285, 1105–11.

Lumb, A.B. 2000a. Carbon Dioxide. In: A.B. Lumb (ed.) *Nunn's Applied Respiratory*

Physiology – Fifth Edition. London: Butterworth-Heinemann, 237–40.

Lumb, A.B. 2000b. Distribution of Pulmonary Ventilation and Perfusion. In: A.B. Lumb (ed.) *Nunn's Applied Respiratory Physiology – Fifth Edition*. London: Butterworth-Heinemann, 192–4.

Lundsgaard, C. and Van Slyke, D.D. 1923. Cyanosis. *Medicine*, 2, 1–76.

Macefield, G. and Burke, D. 1991. Paraesthesiae and tetany induced by voluntary hyperventilation: Increased excitability of human cutaneous and motor axons. *Brain*, 114, 527–40.

McFarland, R.A. and Evans, J.N. 1939. Alterations in dark adaptation under reduced oxygen tensions. *American Journal of Physiology*, 127, 37–50.

Macmillan, A.J.F. 2006. Subatmospheric Decompression Sickness. In: D.J. Rainford and D.P. Gradwell (eds) *Aviation Medicine – Fourth Edition*. London: Arnold, 129–36.

Marshall, J.M. 1999. The integrated response to hypoxia: From circulation to cells. *Experimental Physiology*, 84, 449–70.

Martin, L. 2009. Cyanosis. *Emedicine Pulmonology*. http://emedicine.medscape.com/article/303533-overview

Martin, L. and Khalil, H. 1990. How much reduced hemoglobin is necessary to generate central cyanosis? *Chest*, 97, 182–5.

Matsuoka, T., Saiki, C., and Mortola, J.P. 1994. Metabolic and ventilatory responses to anemic hypoxia in conscious rats. *Journal of Applied Physiology*, 77, 1067–72.

Meah, M.S. and Gardner, W.N. 1994. Post-hyperventilation apnoea in conscious humans. *Journal of Physiology*, 477, 3, 527–38.

Mitchell. R.A., Loeschcke, H.H., Massion, W.H. and Severinghaus, J.W. 1963. Respiratory responses mediated through superficial chemosensitive areas on the medulla. *Journal of Applied Physiology*, 18, 523–33.

Mitchell, R.A. and Singer, M.M. 1965. Respiration and cerebrospinal fluid pH in metabolic acidosis and alkolosis. *Journal of Applied Physiology*, 20, 905–11.

Miyamoto, O. 2000. Hypoxia, hyperoxia, ischemia, and brain necrosis. *Neurology*, 54, 362–70.

Mortazavi, A., Eisenberg, M.J., Langleben, D., Ernst, P. and Schiff, R.L. 2003. Altitude-related hypoxia: Risk assessment and management for passengers on commercial aircraft. *Aviation, Space, and Environmental Medicine*, 74, 922–7.

Nattie, E. 2000. Multiple sites for central chemoreception: Their roles in response sensitivity and in sleep and wakefulness. *Respiration Physiology*, 122, 223–35.

Nicholson, A.N. and Ernsting, J. 1967. Neurological sequelae of prolonged decompression. *Aerospace Medicine*, 38, 389–94.

Nicholson, A.N., Freeland, S.A. and Brierley, J.B. 1970. A behavioural and neuropathological study of the sequelae of profound hypoxia. *Brain Research*, 22, 327–45.

Nicholson, A.N. and Wright, C.M. 1975. Effect of mild hypoxia on delayed differentiation in the monkey (*Mucaca mulatta*). *Experimental Neurology*, 47, 535–43.

Nielsen, M. and Smith, H. 1952. Studies on the regulation of respiration in acute hypoxia. *Acta Physiologica Scandinavica*, 24, 293–313.

Nunn, J.F. and Matthews, R.L. 1959. Gaseous exchange during halothane anaesthesia: The steady respiratory state. *British Journal of Anaesthesia*, 31, 330–40.

Otis, A.B. 1970. Physiology of carbon monoxide poisoning and evidence for acclimatization. *Annals of the New York Academy of Sciences*, 174, 242–5.

Pan, L.G., Forster, H.V., Martino, P., Strecker, P.J., Beales, J., Serra, A. et al. 1998. Important role of carotid afferents in control of breathing. *Journal of Applied Physiology*, 85, 1299–306.

Pavlicek, V., Schirlo, C., Nebel, A., Regard, M., Koller, E.A. and Brugger, P. 2005. Cognitive and emotional processing at high altitude. *Aviation, Space, and Environmental Medicine*, 76, 28–33.

Pearigen, P., Gwinn, R. and Simon, R.P. 1996. The effects *in vivo* of hypoxia on brain injury. *Brain Research*, 725, 184–91.

Pearson, R.G. and Neal, G.L. 1970. Operator performance as a function of drug, hypoxia, individual, and task factors. *Aerospace Medicine*, 41, 154–8.

Peers, C. 2002. Hypoxic regulation of ion channel function and expression. *Experimental Physiology*, 87, 413–22.

Peers, C. and Wyatt, C.N. 2007. The role of maxiK channels in carotid body chemotransduction *Respiratory Physiology & Neurobiology*, 157, 75–82.

Perkin, G.D. and Joseph, R. 1986. Neurological manifestations of the hyperventilation syndrome. *Journal of the Royal Society of Medicine*, 79, 448–50.

Powell, F.L., Milsom, W.K and Mitchell, G.S. 1998. Time domains of the hypoxic ventilatory response. *Respiration Physiology*, 112, 123–34.

Putnam, R.W., Filosa, J.A. and Ritucci, N.A. 2004. Cellular mechanisms involved in CO_2 and acid signaling in chemosensitive neurons. *American Journal of Physiology – Cell Physiology*, 287, C1493–526.

Prefaut, C., Durand, F., Mucci, P. and Caillaud, C. 2000. Exercise-induced arterial hypoxaemia in athletes. *Sports Medicine*, 30, 47–61.

Pretorius, H.A. 1970. Effect of oxygen on night vision. *Aerospace Medicine*, 41, 560–62.

Rafferty, G.F., Saisch, G.N. and Gardner, W.N. 1992. Relation of hypocapnic symptoms to rate of fall of end-tidal PCO_2 in normal subjects. *Respiratory Medicine*, 86, 335–40.

Rahn, H. and Otis, A.B. 1947. Alveolar air during simulated flights to high altitudes. *American Journal of Physiology*, 150, 202–21.

Rahn, H. and Otis, A.B. 1949. Man's respiratory response during and after acclimatization to high altitude. *American Journal of Physiology*, 157, 445–62.

Rahn, H., Otis, A.B., Hodge, M., Epstein, M.A., Hunter, S.W. and Fenn, W.O. 1946. The effects of hypocapnia on performance. *Aviation Medicine*, 17, 164–72.

Raichle, M. and Plum, F. 1972. Hyperventilation and cerebral blood flow. *Stroke*, 3, 566–75.

Rayman, R.B. and McNaughton, G.B. 1983. Hypoxia: USAF experience 1970–80. *Aviation, Space, and Environmental Medicine*, 54, 357–9.

Read, D.J.C. and Leigh, J. 1967. Blood-brain tissue PCO_2 relationships and ventilation during rebreathing. *Journal of Applied Physiology*, 23, 53–70.

Rebuck, A.S., Rigg, J.R.A., Kangalee, M. and Pengelly, L.D. 1974. Control of tidal volume during rebreathing. *Journal of Applied Physiology*, 37, 475–8.

Reivich, M. 1964. Arterial PCO_2 and cerebral hemodynamics. *American Journal of Physiology*, 206, 25–35.

Richardson, D.W., Kontos, H.A., Shapiro, W. and Patterson, J.L. 1966. The role of hypocapnia in the circulatory response to acute hypoxia in man. *Journal of Applied Physiology*, 21, 22–6.

Richardson, D.W., Kontos, H.A., Raper, A.J. and Patterson, J.L. Jr. 1967. Modification by beta-adrenergic blockade of the circulatory responses to acute hypoxia in man. *The Journal of Clinical Investigation*, 46, 77–85.

Richerson, G.B., Wang, W., Hodges, M.R., Dohle, C.I. and Diez-Sampedro, A. 2005. Homing in on the specific phenotype(s) of central respiratory chemoreceptors. *Experimental Physiology*, 90, 3, 259–69.

Risdale, J. 2006. Clinical Management of Decompression Illness. In: D.J. Rainford and D.P. Gradwell (eds) *Aviation Medicine – Fourth Edition*. London: Arnold, 757–66.

Robbins, P.A. 2007. Role of the peripheral chemoreflex in the early stages of ventilatory acclimatization to altitude. *Respiratory Physiology & Neurobiology*, 158, 237–42.

Rumi, E., Passamonti, F., Pagano, L., Ammirabile, M., Arcaini, L., Elena, C. et al. 2009. Blood p50 evaluation enhances diagnostic definition of isolated erythrocytosis. *Journal of Internal Medicine*, 265, 266–74.

Sahn, S.A., Zwillich, C.W., Dick, N., McCullough, R.E., Lakshminarayan, S. and Weil, J.V. 1977. Variability of ventilatory responses to hypoxia and hypercapnia. *Journal of Applied Physiology*, 43, 1019–25.

Saurenmann, P. and Koller, E.A. 1984. The ECG changes due to altitude and to catecholamines. *European Journal of Applied Physiology*, 53, 35–42.

Schneider, E.C. 1918. Medical studies in aviation: II. Physiologic observations and methods. *Journal of the American Medical Association*, 71, 1384–9.

Schneider, E.C. and Truesdell, D. 1921. A study of low oxygen effects during rebreathing. *American Journal of Physiology*, 55, 223–56.

Severinghaus, J.W. 1966. Blood gas calculator. *Journal of Applied Physiology*, 21, 1108–116.

Severinghaus, J.W. 1979. Simple, accurate equations for human blood O_2 dissociation computations. *Journal of Applied Physiology*, 46, 599–602.

Severinghaus, J.W., Mitchell, R.A., Richardson, B.W. and Singer, M.M. 1963. Respiratory control at high altitude suggesting active transport regulation of CSF pH. *Journal of Applied Physiology*, 18, 1155–66.

Shapiro, W., Waserman, A.J., Baker, J.P. and Patterson, J.L. 1970. Cerebrovascular response to acute hypocapnic and eucapnic hypoxia in normal man. *The Journal of Clinical Investigation*, 49, 2362–8.

Shepherd, R.J. 1956. Physiological changes and psychomotor performance during acute hypoxia. *Journal of Applied Physiology*, 9, 343–51.

Simon, R.P. 1999. Hypoxia versus ischemia. *Neurology*, 52, 4–6.

Smith, C.A., Rodman, J.R, Chenuel, B.J.A., Henderson, K.S. and Dempsey, J.A. 2006. Response time and sensitivity of the ventilatory response to CO_2 in unanesthetized intact dogs: Central vs. peripheral chemoreceptors. *Journal of Applied Physiology*, 100, 13–19.

Sola, A. 2008. Oxygen in neonatal anesthesia: Friend or foe? *Current Opinion in Anaesthesiology*, 21, 332–9.

Squires, R.W. and Buskirk, E.R. 1982. Aerobic capacity during acute exposure to simulated altitude, 914 to 2286 meters. *Medicine & Science in Sports & Exercise*, 14, 36–40.

Steinback, C.D. and Poulin, M.J. 2008. Cardiovascular and cerebrovascular responses to acute isocapnic and poikilocapnic hypoxia in humans. *Journal of Applied Physiology*, 104, 482–9.

Swanson, G.D., Whipp, B.J., Kaufman, R.D., Aqleh, K.A., Winter, B. and Bellville, J.W. 1978. Effect of hypercapnia on hypoxic ventilatory drive in carotid body-resected man. *Journal of Applied Physiology*, 45, 971–7.

Tacker, W.A.J., Balldin, U.I., Burton, R.R., Glaister, D.H., Gillingham, K.K. and Mercer, J.R. 1987. *Aviation, Space, and Environmental Medicine*, 58, 69–75.

Teichman, P.G., Donchin, Y. and Kot, R.J. 2007. International aeromedical evacuation. *New England Journal of Medicine*, 356, 262–70.

Timmers, H.J.L.M., Wieling, W., Karemake, J.M. and Lenders, J.W.M. 2003. Denervation of carotid baro- and chemo-receptors in humans. *Journal of Physiology*, 553, 3–11.

Tissandier, M. 1875. In: Fatal ballooning: The sad story of the Zenith. *New York Times*, 2 May 1875.

Torre-Bueno, J.R., Wagner, P.D., Saltzman, H.A., Gale, G.E. and Moon, R.E. 1985.

Diffusion limitation in normal humans during exercise at sea level and simulated altitude. *Journal of Applied Physiology*, 58, 989–95.

United Kingdom Civil Aviation Authority (UK CAA), Aviation Health Unit, 2010. Guidelines for Medical Professionals: Assessing fitness to fly. Available at: http://www.caa.co.uk/docs/923/Fitness%20To%20Fly%20December%202010%20PDF.pdf

Van der Post, J., Noordzij, L.A.W., de Kam, M.L., Blauw, G.J., Cohen, A.F. and van Gerven, J.M.A. 2002. Evaluation of tests of central nervous system performance after hypoxemia for a model for cognitive impairment. *Journal of Psychopharmacology*, 16, 337–43.

Wagner, P.D. 2000. Reduced maximal cardiac output at altitude: Mechanisms and significance. *Respiration Physiology*, 120, 1–11.

Wagner, P.D., Gale, G.E., Moon, R.E., Torre-Bueno, J.R., Stolp, B.W. and Saltzman, H.A. 1986. Pulmonary gas exchange in humans exercising at sea level and simulated altitude. *Journal of Applied Physiology*, 61, 260–70.

Wagner, P.D., Wagner, H.E., Groves, B.M., Cymerman, A. and Houston, C.S. 2007. Hemoglobin P50 during a simulated ascent of Mt. Everest, Operation Everest II. *High Altitude Medicine & Biology*, 8, 32–42.

Wald, G., Harper, P.V. Jr, Goodman, H.C. and Krieger, H.P. 1942. Respiratory effects upon the visual threshold. *The Journal of General Physiology*, 25, 891–903.

Ward, J.P.T and McMurtry, I.F. 2009. Mechanisms of hypoxic pulmonary vasoconstriction and their roles in pulmonary hypertension: New findings for an old problem. *Current Opinion in Pharmacology*, 9, 287–96.

Wasserman, K., Whipp, B.J., Koyal, S.N. and Beaver, W.L. 1973. Anaerobic threshold and respiratory gas exchange during exercise. *Journal of Applied Physiology*, 35, 236–43.

Wasserman, K., Whipp, B.J., Koyal, S.N. and Cleary, M.G. 1975. Effect of carotid body resection on ventilatory and acid-base control during exercise. *Journal of Applied Physiology*, 39, 354–8.

Weil, J.V., Byrne-Quinn, E., Sodal, I.E., Friesen W.O., Underhill, B., Filley, G.F. and Grover, R.F. 1970. Hypoxic ventilatory drive in normal man. *The Journal of Clinical Investigation*, 49, 1061–72.

Weil, J.V. and Zwillich, C.W. 1976. Assessment of ventilatory response to hypoxia. *Chest*, 70, 124–8.

West, J.B. 1990. *Ventilation/Blood Flow and Gas Exchange*. Oxford: Blackwell Scientific.

West, J.B., Lahiri, S., Gill, M.B., Milledge, J.S., Pugh, L.G.C.E. and Ward, M.P. 1962. Arterial oxygen saturation during exercise at high altitude. *Journal of Applied Physiology*, 17, 617–21.

Westerman, R.A. 2004. Hypoxia familiarisation training by the reduced oxygen breathing method. *Australian Defence Force Health Journal*, 5, 11–15.

Westerman, R.A. and Bassovitch, O. 2010. Effectiveness of the GO2Altitude® Hypoxia Training System. *Journal of the Australasian Society of Aerospace Medicine*, 5, 7–12.

Whipp, B.J. 1994. Carotid bodies and breathing in humans. *Thorax*, 49, 1081–4.

Winslow, R.M. 2007. The role of hemoglobin oxygen affinity in oxygen transport at high altitude. *Respiratory Physiology & Neurobiology*, 158, 121–7.

Winslow, R.M., Samaja, M. and West, J.B. 1984. Red cell function at extreme altitude on Mount Everest. *Journal of Applied Physiology*, 56, 109–16.

Woorons, X.P., Mollard, P., Lamberto, C., Letournel, M. and Richalet, J.-B. 2005. Effect of acute hypoxia on maximal exercise in trained and sedentary women. *Medicine & Science in Sports & Exercise*, 37, 147–54.

Yoneda, I. and Watanabe, Y. 1997. Comparisons of altitude tolerance and hypoxia symptoms between nonsmokers and habitual smokers. *Aviation, Space, and Environmental Medicine*, 68, 807–11.

Zavorsky, G.S., Walley, K.R., Hunte, G.S., McKenzie, D.C., Sexsmith, G. and Rissell, J.A. 2003. Acute hypervolaemia improves arterial oxygen pressure in athletes with exercise-induced hypoxaemia. *Experimental Physiology*, 88, 555–64.

Zaugg, M., Kaplan, V., Widmer, U., Baumann, P.C. and Russi, E.W. 1998. Fatal air embolism in an airplane passenger with a giant intrapulmonary bronchogenic cyst. *American Journal of Respiratory and Critical Care Medicine*, 157, 1686–9.

Chapter 7

HYPOBARIC HYPOXIA: ADAPTATION AND ACCLIMATIZATION

John H. Coote and James S. Milledge

The adverse effects of hypoxia on the nervous system are experienced at relatively low altitudes, and the severity increases from that experienced by aircrew in the mild hypoxic environment of the cabins of commercial transport aircraft to that experienced by mountaineers and those who live in the mountains. Aircrew operating transport aircraft may be exposed for several hours to barometric pressures (560 mm Hg: 74.7 kPa) approaching the equivalent of around 8,000 feet (2,450 metres), while mountaineers and those who live in the mountains may stay for many days or years at barometric pressures (460 mm: 61.3 kPa) equivalent to or above 13,000 feet (4,000 metres).

With respect to the mild hypoxia of the cabin environment, the issue is that of subtle changes in behaviour that could potentially prejudice the capability of the aircrew. As far as mountaineers and those who live in the mountains are concerned, the issue is the way in which the adverse effects of severe hypoxia are ameliorated by physiological adaptations and by acclimatization. Studies in mountaineers provide the link between the effects of mild hypoxia experienced in the cabin of transport aircraft and profound hypoxia at extreme altitudes as would be experienced in decompressions in supersonic transport aircraft, particularly with respect to the emergence of permanent brain damage (Chapter 8, Profound Hypoxia: Extreme Altitude and Space).

Part 1: AEROMEDICAL CONSIDERATIONS: MILD HYPOXIA

In view of the known sensitivity of the central nervous system to hypoxia, it is not surprising that there are reports of significant deterioration in memory, cognition, decision making, sleep, mental function (psychiatric disorders), vision and hearing at altitudes above sea level. It is commonly accepted that overt biological effects associated with a lower partial pressure of oxygen occur around 10,000 feet (3,050 metres) where atmospheric pressure is around 523 mm Hg: 69.7 kPa. However, symptoms may appear at elevations as low as 5,000 to 6,000 feet (1,500 to 1,850 metres) (607 to 596 mm Hg: 80.9 to 79.5 kPa) (McFarland and Evans, 1939; Squires and Buskirk, 1982). Such effects are important in the practice of aviation medicine as the cabin altitude of current civil aircraft can exceed 8,000 feet (2,450 metres) (Cummin and Nicholson, 2002). The question arises at what ambient pressure does the partial pressure of arterial oxygen (PaO_2) drop sufficiently to impair brain function.

Early aeromedical studies (Denison *et al.*, 1966) indicated that at altitudes as low as 5,000 feet (1,500 metres) subjects were slower in learning complex tasks. Initially, the conclusion of this study did not appear to be supported by several other studies from different groups using different routines to test task performance. However, an extensive and well-designed study by Farmer *et al.* (1991) confirmed the results. The latter study measured reaction time and the accuracy of the recognition of the position of a manikin whilst observers were exposed either to air at sea level or to a simulated altitude of 8,000 feet (2,450 metres) or while breathing oxygen-enriched air in these two conditions. It was shown that these low levels of hypoxia impaired the learning of a novel task, but there was no effect on the performance of already well-practised tasks. It was, therefore, concluded that the routine cockpit tasks of pilots exposed to the presently agreed maximum cabin pressure of commercial aircraft of 8,000 feet (2,450 metres) could be performed competently provided they have been well learned at ground level.

This appears to be the case at altitudes up to 10,000 feet (3,050 metres). Above this altitude with the partial pressure of alveolar oxygen (P_AO_2) below 55 mm Hg (7.3 kPa), reaction time is affected as well as tasks requiring complex hand–eye coordination such as instrument flying, even if they have been well learned at ground level. At altitudes in excess of 12,000 feet (3,650 metres) where the partial pressure of alveolar oxygen is below 50 mm Hg (6.7 kPa), there is a 10 per cent decrease in the ability of pilots to maintain a given speed, heading or vertical velocity. In unacclimatized subjects this decrement rises from 20 to 30 per cent at altitudes above 15,000 feet (4,500 metres), where the alveolar oxygen tension drops below 40 mm Hg (5.3 kPa). At the higher altitudes psychomotor performance is compromised further by impairment of muscle coordination, hand tremor, hand grip and in writing.

In concert with these motor changes, cognitive functions are also less good in poorly acclimatized subjects. For example, conceptual reasoning, short- and long-term memory including spatial memory (Shukitt-Hale *et al.*, 1994), recall of lists of names (Pelamatti *et al.*, 2003), speed and accuracy of hand–eye coordination (Sharma *et al.*, 1975) show significant impairment (~ 10 per cent) at altitudes even as low as from 8,000 to 10,000 feet (2,450 to 3,050 metres) where alveolar oxygen is around 60 mm Hg (8.0 kPa). This rises to as much as 25 per cent impairment at 15,000 feet (4,500 metres) with the partial pressure of alveolar oxygen around 40 mm Hg (5.3 kPa). In laboratory studies it has been shown that lowering of the partial pressure of alveolar oxygen to 75 mm Hg (10.0 kPa), equivalent to an altitude of 5,000 feet (1,500 metres), impairs light sensitivity of the dark-adapted eye (scotopic or rod vision), and above 12,000 feet (3,650 metres), even in bright light, retinal sensitivity and the integrity of the visual field are impaired (Gradwell, 2006).

There are also concurrent reductions in auditory activity (Klein *et al.*, 1961; Carlile and Paterson 1992).

Part 2:
MOUNTAINEERS – ADAPTATION AND ACCLIMATIZATION

The physiological challenges to mountaineers and those who live in the mountains are not only complex but of serious import, and induce significant changes in the respiratory and circulatory systems that, in due course, may prejudice the function of the central nervous system. However, a degree of acclimatization occurs in lowland visitors, such as trekkers and mountaineers. It involves time-dependent and reversible physiological changes that compensate to some extent for the effect of lower oxygen during an acute or short-term exposure to altitude. Further, adaptation to living and working at low barometric pressure occurs in the substantial human populations that have remained at high altitude over many generations. These processes involve the autonomic nervous system, oxygen sensing, ventilation and gas exchange, and the circulatory and cerebral circulations, and these systems work together to mitigate the potential effects of hypoxia on the nervous system.

Autonomic Nervous System

Acclimatization to hypobaric hypoxia is accompanied by increases in systemic arterial pressure and sympathoadrenal activity (Wolfel *et al.*, 1994). At altitudes around 14,100 feet (4,300 metres) it has been shown that catecholamine levels are raised with arterial adrenaline initially being most marked, whilst noradrenaline levels show a slower increase but become the most obvious feature of a prolonged stay (Mazzeo *et al.*, 1991, 1998; Wolfel *et al.*, 1994; Calbet, 2003). More direct estimates of autonomic nerve activity show that muscle sympathetic nerve activity measured by microneurography is enhanced in visitors staying at altitudes up to 17,250 feet (5,260 metres) (Duplain *et al.*, 1999; Hansen and Sander, 2003).

Acute exposure to high altitude also results in an increase in resting heart rate (Bernardi *et al.*, 1998; Vogel and Harris, 1967) which then returns to sea level values with acclimatization (Vogel and Harris, 1967). Somewhat surprisingly, adrenoreceptors appear to be down-regulated (Richalet *et al.*, 1988a). The increase in heart rate is a consequence of reduction in parasympathetic tone as well as an increase in cardiac sympathetic drive and circulating adrenaline (Duplain *et al.*, 1999; Boushel *et al.*, 2001; Kanai *et al.*, 2001; Clar *et al.*, 2001; Calbet, 2003; Hansen and Sander, 2003; Cornolo *et al.*, 2004; Liu *et al.*, 2007). The arterial baroreceptor reflex control of heart rate and vascular resistance shows a decreased gain in visitors to high altitude (> 11,800 feet: 3,600 metres) without a change in its set point which is consistent with a relatively mild increase in sympathetic activity (Bernardi *et al.*, 1998, 2003; Blaber *et al.*, 2003; Cooper *et al.*, 2005). This is confirmed by hypobaric chamber studies in subjects exposed to simulated altitudes of up to 14,100 feet (4,300 metres) (Sagawa *et al.*, 1997; Sevre *et al.*, 2001).

Healthy high-altitude dwellers in the Andes have high blood levels of catecholamines, suggesting there is a higher level of sympathetic activity, but baroreceptor function curves are similar to those observed at sea level (Bernardi *et al.*, 1998; Moore *et al.*, 2006). Another index of autonomic activity, that of response to orthostatic stress, shows that Ethiopians and Andeans have better tolerance than do residents at sea level (Claydon *et al.*, 2004, 2005a, 2005b). These authors suggest this is most likely due to larger blood volumes in the high-altitude dwellers (Hainsworth *et al.*, 2007). In chronic mountain sickness (CMS) baroreceptor function is impaired (Bernardi *et al.*, 2003) and set point higher (Moore *et al.*, 2006).

Oxygen Sensing and Chemoreceptors

It is generally agreed that the increase in ventilation during acclimatization is initially driven by the peripheral arterial chemoreceptors – most probably primarily those of the carotid body. It is also clear that these receptors continue to make a significant contribution to oxygen homeostasis, even in time-dependent changes in ventilation that are a factor in the adaptation of ventilation in high-altitude dwellers. Almost all cells respond to a lowering of oxygen tension from the sea-level norm by transcription factor activation and second messenger activation or depression. However, the specialized chemoreceptor cells of the carotid body are the most sensitive to the changes in arterial oxygen tension. Carotid body afferent nerve traffic is increased by quite moderate decreases in arterial tensions from 100 to 80 mm Hg (13.3 to 10.7 kPa), whereas an arterial tension below 40 mm Hg (5.3 kPa) is needed to cause changes in cellular responses in most other tissues (Lübbers, 1977).

Carotid Body

The chemoreceptor tissue is composed of two cell types, type I and type II. Type I cells express a variety of neurotransmitters and form synaptic contacts with afferent nerve endings of the carotid branch of the ninth cranial nerve. Type II cells resemble glial cells and are supporting cells. Much of the evidence indicates that type I cells are the initial site of oxygen sensing and they act in concert with the afferent terminals as a 'chemosensing unit'. There are several theories based on experimental evidence that attempt to explain how the type I cell transduces the oxygen stimulus. These are summarized in Figure 7.1. Central to this oxygen sensing is the rapid inhibition of ion channels by a decrease in arterial oxygen tensions leading to depolarization of the type I cell (Lopez-Barneo *et al.*, 1988, 2001).

Although a variety of oxygen-sensitive potassium (K^+) channels have been described, recent evidence favours a major involvement for

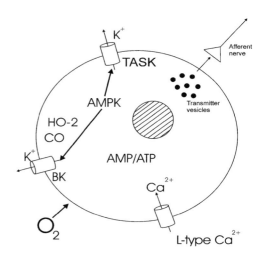

Figure 7.1   Oxygen sensing in the carotid body

Schematic of hypoxia sensing mechanisms in the peripheral chemoreceptor Type 1 cell of the carotid body. BK, large conductance Ca^{2+} activated K^+ channel that helps to maintain the membrane voltage during normoxia with the aid of CO generated by Haem oxygenase (HO-2). TASK, acid sensitive tandem P domain K channel open at resting membrane potential and thus contributes to this. During hypoxia both of these channels are inactivated and associated with a rise in AMP and stimulation of the proteinkinase (AMPK). Consequently the cell depolarises leading to calcium influx and neurosecretion of transmitter (filled circles) which stimulate the afferent nerve ending. Based on Kumar (2007).

the non-inactivating calcium (Ca^{2+}) dependent channels (Peers, 1990). Hypoxia inactivates these channels, so increasing membrane resistance and inducing sufficient cell depolarization to activate voltage-gated calcium entry. The elevation in intracellular calcium levels leads to neurosecretion of transmitter substances from the type I cells that lead to action potential generation in the post-synaptic afferent nerve endings. It appears that the ion channels that conduct potassium through type I cell membranes (BK channels) are not directly oxygen-sensitive, but coupled to a non-membrane sensor located elsewhere in the cell. One proposed mechanism is that an oxygen-dependent enzyme, haemoxygenase-2, which is found in a protein complex associated with various membrane-bound potassium channels, produces carbon monoxide which appears essential for BK channel activation (Williams et al., 2004). In the presence of oxygen and the co-substrates, haem and dihydro-nicotinamide adenine di-nucleotide phosphate (NADPH), the released carbon monoxide increases the open probability of the channels, and when oxygen is reduced in hypoxia there is a reduction of carbon monoxide production leading to inactivation of the BK channel and depolarization. Other more contentious ideas are based on changes in the mitochondrial electron transport chain and oxidative phosphorylation which, by a variety of means, result in potassium channel inactivation (Kumar, 2007; Kemp, 2006; Prabhakar, 2006).

Several of the currently proposed mechanisms for oxygen sensing have favourable points, but none can fully reconcile all of the data. It has, therefore, been suggested that oxygen sensing is so important that several mechanisms may have evolved to ensure that cellular function is never compromised during moderate to severe hypoxia. Once a fall in arterial oxygen tension has been detected at the type I cell, there is a chain of events leading to depolarization and the release of a series of chemical neurotransmitters. Some neurotransmitters, such as acetylcholine, substance P and, most importantly, adenosine triphosphate (ATP), excite afferent terminals, whilst others, such as dopamine and enkephalins, inhibit. It is proposed that the excitatory and inhibitory messengers act in concert like a push–pull mechanism, so that inhibitory messengers prevent a brief over-excitation and allow a sustained stimulation (Prabhakar, 1994, 2006).

Hypoxia-Inducible Factor

All these actions within the carotid body are dependent on another oxygen-sensitive protein, the hypoxia-inducible factor 1 (HIF-1α). It has been shown that an increase in ventilatory drive, measured from activity in the phrenic nerve, induced by an hypoxic stimulus of the carotid body (but not aortic body), is impaired in heterozygous mice bred with a partial deficit in HIF-1α expression (Kline et al., 2002; Peng et al., 2006). The regulatory pathways controlling HIF-1 are illustrated in Figure 7.2. The oxygen-regulated HIF-1α sub-unit is one part of a heterodimeric protein that is also comprised of a constitutively expressed HIF-1β sub-unit. The level of HIF-1α increases with hypoxia due to depression of the oxygen-requiring enzyme prolyl hydroxylase that breaks down HIF-1α when sufficient oxygen is present.

The hypoxia-inducible factors are transcription factors that are a key part of the genomic response to sustained hypoxia (Semenza, 2000). Around 100 directly targeted genes have been reported. These include those for nitric

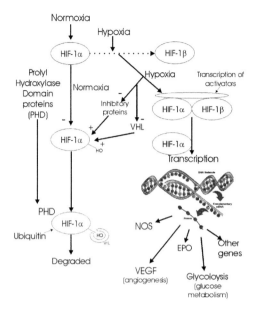

Figure 7.2   Hypoxia-inducible factor pathway (see colour section)

HIF-1 consists of a constituitively expressed β subunit and an oxygen regulated α subunit. Under normoxic conditions HIF-1α is degraded by hydroxylation under the influence of proline hydroxylase and various proteins such as von Hippel Lindau Factor (VHL), indicated by the left hand oxygen dependent pathway.During hypoxia the degradation of HIF-1α is inhibited so that it follows the right hand pathway whereby two transcription activators interact with HIF-1α to enable it to induce transcription of a number of genes. Many are responsible for expression of proteins involved in oxygen homeostasis such as nitric oxide synthase (NOS), vasular endothelial growth factor (VEGF), erythropoietin (EPO).

oxide synthase (cell signalling), vascular endothelial growth factor (VEGF; angiogenesis), erythropoietin (EPO; erythrocytosis), glycolysis and others. The collective activation of these target genes facilitates acclimatization and adaptation to hypoxia. The significance of particular genes activated by HIF-1α for the response of different persons acclimatizing to high altitude or to adaptation in high-altitude dwellers is an area that currently needs research.

Central Receptors

At sea level, ventilation is predominantly (80 per cent) regulated by central

chemoreceptors stimulated by hydrogen ions (H^+) generated from the prevailing tension of arterial carbon dioxide ($PaCO_2$). This stimulus is regulated by the buffering capacity of the cerebrospinal fluid. During acclimatization to hypoxia the buffering capacity of the brain is reduced so that a lower arterial tension of carbon dioxide is sufficient to generate free hydrogen ions at the central chemoreceptor (Figure 7.3). A probable sequence of events is that, initially, cerebrospinal fluid pH is decreased due to lactacidosis, probably in part due to increased production of lactate via the normal brain aerobic glycolytic pathway (Larsen *et al.*, 2008; Schurr, 2006, 2008), but also as a consequence of brain anaerobic glucose metabolism (Milledge, 1979). Later, active or possibly passive transport of the bicarbonate radical (HCO_3^-) out of the brain fluids reduces the buffering capacity. Since the latter events take time, it should be appreciated that initially a robust hypoxia ventilatory response (HVR) mediated by peripheral chemoreceptors is highly beneficial for acclimatization to acute and prolonged exposure of visitors to high altitude. However, there are several reports showing that the actual value of HVR is not necessarily positively correlated with high-altitude performance in each individual (see later).

Ventilation

The lowered pressure of inspired oxygen at altitude makes its transfer and utilization by the tissues more difficult. The main mechanisms have been described in Chapter 6 (Oxygen Delivery and Acute Hypoxia: Physiological and Clinical Considerations), but it is useful to review some of these in order to understand the events involved in acclimatization and adaptation to hypoxia. In Figure

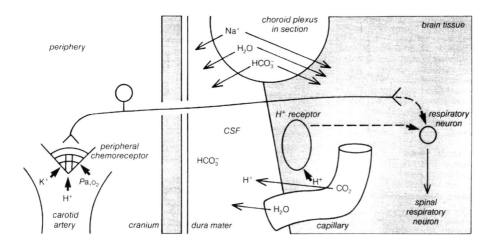

Figure 7.3   Key sites in ventilatory control

Diagram illustrating key sites in the ventilatory control system involved in the response to hypoxia. At sea level around 80% of ventilatory drive to the respiratory neurones arises from the central chemoreceptors (H+ receptor). This responds to free H+ generated by hydration of CO_2 to form carbonic acid which then dissociates. The capillary wall is freely permeable to CO_2 which passes into the brain interstitium. The changes in brain pH are buffered by HCO_3^-, produced mainly from cells of the choroid plexuses. In addition, the H+ and the change in partial pressure of oxygen in arterial blood are detected by peripheral chemoreceptors, providing additional drive to the respiratory neurones in the brain (After Coote, 1991).

7.4 the steps in the cascade of oxygen and carbon dioxide partial pressures in each compartment of the gas exchange system in a resting subject breathing air at sea level (760 mm Hg: 101.3 kPa – solid line) are compared with those that pertain in a subject who has spent two weeks at an altitude of 14,700 feet (4,500 metres) (433 mm Hg: 57.7 kPa – dashed line). For the interstitial fluid and cellular compartments, the values are hypothetical but based on real data from various types of experimental approaches. This diagram is useful because it shows that each step in the oxygen cascade from one compartment to another is reduced in the subject acclimatized to the higher altitude. This would suggest that the resistances opposed to oxygen flux are less at high altitude as far as the oxygen consumption is concerned. How, then, is this achieved?

The large step between the inspired and the alveolar oxygen tensions, which at sea level is around 50 mm (6.7 kPa), is reduced to around 30 mm (4.0 kPa) at the altitude simulated in the diagram (Figure 7.4). This is achieved by an increase in ventilation. Such hyperventilation is of adaptive value, being functionally equivalent to a descent to a lower altitude (Rahn and Otis, 1949). Initially, the increase in ventilation in response to a decrease in ambient oxygen tensions results from the stimulation of carotid body chemoreceptors by the reduction in the tension of oxygen in arterial blood. This can be shown in humans by the use of the Dejours O_2-test (Dejours, 1957), whereby an abrupt inhalation of 100 per cent O_2 in a subject breathing at progressively increased levels of hypoxia leads to a decrease in ventilation. By plotting the steady-state ventilation for each level of hypoxia and observing the ventilation following the Dejours O_2-test, two curves are obtained of ventilation at the different degrees of oxygenation shown in Figure 7.5. The magnitude of the difference between the hypoxia ventilation and that of the few breaths during pure oxygen is a measure of the peripheral chemoreceptor drive (Bouverot *et al.*, 1965; Leitner *et al.*, 1965a, 1965b; Guz *et al.*, 1966).

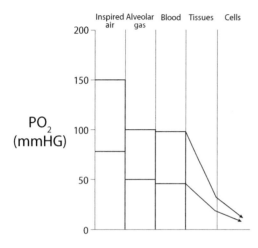

Figure 7.4   Transport   of   oxygen   from inspired air to cells

Schematic showing the expected oxygen tension at each of the stages in the transport of oxygen from inspired air to cells in an idealised individual subject at sea level and after acclimatizing to 14,750 feet (4,500 metres). Blood value is for arterial blood, tissue value is for the interstitium and cell is for the intracellular compartment.

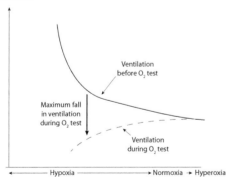

Figure 7.5   Chemoreceptor   drive   with decreasing altitude

Schematic representation of changes in the peripheral chemoreceptor drive with increasing altitude. The graph shows the ventilatory response to hypoxia (solid line) compared with ventilation after switching to breathing pure oxygen at a series of decreasing levels of ambient pressure of oxygen (dotted line: Dejours Test). The maximum fall in ventilation indicated by the vertical distance between the two ventilation curves (arrows) at each level of hypoxia indicates the degree of chemoreceptor drive (based on Bouverot, 1985).

Gas Exchange

The increase in ventilation is a time-dependent process improving over several days in visitors to high altitude. Ventilatory acclimatization is illustrated in Figure 7.6. The upper curve of this figure shows the changes in alveolar oxygen tensions during an acute exposure to increasingly higher altitudes plotted against the alveolar tension of carbon dioxide (an indication of the increase of ventilation). The lower curve shows the relationship of subjects acclimatized over many months at each altitude, and is based on measurements made on miners in the camps around Colorado by Maria FitzGerald (1913). Acclimatization results in ventilation increasing at lower altitudes so that the alveolar oxygen tension is higher. Thus, point A on the upper curve shows the alveolar oxygen tension of an unacclimatized person with an inspired oxygen tension of 90 mm (12.0 kPa) and a small increase in ventilation as indicated by the small reduction in the alveolar tension. Point B shows the situation after two weeks' exposure to the same level of inspired oxygen where the alveolar tension is higher (so reduction from inspired oxygen is less) and the alveolar tension of carbon dioxide is lower as a result of an increase in ventilation (based on Rahn and Otis, 1949).

Thus, during acclimatization the ventilatory response to hypoxia progressively increases and eventually stabilizes. The latter effect is due to a gradual return of the drive from the central chemoreceptors adding to the hypoxia-driven effect of the peripheral chemoreceptors. This is illustrated schematically by the bar chart in Figure 7.7. The differences in ventilation between acute versus prolonged exposure to an hypoxic environment probably result from an initial reduction

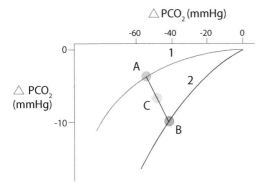

Figure 7.6   Changes in alveolar oxygen tension and carbon dioxide at increasing altitude

The change in carbon dioxide is an indication of the degree of hyperventilation. Top curve (1) is the response of an unacclimatized lowland subject, bottom curve (2) is after acclimatization. Point A and B indicate the values of PCO2 (inversely proportional to ventilation) in subjects at same altitude. Point C is expected ventilation at this same altitude for a life long resident of high altitude. Based on Rahn and Otis (1949) and Bouverot (1985).

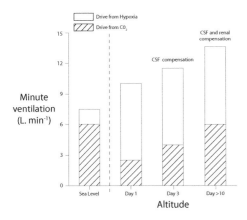

Figure 7.7   Ventilatory acclimatization

Diagram illustrating the way breathing acclimatizes after arrival at high altitude over a period of days. At first ventilation becomes dependent on drive from peripheral chemoreceptors (open columns) stimulated by hypoxia and this results in a reduction in arterial PCO2. Gradually central chemoreceptor drive (hatched columns) returns following acid-base compensation for hypocapnia of blood and cerebrospinal fluid. Final ventilation is the sum of the two respiratory drives. Based on Widdicombe and Davies (1991).

in the central chemoreceptor stimulation because the arterial tension of carbon dioxide ($PaCO_2$) falls during the increased ventilation driven by peripheral chemoreceptors.

It is clear from Figure 7.4 that the difference between arterial and venous blood oxygen tensions decreases at the lower ambient air pressure of altitude. This indicates that an adaptive process must occur in the transport of oxygen by blood that prevents oxygen pressure in the blood flowing through the capillaries from falling too greatly during hypoxia. This is ensured in two main ways. One is a shift in the haemoglobin–oxygen affinity (Hb-O_2 association) and the other is in the amount of haemoglobin. In lowland visitors acclimatized to high altitude, it is now generally agreed that an increase in 2,3-diphosphoglycerol (2,3-DPG) favouring a lower affinity, and therefore a right shifted Hb-O_2 curve, is overwhelmed by the alkalosis induced by hyperventilation so there is a slight leftward shift of the Hb-O_2 curve (Turek et al., 1973; Winslow et al., 1984). At high altitude (above 26,000 feet; 8,000 metres), more severe alkalosis causes a significant left shift in the Hb-O_2 curve, which has considerable benefits for climbers (West et al., 1983) because it provides a greater oxygen delivery to the tissues at the very low arterial pressure of oxygen. A similar picture emerges for high-altitude dwellers of the Andes and Himalayas (Aste-Salazar and Hurtado, 1944; Lenfant and Sullivan, 1971; Winslow et al., 1981).

Haemoglobin

An increase in the number of red blood cells and, therefore, of haemoglobin concentration has long been a consistent finding in lowland visitors to high altitude (Viault 1890; West et al., 2007). Typically, at altitudes up to 18,000 feet (5,500 metres) there is a progressive increase in haemoglobin concentration from sea-level values around 15 gm.100 mL^{-1} to values around 18 to 20 gm.100 mL^{-1} with haematocrit values rising from 45 to over 50 per cent. Above this altitude there is little further increase (Pugh, 1964a; Winslow *et al.*, 1984) suggesting that these peak values are optimal (Guyton and Richardson, 1961). The resultant increase in the concentration of oxygen per millilitre of blood means that more oxygen is carried at a low partial pressure of oxygen so that the curve showing the relationship becomes steeper as illustrated in Figure 7.8. From this graph it can be deduced that, assuming arterial PaO_2, blood flow/cardiac output and oxygen consumption remain unchanged, the arterial and venous concentration end-points are both shifted to the left, that is to a lower PaO_2, but the (a-v) oxygen content difference is maintained constant.

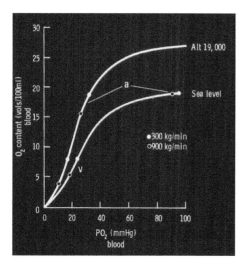

Figure 7.8   Haemoglobin–oxygen association and oxygen delivery at altitude

HbO$_2$ dissociation curves for blood at sea level and at 19,000 feet (5,800 meters) showing the effect of increased haemoglobin concentration on oxygen content (vertical axis) at decreasing blood PO$_2$ (horizontal axis). At high altitude arterial O$_2$ content will move to left and upwards indicating higher delivery at a lower partial pressure of oxygen. This enables similar oxygen delivery when exercising at high altitude to that at sea level as indicated by the arterial a and mixed venous v points at two work rates 300 kg. min^{-1} closed circles and 900 kg. min^{-1} open circles. Based on Pugh (1964b).

Furthermore, because of the shape of the oxygen association curve and the shift of the arterial oxygen point on to the steep part of the curve, the difference between the arterial and venous oxygen tensions is less. The adjustment is apparent at rest and also during exercise, as shown for work rates of 300 kg. min^{-1} and 900 kg. min^{-1} (Pugh, 1964b). These changes accompanying the increased haemoglobin indicate there has been an automatic adjustment of blood oxygen conductance, and so the amount of oxygen delivered to the tissues per litre of blood at a lower oxygen tension is similar to that at sea level. Without such an adaptation, maintenance of the arterial oxygen delivery to the tissues would require an increased cardiac output, an energy-intensive response that is better avoided when ambient oxygen levels are reduced.

However, increases in haematocrit values lead to increases in blood viscosity and this is a potent effector in reducing cerebral blood flow (Thomas *et al.*, 1977a, 1977b; Massik *et al.*, 1987). Thus, a balance needs to be achieved between the increase in number of red blood cells for carriage of oxygen and the extent of the resultant increase in viscosity. This has led to questioning the beneficial role of erythrocytosis for oxygen transport in response to hypoxia of altitude (Winslow and Monge, 1987; Winslow *et al.*, 1985) and suggested there is an optimal haematocrit value (Villafuerte *et al.*, 2004). In high-altitude populations there is a wide variation in the haematocrit value and haemoglobin concentration. Andean male highlanders living above 13,000 feet (4,000 metres) have higher haemoglobin concentrations (around 18 gm.100 mL^{-1}) than Tibetan men with mean values of 17 gm.100 mL^{-1} (Beall *et al.*, 1998). An Ethiopian sample showed they resembled Tibetans (Beall *et al.*, 2002).

Haemoglobin is contained in red blood cells and the concentration of these is controlled principally by a protein, erythropoietin (EPO). It is produced mainly in the kidney and causes differentiation of erythroid progenitor cells in bone marrow that will become haemoglobin-containing red blood cells. Erythropoietin secretion is stimulated by a reduction in oxygen delivery so that it is sensitive to hypoxia, changes in blood flow or anaemia. The oxygen-sensitive protein HIF-1α plays an important part in activation of the erythropoietin gene, as indicated previously. Not surprisingly, the concentration of EPO in the blood is raised in acclimatized visitors. At the same altitude Tibetans have lower values, whereas Andeans have higher values (Beall, 2007; Basu *et al.*, 2007).

High-altitude climbers and residents descending to lower altitudes around sea level experience a rapid reduction in red cell mass. The process is known as neocytolysis, during which young blood cells are selectively haemolyzed. On descent from altitude, arterial oxygen saturation will return to the normal 96 to 98 per cent and this, together with the now inappropriate raised haemoglobin concentration, would be expected to inhibit EPO secretion. Milledge and Cotes (1985) reported that levels were indeed reduced to 66 per cent of control values eight and 20 hours after descent to 4,000 feet (1,200 metres) following two months at or above 14,750 feet (4,500 metres). Risso *et al.* (2007) found serum EPO levels to be only 25 per cent of control values six days after descent, following 53 days at or above 14,750 feet (4,500 metres). The low EPO levels would be expected to reduce the rate of red cell production, but a study by Rice *et al.* (2001) of haematological values of high altitude residents descending to sea level, found evidence also of neocytolysis.

More recent work (reviewed by Rice and Alfrey, 2005) indicates that the process involves selective haemolysis of young red blood cells by the cells of the reticuloendothelium, especially in the spleen. These young cells are recognized by changes in their surface markers. When EPO levels fall below the critical threshold, the markers appear to undergo rapid change, making the young cells appear old. They are then phagocytosed. The process was first observed in astronauts (Alfrey *et al.*, 1996). On entering micro gravity, their plasma volume decreases, triggered by fluid shifts from lower limbs to upper body, and the haematocrit rises. Erythropoietin levels fall to below normal, triggering neocytolysis. This results in a reduction of red cell mass, bringing the haemoglobin concentration back to normal but with a reduced blood volume. The reduced blood volume may cause fainting if the astronaut stands up quickly after arrival on Earth.

Central Nervous System

Cerebral blood flow varies throughout the brain. When neurons in particular regions are more active, there is a higher level of oxidative metabolism and glucose uptake and blood flow increases proportionately in these areas. A main reason for this is increased tissue carbon dioxide (CO_2) associated with more neural activity which dilates brain blood vessels that are more sensitive to changes in CO_2 than any other vascular bed. An elegant example of this was shown in a study by Lennox and Gibbs (1932) who compared the vascular and blood flow changes in the brain with those of the leg of a human being. In addition to this, there is autoregulation, whereby arterial pressure is maintained above a critical level ($\sim$ 60 mm Hg: 8.0 kPa) to ensure there is sufficient blood flow to meet the energy demands. Cardiovascular receptors play a significant role by reflexly adjusting cardiac output and peripheral resistance.

Effect of Carbon Dioxide

The cerebral blood vessels are much more sensitive to changes in carbon dioxide than to changes in oxygen delivery or tension (Häggendal and Winsö, 1975; Lassen and Christenssen, 1976; Poulin et al., 2002). This led to the idea that inhalation of carbon dioxide at altitude may relieve the symptoms of hypoxia. This was first shown as early as 1898 by Angelo Mosso (1898) who administered carbon dioxide–oxygen mixtures to subjects exposed to pressures as low as 250 mm Hg (33.3 kPa), approximately equivalent to 28,900 feet (8,800 metres) in a hypobaric chamber, and was confirmed much later (Henderson, 1938; Douglas et al., 1913). Childs et al. (1935) suggested that inhaled carbon dioxide might be useful in climbing to great altitudes, and there has been interest in its use in aviation to counteract hypoxia in pilots (Nims 1948; Gillies, 1965; Lutz et al., 1943; Gibbs et al., 1943; Gellhorn, 1936). The effect of carbon dioxide was revisited more recently by members of the Birmingham Medical Research Expeditionary Society (Harvey et al., 1988) who showed that inhalation of 3 per cent carbon dioxide not only increased ventilation but improved arterial oxygen tensions (PaO_2) by 40 per cent and cerebral blood flow by as much as 39 per cent as measured by xenon clearance at an altitude of around 17,700 feet (5,400 metres).

It has been suggested that too large an increase in cerebral blood flow may increase the risk of acute mountain sickness or cerebral oedema since Jansen et al. (1999) reported this in a group of subjects with the condition. However, the majority of studies have not found a positive correlation (Reeves et al., 1985; Harvey et al., 1988; Jensen et al., 1990; Baumgartner et al., 1999). The conclusion is that, within limits, an increase in blood flow to the brain will improve oxygen delivery and is, therefore, of benefit in visitors to high altitude.

Effect of Hypoxia

Brain blood flow increases in response to the fall in the partial pressure of oxygen of the environment or arterial oxygen tensions (Lassen and Christensen, 1976; Poulin et al., 2002; Van Mil et al., 2002). The increase varies with altitude, but can be as much as 53 per cent above sea-level value at altitudes above 16,500 feet (5,000 metres) (Severinghaus et al., 1966; Kety and Schmidt, 1948; Jensen et al., 1990). There are no measurements so far reported of cerebral blood flow in mountaineers at high altitude (> 23,000 feet; 7,000 metres). However, studies in anaesthetized rats showed that with eucapnic hypoxia of less than 60 mm Hg (8.0 kPa) P_IO_2 there was a dramatically steep increase in cerebral blood flow, so that at a PaO_2 of 25 mm Hg (3.3 kPa), equivalent to the measured value in a climber on the summit of Everest, it was five times the normal sea-level value (Xu and La Manna, 2006). In humans, a continued stay at high altitude results in a fall from the peak of these initial increases so that the cerebral blood flow returns to values only a little above those at sea level (Severinghaus et al., 1966).

The fall in arterial oxygen tensions, as occurs on exposure to a hypoxic environment, inevitably results in a reduction in the diffusion gradient between capillary and brain parenchyma.

During acclimatization to high altitude, several mechanisms are brought into play to minimize the extent of this effect on brain function. Hyperventilation induced by the carotid body chemoreceptor (eventually reinforced by central chemoreceptor drive) improves alveolar and hence arterial oxygen tensions, so partially alleviating the amount of drop in the driving force for oxygen flux. Also oxygen delivery in terms of molecules of oxygen per minute at the end arteriole is preserved by vasodilatation in response to the fall in oxygen tension.

Vasodilatation occurs despite a fall in the tension of carbon dioxide due to hyperventilation. In time, oxygen delivery is aided by an increase in blood haemoglobin due to erythropoiesis, an effect initiated by the oxygen-sensitive hypoxia inducible factor (Semenza and Wang, 1992). The factor activates a gene expressing vascular endothelial growth factor that initiates capillary angiogenesis. As a consequence, exposure to a hypoxic environment results in an increase in brain capillary density (Diemer and Henn, 1964). There are no studies so far in humans, but recent studies in the rat show that angiogenesis begins within the first week of hypobaric hypoxia (380 mm Hg: 50.7 kPa) (~ 10 per cent inspired oxygen), and by three weeks the remodelling was complete with a 60 per cent increase in capillary density (Pichiule and LaManna, 2002).

The increase in number of capillaries per unit of cerebral tissue ensures that oxygen levels in the environment of brain cells are kept as close as possible to the arteriolar/capillary oxygen tension because it reduces the amount of oxygenated tissue close to that of the venule/capillary (Figure 7.9). This has positive consequences for the many neuronal oxygen-consuming reactions controlled by oxygenases and oxidases

where the reaction velocities become limited when the tension of oxygen falls below 80 mm Hg (10.7 kPa) and are severely limited below 40 mm Hg (5.3 kPa) (Denison, 1981). This may help to explain why hypoxia alters the enhancement of neural signals. This is known as long-term potentiation (LTP) which is explained later in the section dealing with learning and memory. The process depletes the monoamine content and turnover in the brain of rats, and interferes with synaptic transmission long before axonal conduction is affected (Davis and Carlsson, 1973).

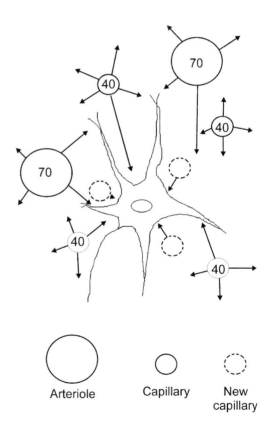

Figure 7.9   Oxygen delivery in the brain
Schematic representation of blood oxygen transfer from arterioles (large circles) and capillaries (small circles) to a neurone in the cerebral cortex in normoxia, and after a period of acclimatization to 18,000 feet (5,500 metres) when there has been an increase of new capillaries (dotted circles) which results in decreased diffusion distances. Based on data from experimental animals. Various sources (see text).

The hypoxia inducible factor also up-regulates, via gene induction, the enzymes involved in anaerobic glycolysis, and so brain glycolysis increases in both acute and chronic hypoxia, but contributes little to the energy needs of the cells. It appears that its significance is in increasing brain lactate and hence acidifying brain tissue and the cerebrospinal fluid, which otherwise would become alkaline due to the decrease in the tension of arterial carbon dioxide caused by hyperventilation. This is one mechanism that enables central chemoreceptor drive to increase during acclimatization. These changes are accompanied by increased transport of glucose across the capillary–brain barrier due to up-regulation of the glucose transporter 1 (GLUT 1). This is due, again, to HIF-1α gene induction. GLUT 1 is responsible for carrier-mediated facilitated diffusion at the capillary endothelium (Harik *et al.*, 1994; Chavez *et al.*, 2000). Therefore, there are several intrinsic and extrinsic mechanisms that allow the brain to function under low-oxygen conditions. Much, though, still needs to be learned about the role of these and other mechanisms in the brain of humans, particularly those adapted to living and working at high altitude.

Tissue Oxygen Distribution and Usage

Brain cells have a high energy usage needed to maintain membrane potential and synaptic transmission, axonal transport and other cellular processes. Adenosine triphosphate (ATP) is the most important source of energy and is liberated through phosphorylating oxidation driven by electron-transfer oxidase acting on the respiratory chain (Krebs cycle) in the mitochondria.

Oxygen is the terminal electron acceptor in the respiratory chain so that a greater energy (ATP) yield is provided when oxygen is available. To provide this energy for normal brain function, the brain uses about 20 per cent of total body oxygen uptake at rest, supplied by about 15 per cent of cardiac output. To aid the oxygen delivery to neurons, there is a branching capillary network that is concentrated in the brain grey matter where it is amongst the densest of any tissue in the body. This ensures that diffusion distance from the blood to neurons is small (Figure 7.9).

In addition, there is a high transfer of oxygen from small arterioles as well as from the capillaries (Figure 7.9), about three times higher than in skeletal muscle (Tsai *et al.*, 2003), so that the perivascular gradient for oxygen is high. Despite this, because of the high metabolism and uptake of oxygen by neurons, the distribution of oxygen tensions within the brain parenchyma is shifted to lower values so there is a high oxygen gradient between the vessel and interstitium. In the rat cerebral cortex, more than 50 per cent of measurements of oxygen tensions are less than 10 mm (1.3 kPa) and only 10 per cent of sites have values around 40 mm Hg (5.3 kPa) (Tsai *et al.*, 2003).

With acute systemic hypoxia, as occurs on ascent to high altitude, the high gradient of oxygen tension from arteriole and capillary to tissue will inevitably decrease and so oxygen delivery is compromised. There are several changes that attempt to limit the effect on brain function, some of which have been referred to earlier. Acutely, cerebral vessel dilatation increases cerebral blood flow and the carotid chemoreceptor-induced hyperventilation reduces the magnitude of decrease in oxygen tension in the blood supplying the brain.

During acclimatization, oxygen delivery is further improved by an increase in the number of red blood cells due to hypoxia-induced release of erythropoietin which stimulates erythropoiesis. Perhaps most importantly, the oxygen environment close to neurons is improved by a lessening of the diffusion distance by angiogenesis leading to an increase in the number of capillaries and small arterioles (Figure 7.9). According to studies on experimental animals exposed to hypoxia for three weeks, the number of capillaries in the cortex may double (LaManna *et al.*, 2004; LaManna, 2007). The target genes for erythropoiesis and for angiogenesis are activated by the hypoxia-sensitive transcription factor HIF-1α, as described in a previous section.

Although these structural and functional changes limit the impact of the fall in oxygen delivery, they cannot entirely compensate, so that some alterations in brain function do occur at quite low altitudes. Part of the reason is that the velocity of action of any oxygen-consuming process is a function of the partial pressure of oxygen in solution. This is usually expressed by the Michaelis constant (K_M) of a reaction which is the pressure (concentration) at which the reaction proceeds at half its maximum velocity. To illustrate, a series of curves for different oxygen dependent reactions is given in Figure 7.10. Oxidative phoshorylation has a low K_M or high affinity, so that ATP-dependent neuronal processes such as membrane potential and conduction are unaffected until oxygen pressure falls to quite low levels. However, neuronal mechanisms controlled by oxygenases and oxidases that use chemical bonding with molecular oxygen have a higher K_M.

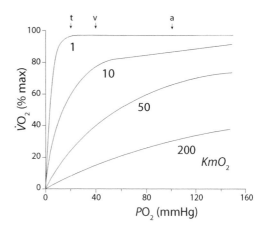

Figure 7.10 Effect of oxygen partial pressure on rate of different oxygen-consuming reactions

Schematic illustration of Michaelis curves for a series of 4 hypothetical oxygen consuming reactions with K_M values of 1, 10, 50, 200 mm Hg, encompassing oxidative phosporylation (high affinity, low K_M < 1mm Hg) to oxygenation and oxidative reactions (lower affinity, K_M > 5 mm Hg), that are known to participate in cell function. Oxygen consumption on ordinate and partial pressure of oxygen (linearly related to substrate concentration) on abscissa. (a, arterial PO2; v, venous PO_2; t, brain parenchyma PO_2 during normoxia).

Learning and Memory

Such reactions are involved in learning and memory which involve the neocortex and structures in the medial temporal lobe including the hippocampus. In the hippocampus, transmission has been shown to be enhanced for a long time following a brief burst of stimuli in a process termed long-term potentiation (LTP). Long-term potentiation is thought to be a neural process underlying learning and memory, and such an event at the synapse includes activation of a type of glutamate receptor known as the N-methyl-D-aspartate (NMDA) receptor on the post-synaptic membrane. After activation by a neurotransmitter, this receptor only allows a limited amount of calcium entry into the post-synaptic cell, initially causing a small membrane depolarization that then leads to activation of a second class of glutamate receptor, the α-amino-3-hydroxy-5-methyl-4-isoxazolepropionic acid (AMPA) receptor. As a consequence, more calcium channels open and there is a large increase in calcium-dependent post-synaptic currents, a strong depolarization of the membrane and action potential generation.

The rise in intracellular calcium activates two protein kinases, protein kinase C and calcium calmodulin-dependent protein kinase II (CaMKII), which phosphorylate the AMPA receptors and so increase the ionic conductance of the channel for calcium entry. In addition, activation of the kinases leads to insertion of new AMPA receptors into the post-synaptic membrane. The biochemical pathways involving the kinases require molecular oxygen. Thus, the change in the synapse associated with LTP is very vulnerable to hypoxia. This has been shown by *in vitro* studies on mice and rat hippocampi where lowering the oxygen levels reduces LTP and leads to irreversible impairment of synaptic transmission (Arai *et al.*, 1990; Tsien *et al.*, 1995; Sekhon *et al.*, 1998; Huang and Hsu, 2001). In accord with these experimental approaches are data from humans showing that various measures of short-term memory are decreased after exposure to acute hypobaric hypoxia for as little as one hour (Du *et al.*, 1999). The maintained modification of the synapse that is needed for memory consolidation is also going to be affected by hypoxia since it is dependent on the synthesis of new protein. This occurs via generation of gene expression by a transcription factor (cAMP response element binding (CREB) protein) that is activated by phoshorylation by a protein kinase again using pathways that involve oxygen. Hence, a reduction in reaction velocity due to decreased pressure of oxygen is a likely explanation for the reported inability to memorize novel information at high altitude.

Longer-term disruption in brain function in low-oxygen environments is likely also to be a consequence of impairment of synthesis of neurotransmitters. For example, the synthesis of brain monoamines are rate-limited by the enzyme tyrosine hydroxylase in the case of dopamine, noradrenaline and adrenaline or tryptophan hydroxylase in the case of serotonin, both enzymes requiring molecular oxygen (Siesjo, 1978). In support of this are data from rats showing that measures that improve the synthesis of brain amines protect against the deleterious effects of hypobaric hypoxia (Boismare *et al.*, 1980). Also, the re-uptake of glutamate and formation of the gaseous transmitter nitric oxide, which participate in new tasks, are processes requiring oxidation, and these transmitters are involved in numerous brain pathways. These reactions are severely impaired when the oxygen tensions are reduced to around 50 mm Hg (6.7 kPa). Proof of this has come from experimental animal studies showing that hypoxia altered the content of neurotransmitters, their turnover and synaptic transmission long before axonal conduction was affected (Siesjo, 1978; LaManna, 2007). The high sensitivity (K_M – see Figure 7.10) of the oxygen-consuming processes involved in LTP is a likely explanation for the learning deficits demonstrated in subjects exposed to a mild hypoxia of 8,000 feet (2,500 metres) (Denison, 1981), confirmed by Farmer *et al.* (1991), where the partial pressure of oxygen in the blood will be around 50 mm Hg (6.7 kPa). It is also very likely that this contributes to the marked disturbances of cognitive and psychomotor behaviour reported during exposure to altitudes above 13,000 feet (4,000 metres).

As well as these transient effects of hypoxia, there is much evidence from studies on rats and mice suggesting how long-term or permanent brain damage may occur. Severe hypoxia causes irreversible neuronal injury and neurodegeneration (Tsien *et al.*, 1995; Furling *et al.*, 2000; Titus *et al.*, 2007; Jayalakshmi *et al.*, 2007; Barhwal *et al.*, 2007). The likely explanation for the neuronal damage is that oxidative stress induced by a low partial pressure of oxygen at altitude will lead to generation of oxygen free radicals that react rapidly with many biological molecules. These include DNA and certain cell proteins, leading to apoptosis; also polyunsaturated fatty acids of membrane lipids leading to disruption of membrane integrity and triggering calcium overflow into the neuron (Musleh *et al.*, 1994; Barhwal *et al.*, 2007; Jayalakshmi *et al.*, 2007). The neuropathology of permanent brain damage induced by the hypobaric hypoxia of extreme altitudes is dealt with in Chapter 8 (Profound Hypoxia: Extreme Altitude and Space).

Part 3:
LOWLAND VISITORS AND HIGH-ALTITUDE RESIDENTS

It is surprising that those adapted to lifelong hypoxia have less of an hypoxic ventilatory response (HVR) than do visitors (Moore, 2000). The functional consequence is illustrated schematically in Figure 7.6, where ventilation in an adapted highlander in response to a similar degree of hypoxia to that of an acclimatized person would result in an alveolar oxygen tension at point C somewhere between that of the acute (A) and prolonged exposed visitor (B). The actual value at point C will depend on the HVR. However, there are distinct differences between high-altitude populations resident on the Tibetan plateaux and the Andes of South America. A comparative analysis of residents at an average altitude of 12,900 feet (3,900 metres) found that the mean HVR of Tibetans was around double that of Andeans (Beall, 2001). Thus, it was found that Tibetans had a higher resting ventilation of around 15.0 litres min^{-1} compared with 10.5 litres min^{-1} for the Andeans. Despite this, the value of the arterial oxygen tension and haemoglobin saturation in Tibetans was found to be lower than in a sample of Andeans living at a similar altitude (Beall *et al.*, 1997, 1999). Since both groups have a similar basal metabolic rate (BMR) and maximum oxygen consumptions (VO_2max), it appears that the higher ventilatory sensitivity to hypoxia in Tibetans is necessary for them to achieve this, whilst Andeans manage to do so with a lower HVR.

Importantly, this suggests there are differences in the way mechanisms involved in the oxygen transport cascade are engaged to sustain a similar aerobic metabolism between the two highland groups. Thus, although hyperventilation is an important feature of life at high altitude, the extent is dissimilar not only amongst well-acclimatized visitors, but also across different populations of high-altitude dwellers. Furthermore, for those adapted residents, levels of ventilation reached at exercise using identical oxygen consumption to lowlanders at the same altitude is less. For example, in one study in Sherpas, it was 20 to 30 per cent decreased, and the maximal oxygen consumption (VO_2max) was higher compared with acclimatized lowlanders (Pugh *et al.*, 1964; Lahiri *et al.*, 1972). This adaptive feature in Sherpas would ensure that more of the oxygen taken up is delivered to limb muscles and vital tissues other than respiratory muscles.

In contrast with high-altitude dwellers, lowland visitors, in the first few weeks at altitude, have an increased basal metabolic rate (BMR) and therefore require more oxygen at rest. Also, at the other extreme of energy expenditure, maximum work ($\dot{V}O_2$max) is decreased. Thus, the range for increasing oxygen uptake above basal levels is decreased compared with sea level, unlike that of high-altitude residents. This suggests that acclimatization would be better in lowlanders who have a high $\dot{V}O_2$max to start with. Richalet et al. (1988b) provided strong evidence for this in a prospective study of 128 climbers taking part in expeditions to extreme altitudes, whose $\dot{V}O_2$max measured at sea level correlated positively with the height achieved.

It might then be presupposed that endurance athletes with known high $\dot{V}O_2$max would perform better at altitude than non-athlete mountaineers. However, when a group of high-performance endurance athletes was compared with a group of mountaineers, this proved not to be the case (Schoene, 1982). A reason might be that highly trained endurance athletes generally develop a lower HVR (Byrne-Quinn et al., 1971), a training-conditioned change considered important to high performance at sea level. Thus, it would seem advantageous for good performance at high altitude that a high $\dot{V}O_2$max and a brisk HVR in response to a decreased level of oxygen are prerequisite in lowland visitors. However, within those so advantaged there are differences in their respiratory efficiency that enable some to perform better at extreme altitude. For example, there are several reports that some elite climbers with a lower HVR than fellow climbers have performed better at high altitudes (Milledge et al., 1983; Schoene et al., 1987; Oelz et al., 1986; Bernardi

et al., 2008). Also Richalet et al. (1988b) found that HVR did not correlate positively with height reached in a group of climbers who had been on various expeditions to high altitudes. Strikingly, of the two Europeans to reach the summit of Mount Everest first without supplementary oxygen, one had a lower HVR (Schoene et al., 1987).

An explanation is provided by Bernardi et al. (2008) who, in a carefully conducted study, found that of 11 climbers on Mount Everest and on K2 (the second highest mountain after Mount Everest) the five climbers who were successful in reaching the summits without supplementary oxygen all had lower HVR as well as lower minute ventilation relative to those who required supplementary oxygen or did not succeed. Furthermore, at lower altitudes the difference between resting ventilation and maximum voluntary ventilation was greater in the five summiteers. This would mean that at any given altitude less of the oxygen taken up would be needed for supplying the respiratory muscles. Significantly, the lower ventilation at rest in the more successful group did not compromise their arterial oxygen saturation relative to that of the other climbers, indicating that they adapted with a better respiratory efficiency. Thus, it was suggested that a relatively less sensitive hypoxic response of the five summiteers increased their ventilatory reserve (extent to which ventilation can increase) and allowed a sustainable ventilation in the severe hypoxia at the summits. Therefore, although changes in ventilation and its control are significant factors in acclimatization and adaptation, the main factor is oxygen uptake and delivery to the tissues. This has been achieved in different ways and by different mechanisms in humans and across the animal kingdom.

Central Nervous System

Important to brain function in those living permanently at high altitude is the responsiveness of cerebral blood flow to hypoxia and changes in arterial carbon dioxide tensions. This is less in Andeans compared with Tibetans and with visitors (Norcliffe *et al.*, 2005; Appenzeller *et al.*, 2004; Sun *et al.*, 1996; Jansen *et al.*, 2000), as referred to earlier. Despite the difference in responsiveness, in general, at rest cerebral blood flow in high-altitude residents has a similar range of values to those of sea-level residents with similar haematocrits. However, there is a linear decrease in blood flow with increasing haematocrit in those living at high altitude (Milledge and Sorensen, 1972; McVergnes *et al.*, 1973; Sorensen *et al.*, 1974). This has significant consequences for those high-altitude residents with excessive erythrocytosis (Sun *et al.*, 1996; Norcliffe *et al.*, 2005), a condition known as chronic mountain sickness (CMS) (Monge, 1942), in which the resulting increase in blood viscosity adds to the impairment of the normal compensatory increases in brain blood flow during sleep.

Features of the condition are described in detail by Winslow and Monge (1987) and by Heath and Williams (1989). Those affected typically appear cyanotic and have rather vague neuropsychological complaints including headache, dizziness, paraesthesia, somnolence, fatigue, difficulty in concentration and loss of mental acuity. They may also be irritable, depressed and hallucinate. Dyspnoea on exertion is not a common complaint, but poor exercise tolerance is common and they may gain weight. A characteristic feature of the disease is that symptoms disappear on returning to sea level, only to reappear on return to altitude (West *et al.*, 2007).

Chronic mountain sickness is prevalent in the Quechua and Aymara Indians of the Andes, but has been described in Caucasians in the North American Rockies, in Han Chinese living on the Tibet plateau, in Ethiopian highlanders and in mountain dwellers of the south-western heights (Asir) of Saudi Arabia.

Those with chronic mountain sickness have a blunted hypoxia ventilatory response, and, since breathing during sleep is shallower, periods of severely low oxygen saturation can occur without arousal (Weil *et al.*, 1978; Coote *et al.*, 1992, 1993; Sun *et al.*, 1996; Spicuzza *et al.*, 2004). Therefore, it has been proposed that sleep-related hypoxaemia may be a strong stimulus to erythrocytosis and worsen or even be a cause of the polycythaemia (Beall *et al.*, 1983; Coote, 1994; Sun *et al.*, 1996; Spicuzza *et al.*, 2004). It appears that the situation is made worse by an impaired autoregulation of cerebral blood vessels (Roach *et al.*, 2001; Claydon *et al.*, 2005b).

Sleep

At sea level, normal sleep consists of two different states that are recognizable by the pattern of neuronal activity of the cerebral cortex recorded electroencephalographically. The two states are commonly known as non-rapid eye movement (NREM) and rapid eye movement (REM) sleep. NREM sleep is made up of four stages, progressing from light sleep (stage 1) to deep sleep (stage 4) with REM periods of so-called 'active sleep' interposed – as indicated in a time plot of these stages (hypnogram) for a subject sleeping at sea level (Figure 7.11a). Anyone who has stayed at altitude as low as 3,000 metres knows that sleep is often disrupted and of poor quality (Coote, 1994; Jafarian *et al.*, 2008).

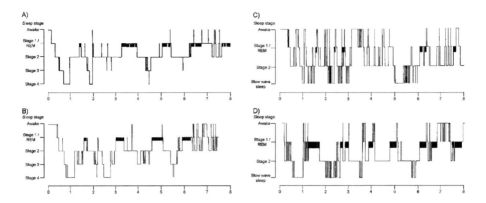

Figure 7.11 Hypnograms showing effect of altitude on sleep structure
A) hypnogram of lowland subject sleeping at < 600 feet (200 metres). The graph shows on vertical axis stages of sleep 1–4 and REM(thick line) and wakefulness plotted throughout the night (hrs, horizontal axis) from records obtained with a Medilog recorder. (from Coote et al., 1992 with permission). B) hypnogram showing typical sleep pattern of a young healthy high altitude Andean sleeping at 14,300 feet (4,330 metres) (from Coote et al., 1992). C) hypnogram of lowland subject sleeping at >14,300 feet (4,330 metres) after ingesting a placebo pill, showing sleep is much more disturbed with numerous awakenings, a reduction in both REM and non-REM. D) hypnogram of lowland subject sleeping at same altitude as in C but after ingesting temazepam (10mg). Here there is more REM sleep, and fewer awakenings. (from Nicholson *et al.*, 1988 with permission).

During sleep the brain is active and requires increased amounts of oxygen and nutrients. To supply these, brain blood flow increases. This occurs against a background of other autonomic changes. Studies in sleeping animals, such as cats and rats, under normoxic conditions indicate that there is a non-uniform distribution of cardiac output that is finely tuned by the peripheral arterial chemoreceptors. These receptors ensure a balance of vasodilatation and vasoconstriction in organs throughout the body, so that the increase in brain blood flow is maintained throughout the sleep period (Mancia and Zanchetti, 1980; Coote, 1982). It is likely that similar cardiovascular events occur in humans (Lassen and Christensen, 1976; Jones *et al.*, 1982) which help to ensure a suitable level of oxygen availability to neurons and other cells of the brain.

Disordered Breathing

Sleep at sea level is also associated with marked changes in ventilation. During non-rapid eye movement (NREM) sleep, there is a decrease in minute volume, P_ACO_2 rises by up to 6 mm (0.8 kPa) and P_AO_2 can fall by as much as 9 mm Hg (1.2 kPa) (Coote, 1982, 1994; Douglas and Haldane, 1909). At sea level, these blood gas and ventilatory changes have little effect on arterial saturation of oxygen because they lie on the flat part of the haemoglobin–oxygen association curve. However, at the low barometric pressures of altitude, the decreases in ventilation during sleep will result in significant falls in arterial oxygen saturation (Reed and Kellog, 1960) because the arterial value now lies on the steep part of the oxygen saturation curve. Thus, at altitude, changes in blood flow to the brain and/or in ventilation could affect oxygen delivery and disturb sleep and associated brain activity. Detailed accounts of the changes during sleep at altitude are provided in reviews by Coote (1994) and West *et al.* (2007). A brief summary appears here.

Based on hypobaric chamber studies (Millar and Horvath, 1977a, 1977b) and of European lowland residents sleeping high in the Swiss Alps (Smith *et al.*, 1989), sleep efficiency (ratio of total sleep time over time in bed) is first seen to be reduced by about 10 per cent at 11,500 to 12,500 feet (3,500 to 3,800 metres). In accord, a recent hypobaric chamber study simulating the cabin altitude (8,000 feet; 2,438 metres) experienced by crew members on ultra-long commercial flights, found no significant changes in any aspect of sleep, compared with ground-level sleep (Muhm *et al.*, 2009). Sleep onset is slower, stage 1 sleep and the number of awakenings are increased, and there is a small reduction in the amount of NREM and REM sleep. A similar picture emerged in a study of lowland residents of northern India (Ladakh) who slept at 11,500 feet (3,500 metres) (Selvamurthy *et al.*, 1986). It is, therefore, generally agreed that there is an altitude threshold for sleep disturbance and that some lowlanders are affected around 10,000 to 11,500 feet (3,000 to 3,500 metres). Above 13,000 feet (4,000 metres) it is clear that sleep of virtually all visitors becomes unequivocally disturbed as shown in the hypnogram (Figure 7.11c). At this and high altitudes (> 19,700 feet; 6,000 metres) visitors have difficulty falling asleep, sleep efficiency is reduced by more than 30 per cent, awake activity increases by five times or more, NREM sleep decreases by 40 per cent or more, and REM sleep is decreased by 45 per cent or more. These disturbances persist during stays at these altitudes, although robust measurements have only been made for eight days up to 19,700 feet (6,000 metres) (Nicholson *et al.*, 1988; Smith *et al.*, 1989; Coote *et al.*, 1993; Finnegan *et al.*, 1985). Temazepam (10mg orally) improves the structure and quality of sleep (Figure 7.11d) and next-day performance is better (Nicholson *et al.*, 1988; Nickol *et al.*, 2006).

Circulatory Events

In visitors to high altitude, the initial increase in cerebral blood flow in the awake subject returns to normal sea-level values within a few days of ascent (Severinghaus *et al.*, 1966). No studies have so far been made of cerebral blood flow in visitors or high-altitude residents during sleep at altitude. However, cerebrovascular responses are impaired in high-altitude Andean residents (Norcliffe et al., 2005) and can be deficient in those with chronic mountain sickness (Sun *et al.*, 1996) where there is also a measurable degree of sleep-related hypoxaemia (Spicuzza *et al.*, 2004). Part of the reason for disturbed sleep at high altitude is due to changes in ventilation. In lowland visitors to high altitude one of the most characteristic features of sleep is the development of periodic breathing with apnoea. The ventilatory patterns take the form of three or four increasingly larger breaths in quick succession followed by a cessation of breathing for ten seconds or more. Much has been written about this and there are excellent summaries by Heath and Williams (1989) and West *et al.* (2007). A recent hypobaric chamber study simulating the airline cabin altitude of 8,000 feet (2,438 metres) reported that baseline blood oxygen saturation remained relatively stable throughout the sleep period (Muhm *et al.*, 2009), which would suggest that ventilatory apnoeas were sparse at this altitude. Above this altitude, episodic apnoeas increase markedly, as was shown in a study of climbers sleeping between 9,000 feet (2,750 metres) to 11,975 feet (3,650 metres) in the Himalayas (Nicholson *et al.*, 1988). Thereafter, the incidence of apnoeas during sleep increases with altitude varying from a mean of 10 per night at sea level to more than 200 per night at 5,400 metres and higher (Weil et al., 1978; West et al., 1986; Coote et al., 1993; Coote, 1994). Apnoeas can occur in any stage of sleep, but are usually more frequent during drowsy sleep (stage 1) and early NREM sleep (stage 2).

Pronounced fluctuations in arterial oxygen saturations amounting from 5 to 15 per cent occur during periodic breathing at altitude (Lahiri and Barnard, 1983; West et al., 1986; Normand et al., 1990; Coote et al., 1993; Coote, 1994). The more severe levels of desaturation result in awakening and hence the number of awakenings increases with higher altitudes. On awakening, ventilation increases and oxygen saturation increases so that arousal protects against too great a degree of hypoxaemia. Thus, for improved sleep, a relatively brisk HVR reflecting increased peripheral chemoreceptor responsiveness is advantageous to climbers who consequently have a higher PaO_2 and are able to attain and spend many nights at high altitude (> 26,000 feet; 8,000 metres) (Eichenberger et al., 1996; Schoene et al., 1984; Matsuyama et al., 1986). The same is true even at a moderate altitude around 16,500 feet (5,000 metres), as found in a study by the Birmingham Medical Research Expeditionary Society to Gondokoro (18,500 feet; 5,620 metres) in the Karakorum, as reported by Coote (1994). These studies revealed that in general those who did not acclimatize well had a poorer HVR associated with lower SaO_2 and hence lower respiratory efficiency. See earlier discussion of HVR and the study by Bernardi et al. (2008).

Administration of oxygen stabilizes the breathing pattern during sleep at altitude (Douglas and Haldane, 1909; Lahiri and Barnard, 1983; Lahiri et al., 1983). This is most likely because as oxygen saturation increases (from

around 75–100 per cent in the latter studies), stimulation of peripheral chemoreceptors is diminished. The resulting fall in ventilation would then allow the P_ACO_2 to increase which would enhance stimulation of central chemoreceptors and ventilation (Figure 7.3). This explanation is supported by the observation of Lahiri et al. (1983) that adding carbon dioxide (5 per cent) to the inspired air in sleeping subjects also eliminates apnoeas. Thus, in lowland visitors who acclimatize well to high altitude, respiratory control is a highly unstable control system (Berssenbrugge et al., 1983). Damping down the sensitivity of the system limits acclimatization.

In contrast with lowland visitors, in those born and living at altitudes between 13,000 and 19,700 feet (4,000 and 6,000 metres) adaptation has resulted in lower HVR, less periodic breathing and a better sleep structure. Peruvian residents of Cerro de Pasco (13,100 feet; 4,300 metres) have more NREM and REM sleep compared with visitors sleeping at same altitude, as well as more total sleep time and fewer awakenings. However, compared with a group of Europeans sleeping at sea level in England, sleep efficiency was less (Coote et al., 1992, 1993; Coote, 1994). In the Himalayas, high-altitude residents of Ladakh show similar features of sleep structure to Andeans (Selvamurthy et al., 1986). Periodic breathing is present in most high-altitude residents so far studied – Andeans (Coote, 1994), Ladakhis (Selvamurthy et al., 1986) and Nepalese (Coote, unpublished observations). However, of seven Sherpas studied by Lahiri (Lahiri et al., 1983; Lahiri and Barnard 1983) sleeping at 18,000 feet (5,500 metres), one displayed some periodic breathing whilst the other six had a regular pattern of breathing.

Behaviour and Performance

The sensitivity of the brain to hypoxia has led to speculation regarding the degree of short- and long-term impairment in cerebral function. Decrements in neuropsychological function and in sensory and motor systems are observed at and after visits to high altitude (Virués-Ortega *et al.*, 2004). As already described, even at quite low altitude around 8,000 feet (2,500 metres), learning of complex mental tasks is slowed or is poor. At higher altitudes, reaction time, hand–eye coordination and higher cerebral cognitive function such as memory and language expression are not as good as at sea level. Psychopathological symptoms have been diagnosed in some members of expeditions to altitudes in excess of 12,800 feet (3,800 metres) and are especially manifest after stays at high altitudes. Depending on the altitude and duration of stay, mental disturbances took the form of the neurasthenic syndrome at 10,000 to 13,000 feet (3,000 to 4,000 metres), the cyclothymic syndrome at 13,000 to 16,500 feet (4,000 to 5,000 metres) and the acute organic brain syndrome at altitudes above 23,000 feet (7,000 metres). In one study, in 35 per cent of cases there were psychotic disturbances with profound disturbances of consciousness and orientation (Ryn, 1979, 1988), though whether this was in part due to trauma and stress in the subjects was not eliminated. Detailed accounts of cerebral dysfunction on ascent to high altitude, including changes in neuropsychological function, can be found in recent reviews (Basnyat *et al.*, 2000; Virues-Ortega *et al.*, 2004; Wilson *et al.*, 2009).

Transient Neurological Disturbances

These have been reported in persons ascending to altitude, particularly above 23,000 feet (7,000 metres) (Cauchy *et al.*, 2002). Symptoms include intense migraine-like headache, hyperventilation, sweating, paraesthesia, ataxia and dysphagia. The underlying mechanisms are unclear since there is usually a complete resolution of symptoms without sequelae and with a normal magnetic resonance image after return to sea level. Focal hypocapnic vasoconstriction or gas and/or clot embolism are possible, but unconfirmed, explanations. Transient cerebral oedema is another possible cause (Wohns, 1981), though in its more severe form it is usually fatal. The cerebral effects of mild hypoxia can be alleviated by the addition of carbon dioxide (3 per cent) in the inspired air. A recent study by Van Dorp *et al.* (2007) used standard aviation vigilance and tracking task performance tests. Brain oxygenation was measured with two near infrared sensors placed one either side of the midline on the forehead. Subjects were exposed either to sham hypoxia (end tidal partial pressure (PaO_2) 103 mm (13.7 kPa) without CO_2), isocapnic hypoxia (PaO_2 40 mm Hg (5.3 kPa) P_ACO_2 4 mm Hg (0.5 kPa) higher than resting values), and hypocapnic hypoxia (PaO_2 40 mm Hg (5.3 kPa) without added CO_2). Performance was worst on the hypocapnic hypoxia protocol.

In mountaineers and trekkers who ascend more slowly to moderate or high altitude, the cerebral effects of hypoxia are partly alleviated by acclimatization, slow ascent being important (McFarland, 1937a, 1937b, 1938). However, there is still some impairment even after a long stay at altitude. Members of the

Silver Hut Expedition (1960–1961) who spent three months at 19,000 feet (5,800 metres) found that mental efficiency of sorting playing cards was poor, it taking longer to place cards in correct bins, although interestingly accuracy was not impaired (Gill et al., 1964). A similar effect was noted by Cahoon (1972). Members of the 1981 American Medical Research Expedition to Mount Everest (AMREE) found that finger tapping was slowed at 20,700 feet (6,300 metres) (Townes et al., 1984). There is an indication that with very prolonged stays at high altitude the initial impairment is overcome and recovery occurs. This was apparent in Indian troops who undertook hand–eye coordination tests when on service at an altitude of 13,000 feet (4,000 metres) in Ladakh (Western Himalayas). Psychomotor efficiency decreased up to ten months and then progressively recovered to previous sea-level performance, over the ensuing 13 months (Sharma et al., 1975).

Nonetheless, at higher altitudes of 19,700 feet (6,000 metres) and more, there is evidence that certain cerebral functions are permanently damaged. In the American expedition of 1981 to Mount Everest (Townes et al., 1984), 21 members undertook a Halstead–Wepman aphasia screening test, a digit vigilance task and a verbal passage of the Wechsler memory scale. These tests were carried out at sea level before and a year after the expedition, in which members had spent time at altitudes from 21,000 to 26,000 feet (6,300 to 8,000 metres). Verbal learning and memory showed significant decline, and in the aphasia test, expressive language errors increased. Later studies by other groups have also found persistent abnormalities in similar aspects of cerebral function after ascents to various altitudes, in Polish climbers after ascent to 18,000 feet (5,500 metres) (Ryn, 1970, 1971), in seven climbers after ascents to 23,000 feet (7,075 metres) without supplementary oxygen (Cavaletti et al., 1987) and in five world-class mountaineers who had reached summits over 28,000 feet (8,500 metres) (Regard et al., 1989). However, this has not been a consistent finding in all published studies.

Tests on climbers who have spent time at altitude between 18,000 feet (5,500 metres) and around 19,700 feet (6,000 metres) have been less consistent, suggesting that there is a threshold below which levels of hypoxia become damaging to the brain. On the one hand, there are two studies on climbers who have ascended to 16,000 to 18,000 feet (5,000 to 5,500 metres) in which long-term impairment in memory tests and electroencephalographic abnormalities have been documented (Ryn, 1970, 1971; Zhongyuan et al., 1983; Cavaletti and Tredici, 1993). In addition, there are many studies concerned with the possibility of neurological impairment at altitude that have shown decrements in various aspects of brain function (see later). Nevertheless, in contrast, 22 mountaineers tested between 16 and 221 days after ascending above 16,700 feet (5,100 metres) showed no cognitive deficits (Clark et al., 1983). Similarly, Anooshiravani et al. (1999) were unable to demonstrate changes in cognitive performance in eight climbers from five to ten days after return to sea level following ascent to over 19,700 feet (6,000 metres). Imaging (magnetic resonance) was also unexceptional, though it is doubtful that these were sensitive enough to discern small changes at synapses relevant to cognition or memory. The reason why there are these differences in the degree of impact that low-oxygen environment has on individuals may be related to oxygen delivery and oxygen usage by the brain.

Residual Neurological Impairment

There are several studies showing that after return from high altitudes (> 23,000 feet; 7,000 metres) a high proportion of mountaineers have clear deterioration of mental tasks, including memory, electroencephalographic abnormalities, deficits in concentration, slowness in switching from one task to another, cortical atrophy and abnormal imaging of the brain (Ryn, 1970, 1979, 1988; Townes *et al.*, 1984; Regard *et al.*, 1989; Hornbein *et al.*, 1989; Cavaletti *et al.*, 1987; Cavalletti and Tredici, 1993; Garrido *et al.*, 1993, 1995, 1996; Fayed *et al.*, 2006). After recovery from high-altitude cerebral (o)edema (HACE), significant personality changes associated with lesions of the globus pallidus have been reported (Jeong *et al.*, 2002), and in two cases there was evidence of irreversible subcortical dementia and severe neuropsychiatric symptoms (Usui *et al.*, 2004). One imaging study has found abnormalities in the corpus callosum (Hackett *et al.*, 1998). In contrast, many climbers who have ascended to high altitude (> 7,000 metres) return healthily with no subsequent imaging changes or lasting cerebral dysfunction as measured by a battery of neuropsychological tests (Clark *et al.*, 1983; Anooshiravani *et al.*, 1999; Jason *et al.*, 1989).

Some of the cases with neurological symptoms may have a vascular origin such as vessel spasm, thrombosis, embolus or even haemorrhage (Cauchy *et al.*, 2002). Migraine with ophthalmoplegia has been reported following ascent to high altitude. There are also cases of high-altitude global amnesia and of rectus palsy due to sixth nerve ischaemia or vascular events in the sixth nerve nucleus – both resulting in diplopia. Transient ischaemic amnesia has been reported,

as well as transient blindness and retinal haemorrhage (Hackett 1987; Wohns, 1987; Sutton, 1982; McFadden *et al.*, 1981; Clarke, 2006). The nature of the cerebral pathology observed in climbers has similarities with that observed after decompressions to altitudes above 30,000 feet (10,000 metres), and is discussed further in Chapter 8 (Profound Hypoxia: Extreme Altitude and Space).

Conclusion

Hypobaric hypoxia presents significant challenges to aviation medicine and to environmental physiology, and it is studies related to the mild hypoxia of aircraft cabins, to adaptation and acclimatization at high altitudes and to decompressions at extreme altitudes that have provided the spectrum of present-day knowledge. The effects of hypobaric hypoxia range from the subtle findings in mild hypoxia that may transiently impair higher nervous function to serious disturbances of the cerebral circulation that may lead to residual neurological and behavioural impairment. The effects of mild hypoxia are specially relevant to aeromedical practice as permitted cabin altitudes would appear to be at the border of acceptable limits in terms of the potential to impair the functions of aircrew that are not learned. However, this is well appreciated and the operating cabin altitudes of future aircraft may well be kept somewhat below that of the maximum cabin altitude of 8,000 feet that is currently recommended.

Understanding the complexities of the adaptation of the central nervous system to hypoxia has been the province of the environmental physiologist. It has involved studies on residents at altitude and on mountaineers coping with even higher altitudes. These studies, supported by laboratory investigations both fundamental and applied, provide the link with aviation physiology, not only with respect to the effects of the mild hypoxia of transport aircraft, but also in defining the circumstances that could lead to permanent brain damage. Neurological and behavioural disorders are experienced transiently by some climbers, and with expeditions above 22,500 feet (7,000 metres) there may be residual impairments, not necessarily of a subtle nature. Permanent brain damage is explored further in Chapter 8 concerned with exposures to extreme altitudes that could occur in certain circumstances during a decompression in transport aircraft and in space. It would appear that the neurological disturbances that have been described in climbers are of similar aetiology to that of the permanent brain damage observed in non-human primates exposed to such decompressions.

References

Alfrey, C.P., Udden, M.M., Leach-Huntoon, C., Driscoll, T. and Pickett, M.H. 1996. Control of red blood cell mass in space flight. *Journal of Applied Physiology*, 81, 98–104.

Anooshiravani, M., Dumont, L., Mardirossof, C., Soto-Debouj, G. and Delavelle, J. 1999. Brain magnetic resonance imaging [MRI] and neurological changes after a single high altitude climb. *Medicine & Science in Sports & Exercise*, 31, 969–72.

Appenzeller, O., Passino, C., Roach, R., Gamboa, J., Gamboa, A., Bernardi, L. et al. 2004. Cerebral vasoreactivity in Andeans and headache at sea level. *Journal of the Neurological Sciences*, 219, 101–6.

Arai, A., Larson, J. and Lynch, G. 1990. Anoxia reveals a vulnerable period in the development of long-term potentiation. *Brain Research*, 511, 353–7.

Aste-Salazar, H. and Hurtado, A. 1944. The affinity of haemoglobin for oxygen at sea level and at high altitude. *American Journal of Physiology*, 142, 733–43.

Barhwal, K., Singh, S.B., Hota, S.K., Jayalakshmi, K. and Ilavazhagan, G. 2007. Acetyl-L-carnitine ameliorates hypobaric hypoxic impairment and spatial memory deficits in rats. *European Journal of Pharmacology*, 570, 97–107.

Basnyat, B., Cumbo, T.A. and Edelman, R. 2000. Acute medical problems in the Himalayas outside the setting of altitude sickness. *High Altitude Medicine & Biology*, 1, 167–74.

Basu, M., Malhotra, A.S., Pal, K., Prasad, R., Kumar, R., Prasad, B.A.K. and Sawhney, R.C. 2007. Erythropoietin levels in lowlanders and high-altitude natives at 3450m. *Aviation, Space, and Environmental Medicine*, 78, 963–7.

Baumgartner, R.W., Spyridopoulos, I., Bartsch, P., Maggiorini, M. and Oelz, O. 1999. Acute mountain sickness is not related to cerebral blood flow: A decompression chamber study. *Journal of Applied Physiology*, 86, 1578–82.

Beall, C.M. 2001. Adaptations to altitude: A current assessment. *Annual Review of Anthropology*, 30, 423–46.

Beall, C.M. 2007. Two routes to functional adaptation: Tibetan and Andean high-altitude natives. *Proceedings of the National Academy of Sciences of the United States of America*, 104, Suppl. 1, 8655–60.

Beall, C.M., Almasy, L.A., Blangero, J., Williams-Blangero, S., Brittenham, G.M., Strohl, K.P. et al. 1999. Percent of oxygen saturation of arterial hemoglobin among Bolivian Aymara at 3,900–4,000m. *American Journal of Physical Anthropology*, 108, 41–51.

Beall, C.M, Brittenham, G.M., Strohl, K.P., Blangero, J., Williams-Blangero, S., Goldstein, M.C. et al. 1998. Hemoglobin concentration of high-altitude Tibetans and Bolivian Aymara. *American Journal of Physical Anthropology*, 106, 385–400.

Beall, C.M., Decker, M.J., Brittenham, G.M., Kushner, I., Gebremedhim, A. and Strohl, K.P. 2002. An Ethiopian pattern of human adaptation to high-altitude hypoxia. *Proceedings of the National Academy of Sciences of the United States of America*, 99, 17215–8.

Beall, C.M., Strohl, K.P., Blangero, J., Williams-Blangero, S., Almasy, L.A., Decker, M.J. *et al.* 1997. Ventilation and hypoxic ventilatory response of Tibetan and Aymara high altitude natives. *American Journal of Physical Anthropology*, 104, 427–47.

Beall, C.M., Strohl, K.P. and Brittenham, G.M. 1983. Reappraisal of Andean high altitude erythrocytosis from a Himalayan perspective. *Seminars in Respiratory Medicine*, 5, 195–201.

Bernardi, L., Passino, C., Spadacini, G., Calciali, A., Robers, R., Green, R. *et al.* 1998. Cardiovascular autonomic modulation and activity of carotid baroreceptors at altitude. *Clinical Science*, 95, 565–73.

Bernardi, L., Roach, R.C., Key, C., Spicuzza, L., Passino, C., Bonfichi, M. *et al.* 2003. Ventilation, autonomic function, sleep and erythropoietin: Chronic mountain sickness of Andean natives. *Advances in Experimental Medicine and Biology*, 543, 161–75.

Bernardi, L., Schneider, A., Pomodori, L., Paullucci, E. and Cogo, A. 2008. Hypoxic ventilatory response in successful extreme altitude climbers. *European Respiratory Journal*, 27, 165–71.

Berssenbrugge, A., Dempsey, J., Iber, C., Skatral, J. and Wilson, P. 1983. Mechanisms of hypoxia-induced periodic breathing during sleep in humans. *Journal of Physiology*, 343, 507–26.

Blaber, A.P., Hartley, T. and Pretorius, P.J. 2003. Effect of acute exposure to 3660 m altitude on orthostatic responses and tolerance. *Journal of Applied Physiology*, 95, 591–601.

Boismare. F., Le Poncin-Lafitte, M. and Rapin, J.R. 1980. Blockade of the different enzymatic steps in the synthesis of brain amines and memory (CAR) in hypobaric hypoxic rats treated and untreated with L-dopa. *Aviation, Space, and Environmental Medicine*, 51, 126–8.

Boushel, R., Calbert, J.A., Radegran, G., Sondergaard, H., Wagner, P.D. and Saltin, B. 2001. Parasympathetic neural activity accounts for the lowering of exercise heart rate at high altitude. *Circulation*, 104, 785–91.

Bouverot, P., Flandrois, R., Puccinelli, R. and Dejours, P. 1965. Étude du rôle des chemoréceptuers artériels dans la régulation de la respiration pulmonaire chez le chien éveillé. *Archives Internationales de Pharmacodynamie et de Thérapie*, 157, 253–71.

Byrne-Quinn, E., Weil, S.V., Sodal, I.E., Filley, G.F. and Grover, R.F. 1971. Ventilatory control in athletes. *Journal of Applied Physiology*, 30, 91–8.

Cahoon, R.L. 1972. Simple decision making at high altitude. *Ergonomics*, 15, 157–63.

Calbet, J.A. 2003. Chronic hypoxia increases blood pressure and noradrenaline spillover in healthy humans. *Journal of Physiology*, 551, 379–86.

Carlile, S. and Paterson, D.J. 1992. The effects of chronic hypoxia on human auditory system sensitivity. *Aviation, Space, and Environmental Medicine*, 63, 1093–7.

Cauchy, E., Larmignat, P., Boussuges, A., Le Roux, G., Charnoit, J.-C., Dumas, J.-L. and Richalet, J.-P. 2002. Transient neurological disorders during simulated ascent of Mount Everest. *Aviation, Space, and Environmental Medicine*, 73, 1224–9.

Caveletti, G., Moroni, R., Garavaglia, P. and Tredici, G. 1987. Brain damage after high-altitude climbs without oxygen. *Lancet*, 1, 101.

Caveletti, G. and Tredici, G. 1993. Long-lasting neuropsychological changes after a single high altitude climb. *Acta Neurologica Scandinavica*, 87, 103–5.

Chavez, J.C., Agani, F., Pichiule, P. and LaManna, J.C. 2000. Expression of hypoxic inducible factor 1a in the brain of rats during chronic hypoxia. *Journal of Applied Physiology*, 89, 1937–42.

Childs, S.B., Hamlin, H. and Henderson, Y. 1935. Possible value of inhalation of carbon dioxide in climbing great altitudes. *Nature*, 135, 457–8.

Clar, C., Dorrington, K.L., Fatemian, M. and Robbins, P.A. 2001. Effects of 8h of isocapnic hypoxia with and without muscarinic blockade on ventilation and heart rate in humans. *Experimental Physiology*, 86, 529–38.

Clark, C.F., Heaton, R.K. and Wiens, A.N. 1983. Neuropsychological function after prolonged high altitude exposure in mountaineering. *Aviation, Space, and Environmental Medicine*, 54, 202–7.

Clarke, C. 2006. Neurology at high altitude. *Practical Neurology*, 6, 230–37.

Claydon, V.E., Gulli, G., Slessarev, M., Huppert, T.J., Asseja, T., Gebru, S., Appenzeller, O. and Hainsworth, R. 2005a. Blood and plasma volumes in Ethiopian high altitude dwellers. *Clinical Autonomic Research*, 15, 325.

Claydon, V.E., Norcliffe, L.J., Moore, J.P., Rivera, M, Leon-Velarde, F., Appenzeller, O. and Hainsworth, R. 2005b. Cardiovascular responses to orthostatic stress in healthy altitude dwellers and altitude residents with chronic mountain sickness. *Experimental Physiology*, 90, 103–10.

Claydon, V.E., Norcliffe, L.J., Moore, J.P., Rivera-Ch, M., Leon-Velarde, F., Appenzeller, O. and Hainsworth, R. 2004. Orthostatic tolerance and blood volumes in Andean high altitude dwellers. *Experimental Physiology*, 89, 565–71.

Cooper, V.L., Pearson, S.B., Bowker, C.M., Elliot, M.W. and Hainsworth, R. 2005. Interaction of chemoreceptor and baroreceptor reflexes by hypoxia and hyperventilation. *Journal of Physiology*, 568, 677–87.

Coote, J.H. 1982. Respiratory and circulatory control during sleep. *Journal of Experimental Biology*, 100, 223–44.

Coote, J.H. 1994. Sleep at High Altitude. In: R. Cooper (ed.) *Sleep*. London: Chapman Hall Medical, 243–64.

Coote, J.H., Stone, B.M. and Tsang, G. 1992. Sleep of high altitude natives. *European Journal of Applied Physiology*, 64, 178–81.

Coote, J.H., Tsang, G., Baker, A. and Stone, B.M. 1993. Respiratory changes and quality of sleep in young high-altitude dwellers in the Andes of Peru. *European Journal of Applied Physiology*, 66, 249–53.

Cornolo, J., Mollard, P., Brugniaux, J.V., Robach, P. and Richalet, J.P. 2004. Autonomic control of the cardiovascular system during acclimatization to high altitude: Effects of sildenafil. *Journal of Applied Physiology*, 97, 935–40.

Cummin, A.R.C. and Nicholson, A.N. 2002. *Aviation Medicine and the Airline Passenger*. London: Arnold.

Davis, J.N. and Carlsson, A. 1973. Effect of hypoxia on tyrosine and tryptophan hydroxylation in unanaesthetized rat brain. *Journal of Neurochemistry*, 20, 913–5.

Dejours, P. 1957. Intérêt méthodologique de l'étude d'un organisme vivant a la phase initiale de rupture d'un équilibre physiologique. *Comptes-rendus des séances de l'academie des sciences, Série D, Sciences Naturelles*, 245, 1946–8.

Denison, D. 1981. High Altitude and Hypoxia. In: O.G. Edholm and J.S. Weiner (eds) *The Principles and Practice of Human Physiology*. London: Academic Press, 241–307.

Denison, D.M., Ledwith, F. and Poulton, E.C. 1966. Complex reaction times at simulated cabin altitudes of 5000 feet and 8000 feet. *Aerospace Medicine*, 37, 1010–13.

Diemer, K. and Henn, R. 1964. The capillary density in the frontal lobe of mature and premature infants. *Biologia Neonatorum*, 7, 270–79.

Douglas, C.G. and Haldane, J.S. 1909. The causes of periodic or Cheyne-Stokes breathing. *Journal of Physiology*, 38, 401–19.

Douglas, C.G., Haldane, J.S., Henderson, Y. and Schneider, E.F. 1913. Physiological observations made on Pike's Peak. *Philosophical Transactions of the Royal Society of London – Series B*, 203, 185–318.

Du, J.Y., Li, X.Y., Zhuang, Y., Wu, X.Y. and Wang, T. 1999. Effects of acute mild and moderate hypoxia on human short memory. *Space Medicine and Medical Engineering (Beijing)*, 12, 270–73.

Duplain, H., Vollenweider, L., Delabays, A., Nicod, P., Bartsch, P. and Scherrer, U. 1999. Augmented sympathetic activation during short-term hypoxia and high-altitude exposure in subjects susceptible to high altitude pulmonary edema. *Circulation*, 99, 1713–8.

Eichenberger, U., Weiss, E., Rieman, D., Oelz, O. and Bartsch, P. 1996. Nocturnal periodic breathing and the development of acute high altitude illness. *American Journal of Respiration and Critical Care Medicine*, 154, 1748–54.

Farmer, E.W., Lupa, H.T., Dunlop, F. and McGowan, J.F. 1991. Task Learning Under Mild Hypoxia. In: J.R. Sutton, G. Coates and C.S. Houston (eds) *Hypoxia and Mountain Medicine: Advances in the Biosciences*, 84, 1–8.

Fayed, N., Modrego, P.J. and Morales, H. 2006. Evidence of brain damage after high-altitude climbing by means of magnetic resonance imaging. *American Journal of Medicine*, 119, 68, e1–6.

Finnegan, T.P., Abraham, P. and Docherty, T.B. 1985. Ambulatory monitoring of the electroencephalogram in high altitude mountaineers. *Electroencephalography and Clinical Neurophysiology*, 60, 220–4.

FitzGerald, M.P. 1913. The changes in breathing and blood at various altitudes. *Philosophical Transactions of the Royal Society of London – Series B*, 203, 351–71.

Furling, D., Ghribi, O., Lahsaini, A., Mirault, M.E. and Massicotte, G. 2000. Impairment of synaptic transmission by transient hypoxia in hippocampal slices: Improved recovery in glutathione peroxidase transgeric mice. *Proceedings of the National Academy of Sciences of the United States of America*, 11, 4351–6.

Garrido. E., Castello, A., Ventura, J.L., Capdevila, A. and Rodriguez, F.A. 1993. Cortical atrophy and other brain magnetic resonance imaging (MRI) changes after extremely high-altitude climbs without oxygen. *International Journal of Sports Medicine*, 14, 232–4.

Garrido, E., Segura, R., Capdevila, A., Aldomá, J., Rodriguez, F.A., Javierra, C. and Ventura, J.L. 1995. New evidence from magnetic resonance imaging of brain changes after climbs at extreme altitude. *European Journal of Applied Physiology*, 70, 447–81.

Garrido, E., Segura, R., Capdevila, A., Pujol, L., Javierre, C. and Ventura, J.L. 1996. Are Himalayan Sherpas better protected against brain damage with extreme altitude climbs? *Clinical Science*, 90, 81–5.

Gellhorn, E. 1936. Value of carbon dioxide in counteracting oxygen lack. *Nature*, 137, 700–701.

Gibbs, F.A., Gibbs, E.L., Lennox, W.G. and Nims, L.F. 1943. The value of carbon dioxide in counteracting the effects of low oxygen. *Journal of Aviation Medicine*, 14, 250–61.

Gill, M.B., Poulton, E.C., Carpenter, A., Woodhead, M.M. and Gregory, M.H.P. 1964. Falling efficiency at sorting cards during acclimatization at 19,000 ft. *Nature*, 203, 436.

Gillies, J.A. 1965. (ed.) *A Textbook of Aviation Physiology*. Oxford: Pergamon, 250–60.

Gradwell, D.P. 2006. Hypoxia and Hyperventilation. In: D.J. Rainsford and D.P. Gradwell (eds) *Aviation Medicine – Fourth Edition*. London: Hodder Arnold, 41–56.

Guyton, A.C. and Richardson, T.Q. 1961. Effect of hematocrit on venous return. *Circulation Research*, 9, 157–64.

Guz, A., Noble, M.I.M., Widdecombe, J.G., Trenchard, D. and Mushin, W.W. 1966. Peripheral chemoreceptors in man. *Respiration Physiology*, 1, 38–40.

Hackett, P.H. 1987. Cortical Blindness in High Altitude Climbers and Trekkers: A Report of Six Cases (Abstract). In: J.R. Sutton, C.S. Houston and G. Coates (eds) *Hypoxia and Cold*. New York, NY: Praeger, 536.

Hackett, P.H., Yarnell, P.R., Hill, R., Reynard, K., Heit, J. and McCormick, J. 1998. High-altitude cerebral edema evaluated with magnetic resonance imaging. *Journal of the American Medical Association*, 280, 1920–25.

Häggendal, E. and Winsö, I. 1975. The influence of carbon dioxide tension on cerebrovascular responses to arterial hypoxia and hemodilution. *Acta Anaesthesiologica Scandinavica*, 19, 134–45.

Hainsworth, R., Drinkhill, M.J. and Rivera-Chiva, M. 2007. The autonomic nervous system at high altitude. *Clinical Autonomic Research*, 17, 13–19.

Hansen, J. and Sander, M. 2003. Sympathetic neural overactivity in healthy humans after prolonged exposure to hypobaric hypoxia. *Journal of Physiology*, 546, 921–9.

Harik, S.I., Behmand, R.A. and LaManna, J.C. 1994. Hypoxia increases glucose transport at blood-brain barrier in rats. *Journal of Applied Physiology*, 77, 896–901.

Harvey, T.C., Winterborn, M.H., Lassen, N.A., Raichle, M.E., Jensen, J., Richardson, N.V. and Bradwell, A.R. 1988. Effect of carbon dioxide in acute mountain sickness: A rediscovery. *Lancet*, 2, 639–41.

Heath, D. and Williams, D.R. 1989. *High-Altitude Medicine and Pathology*. London: Butterworth.

Henderson, Y. 1938. *Adventures in Respiration*. London: Bailliere, Tyndall and Cox, 103–140.

Hornbein, T.F., Townes, B.D., Schoene, RB., Sutton, J.R. and Houston, C.S. 1989. The cost to the central nervous system of climbing to extremely high altitude. *New England Journal of Medicine*, 321, 1714–9.

Huang, C.C. and Hsu, K.S. 2001. Progression in understanding the factors regulating the reversibility of long-term potentiation. *Reviews in the Neurosciences*, 12, 51–68.

Jafarian, S., Gorouhi, F., Taghva, A. and Lotfi, J. 2008. High-altitude sleep disturbance: Results of the Groningen Sleep Quality Questionnaire survey. *Sleep Medicine*, 9, 446–9.

Jansen, G.F., Krins, A. and Basnyat, B. 1999. Cerebral vasomotor reactivity at high altitude in humans. *Journal of Applied Physiology*, 86, 681–6.

Jansen, G.F., Krins, A., Basnyat, B., Bosch, A. and Odoom, J.A. 2000. Cerebral autoregulation in subjects adapted and not adapted to high altitude. *Stroke*, 31, 2314–8.

Jason, G.W., Pajurkova, E.M. and Lee, R.G. 1989. High-altitude mountaineering and brain function: Neurophysiological testing of members of a Mount Everest expedition. *Aviation, Space, and Environmental Medicine*, 60, 170–73.

Jayalakshmi, K., Singh, S.B., Kalpana, B., Sairam, M., Muthuraju, S. and Ilavazhagen, G. 2007. N-acetyl cysteine supplementation prevents impairment of spatial working memory functions in rats following exposure to hypobaric hypoxia. *Physiology and Behaviour*, 92, 643–50.

Jensen, J.B., Wright, A.D., Lassen, N.A., Harvey, T.C., Winterborn, M.H., Raichle, M.E. and Bradwell, A.R. 1990. Cerebral blood flow in acute mountain sickness. *Journal of Applied Physiology*, 69, 430–33.

Jeong, J.H., Kworn, J.C., Chin, J., Yoon, S.J. and Na, D.L. 2002. Globus pallidus lesions associated with high mountain climbing. *Journal of Korean Medical Science*, 17, 861–3.

Jones, J.V., Sleight, P. and Smyth, H.S. 1982. Haemodynamic Changes During Sleep in Man. In: D. Ganten and D.W. Pfaff (eds) *Topics in Neuroendocrinology*, 1, 105–126.

Kanai, M., Nishihara, F., Shiga, T., Shimada, H. and Saito, S. 2001. Alterations in autonomic nervous control of heart rate among tourists at 2700 and 3700 m above sea level. *Wilderness and Environmental Medicine*, 12, 8–12.

Kemp, P.J. 2006. Detecting acute changes in oxygen: Will the real sensor stand up? *Experimental Physiology*, 91, 827–32.

Kety, S.S. and Schmidt, C.F. 1948. Effects of altered arterial tensions of carbon dioxide and oxygen in cerebral blood flow and cerebral oxygen consumption in young men. *Journal of Clinical Investigation*, 27, 484–92.

Klein, S.J., Mendelson, E.S. and Gallagher, T.J. 1961. The effects of reduced oxygen intake on auditory threshold shifts in a quiet environment. *Journal of Comparative and Physiological Psychology*, 54, 401.

Kline, D.D., Peng, Y.J, Manalo, D.J., Semenza, G.L. and Prabhakar, N.R. 2002. Defective carotid body function and impaired ventilatory responses to chronic hypoxia in mice partially deficient for hypoxia-inducible factor 1a. *Proceedings of the National Academy of Sciences of the United States of America*, 99, 821–6.

Kumar, P. 2007. Translating blood-borne stimuli: Chemotransduction in the carotid body. *Acta Physiologica Sinica*, 59, 128–32.

Lahiri, S. and Barnard, P. 1983. Role of Arterial Chemoreflexes in Breathing During Sleep at High Altitude. In: J.S. Sutton, C.S. Houston and N.L. Jones (eds) *Hypoxia, Exercise and Altitude*. New York, NY: Liss, 75–85.

Lahiri S., Maret, K. and Sherpa, M.G. 1983. Dependence of high altitude sleep apnea on ventilatory sensitivity to hypoxia. *Respiration Physiology*, 52, 281–301.

Lahiri, S., Milledge, J.S. and Sorensen, S.C. 1972. Ventilation in man during exercise at high altitude. *Journal of Applied Physiology*, 32, 766–9.

LaManna, J.C. 2007. Hypoxia in the central nervous system. *Essays in Biochemistry*, 43, 139–51.

LaManna, J.C., Chavez, J.C. and Pichiule, P. 2004. Structural and functional adaptation to hypoxia in the rat brain. *Journal of Experimental Biology*, 207, 3163–9.

Larsen, T.S., Rasmussen, P., Overgaard, M., Secher, N.H. and Nielsen, H.B. 2008. Non-selective beta-adrenergic blockade prevents reduction of the cerebral metabolic ration during exhaustive exercise in humans. *Journal of Physiology*, 586, 2807–15.

Lassen, N.A. and Christensen, M.S. 1976. Physiology of cerebral blood flow. *British Journal of Anaesthesia*, 48, 719–34.

Leitner, L.M., Pagès, B., Puccinelli, R. and Dejours, P. 1965a. [Simultaneous study of ventilation and glomus caroticum chemoreceptor impulses in cats. I. During brief inhalation of pure oxygen.] *Archives Internationales de Pharmacodynamie et de Thérapie*, 154, 421–6.

Leitner, L.M., Pagès, B., Puccinelli, R. and Dejours, P. 1965b. [Simultaneous study of ventilation and glomus caroticum chemoreceptor impulses in cats. II. During brief inhalation of carbon dioxide.] *Archives Internationales de Pharmacodynamie et de Thérapie*, 154, 427–33.

Lenfant, C. and Sullivan, K. 1971. Adaptation to high altitude. *New England Journal of Medicine*, 284, 1298–309.

Lennox, W.G. and Gibbs, E.L. 1932. The blood flow in the brain and the leg of man, and changes induced by alteration of blood gases. *Journal of Clinical Investigation*, 11, 1155–77.

Liu, C., Smith, T.G., Balanos, G.M., Brooks, J., Crosby, A., Herigstad, M., Dorrington, K.L. and Robbins, P.A. 2007. Lack of involvement of the autonomic nervous system in early ventilatory and pulmonary vascular acclimatization to hypoxia in humans. *Journal of Physiology*, 579, 215–25.

Lopez-Barneo, J., Lopez-Lopez, J.R., Urena, J. and Gonzalez, C. 1988. Chemotransduction in the carotid body: K+ current modulated by PO_2 in type 1 chemoreceptor cells. *Science*, 241, 580–82.

Lopez-Barneo, J., Pardel, R. and Ortega-Saenz, P. 2001. Cellular mechanisms of oxygen sensing. *Annual Review of Physiology*, 63, 259–87.

Lübbers, D.W. 1977. Quantitative Measurement and Description of Oxygen Supply to the Tissue. In: F.F. Jobsis (ed.) *Oxygen and Physiological Function*. Dallas, TX: Professional Information Library, 254–76.

Lutz, W., Wendt, H.J., van Werz, R. and Zirngibi, M. 1943. Über die Wirkung von Kohlensäure auf die erholung aus Sauerstoffmangel. *Luftfahrt Medizin*, 8, 249–55.

McFadden, D.M., Houston, C.H., Sutton, J.R., Powles, A.C.P., Gray, G.W. and Roberts, R.S. 1981. High-altitude retinopathy. *Journal of the American Medical Association*, 245, 581–6.

McFarland, R.A. 1937a. Psycho-physiological studies at high altitude in the Andes: I. The effects of rapid ascents by aeroplane and train. *Comparative Psychology*, 23, 191–225.

McFarland, R.A. 1937b. Psycho-physiological studies at high altitude in the Andes: II. Sensory and motor responses during acclimatization. *Comparative Psychology*, 23, 227–58.

McFarland, R.A. 1938. Psycho-physiological studies at high altitude in the Andes III: Mental and psychosomatic responses during gradual adaptation. *Comparative Psychology*, 24, 147–88.

McFarland, R.A. and Evans, J.N. 1939. Alterations in dark adaptation under reduced oxygen tensions. *American Journal of Physiology*, 127, 37–50.

McVerges, J.P., Blayo, M.D., Coudert, J., Autezani, G., Dediu, P. and Duvand, J. 1973. Cerebral blood flow and metabolism in high altitude residents. *Stroke*, 4, 345–50.

Mancia, G. and Zanchetti, A. 1980. Cardiovascular Regulation during Sleep. In: J. Orem and C.D. Barnes (eds) *Physiology in Sleep*. New York, NY: Academic Press, 1–55.

Massik, J., Tang, Y.L., Hudak, M.L., Koehler, R.C., Traystman, R.J. and Jones, M.D. 1987. Effect of haematocrit on cerebral blood flow with induced polycythaemia. *Journal of Applied Physiology*, 62, 1090–96.

Matsuyama, S., Kimura, H., Sugita, T., Kuriyama, T., Tatsumi, K., Kunitomo, F. *et al.* 1986. Control of ventilation in extreme altitude climbers. *Journal of Applied Physiology*, 61, 500–506.

Mazzeo, R.S., Bender, P.R., Brooks, G.A., Butterfield, G.E., Groves, B.M., Sutton, J.R. *et al.* 1991. Arterial catecholamine responses during exercise with acute and chronic high-altitude exposure. *American Journal of Physiology*, 261, E419–24.

Mazzeo, R.S., Child, A., Butterfield, G.E., Mawson, J.T., Zamudio, S. and Moore, L.G. 1998. Catecholamine response during 12 days of high altitude exposure (4,300m) in women. *Journal of Applied Physiology*, 84, 1151–7.

Milledge, J.S. 1979. Acid-base changes associated with respiratory acclimatization to altitude. *Postgraduate Medical Journal*, 55, 468–70.

Milledge, J.S. and Cotes, P.M. 1985. Serum erythropoietin in humans at high altitude and its relation to plasma renin. *Journal of Applied Physiology*, 59, 360–64.

Milledge, J.S. and Sorensen, S.C. 1972. Cerebral arteriovenous oxygen difference in man native to high altitude. *Journal of Applied Physiology*, 32, 687–9.

Milledge, J.S., Ward, M.P., Williams, E.S. and Clarke, C.R.A. 1983. Cardiorespiratory response to exercise in men repeatedly exposed to extreme altitude. *Journal of Applied Physiology*, 55, 1379–85.

Miller, J.C. and Horvath, S.M. 1977a. Sleep at altitudes. *Aviation, Space, and Environmental Medicine*, 48, 615–20.

Miller, J.C. and Horvath, S.M. 1977b. Cardiac output during sleep at altitude. *Aviation, Space, and Environmental Medicine*, 48, 621–4.

Monge, M.C. 1942. Life in the Andes and chronic mountain sickness. *Science*, 95, 79–84.

Moore, J.P., Claydon, V.E., Norcliffe, L.J., Rivera-Ch, M.C., Leon-Velarde, F., Appenzeller, O. and Hainsworth, R. 2006. Carotid baroreflex regulation of vascular resistance in high-altitude Andean natives with and without chronic mountain sickness. *Experimental Physiology*, 91, 907–14.

Moore, L.G. 2000. Comparative human ventilatory adaptation to high altitude. *Respiration Physiology*, 121, 257–76.

Mosso, A. 1898. *A Life of Man on the High Alps*. London: Fisher Unwin.

Muhm, J.M., Signal, T.L., Rock, P.B., Jones, S.P., O'Keefe, K.M., Weaver, M.R. *et al.* 2009. Sleep at simulated 2438m: Effects on oxygenation, sleep quality, and postsleep performance. *Aviation, Space, and Environmental Medicine*, 80, 691–7.

Musleh, W., Bruce, A., Malfroy, B. and Baudry, M. 1994. Effects of EUK-8, a synthetic catalytic superoxide scavenger, on hypoxia and acidosis-induced damage in hippocampal slices. *Neuropharmacology*, 33, 929–34.

Nicholson, A.N., Smith, P.A., Stone, B.M., Bradwell, A.R. and Coote, J.H. 1988. Altitude insomnia during an expedition to the Himalayas. *Sleep*, 11, 354–61.

Nickol, A.H., Leverment, J., Richards, P., Seal, P., Harris, G.A., Cleland, J. *et al.* 2006. Temazepam at high altitude reduces periodic breathing without impairing next-day performance: A randomized cross-over double-blind study. *Journal of Sleep Research*, 15, 445–54.

Nims, L.F. 1948. Anoxia in aviation. *Annual Review of Physiology*, 10, 305–14.

Norcliffe, L.J., Rivera-Ch, M., Claydon, V.E., Moore, J.P., Leon-Velarde, F., Appenzeller, O. and Hainsworth, R. 2005. Cerebrovascular responses to hypoxia and hypocapnia in high altitude dwellers. *Journal of Physiology*, 566, 287–94.

Normand, H., Barragan, M., Benoit, M., Bailliart, O. and Raynaud, J. 1990. Periodic breathing and O_2 saturation in relation to sleep stages at high altitude. *Aviation, Space, and Environmental Medicine*, 61, 229–35.

Oelz, O., Howard, H., Di Prampero, P.E., Hoppeler, H., Claassen, H., Jenni, R. *et al.* 1986. Physiological profile of world-class high-altitude climbers. *Journal of Applied Physiology*, 60, 1734–42.

Peers, C. 1990. Hypoxic suppression of K+ currents in type 1 carotid-body cells: Selective on the Ca2+ activated K+ currents. *Neuroscience Letters*, 119, 253–6.

Pelamatti, G., Pascotto, M. and Semenza, C. 2003. Verbal free recall in high altitude: Proper names vs common names. *Cortex*, 39, 97–103.

Peng, Y-J., Yuan, G., Ramakrishnan, D., Sharma, S.D., Bosch-Marce, M., Kumar, G.K. *et al.* 2006. Heterozygous HIF-1alpha deficiency impairs carotid body-mediated systemic responses and reactive oxygen species generation in mice exposed to intermittent hypoxia. *Journal of Physiology*, 577, 705–16.

Pichiule, P. and LaManna, J.C. 2002. Angiopoietin-2 and rat brain capillary remodelling during adaptation and de-adaptation to prolonged mild hypoxia. *Journal of Applied Physiology*, 93, 1131–9.

Poulin, M.J., Fatemian, M., Tansley, J.G., O'Connor, D.F. and Robbins, P.A. 2002. Changes in cerebral blood flow during and after 48h of both isocapnic and poikilocapnic hypoxia in humans. *Experimental Physiology*, 87, 633–42.

Prabhakar, N.R. 1994. Neurotransmitters in the carotid body. *Advances in Experimental Medicine and Biology*, 360, 57–69.

Prabhakar, N.R. 2006. Oxygen sensing at the mammalian carotid body: Why multiple O_2 sensors and multiple transmitters? *Experimental Physiology*, 91, 17–23.

Pugh, L.G.C.E. 1964a. Blood volume and haemoglobin concentration at altitude above 18,000 ft (5,000 m). *Journal of Physiology*, 170, 344–54.

Pugh, L.G.C.E. 1964b. Cardiac output in muscular exercise at 5,800 m (19,000 ft). *Journal of Applied Physiology*, 19, 441–7.

Pugh, L.G.C.E., Gill, M.B., Lahiri, S., Milledge, J.S., Ward, M.P. and West, J.B. 1964. Muscular exercise at great altitudes. *Journal of Applied Physiology*, 19, 431–40.

Rahn, H. and Otis, A.B. 1949. Man's respiratory response during and after acclimatization to high altitude. *American Journal of Physiology*, 157, 445–62.

Reed, D.J. and Kellog, R.H. 1960. Effect of sleep on CO_2 stimulation of breathing in acute and chronic hypoxia. *Journal of Applied Physiology*, 15, 1135–8.

Reeves, J.T., Moore, L.G., McCullough, R.E., McCullough, R.G., Harrison, G., Tranmer, B.I. *et al.* 1985. Headache at high altitude is not related to internal carotid arterial blood velocity. *Journal of Applied Physiology*, 59, 909–15.

Regard, M., Oelz, O., Brugger, P. and Landis, T. 1989. Persistent cognitive impairment in climbers after repeated exposure to extreme altitude. *Neurology*, 39, 210–13.

Richalet J.-P., Keromes, A. and Dersch, B. 1988b. Caractéristiques physiologiques des alpinistes de haute altitude. *Science and Sports*, 3, 89–108.

Richalet, J.-P., Larmignat, P., Rathat, C., Keromes, A., Baude, P. and Lhoste, F. 1988a. Decreased cardiac response to isoprotorenol infusion in acute and chronic hypoxia. *Journal of Applied Physiology*, 65, 1957–61.

Rice, L. and Alfrey, C.P. 2005. The negative regulation of red cell mass by neocytolysis: Physiological and pathophysiological manifestations. *Cellular Physiology and Biochemistry*, 15, 245–50.

Rice, L., Ruiz, W., Driscoll, T., Whitley, C.E., Tapia, R., Hachey, D.L. *et al.* 2001. Neocytolysis on descent from altitude: A newly recognized mechanism for the control of red cell mass. *Annals of Internal Medicine*, 134, 652–6.

Risso, A., Turello, M., Biffoni, F. and Antonutto, G. 2007. Red blood cell senescence and neocytolysis in humans after high altitude acclimatization. *Blood Cells and Molecular Disease*, 38, 83–92.

Roach, R., Passino, C., Bernardi, L., Gamboa, A. and Appenzeller, O. 2001. Cerebrovascular reactivity to CO_2 at high altitude and sea level in Andean natives. *Clinical Autonomic Research*, 11, 183.

Ryn, Z. 1970. Mental disorders in alpinists under conditions of stress at high altitudes. Doctoral thesis, University of Cracow, Poland.

Ryn, Z. 1971. Psychopathology in alpinism. *Acta Medica Polona*, 12, 453–67.

Ryn, Z. 1979. Nervous system and high-altitude syndrome of high-altitude asthenia. *Acta Medica Polona*, 20, 155–69.

Ryn, Z. 1988. Psychopathology in mountaineering: Mental disturbances under high-altitude stress. *International Journal of Sports Medicine*, 9, 163–9.

Sagawa, S., Torii, R., Nagaya, K., Wada, F., Endo, Y. and Shiraki, K. 1997. Carotid baroreflex control of heart rate during acute exposure to simulated altitudes of 3,800 m and 4,300 m. *American Journal of Physiology*, 273, R1219–23.

Schoene, R.B. 1982. Control of ventilation in climbers to extreme altitude. *Journal of Applied Physiology*, 53, 886–90.

Schoene, R.B., Hackett, P.H. and Roach, R.C. 1987. Blunted Hypoxic Chemosensitivity at Altitude and Sea Level in an Elite High-Altitude Climber. In: J.R. Sutton, C.S.

Houston and G. Coates (eds) *Hypoxia and Cold.* New York, NY: Praeger, 532.

Schoene, R.B., Lahiri, S., Hackett, P.B., Peters, R.M., Milledge, J.S., Pizzo, C.J. *et al.* 1984. Relationship of hypoxic ventilatory response to exercise performance on Mount Everest. *Journal of Applied Physiology*, 56, 1478–83.

Schurr, A. 2006. Lactate: The ultimate cerebral oxidative energy substrate. *Journal of Cerebral Blood Flow and Metabolism*, 26, 142–52.

Schurr, A. 2008. Lactate: A major and crucial player in normal function of both muscle and brain. Perspectives. *Journal of Physiology*, 586, 2665–6.

Sekhon, L.H., Spence, I., Morgan, M.K. and Weber, N.C. 1998. Long-term potentiation saturation in chronic cerebral hypoperfusion. *Journal of Clinical Neuroscience*, 5, 323–8.

Selvamurthy, W., Raju, V.R.K., Ranganathan, S., Hegde, K.S. and Ray, U.S. 1986. Sleep patterns at altitude of 3500 meters. *International Journal of Biometeorology*, 30, 123–35.

Semenza, G.L. 2000. HIF-1: Mediator of physiological and pathophysiological responses to hypoxia. *Journal of Applied Physiology*, 88, 1474–80.

Semenza, G.L. and Wang, G.L. 1992. A nuclear factor induced by hypoxia via de nova protein synthesis binds to the human erythropoietin gene enhancer at a site required for transcriptional activation. *Molecular and Cellular Biology*, 12, 5447–54.

Severinghaus, J.W., Chiodi, H., Eger, E.I., Brandstater, B. and Hornbein, T.F. 1966. Cerebral blood flow in man at high altitude. *Circulation Research*, 19, 274–82.

Sevre, K., Bendz, B., Hanko, E., Nakstad, A.R., Hauge, A., Kasin, J.I. *et al.* 2001. Reduced autonomic activity during stepwise exposure to high altitude. *Acta Physiologica Scandinavica*, 173, 409–17.

Sharma, V.M., Malhotra, M.S. and Baskaran, A.S. 1975. Variations in psychomotor efficiency during prolonged stay at high altitude. *Ergonomics*, 18, 511–6.

Shukitt-Hale, B., Stillman, A.J., Welch, D.I., Levy, A., Devine, J.A. and Lieberman, H.R. 1994. Hypobaric hypoxia impairs spatial memory in an elevation-dependent fashion. *Behavioural and Neural Biology*, 62, 244–52.

Siesjo, B.K. 1978. *Brain Energy Metabolism.* Chichester: Wiley & Sons.

Smith, P.A., Coote, J.H., Nicholson, A.N. and Stone, B.M. 1989. Sleep during an alpine expedition. *Aviation, Space, and Environmental Medicine*, 59, 478.

Sorensen, S.C., Lassen, N.A., Severinghaus, J.W., Coudert, J. and Zamora, M.P. 1974. Cerebral glucose metabolism and cerebral blood flow in high-altitude residents. *Journal of Applied Physiology*, 37, 305–10.

Spicuzza, L., Casiraghi, N., Gamboa, A., Key, C., Schneider, A., Mori, A. *et al.* 2004. Sleep-related hypoxaemia and excessive erythrocytosis in Andean high-altitude natives. *European Respiratory Journal*, 23, 41–6.

Squires, R.W. and Buskirk, E.R. 1982. Aerobic capacity during acute exposure to simulated altitude, 914–2286 metres. *Medicine & Science in Sports & Exercise*, 14, 36–40.

Sun, S., Oliver-Pickett, C., Ping, Y., Micco, A.J., Droma, T., Zamudio, S., Zhuang, J. *et al.* 1996. Breathing and brain blood flow during sleep in patients with chronic mountain sickness. *Journal of Applied Physiology*, 81, 611–8.

Sutton, J.R. 1982. Medical problems at high altitude. *Australian Journal of Sports Medicine and Exercise Sciences*, 14, 87–91.

Thomas, D.J., du Boulay, G.H., Marshall, J., Pearson, T.C., Ross-Russell, R.W., Symon, L. and Zilkha, E. 1977a. Cerebral blood flow in polycythaemia. *Lancet*, 8030, 161–3.

Thomas, D.J., Marshall, J., Ross-Russell, R.W., Wetherley-Mein, G., du Boulay, G.H., Pearson, T.C. *et al.* 1977b. Effect of haematocrit on cerebral blood in man. *Lancet*, 2, 941–3.

Titus, A.D., Shankaranarayana Rao, B.S., Harsha, H.N., Ramkumar, K., Srikumar, B.B., Singh, S.B. *et al.* 2007. Hypobaric hypoxia-induced dendritic atrophy of hippocampal neurons is associated with cognitive impairment in adult rats. *Neuroscience*, 145, 265–78.

Townes, B.D., Hornbein, T.F., Schoene, R.B., Sanquist, F.H. and Grant, I. 1984. Human Cerebral Function at Extreme Altitude. In: J.B. West and S. Lahiri (eds) *High Altitude and Man*. Bethesda, MD: American Physiological Society, 32–6.

Tsai, A.G., Johnson, P.C. and Intagletta, M. 2003. Oxygen gradients in the microcirculation. *Physiological Reviews*, 83, 933–63.

Tsien, W.R., Lipscombe, D., Madison, D., Bley, K. and Fox, A. 1995. Reflections on Ca^{2+}-channel diversity, 1988–1994. *Trends in Neurosciences*, 18, 52–4.

Turek, Z., Kreuzer, F. and Hoofd, L.J.C. 1973. Advantage or disadvantage of a decrease of blood oxygen affinity for tissue oxygen supply at hypoxia: A theoretical study comparing man and rat. *Pflügers Archives*, 342, 185–97.

Usui, C., Inoue, Y., Kimura, M., Kirino, E., Naguoka, S., Abe, M. *et al.* 2004. Irreversible subcortical dementia following high altitude illness. *High Altitude Medicine and Biology*, 5, 7781.

Van Dorp, E., Los, M., Dirven, P., Sarton, E., Valk, P., Teppema, L., Stienstra, R. and Dahan, A. 2007. Inspired carbon dioxide during hypoxia: Effects on task performance and cerebral oxygen saturation. *Aviation, Space, and Environmental Medicine*, 78, 666–72.

Van Mil, A.H., Spilt, A., Buchan, M.A., Bollenn, E.L., Teppema, L., Westendorp, R.G. and Blauw, G.J. 2002. Nitric oxide mediates hypoxia-induced cerebral vasodilation in humans. *Journal of Applied Physiology*, 92, 962–6.

Viault, F., 1890. Sur l'augmentation considerable de nombre des globules rouges dans le sang chez les habitants des haut plateaux del'Amerique du Sud. *Comptes-rendus des Séances de l'Academie des Sciences, Série D, Sciences Naturelles*, 111, 917–8.

Villafuerte, F.C., Cardenas, R. and Monge, C.C. 2004. Optimal hemoglobin concentration and high altitude: A theoretical approach for Andean men at rest. *Journal of Applied Physiology*, 96, 1581–8.

Virues-Ortega, J., Buela-Casai, G., Garrido, E. and Alcazar, B. 2004. Neuropsychological functioning associated with high-altitude exposure. *Neuropsychology Review*, 14, 197–224.

Vogel, S.A. and Harris, C.W. 1967. Cardiopulmonary response of resting man during early exposure to high altitude. *Journal of Applied Physiology*, 22, 1124–8.

Weil, J.V., Kryger, M.H. and Scoggin, C.H. 1978. Sleep and Breathing at High Altitude. In: C. Guilleminault and W.C. Dement (eds) *Sleep Apnea Syndromes*. New York, NY: Liss, 119–36.

West, J.B., Hackett, P.H., Maret, K.H., Milledge, J.S., Peters, R.M. Jr, Pizzo, C.J. and Winslow, R.M. 1983. Pulmonary gas exchange on the summit of Mount Everest. *Journal of Applied Physiology*, 55, 678–87.

West, J.B., Peters, R.M. Jr, Aksnes, G., Maret, K.H., Milledge, J.S. and Schoene, R.B. 1986. Nocturnal periodic breathing at altitude of 6,300 and 8,050 m. *Journal of Applied Physiology*, 41, 280–87.

West, J.B., Schoene, R.B. and Milledge, J.S. 2007. *High Altitude Medicine and Physiology – Fourth Edition*. London: Hodder Arnold.

Widdicombe, J. and Davies, A. 1991. *Respiratory Physiology – Second Edition*. London: Edward Arnold.

Williams, S.E., Wooten, P., Mason, H.S., Bould, J., Iles, D.E., Ricardi, D. *et al.* 2004. Haemoxygenase-2 is an oxygen sensor for a calcium-sensitive potassium channel. *Science*, 306, 2093–7.

Wilson, M.H., Newman, S. and Imray, C.H. 2009. The cerebral effects of ascent to high altitudes. *Lancet Neurology*, 8, 175–91.

Winslow, R.M. and Monge, C.C. 1987. *Hypoxia, Polycythemia, and Chronic Mountain Sickness*. Baltimore, MD: John Hopkins University Press.

Winslow, R.M., Monge, C.C., Statham, N.J., Gibson, C.G., Charache, S., Whittembury, J. *et al*. 1981. Variability of oxygen affinity of blood: Human subjects native to high altitude. *Journal of Applied Physiology*, 51, 1411–6.

Winslow, R.M., Samaja, M. and West, J. 1984. Red cell function at extreme altitude on Mount Everest. *Journal of Applied Physiology*, 56, 109–16.

Winslow, R.M., Monge, C.C., Brown, E.G., Klein, H.G., Sarnquist, F., Winslow, N.J. and McKneally, S.S. 1985. Effects of hemodilution on O_2 transport in high-altitude polycythemia. *Journal of Applied Physiology*, 59, 1495–502.

Wohns, R.N.W. 1981. High altitude cerebral edema: A pathophysiological review. *Critical Care Medicine*, 9, 880–82.

Wohns, R.N.W. 1987. Transient Ischemic Attacks at High Altitude. In: J.R. Sutton, C.S. Houston and G. Coates (eds) *Hypoxia and Cold*. New York, NY: Praeger, 536.

Wolfel, E.E., Selland, M.A., Mazzeo, R.S. and Reeves, J.T. 1994. Systemic hypertension at 4,300m is related to sympathoadrenal activity. *Journal of Applied Physiology*, 76, 1643–50.

Xu, K. and LaManna, J.C. 2006. Chronic hypoxia and the cerebral circulation. *Journal of Applied Physiology*, 100, 725–30.

Zhongyuan, S., Deming, Z., Changming, L. and Miaoshen, Q. 1983. Changes of electroencephalogram under hypoxia and relationship between tolerant ability to hypoxia and adaptation ability to high altitudes. *Scientia Sinica*, 26, 58–69.

Chapter 8

PROFOUND HYPOXIA: EXTREME ALTITUDE AND SPACE

Anthony N. Nicholson

During the early 1960s the possibility of extravehicular activity during space operations and the requirement for supersonic transport aircraft to operate at extreme altitudes raised questions concerning survival in near vacuum and the well-being of passengers exposed to prolonged decompressions. Spaceflight had been initiated by Yuri Gagarin in Vostok 1 (12 April 1961) and by Alan Shepard in Freedom 7 (5 May 1961), and these ventures were to lead to the extravehicular forays of Alexei Leonov from Voskhod 2 (18 March 1965) and of Edward White from Gemini 4 (3 June 1965). The first flights of a supersonic transport aircraft (Concorde) were handled by André Turcat (2 March 1969) and by Brian Trubshaw (9 April 1969), and Mach 2 operations were achieved during November 1970.

At that time information was not available concerning survival in a near vacuum, though such data could have been useful in deciding whether immediate recompression would be of high priority. Similarly, as far as supersonic transport operations were concerned, there was little information concerning the sequelae of prolonged decompressions at an extreme altitude, though such information proved to be critical in the development of Concorde with respect to acceptable decompression profiles, largely influenced by emergency rates of descent and window size. These concerns led to studies on the effects of decompressions to near vacuum by the United States Air Force School of Aviation Medicine, San Antonio, and on the effects of decompressions relevant to transport aircraft operating at extreme altitude by the Royal Air Force Institute of Aviation Medicine, Farnborough.

The outcomes of the decompression profiles related to extravehicular activity and to supersonic transport aircraft proved to be markedly different. The former involved a sudden exposure to near vacuum, and the issue was the duration of the decompression compatible with survival. The decompression profiles related to supersonic transports were of a triangular profile, and it transpired that, in certain circumstances, they could lead to permanent brain damage in survivors. The studies, in many ways complementary, brought skills from the disciplines of animal behaviour and experimental neuropathology to the practice of aerospace medicine, and it is the contribution of these neurosciences to understanding the operational implications of such decompressions that is explored in this chapter. Further, the studies, together with observations on mountaineers (Chapter 7: Hypobaric Hypoxia: Adaptation and Acclimatization), defined the altitudes and durations of exposure that lead to permanent brain damage at high and extreme altitudes.[1]

Exposure to Near Vacuum

Studies had been carried out many years before the era of space flight on the effects of rapid decompression to an ambient pressure of 30 mm Hg absolute (Edelmann et al., 1946; Edelmann and Hitchcock, 1952), though these were not primarily concerned with the duration of exposures compatible with survival or the possibility of brain damage. Later, decompressions on dogs exposed to near vacuum (Bancroft and Dunn, 1965) were concerned with these issues. The decompressions took place in an oxygen-rich environment from 35,000 feet (10,650 metres; 180 mm Hg: 24.0 kPa) to less than 2 mm Hg (0.3 kPa) within 2 seconds, and the duration of the exposures to near vacuum ranged from 4 to 180 seconds. Recompression to 35,000 feet occurred within 5 or 30 seconds. All animals exposed to the near vacuum for less than 90 seconds survived, but mortality reached 80 per cent of those exposed as durations approached 180 seconds. In only one animal was there evidence of a residual neurological impairment (hemiparesis).

Pathological examinations were carried out on the animals that died and at various intervals after decompression

in those that survived (Dunn et al., 1965). Microscopic examinations of the brain used cresyl violet, Weils' myelin and van Gieson stains. There were no haemorrhages in the brain or in the coverings, and there were no microscopic changes, even in the single animal with temporary neurological impairment that survived for 87 days. It would appear that in these studies the exposure of the brain to hypotension and/or hypoxaemia was of insufficient duration to initiate an irreversible cascade leading to necrosis.

Behavioural Studies in Primates

Although the dogs that survived exposure to vacuum were essentially free of neurological impairment or neuropathological changes, the question arose whether such decompressions could lead to subtle behavioural impairments, temporary or permanent. In these studies, 'learning set' was used as the behavioural task (Harlow, 1949) as it was considered likely to be sensitive to progressive loss of ability related to cortical damage. The studies (Rumbaugh and Ternes, 1968) were carried out in the squirrel monkey (Saimiri sciureus). The decompression profile was similar to that used in the dogs, with a limit to the duration of the exposure at near vacuum of 90 seconds. All animals that survived recovered their pre-exposure performance on the learning set within six days of the decompression. There was no evidence from these behavioural studies to suspect that brain damage had occurred.

Further information relevant to the likelihood of recovery of humans from a decompression in space came later from studies on apes (Koestler and Reynolds, 1968). The study was carried out in chimpanzees (Pan satyrus) with estimated ages between 53 and 81 months. They

---

1   In this text, extreme altitudes refer to altitudes that could be experienced in the event of a decompression in a transport aircraft, an ejection from a high-performance aircraft, and loss of pressurization of a space capsule or of a space suit during extravehicular activity.

were trained on a schedule that involved avoidance and discriminatory behaviour and reaction times to visual and auditory stimuli. Each animal was exposed to a single decompression from a holding pressure of 179 mm Hg (23.9 kPa), breathing 100 per cent oxygen to less than 2 mm Hg (0.3 kPa) within 2 seconds. They were kept in a near vacuum from periods varying between 5 and 210 seconds, and recompression took place in 30 seconds. One animal died, but there was evidence of pre-existing cardiac pathology. All the other six chimpanzees survived (including all of those that were held at near vacuum for periods between 120 and 210 seconds) and were able to perform the schedule at the pre-exposure level within four hours of recompression.

Simulated Decompression in Transport Aircraft

The initial studies concerned with the sequelae of decompression in supersonic transport aircraft assumed an aircraft operating up to 60,000 feet (18,300 metres) with a cabin volume of 10,000 cubic feet held at an altitude of 6,000 feet (1,830 metres). In the event of a decompression, it was anticipated that an emergency descent of the aircraft would be initiated within one minute at the rate of 5,000 feet per minute, and that the average mass flow of air into the cabin would be 100 pounds per minute. The decompression profiles experienced by the occupants would then be determined by the size of the defects in the cabin wall. Calculations on the effect of a small circular defect (such as the loss of a window) showed that a relatively small increase in the size of the defect produced a considerable increase in the maximum cabin altitude attained

and in the duration of the exposure to altitude (Figure 8.1).

Using these assumptions, it was calculated that a defect in the cabin wall, such as the loss of a window of 8 inch (20 centimetre) diameter, would lead to a cabin altitude exceeding 45,000 feet (13,700 metres). The decompression would be of such duration, over 7 minutes above 25,000 feet (7,600 metres), that, even if occupants were breathing oxygen, the decompression may well prove to be fatal. In the case of a 6 inch (15 centimetre) diameter defect, the outcome was less certain. The cabin altitude would not exceed 45,000 feet so that, provided oxygen was breathed, the outcome may not prove to be fatal in healthy passengers, although

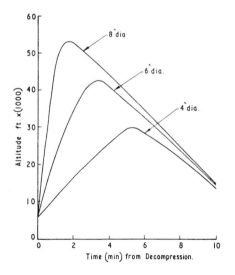

Figure 8.1   Calculated profiles of the cabin altitude during a decompression in a transport aircraft operating at 60,000 feet with an emergency descent rate of 5,000 feet per minute

The three profiles relate to defects in the cabin wall that range from 4 to 8 inch diameter.

Source: Brierley, J.B. and Nicholson, A.N. 1969. Neurological correlates of neurological impairment following prolonged decompression. *Aerospace Medicine*, 40, 148–152. Copyright: Aerospace Medical Association.

unconsciousness would not be averted. A cabin altitude of 25,000 feet would be reached around a minute after the decompression, so the occupants would be able to don oxygen masks. With a 4 inch (15 centimetre) diameter defect involving a maximum cabin altitude of 30,000 feet (9,100 metres) with 3 minutes above 25,000 feet, there would be only a transient loss of consciousness in healthy passengers, even if they were not breathing oxygen.

From these considerations it was apparent that certain cabin altitudes anticipated in the event of a decompression in a transport aircraft could prove to be fatal, even in healthy passengers breathing oxygen. However, decompressions in which the maximum cabin altitude and duration of the decompression over a critical altitude were limited by reducing the size of a possible defect (smaller window size) could be compatible with survival, though the possibility existed that such a prolonged exposure to hypoxia could lead to brain damage. Studies in baboons (*Papio cynocephalus*) confirmed this possibility (Nicholson and Ernsting, 1967; Brierley and Nicholson, 1969a, 1969b; Nicholson, 1971). Exposures simulating a 4 inch diameter defect in which the maximum altitude was within 30,000 feet (9,100 metres) were compatible with survival, exposures simulating a 6 inch diameter defect where the maximum altitudes were around 40,000 feet (12,200 metres) led to gross neurological disturbances, and exposures simulating an 8 inch diameter defect with a maximum altitude above 50,000 feet (15,200 metres) proved to be fatal.

Neuropathology

The neurological disturbances observed in animals after decompressions that

related to a 6 inch diameter defect indicated that severe cortical damage had been inflicted (Magnus and de Kleijn, 1912). Three animals out of four survived the decompression. They were motionless and adopted characteristic postures. In the lateral position their hind limbs were extended and their forelimbs were flexed, and when supine the forelimbs were also flexed. Tonic neck reflexes were present. The resting posture was changed by rotation of the neck with the 'skull' limbs flexed and the 'jaw' limbs extended. Two of the animals died after a few days, but the remaining baboon made a surprising, though partial, recovery. The animal had difficulty in maintaining the upright posture, and there was unsteadiness and impaired gait as well as lack of dexterity. The cerebral damage inflicted by the decompressions that were compatible with immediate survival was investigated by microscopic examinations using cresyl violet, cresyl violet with luxol fast blue, haematoxylin and eosin and with Mallory's phosphotungstic acid haematoxylin stains.

Damage was most prominent in the neocortex (Brierley and Nicholson, 1969a). It was symmetrical and decreased forward from the occipital to the frontal lobes. It was centred upon the boundary zones between the territories supplied by the major cerebral arteries, and was most severe where the gyri were crossed by the anterior and middle cerebral arteries and by the middle and posterior cerebral arteries. In the occipital lobes, no portion of the cortex was normal. There was well-defined laminar necrosis based on the third layer and extended downwards and forwards into the superior and inferior temporal gyri and upwards from the first temporal gyrus into the insula. Necrosis was accentuated over each dorsal convexity within parallel bands lying 2–3 centimetres from the midline, decreasing forwards to die out a few centimetres behind the frontal pole. There was bilateral necrosis in the hippocampus, with almost total necrosis of the Somner section. There was cell loss in the anterior nuclei of the thalami, the caudate nuclei and putamina, with loss of Purkinje cells in the cerebellum (Figure 8.2). Similar pictures of necrosis in cerebral arterial boundary zones had been observed in monkeys in which precipitate falls in blood pressure were induced while normal levels of arterial oxygen tension were maintained (Brierley and Excell, 1966; Brierley et al., 1969). It was concluded from the decompression studies that the brain damage was likely to have arisen from both reduced cerebral blood flow and reduced arterial oxygenation.

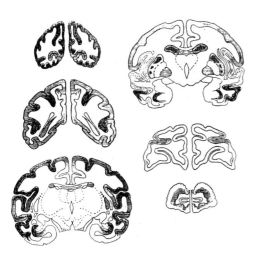

Figure 8.2   Distribution and intensity (as indicated by shading) of neuronal loss in the baboon (Papio cynocephalus) that exhibited decorticate behaviour

Source: Brierley, J.B. and Nicholson, A.N. 1969. Neuropathological correlates of neurological impairment following prolonged decompression. *Aerospace Medicine*, 40, 148–152. Copyright: Aerospace Medical Association.

Experimental Decompressions with Square Wave Profiles

The studies that concerned simulated decompressions in supersonic transport aircraft operating at altitudes approaching 60,000 feet (18,300 metres) showed that in certain circumstances such decompressions may lead to severe neurological impairment. These observations raised the question whether decompressions of less severity could give rise to less severe impairments, perhaps of a subtle behavioural nature. It was, therefore, considered that studies using square wave profiles may provide a steady state that could be used to explore in greater detail the physiopathology and behavioural sequelae of decompressions (Nicholson *et al.*, 1970; Blagbrough *et al.*, 1973). The studies were carried out in the monkey (*Macaca mulatta*). Decompressions at 42,500 feet (13,000 metres) of between 3 and 6 minutes' duration (until spontaneous respiration was about to cease) were found to lead either to death or survival without any evidence of brain damage. In that way, there were similarities with the studies in dogs exposed to near vacuum. On the other hand, square wave decompressions at 37,500 feet (11,400 metres) of between 10 and 16 minutes (also terminated when spontaneous respiration was about to cease) reliably led to permanent brain damage.

Behavioural Studies

In the decompressions to 37,500 feet (11,400 metres), the animals were trained on object and two-dimensional pattern discrimination and spatial alternation. Performance was often at criterion level on at least some of the tasks for a day or two after the decompression, but the animals would then fail to respond to such tasks for several days. Performance on the tasks gradually recovered (Figure 8.3). It was only when the exposure had led to brain damage that such a pattern of disturbed learned behaviour appeared. Even transient neurological or behavioural disturbances after decompression were always associated with microscopic evidence of brain damage. Evidently, the loss of learned behaviour was related to the appearance of permanent neuronal loss, and so the recovery was probably related to the recovery of function of adjacent cells that had not been permanently damaged by the decompression.

Neuropathology

In the studies that involved square wave decompressions at 37,500 feet, neuronal damage was either predominantly cortical or predominantly subcortical. The former involved the boundary zones between the cerebral arteries and spread across the parietal, temporal and frontal cortices, and the latter affected the thalamus and basal ganglia. An example of the necrosis observed in animals that was predominantly cortical is given in Figure 8.4. In the occipital lobes, necrosis was marked around each parieto-occipital sulcus involving principally the third layer. Necrosis extended over the dorsal aspect of the hemispheres as two paramedian bands 9 to 12 millimetres wide and 15 to 18 millimetres from the midline. Necrosis was limited in the temporal gyri, hippocampi, basal ganglia and cerebellum. An example of the necrosis observed in animals with a predominantly subcortical distribution is given in Figure 8.5. Subcortical necrosis affected the caudate nucleus, putamen, globus pallidus, thalamus and cerebellum, but there was only slight loss of neurons in the occipital cortex along two paramedian bands 5 to 7 millimetres wide lying 15 to 18 millimetres from the midline.

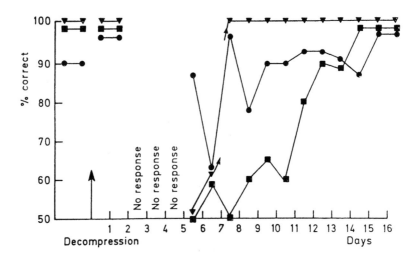

Figure 8.3   Performance in the monkey (*Macaca mulatta*) on various tasks after a decompression to 37,500 feet that involved permanent brain damage

Source: Reprinted with permission from Elsevier from Nicholson *et al.*, 1970. A behavioural and neuropathological study of the sequelae of profound hypoxia. *Brain Research*, 22, 327–345.

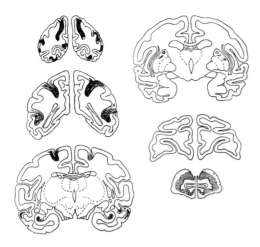

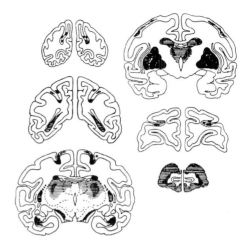

Figure 8.4   Distribution and intensity (as indicated by shading) of neuronal loss that was predominantly cortical. The animal (*Macaca Mulatta*) exhibited locomotor impairment. The neuropathological examination was carried out about 8 months after the decompression

Source: Reprinted with permission of Elsevier from Nicholson *et al.*, 1970. A behavioural and neuropathological study of the sequelae of profound hypoxia. *Brain Research*, 22, 327–34.

Figure 8.5   Distribution and intensity (as indicated by shading) of neuronal loss that was predominantly subcortical. There was gross neurological impairment and the animal (*Macaca Mulatta*) died seven days later

Source: Reprinted with permission of Elsevier from Nicholson *et al.*, 1970. A behavioural and neuropathological study of the sequelae of profound hypoxia. *Brain Research*, 22, 327–345.

Ascents and Simulated Mountain Ascents

Transient neurological and residual cognitive impairments are observed in some climbers as well as in subjects undergoing simulated ascents. In Chapter 7 (Hypobaric Hypoxia: Adaptation and Acclimatization), Coote and Milledge have reviewed the data on both transient events and residual sequelae, and it would appear that exposures for several days to high altitudes may lead not only to transient neurological and residual cognitive impairments, but also to permanent brain damage. Indeed, there is some evidence from imaging studies to link impaired cognitive function with cerebral pathology (Gunning-Dixon and Raz, 2000; MacLullich *et al.*, 2004).

In the context of residual impairments in high-altitude climbers, the advent of imaging techniques has made possible retrospective studies related to the possibility of brain damage. Fayed *et al.* (2006) examined climbers who had been involved in expeditions to Mount Everest (up to 8,848 metres: 29,029 feet), Mount Aconcagua (up to 6,959 metres: 22,831 feet), Mount Kilimanjaro (up to 5,895 metres: 19,341 feet) and Mont Blanc (4,810 metres: 15,781 feet). There was clear evidence of cortical atrophy in the climbers involved in the Mount Everest and Mount Aconcagua expeditions. In view of those findings, it was considered that the concomitant changes in the extensions of the subarachnoid space that surround penetrating arteries (Virchow–Robin spaces) may also have indicated cerebral pathology. The reader is also referred to other studies with respect to the use of imaging techniques (Garrido *et al.*, 1993; Anooshiravani *et al.*, 1999; Groeschel *et al.*, 2006).

From the studies on climbers to high altitudes using cerebral imaging techniques and from the studies on decompressions in primates using microscopy for the examination of the brain tissues, it is therefore possible to indicate the range of exposures to a hypobaric environment that may lead to permanent brain damage. The studies in climbers suggest that permanent brain damage is a possibility in humans that attain altitudes even below 7,000 metres (say, 22,500 feet) for several hours or even days, while the studies in primates show that permanent brain damage may occur in animals after exposures to 37,500 feet (say, 11,500 metres) for several minutes. It would appear that exposures significantly above 37,500 feet are unlikely to lead to permanent brain damage as the period of survival is not long enough to induce the necrotic process.

Considerations of the clinical, imaging and pathological data lead to a broad consensus on the nature of brain damage that arises in a hypobaric hypoxic environment. Residual cognitive impairments suggest changes at the cortical level, and the transient neurological disorders observed in simulated ascents suggest that watershed areas, such as those of the vertebrobasilar and carotid arteries may be involved (Cauchy *et al.*, 2002). The neuropathological data gathered from the decompressions in both baboons and monkeys demonstrate both cortical and subcortical ischaemia based on boundary zone lesions.

Genesis of Brain Damage

Questions arise from these studies concerning the pathophysiological mechanisms underlying the appearance of brain damage – particularly with respect to the necrosis related to the zones linked to the boundaries between the main cerebral arteries. There is microscopic evidence from studies in which hypoxaemia was avoided that a precipitate and prolonged hypotension alone can lead to boundary zone lesions (Brierley and Excell, 1966; Brierley *et al.*, 1969), but there is insufficient experimental evidence to claim that hypoxia alone, in the absence of reduced cerebral perfusion, leads to neuronal loss.

Studies in monkeys exposed to an environmental pressure of 160 mm Hg (21.3 kPa) absolute (an exposure known to lead consistently to brain damage) have shown that arterial pressure is maintained above 50 mm Hg (6.7 kPa) for up to a minute or so before cessation of respiration (Ernsting and Nicholson, 1971). The arterial gas tensions were relatively consistent between animals, with arterial oxygen values falling to about 8 to 12 mm Hg (1.1 to 1.6 kPa) and arterial carbon dioxide levels falling to between 10 and 15 mm Hg (1.3 to 2.0 kPa). It would appear that brain damage can occur during arterial hypoxaemia in the absence of systemic hypertension, but that would not exclude the possibility that local cerebral perfusion was compromised.

Essentially, experimental evidence supports the position that boundary zone necrosis can arise during hypotension when hypoxaemia is avoided and during hypoxaemia in the absence of systemic hypotension. In the latter case, however, impaired perfusion at the cortical level related in part to hypocapnia cannot be excluded. It is likely that reduced cerebral blood flow was essential to the appearance of boundary zone necrosis in both the hypotensive and decompression studies. That would also accord with the conclusion from the observations on transient neurological disorders observed in the simulated ascents of Mount Everest. Cauchy *et al.* (2002) considered that the most likely explanation for the symptoms were hypocapnic vasoconstriction associated with cerebral hypoxia and affecting areas with the weakest perfusion.

Space and Transport Operations: Operational Considerations

The operational conclusion that can be drawn from the studies in the squirrel monkey (*Saimiri sciureus*) concerned with decompression to near vacuum was that, in humans, survival from an exposure to space may be possible if recompression, possibly in an oxygen-rich environment, occurred within 90 seconds. The studies in the chimpanzee (*Pan satyrus*) supported this observation with survival from exposures to near vacuum extended to 210 seconds. In the context of these findings it is relevant to consider the circumstances in which such a decompression occurred during the re-entry of Soyuz 11 in 1971. The Soyuz craft was not designed to accommodate three cosmonauts each wearing a pressurized garment, and when the sealing of the capsule was lost during re-entry, the outcome was fatal for all the occupants.

In subsequent flights the number of occupants was reduced to two, both wearing space suits, and so, even if the suits were not pressurized, emergency pressurization of the suits could be a life-saving procedure. However, though permanent brain damage would be highly unlikely in survivors who experienced an emergency pressurization from a near-vacuum environment, performance is likely to be impaired for, at least, several hours. Clearly, from an operational point of view, successful outcomes of emergency pressurizations from space would be few and far between. A successful outcome could be envisaged during an orbital phase of a mission as there would be time for recovery before a critical phase of the mission, but that would be highly unlikely during the urgency of a re-entry. It is of interest that, against advice, the crew of Apollo 7 (1968), though admittedly suffering from an upper respiratory tract infection, had not worn helmets during re-entry (Berry *et al.*, 2009).

The studies on decompressions linked to the operation of supersonic transports, on experimental square decompressions to 37,500 feet (11,430 metres) and observations on simulated ascents of mountains have shown that neurological disturbances can occur when there is a sufficient degree of hypoxia sustained for a sufficient period of time. Such exposures are possible within a range that involves 'long' stays even below 22,500 feet (6,700 metres) to exposures of a few minutes at 37,500 feet (11,400 metres). The triangular profiles of the cabin altitudes related to an aircraft decompression would be largely contained within these limits. Such information may help to predict the likelihood of brain damage in decompression profiles that could, in some circumstances, arise in other and future aircraft. Present-day long-haul aircraft may operate up to 45,000 feet (13,700 metres), subsonic aircraft of the future may be designed to operate around 50,000 feet (15,200 metres) and further developments in supersonic transport operations are possible.

It would be advantageous if calculated cabin altitudes could be used to predict the relative safety of decompression profiles that could arise in future aircraft, but that is problematical. It is doubtful whether it would be possible to calculate with sufficient accuracy, to be of practical use, the alveolar and arterial gas tensions with an ever-changing cabin pressure. The tensions would, in any case, vary between individuals. Further, little is known about gas exchange at such altitudes. Even if an estimate could be made of the relation between the cabin pressure and the alveolar gas tensions, the exact influence of the arterial gas tensions on cerebral blood flow could not be predicted. The cascade leading to brain damage is determined not only by the hypoxaemia but also by the modulation of cerebral blood flow, and cerebral blood flow, itself, is influenced by both systemic and local factors.

Certainly, existing knowledge on the neurological sequelae of decompressions provides much useful data, but the information is only likely to be predictive and, therefore, of practical application in the assessment of profiles similar to those that have been studied experimentally. With the likelihood that calculated respiratory data would not be adequate, neurological, behavioural and neuropathological data may be needed to confirm the safety of decompression profiles in future transport aircraft. Indeed, that approach was needed to determine the maximum possible window size in Concorde when all other factors that influenced the cabin altitude during a decompression had been optimized and had been taken into consideration.

In the calculations related directly to a potential decompression in Concorde, the average emergency descent rate was taken as 7,000 feet per minute. With window sizes from 6 to 8 inch diameter, all the animals survived and there was no evidence of neurological impairment or brain damage. The studies were supported by recordings of the electrocorticogram. Isoelectric periods or even cessation of the electrical activity of the brain were observed, but only when the defect exceeded 6 inch diameter. It appeared that the descent rate of the aircraft was a critical factor in the appearance of permanent brain damage, and that with triangular decompression profiles gross changes in the electrical activity of the brain would only be expected if the cabin altitude reached 35,000 feet (Brierley and Nicholson, 1969b). It was concluded that a decompression profile bearing in mind these parameters could be defined that would not lead to permanent brain damage in healthy passengers, even while breathing air, provided pulmonary ventilation was maintained (Figure 8.6). These observations influenced the final decision on the window size of Concorde.

Addendum

The studies that have involved observations on humans, both as mountaineers and as experimental subjects, and decompressions in animals to high and extreme altitudes respectively have shown that brain damage may occur between 22,500 feet (say, 7,000 metres) and 37,500 feet (say, 11,500 metres), provided that survival is long enough for the process of necrosis to be initiated. The decompression profiles are brought together in Figure 8.7. The horizontal bars indicate the durations of exposures to near vacuum

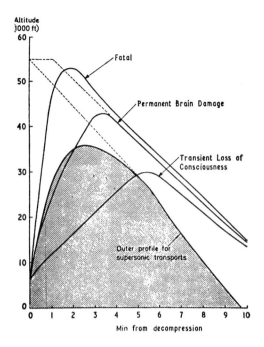

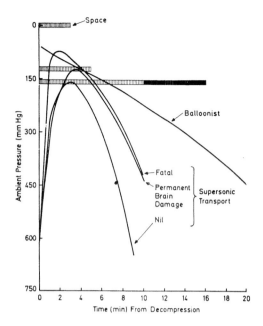

Figure 8.6   Calculated decompression profile (hatched) in a supersonic transport aircraft with an emergency descent rate of 7,000 feet per minute with a defect in the cabin wall of 6 inch diameter

The other profiles relate to an average emergency descent rate of 5000 feet per minute (dotted line) with defects of diameters of 4 inch (transient loss of consciousness), 6 inch (permanent brain damage) and 8 inch (fatal). Copyright: Aerospace Medical Association

Figure 8.7   Profiles of decompressions that relate to brain damage

kPa) occurred without breathing oxygen. On landing, the balloonist was alive, but died six months later. Neuropathological examination revealed decortication.

References

Anooshiravani, M., Dumont, L., Mardirosoff, C., Soto-Debeuf, G. and Dellevelle, J.M. 1999. Brain magnetic resonance imaging (MRI) and neurological changes after a single high altitude climb. *Medicine & Science in Sports & Exercise*, 31, 969–72.

Bancroft, R.W. and Dunn, J.E. 1965. Experimental animal decompressions to a near-vacuum environment. *Aerospace Medicine*, 36, 720–25.

Berry, C.A., Hoffler, G.W., Jernigan, C.A., Kerwin, J.P. and Mohler, S.R. 2009. History of space medicine: The formative years at NASA. *Aviation, Space, and Environmental Medicine*, 80, 345–52.

(< 2 mm Hg) and to ambient pressures of 124 mm Hg (16.5 kPa: 42,500 feet; 12,950 metres) and 160 mm Hg (21.3 kPa: 37,500 feet; 11,430 metres). The profiles of the cabin pressures related to calculated decompressions in a transport aircraft operating at 60,000 feet (18,300 metres) with defects of 4, 6 and 8 inch diameters were without residua, led to permanent brain damage or were fatal without evidence of brain damage respectively. The descent profile of the balloonist that led to decortication is also depicted. The descent from 55,000 feet (16,760 metres: 68.5 mm Hg; 9.1

Blagbrough, A.E., Brierley, J.B. and Nicholson, A.N. 1973. Behavioural and neurological disturbances associated with hypoxic brain damage. *Journal of Neurological Sciences*, 18, 475–88.

Brierley, J.B., Brown, A.W., Excell, B.W. and Meldrum, B.S. 1969. Brain damage in the rhesus monkey resulting from profound arterial hypotension: Its nature, distribution and general physiological correlates. *Brain Research*, 123, 80–101.

Brierley, J. and Excell, B.J. 1966. The effects of profound systemic hypotension upon the brain of M. rhesus: Physiological and pathological observations. *Brain*, 89, 269–98.

Brierley, J.B. and Nicholson, A.N. 1969a. Neuropathological correlates of neurological impairment following prolonged decompression. *Aerospace Medicine*, 40, 148–52.

Brierley, J.B. and Nicholson, A.N. 1969b. Neurological study of simulated decompression in supersonic transport aircraft. *Aerospace Medicine*, 40, 830–33.

Cauchy, E., Larmignat, P., Boussuges, A., Le Roux, G., Charniot, J.C., Dumas, J.L. *et al.* 2002. Transient neurological disorders during a simulated ascent to Mount Everest. *Aviation, Space, and Environmental Medicine*, 73, 1224–9.

Dunn, J.E., Bancroft, R.W., Haymaker, W. and Foft, J.W. 1965. Experimental animal decompressions to less than 2 mm Hg absolute (pathologic effects). *Aerospace Medicine*, 36, 725–32.

Edelmann, A. and Hitchcock, F.A. 1952. Observations on dogs exposed to an ambient pressure of 30 mm Hg. *Journal of Applied Physiology*, 4, 807–12.

Edelmann, A., Whitehorn, W.V., Lein, A. and Hitchcock, F.A. 1946. Pathological lesions produced by explosive decompression. *Journal of Aviation Medicine*, 17, 596.

Ernsting, J. and Nicholson, A.N. 1971. Respiratory and cardiovascular status of Rhesus monkeys exposed to an environmental pressure of 160 mm Hg abs (11,430 m). *Clinical and Developmental Medicine*, 39/40, 162–9.

Fayed, N., Modrego, P.J. and Morales, H. 2006. Evidence of brain damage after high-altitude climbing by means of magnetic resonance imaging. *American Journal of Medicine*, 119, 168, e1–6.

Garrido, E., Castelló, A., Venturta, J.L., Capdevila, A. and Rodriguez, F.A. 1993. Cortical atrophy and other brain magnetic resonance imaging (MRI) changes after extremely high-altitude climbs without oxygen. *International Journal of Sports Medicine*, 14, 232–4.

Groeschel, S., Chong, W.K., Surtees, R. and Hanefield, F. 2006. Virchow-Robin spaces on magnetic resonance images: Normative data, their dilatation, and a review of the literature. *Neuroradiology*, 48, 745–54.

Gunning-Dixon, F.M. and Raz, N. 2000. The cognitive correlates of white matter abnormalities in normal aging: A quantitative review. *Neuropsychology*, 14, 224–32.

Harlow, H.F. 1949. The formation of learning sets. *Psychological Reviews*, 56, 51–65.

Koestler, A.G. and Reynolds, H.H. 1968. Rapid decompression of chimpanzees to a near vacuum. *Journal of Applied Physiology*, 25, 153–8.

MacLullich, A.M., Wardlow, J.M., Ferguson, K.J., Starr, J.M., Seckl, J.R. and Deary, I.J. 2004. Enlarged perivascular spaces are associated with cognitive function in healthy elderly men. *Journal of Neurology, Neurosurgery and Psychiatry*, 75, 1519–23.

Magnus, R. and de Kleijn, A. 1912. Die Abhängigkeit des Tonus de Extremitätemuskeln von der Kopfstellung. *Pflügers Archiv – European Journal of Physiology*, 45, 455–8.

Nicholson, A.N. 1971. Neurological and behavioural studies on the sequelae of profound hypoxia. *Clinical and Developmental Medicine*, 39/40, 152–61.

Nicholson, A.N. and Ernsting, J. 1967. Neurological sequelae of prolonged decompression. *Aerospace Medicine*, 38, 389–94.

Nicholson, A.N., Freeland, S.A. and Brierley, J.B. 1970. A behavioural and neuropathological study of the sequelae of profound hypoxia. *Brain Research*, 22, 327–45.

Rumbaugh, D.M. and Ternes, J.W. 1968. Learning-set performance of squirrel monkeys after rapid decompression to vacuum. *Aerospace Medicine*, 36, 8–12.

Chapter 9

THE NEUROLOGICAL EXAMINATION: AEROMEDICAL CONSIDERATIONS

Michael D. O'Brien

The functional integrity of the nervous system of aircrew may be compromised by the demands and physical nature of the working environment and by clinical disorders of the nervous system. The manner in which such impairments may present have much in common. Disturbed sleep and impaired wakefulness are inevitable sequelae of most air operations, orientation and awareness may be impaired by conflicting sensory information during flight, and cognition may be threatened by inadequacies of the air quality of the cabin environment. From the clinical perspective, the sleep–wakefulness continuum is subject to many neurological disorders, orientation and awareness are dependent on the integrity of the vestibular and visual systems, and there is always the possibility of a developing neurodegenerative condition with the subtleties of impaired cognition. In aircrew with complaints referred to the nervous system, the working environment and the clinical picture have to be considered together.

Understanding impairment of the nervous system, whether arising from working in the air domain or due to the existence of a clinical disorder, has advanced considerably in recent years, and, as far as aviation medicine is concerned, there has been a valuable synergy between the disciplines of physiology and clinical medicine. For example, similar techniques have been developed to measure the effects of sleep deprivation and of narcolepsy on daytime function, the investigation of aircrew with difficulties in coping with a force environment have much in common with the clinical investigation of disorders of the vestibular system, and determination of visual standards for operational aircrew have related to clinical experience. Such interactions have had much beneficial influence on the practice of aviation medicine, but at the same time have emphasized the challenges faced by aeromedical practitioners in the assessment of the nervous system in potential and operational aircrew.

Aeromedical Approach

So far this volume has been concerned with impairments of neurological function that may arise from the interaction of aircrew with the air domain. The remaining chapters are concerned with clinical disorders of the nervous system that may also compromise effectiveness. In this matter the role of the aeromedical practitioner is crucial as they bring to the assessment of aircrew both physiological and clinical skills. Assessments may involve potential aircrew with a history of a neurological problem and aircrew who develop a neurological problem, as well as potential aircrew without any history of a neurological condition or of neurological symptoms and established aircrew attending for renewal of their medical certificate. Most of those with a history or a current neurological problem will have already been fully investigated, and in many cases it is possible to reach a conclusion concerning their suitability as aircrew. However, when the available information is inadequate, most commonly due to a poor or inconsistent history, further investigation may be needed. These applicants may be divided into those with an ongoing deficit and those who have fully recovered from a single event or series of events affecting the nervous system.

In those with an ongoing neurological deficit, the nature of the deficit and the risk of progression or complications must be considered. The persisting deficit can be readily assessed and sometimes best achieved in a simulator. It is also necessary to assess the risk of progression and, if present, the likely rate of progression. Similarly, the risk of complications should be considered and whether this is likely to occur suddenly and cause a problem in flight, or progress so slowly that an in-flight emergency would be very unlikely.

Examples of neurological deficits without risk of progression are some cases of subarachnoid haemorrhage, some cases of head injury, spinal cord and peripheral nerve injuries, and some cases of dystonia, as well as some individuals who have undergone neurosurgery. However, in some cases of subarachnoid haemorrhage and of head injury there is the risk of progression or complications, as there is with multiple sclerosis, cervical myelopathy and cerebral angiomas. Neurodegenerative conditions are progressive, and conditions such as motor neuron disease and dementia preclude a medical certificate once diagnosed, but some neurodegenerative diseases, such as Parkinson's disease, usually progress very slowly, an in-flight emergency is unlikely and a restricted medical certificate may be allowed. It is usually the need for disqualifying medication that limits a pilot's flying career.

In those applicants who have fully recovered from a neurological event, it is the risk of recurrence which might cause incapacity in flight that determines the acceptability of the individual as aircrew. Extradural and subdural haemorrhages are unlikely to reoccur, but migraine, cluster headaches, cough headaches, epilepsy, syncope, transient ischaemic attacks, transient global amnesia, paroxysmal vertigo and narcolepsy/ cataplexy are conditions that are likely to compromise the integrity of aircrew sometime in the future. Some of these conditions, such as a history of epilepsy over the age of five years, preclude employment as aircrew. There may be exceptions. A single provoked attack may be considered, after a detailed assessment and a period without medication, as unlikely to reoccur.

In aeromedical practice the vast majority of individuals have neither a history nor symptoms of a neurological condition. They may be applicants for aircrew training, and, in that case, it must be borne in mind that they may have started training as potential aircrew without medical approval, though they will need such approval from the regulatory body before they fly solo. Many individuals will be currently employed as aircrew and so are required to undergo a periodic medical assessment. The question arises as to what neurological screening should be done to exclude neurological conditions that are asymptomatic or are sufficiently insignificant to the applicant that the symptoms have not been disclosed. It is unusual to conceal completely a significant neurological problem, but quite common for the problem to be minimized and the history to be modified, especially if the applicant realizes the potential effect on their employment. In general, if there are any neurological symptoms, then a detailed examination of the system affected and related systems is necessary. Otherwise, the neurological examination can be quite selective, though always tailored to the individual.

Asymptomatic Aircrew

The neurological examination of asymptomatic applicants should involve consideration of cognitive abilities, the functions served by the cranial nerves and the cerebellum, the mobility of the cervical spine, and the integrity of the motor and sensory systems. As far as cognition is concerned, a subtle impairment of higher mental function is difficult to determine clinically, and a formal psychometric assessment is seldom appropriate as it does not test the

skills required of aircrew. An exception would be after a head injury, particularly if there is radiological evidence of frontal contusion. If cognitive impairment is suspected, the individual is best assessed in a simulator.

Olfaction is not usually a routine part of the neurological examination, though it is the only cranial nerve in the anterior fossa. The sense of smell may be lost after a head injury and impairment may be a very early sign in Parkinson's and Alzheimer's diseases. Vision must be assessed fully in all applicants. Colour vision is tested with Ishihara charts. Corrected visual acuity is tested in each eye separately with a Snellen chart at 6 metres, using a pinhole if necessary. The disc head, macula, periphery and the arteries and veins of the retina must be inspected by fundoscopy. Asymptomatic subjects are very unlikely to have a recently acquired monocular field defect and so it is, therefore, only necessary to test for an hemianopic attention defect, both within and outside binocular vision, using minimal stimuli. If there is any suggestion of a defect, this can be explored in each eye separately with a 3 mm white pin or a 5–10 mm red pin which gives a good qualitative indication of the field defect. Quantification with formal perimetry is then necessary.

As far as eye movements are concerned (III, IV and VI nerves), it is necessary to test for the full range looking for smooth pursuit and pausing at the end in each direction of gaze to ascertain the presence or absence of nystagmus. The integrity of the pupillary response to light must also be established as well as convergence. The practitioner should test for the corneal reflex (V), look for ptosis and ensure that movements of the upper and lower face are not impaired (VII). The tympanic membrane should be inspected, and audition tested (VIII). The latter requires either a simple test of auditory acuity or an audiogram depending on the medical standards required of the individual being examined. The movement of the uvula should be observed, and the tongue inspected at rest, on protrusion and with rapid side-to-side movements (IX and X). With respect to cerebellar function, the practitioner is looking for nystagmus, dysarthria, ataxia and loss of equilibrium. Limb ataxia is tested by the finger to nose test and by rapid alternations of hand movements involving pronation and supination. There is no need to test coordination in the legs, but tandem gait should be observed to detect disequilibrium.

The aeromedical practitioner should always look for abnormalities in the sensory and motor systems. That includes posture and deformity of the limbs as well as focal wasting, fasciculation and unwanted movements at rest and on a maintained posture. The cervical spine should be checked for a full range of passive movement (flexion, extension, rotation to left and right, and lateral flexion). Tone should be examined using pronation and supination of the forearms, and power in the upper limbs by assessing the strength of shoulder and finger (first dorsal interosseous) abduction. As far as the lower limbs are concerned, the strength of hip flexion and ankle dorsiflexion should be ascertained. These four movements are preferentially affected in upper motor neuron lesions and, when normal, exclude the possibility of such

weakness in the arms and legs. The integrity of the main reflexes should be confirmed (biceps C5/6, supinator C6, triceps C7, digital C8, knee L3/4, ankle S1/2), together with that of the plantar response. In the absence of cutaneous sensory symptoms, it is only necessary to test joint position sense at the terminal phalanx of the index fingers and at the big toes and to test vibration sense at both ankles.

Conclusion

These are the clinical imperatives in the neurological assessment of potential aircrew and in the periodic examinations of operational aircrew. Essentially, the crucial role of the aeromedical practitioner is the detection of a neurological disorder from the history and by a clinical examination. If any abnormality is suspected, the applicant should be referred to a neurologist. The remaining chapters of this volume deal with specific neurological disorders that are considered to be particularly relevant to the practice of aviation medicine. They are concerned with the pathophysiology of transient and episodic conditions, the associated prognoses and implications for training as potential aircrew and for continued employment. A bibliography of case reports of neurological disorders in individual aircrew has been compiled from the pages of *Aviation, Space, and Environmental Medicine* and can be found in Appendix I.

Chapter 10

INVESTIGATION

OF

SLEEP AND WAKEFULNESS IN

AIRCREW

Anthony N. Nicholson

In the investigation of aircrew with difficulties in coping with the irregularity of their rest and activity or with the possibility of a sleep disorder, it may be appropriate to assess, in some detail, the quality of their sleep and the possibility of impaired wakefulness. Initially, much useful information can be gathered from the clinical history together with sleepiness scales, sleep diaries and actigraphy. In due course the investigation may require the facilities of a sleep centre carrying out studies on the sleep–wakefulness continuum. However, the aeromedical practitioner can make a significant contribution by bringing together familiarity with the nature of the work of aircrew and the clinical picture. This chapter is intended as a guide to the aeromedical practitioner in the initial stage of an investigation and in deciding whether it would be appropriate to refer the individual to a respiratory physician or a neurologist with experience in sleep disorders. The scope is, therefore, limited, and for a detailed account of the investigation of disturbed sleep and wakefulness, the reader is referred to texts such as that by Chokroverty, Thomas and Bhatt (2005).

Clinical History

As well as the information that is usually gathered in a clinical history, the aeromedical practitioner should document the pattern of the sleep and wakefulness when the individual is off duty. These data include the estimated hours of sleep each night with times of going to bed and of waking up related to the week, weekends and holidays; the quality of sleep (whether there is difficulty in falling asleep and whether there are awakenings during the night); and how alert the individual feels in the morning. The alertness of the individual during the day is an essential feature of the assessment of the sleep–wakefulness continuum. It is also important to obtain information on the occurrence of naps during the day. Some indication of undue sleepiness may be provided by enquiries concerning the part of the day during which that the individual would undertake an important task or under what circumstances they may experience drowsiness while driving or being driven. The clinical history may also indicate the possibility of sleep pathology, and these aspects are dealt with in Chapter 11 (Excessive Daytime Sleepiness: Clinical Considerations).

Sleepiness Scales

Three scales are used in the investigation of sleepiness. They are the Stanford Sleepiness (Hoddes *et al.*, 1973), the Epworth Sleepiness (Johns, 1991) and the Karolinska Sleepiness (Akerstedt and Gilberg, 1990) Scales, as given below. Their appropriateness in the investigation of aircrew is discussed in Chapter 11 (Excessive Daytime Sleepiness: Clinical Considerations). In aeromedical practice the initial requirement is some information on the implications of the potential sleep disturbance, and the Epworth Sleepiness Scale is a useful approach.

Stanford Sleepiness Scale

Check the one statement that best describes you at present:

1. Feeling active, vital, alert or wide awake.
2. Functioning at a high level, but not at peak; able to concentrate.
3. Awake, but relaxed; responsive, but not fully alert.
4. Somewhat foggy, let down.

5. Foggy; losing interest in remaining awake; slowed down.
6. Sleepy, woozy, fighting sleep; prefer to lie down.
7. No longer fighting sleep, sleep onset soon; having dreamlike thoughts.

Epworth Sleepiness Scale

On a scale of 0–3, how likely are you to dose off or fall asleep in each of the following situations (0 = No Chance; 1 = Slight Chance; 2 = Moderate Chance; 3 = High Chance):

> Sitting and reading
> Watching television
> Sitting, inactive, in a public place (theatre or meeting)
> As a passenger in a car for one hour without a break
> Lying down in the afternoon to rest when circumstances permit
> Sitting and talking to someone
> Sitting quietly after lunch without alcohol
> In a car, while stopped for a few minutes in traffic

The total score (out of 24) gives an indication of the severity of sleepiness. A score in excess of 10 may indicate undue background sleepiness.

Karolinska Sleepiness Scale

Rate your level of sleepiness according to the scale below:

> 1 = Very alert
> 2 =
> 3 = Alert
> 4 =
> 5 = Neither alert nor sleepy
> 6 =

7 = Sleepy, but not strenuous to stay awake

8 =

9 = Very sleepy, great effort to stay awake or fighting sleep

Sleep Diaries

In aviation medicine, sleep diaries are usually concerned with the analysis of the work and rest patterns of aircrew, but they are also helpful in dealing with a suspected disorder of sleep – particularly a disturbance of the circadian rhythm. Diaries should provide day-to-day details of duty, including time-zone changes, and daily estimates, though subjective, of the quality of sleep. Much thought has been given to their format, and, when designed carefully and the information analyzed appropriately, they provide much useful information. As far as field studies are concerned, it is necessary to design a diary specifically for the particular study, and the practitioner should seek statistical advice on both the design and analysis of the data. The use of diaries, together with actigraphs, has worked well when looking at large numbers of aircrew operating similar routes (Chapter 3: Aircrew and Alertness), and the diary can be used again once remedial action on the schedule had been taken to assess whether there has been any general improvement.

Actigraphy

The principle behind actigraphy is that increased movement occurs during wakefulness, whereas decreased movement, or even no movement at all, occurs during sleep – except movement due to changes in posture. The technique differentiates between the states of sleep and wakefulness, but does not identify the depth of sleep or accurately reflect arousals. It is also considered that actigraphy is not suitable for estimations of sleep efficiency or latency (Signal *et al.*, 2005). Nevertheless, actigraphy, together with a diary, is the initial approach in the assessment of circadian disorders and may prove useful in the investigation of excessive daytime sleepiness. The reader is referred to the report from the American Academy of Sleep Medicine (2007) for details on the use of the technique in clinical practice (Littner *et al.*, 2003). As far as aviation medicine is concerned, it has been used in the investigation of the rest and activity patterns of operational aircrew (Chapter 3: Aircrew and Alertness).

Sleep Electroencephalography

The step from actigraphy to electroencephalography should not be taken lightly, and the practitioner should consider whether such recordings are necessary. Such an investigation usually requires the facilities of a centre carrying out studies on the sleep–wakefulness continuum or of a sleep clinic, and is expensive as it involves overnight staffing. Further, the value placed on electroencephalography in the assessment of sleep varies from physician to physician. Indeed, its use depends to a considerable extent on the approach and clinical experience of the physician involved and of the facilities to hand. Certainly, electroencephalography provides the complete picture of the sleep process and of sleep disturbance, but such detail may not be required. It is, therefore, necessary for the aeromedical practitioner to have some familiarity with recordings of the sleep–wakefulness continuum so that they can exercise an informed opinion concerning the potential relevance of the recordings to the individual aviator in question

Sleep Stages and the Hypnogram

Sleep electroencephalography involves recordings from the frontal, parietal and occipital areas, together with the electro-oculogram for the detection of conjugate eye movements and the submental electromyogram to indicate muscle tone. With these recordings it is possible to trace the development of the sleep process from wakefulness through drowsiness to sleep onset, the deepening of sleep with slow-wave activity, the cyclical appearance of rapid eye movement sleep and to identify periods of wakefulness. During wake activity (Figure 10.1), the alpha rhythm often predominates with obvious activity in the submental myogram. The onset of sleep is usually taken as the first appearance of a spindle or a K-complex (Figure 10.2).

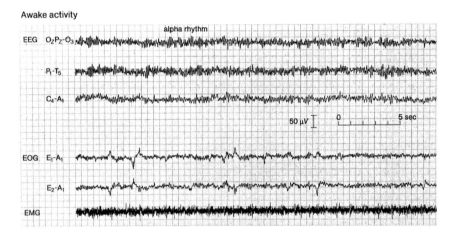

Figure 10.1 Awake activity

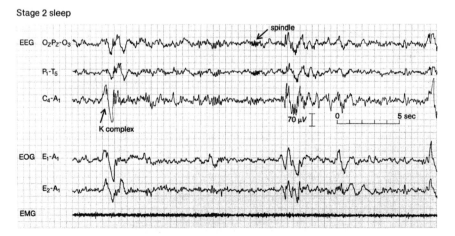

Figure 10.2 Stage 2: The onset of sleep

Slow-wave sleep is the predominant feature of the first third of the night (Figure 10.3), and the feature of the latter two-thirds of the night is the cyclical periods of rapid eye movement sleep, with each episode increasing in duration. In rapid eye movement sleep, there is low-amplitude activity in the electroencephalogram, conjugate eye movements and little muscle activity in the submental channel (Figure 10.4). The first period of rapid eye movement sleep is short and usually appears within the early changes in sleep that involve slow-wave activity. Sometimes this brief period of rapid eye movement sleep is absent.

These definitions of the sleep stages, analyzed by 30-second epochs, are based mainly on a manual published by the Brain Information Service, Los Angeles, in 1968, revised by the American Academy of Sleep Medicine in 2007. The stages are brought together in a time-based hypnogram (Figure 10.5) so that the sleep process can be

Stage 4 – slow wave sleep

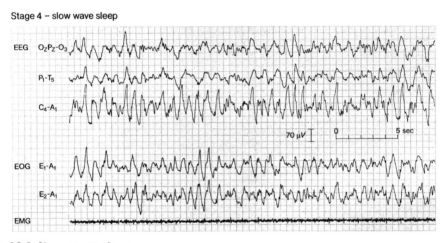

Figure 10.3 Slow-wave sleep

REM sleep

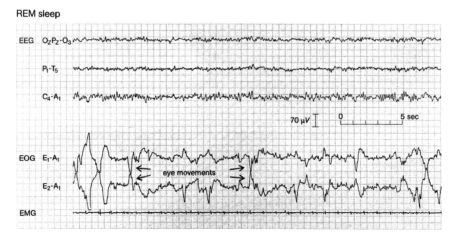

Figure 10.4 Rapid eye movement sleep

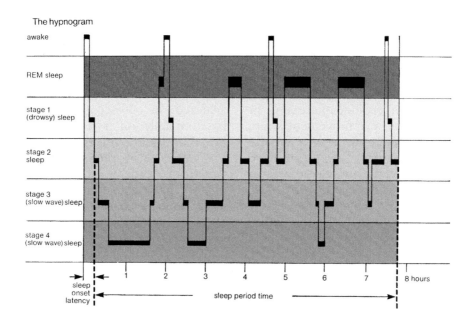

Figure 10.5 Hypnogram

easily visualized. In the interpretation of the sleep process, inspection of the individual epochs of the hypnogram is the initial approach. The time to the onset of the first period of stage 2 sleep and the total sleep time within a period of rest provide data that are related to the efficiency of the sleep process, and are used often in studies concerned with the effect of aircrew schedules on sleep. The electroencephalogram also provides valuable information on the continuity of sleep, particularly the existence of arousals. Arousals may be important in understanding the adverse effects of the environment on sleep and the complaint of daytime sleepiness, but such events have to be identified on the original recordings.

Polysomnography

Additional physiological recordings are required where there is the possibility of

a sleep disorder, and that constitutes a polysomnogram. Attention is directed to peripheral events, such as apnoeas and leg movements, and the recordings provide data on the frequency and severity of arousals linked to such disturbances. The atlas by Chockraverty *et al.* (2005) is recommended if the practitioner requires more information on recording techniques, the electroencephalographic correlates of the sleep process or on recordings that indicate sleep pathology.

In sleep-disordered breathing (Figures 10.6, a and b) the recordings include respiratory effort, airflow and arterial oxygen saturations as, in obstructive sleep apnoeas, there may be cessation of airflow through the nose, though abdominal movements associated with respiration continue, and the apnoeic episode may be accompanied by a fall in arterial saturation. Such information is useful in making the diagnosis and may help in the follow-up of the effectiveness of the treatment. In the periodic leg movement disorder (Figure 10.7), recordings from the anterior tibialis muscle demonstrate the periodicity of the disorder, and, again, the electroencephalogram may link these events to arousals.

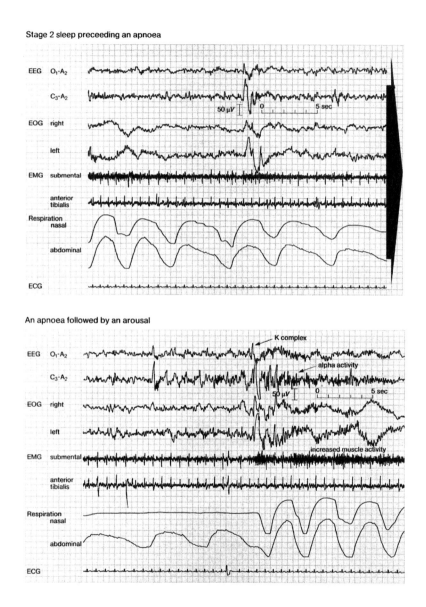

Figure 10.6 a) Stage 2 sleep immediately preceding the apnoea and b) The apnoea with an arousal

Daytime Recordings

Multiple Sleep Latency Test

The multiple sleep latency test (Carskadon and Dement, 1978; Richardson *et al.*, 1978) measures the rate of falling asleep. It is concerned with the tendency at particular times of the day and in particular circumstances to dose off or fall asleep, and so enter stage 1 sleep (Figure 10.8). The test consists of four to six naps taken at two-hourly intervals from around an hour after awakening. The subjects are encouraged to fall asleep in a darkened room, and the electroencephalogram and electro-oculogram are used to determine the latency to the first epoch of sleep observed on each occasion.

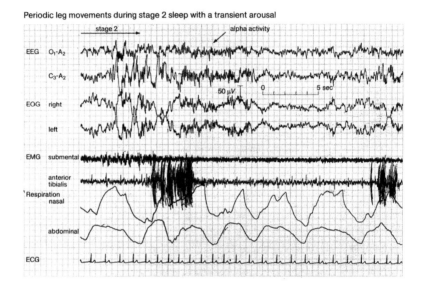

Figure 10.7 Periodic leg movements during stage 2 sleep with an arousal

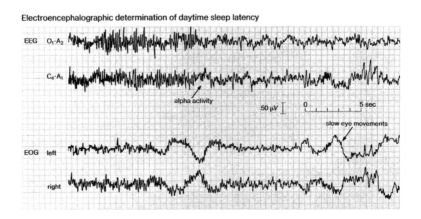

Figure 10.8 Daytime sleep latency

The sleep latencies are particularly sensitive to the time of day. They have a characteristic pattern – reducing during the morning, presumably linked to the decreasing influence of the previous nocturnal sleep, and increasing during the afternoon, presumably linked to the rising circadian rhythm of alertness (Figure 10.9). The appropriateness of this test in the investigation of aircrew is discussed in Chapter 11 (Excessive Daytime Sleepiness: Clinical Considerations).

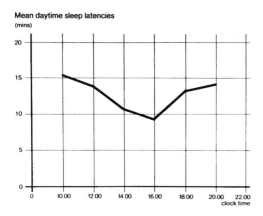

Mean daytime sleep latencies
(mins)

Figure 10.9 Mean daytime sleep latencies

Maintenance of Wakefulness Test

The maintenance of wakefulness test (Mittler *et al.*, 1982), as the title implies, is concerned with the ability to maintain wakefulness at the time of the assessment. Subjects, at two-hourly intervals, sit upright in a darkened room and remain awake as long as they can. The assessment takes place within a specified period of time, say 20 or 40 minutes, and the time to the first epoch of any stage of sleep recorded. The normative study carried out by Doghramji *et al.* (1997) indicated that the lower limits for the time to fall asleep (taken as two standard deviations below the mean) were 10.9 minutes with the 20-minute test and 19.4 minutes with the 40-minute test. Both

the maintenance of wakefulness and the multiple sleep latency tests measure sleep latencies, though in different circumstances, and do not necessarily indicate a pervasive ongoing excessive sleepiness. The maintenance test is useful when there are concerns about the ability to sustain attention.

Oxford Sleep Resistance (OSLER) Test

The maintenance of wakefulness test, as with the multiple sleep latency test, requires electroencephalographic recordings, and so presents logistic problems in routine clinical practice. The recording of the electroencephalogram is avoided in the Oxford Sleep Resistance (OSLER) test. The test requires subjects to press a switch in response to a light that is illuminated for 1 second in every 3 seconds. When the subject fails to respond for 21 seconds, sleep it is concluded to have occurred (Bennett *et al.*, 1997). It would appear that the test is a reliable and useful method to assess daytime somnolence.

Summary

It is important to stress that much useful information on the sleep and wakefulness of aircrew having difficulty in coping with schedules or with a potential sleep disorder can be gathered through the history, sleepiness scales, diaries and actigraphy, and these approaches are within the scope of the aeromedical practitioner. Indeed, with our current understanding of work and rest, electroencephalography may not be needed in the investigation of the adverse effects of schedules. Careful design of diaries and adequate attention to the analysis of the data, together with actigraphic patterns of activity in some cases, may suffice in most field studies.

On the other hand, the full panoply of polysomnography is likely to be necessary when there is the possibility of a potential disorder of sleep in a particular individual. It is often argued that electroencephalography is not needed for the diagnosis of many sleep disorders, and that may be true in day-to-day clinical practice. However, a sleep problem in aircrew may have implications for their employability, and so an adequate assessment is essential. Electroencephalography provides data on the frequency and severity of brief disturbances of sleep (arousals) that may arise from the peripheral events of sleep disorders. Arousals may relate to the complaint of daytime sleepiness, and so could be relevant in the assessment of aircrew and in tracking the success of treatment.

Acknowledgement

The polysomnograms were initially published in A.N. Nicholson and I.B. Welbers (eds) *Sleep and Wakefulness: Physiology, Pathology and Pharmacology* (1984) Ingelheim, Boehringer. Reprinted with permission.

References

Akerstedt, T. and Gilberg, M. 1990. Subjective and objective sleepiness in the active individual. *International Journal of Neuroscience*, 52, 29–37.

American Academy of Sleep Medicine. 2007. *Manual for the Scoring of Sleep and Associated Events: Rules, Terminology and Technical Specifications*, edited by C. Iber, S. Ancoli-Israel and S.F. Quan. Westchester, IL: American Academy of Sleep Medicine.

Bennett, L.S., Stradling, J.R. and Davies, R.J.O. 1997. A behavioural test to assess daytime sleepiness in obstructive sleep apnoea. *Journal of Sleep Research,* 6, 142–5.

Brain Information Service 1968. *A Manual of Standardized Terminology: Techniques and Scoring System for Sleep Stages of Human Subjects*, edited by A. Rechtscaffen and A. Kales. Los Angeles, CA: Brain Information Service.

Carskadon, M.A. and Dement, W.C. 1978. Sleep tendency: An objective measure of sleep loss. *Sleep Research*, 7, 200.

Chokroverty, S., Thomas, R.J. and Bhatt, M. 2005. *Atlas of Sleep Medicine*. Philadelphia, PA: Elsevier.

Doghramji, K., Mittler, M.M., Sangal, R.B., Shapiro, C., Taylor, S., Walseben, J. *et al.* 1997. A normative study of the maintenance of wakefulness test (MWT). *Electroencephalography and Clinical Neurophysiology*, 103, 554–62.

Hoddes, E., Zarcone, V., Smythe, H., Phillips, R. and Dement, W.C. 1973. Quantification of sleepiness: A new approach. *Psychophysiology*, 10, 431–6.

Johns, M.W. 1991. A new method for measuring daytime sleepiness: The Epworth Sleepiness Scale. *Sleep*, 14, 540–45.

Littner, M., Kushida, C.A., Anderson, W.M., Bailey, D., Berry, R.B., Davila, D.G. *et al.* 2003. Practice parameters for the role of actigraphy in the study of sleep and circadian rhythms. *Sleep*, 26, 337–41.

Mittler, M.M., Gujavarty, K.S. and Browman, C.P. 1982. Maintenance of wakefulness test: A polysomnographic technique for evaluating treatment of efficacy in patients with excessive somnolence. *Electroencephalography and Clinical Neurophysiology*, 53, 658–61.

Richardson, G.S., Carskadon, M.A., Flagg, W., van den Hoed, J., Dement, W.C. and Mittler, M.M. 1978. Excessive daytime sleepiness in man: Multiple sleep latency measures in narcoleptic and control subjects. *Electroencephalography and Clinical Neurophysiology*, 45, 621–7.

Signal, T.L., Gale, J. and Gander, H. 2005. Sleep measurement in flight crew: Comparing actigraphic and subjective estimates to polysomnography. *Aviation, Space, and Environmental Medicine*, 76, 1058–63.

Figure 1.1a

Figure 1.1a

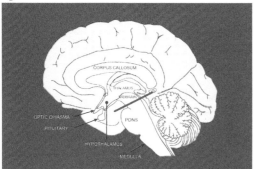

Figure 1.1b

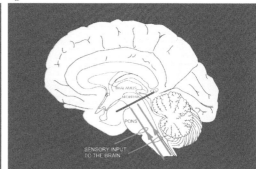

Figure 1.1c

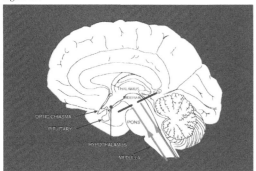

Figure 1.1d

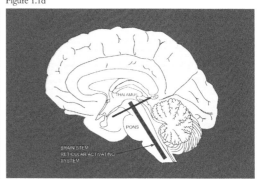

Figure 1.1   Schematic depiction of the studies by Bremer (1935, 1938) and Moruzzi and Magoun (1949)

1.1a and 1.1b: Transection of the brain at the boundary between the cerebrum and brain stem led to sleepiness (Figure 1.1a). The transection severed the connection of the ascending sensory pathways with the cerebrum, but connections with the cerebrum still existed with the visual and olfactory sensory systems (Figure 1.1b). That cast some doubt on the concept that sleepiness induced by the transection was due to loss of sensory inputs alone, and, in turn, that wakefulness was dependent on the input of the ascending sensory pathways.

1.1c and 1.1d: Transections that spared the core of the medulla, but still severed the ascending sensory pathways, did not lead to sleepiness (Figure 1.1c). It was the section of the central core of the brain stem that had led to sleepiness (Figure 1.1d), and so sleepiness observed with complete transections of the brain stem was not due to the loss of the influence of the ascending sensory inputs. These experiments led to the concept of the Reticular Activating System in the control of sleep and wakefulness.

Source: Nicholson, A.N. 1998. *The Neurosciences and Aviation Medicine: A Century of Endeavour. International Academy of Aviation and Space Medicine*, Auckland: Uniprint (L.J. Thompson (ed.) with permission from the Academy).

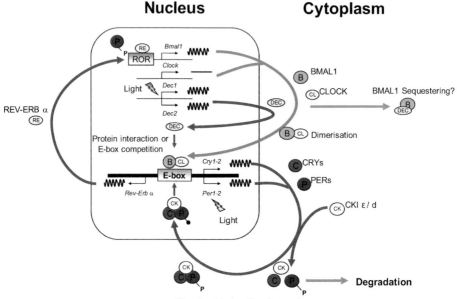

Figure 2.4   Mammalian Molecular Clock

The mammalian molecular clock is based upon a transcriptional drive produced by CLOCK:BMAL1 heterodimers Clock is constitutively expressed, whereas Bmal1 is rhythmically expressed. The CLOCK:BMAL1 heterodimers bind to E-box enhancers in the Period and Cryptochrome promoters, producing rhythmic Per and Cry expression. Per1 and Per2 have a well documented role in this feedback loop, whilst Per3's role is less clear. The resulting PER proteins are phosphorylated by CK1e/d and interact with CRY proteins to form a phosphorylated multimeric complex. This complex enters the nucleus and produces a negative feedback by inhibiting CLOCK:BMAL1-mediated transcription. An additional loop is produced via Rev-erba, which also possesses an E-box enhancer activated by CLOCK:BMAL1. Rev-erba acts via a ROR element in the Bmal1 promoter to inhibit Bmal1 transcription, thus feeding back to remove the positive drive produced by CLOCK and BMAL1. As the PER/CRY/CK1e/d complex re-enters the nucleus and inhibits the CLOCK:BMAL1 drive on the E-box, Rev-erba expression is also reduced. This leads to a disinhibition (activation) of Bmal1, thus restarting the molecular cycle. The newly identified components Dec1 and Dec2 may modulate the CLOCK:BMAL1 drive by competing for E-box binding or sequestering BMAL1. Light detection by photosensitive retinal ganglion cells (pRGCs) ultimately alters the expression levels of Per1-2 and possibly Dec1. Altered levels of these proteins act to advance or delay the molecular feedback loops and so aligns the molecular clock to the light/dark cycle.

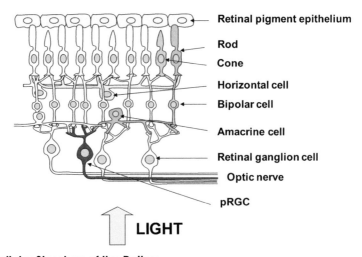

Figure 2.5   Cellular Structure of the Retina

The rods and cones of the retina detect light and convey visual information to the ganglion cells via the second order bipolar cells. At the first synaptic layer, horizontal cells facilitate lateral connectivity and feedback to the photoreceptors. At the second synaptic layer in the inner retina, amacrine cells allow lateral connections between bipolar and ganglion cells. The optic nerve is formed from the axons of all the ganglion cells. A subset of ganglion cells, the photosensitive retinal ganglion cell (pRGC) also detect light directly; utilising the photopigment melanopsin. Thus photodetection occurs both within the outer and inner retina. Note: In the vertebrate retina, light passes through the transparent ganglion layer to reach the rods and cones of the image forming pathway, as indicated by the white arrow.

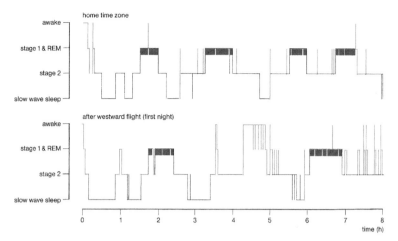

Figure 3.2   Sleep patterns (hypnogram) after a westward flight with a time-zone change of five hours

The recovery of the sleep process after five time-zone transitions is quicker after westward than after eastward flights. After a westward flight, subjects tend to fall asleep quickly and sleep more deeply as the rest period is delayed, but there is less sleep during the later part of the rest period (Figure 3.2). The normal pattern of sleep is re-established within a couple of days. After an eastward flight, sleep is delayed and disturbed for several days, with a delay also in the cyclical appearance of rapid eye movement sleep (Figure 3.3).

Source: A.N. Nicholson and I.B.Welbers (eds.) 1986. *Sleep and Wakefulness: Physiology, Pathology and Pharmacology*. Ingelheim, Boehringer (reprinted with permission).

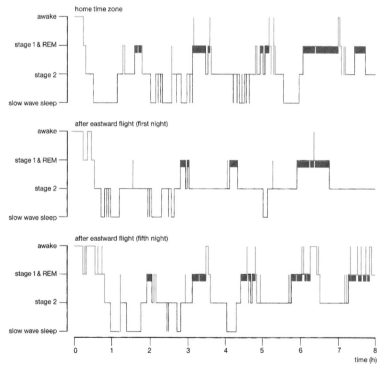

Figure 3.3   Sleep patterns (hypnogram) after an eastward flight with a time-zone change of five hours

The recovery of the sleep process after five time-zone transitions is quicker after westward than after eastward flights. After a westward flight, subjects tend to fall asleep quickly and sleep more deeply as the rest period is delayed, but there is less sleep during the later part of the rest period (Figure 3.2). The normal pattern of sleep is re-established within a couple of days. After an eastward flight, sleep is delayed and disturbed for several days, with a delay also in the cyclical appearance of rapid eye movement sleep (Figure 3.3).

Source: A.N. Nicholson and I.B.Welbers (eds.) 1986. *Sleep and Wakefulness: Physiology, Pathology and Pharmacology*. Ingelheim, Boehringer (reprinted with permission).

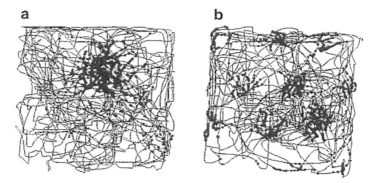

Figure 4.1   The pattern of activity in a) a place cell in the hippocampus and b) a grid cell in the entorhinal cortex

Black lines represent the movement of the experimental animal within its square enclosure. Whereas the place cell fires predominantly in one location, the grid cell fires at multiple locations forming a triangular pattern across the entire area of the enclosure (from Moser *et al.*, 2008 with permission '*Annual Reviews*').

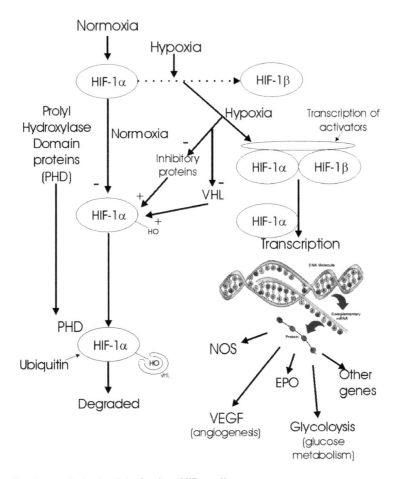

Figure 7.2.   The hypoxia inducible factor (HIF) pathway

HIF-1 consists of a constituitively expressed b subunit and an oxygen regulated a subunit. Under normoxic conditions HIF-1a is degraded by hydroxylation under the influence of proline hydroxylase and various proteins such as von Hippel Lindau Factor (VHL), indicated by the left hand oxygen dependent pathway.During hypoxia the degradation of HIF-1a is inhibited so that it follows the right hand pathway whereby two transcription activators interact with HIF-1a to enable it to induce transcription of a number of genes. Many are responsible for expression of proteins involved in oxygen homeostasis such as nitric oxide synthase (NOS), vasular endothelial growth factor (VEGF), erythropoietin (EPO).

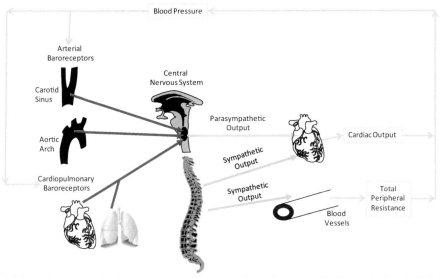

Figure 13.1 Scheme outlining autonomic neural pathways that control arterial blood pressure

The autonomic nervous system has a central role in the regulation of blood pressure. Normal physiologic feedback mechanisms work through cranio-sacral parasympathetic and thoraco-lumbar sympathetic neural pathways to maintain blood pressure, and thus adequate cerebral perfusion.

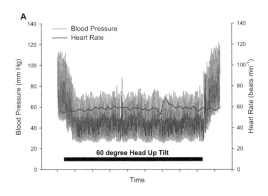

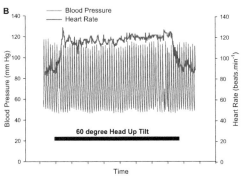

Figure 13.5 Continuous blood pressure and heart rate tracings of orthostatic hypotension in an autonomic failure patient (A) and postural tachycardia in a PoTS patient during 60 degree head up tilt tests. From Mathias (2009)

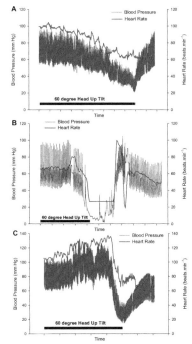

Figure 13.6 Continuous blood pressure and heart rate tracings during the predominantly vasodepressor (A), cardio-inhibitory (B) and mixed (cardio-inhibitory and vasodepressor, C) forms of vasovagal syncope during 60 degree head up tilt tests. From Mathias (2009)

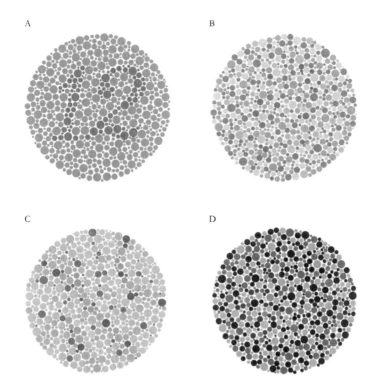

Figure 17.3 Examples of plates found in the Ishihara test book

A. This is a control plate. No colour vision is required to read the '12' but the subject needs adequate visual acuity and be able to distinguish the 'Figure' (dots making up the number) from the "ground" (dots making up the background).
B. A trichromat will read '6' whereas a dichromat may see nothing or read a different number.
C. A trichromat cannot read a number. A dichromat may or may not read a number '2'.
D. A trichromat will read '42'. A protanope will not see the '4' and a deuteranope will not see the '2'

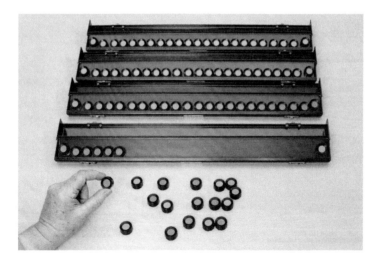

Figure 17.4 The Farnsworth–Munsell 100-hue test

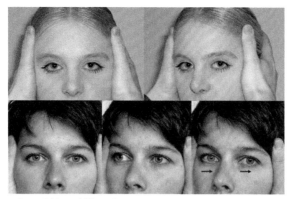

Figure 18.2 Doll's Head and Head Thrust

The horizontal vestibulo-optic reflex is assessed by asking the patient to fix their gaze on the bridge of the examiner's nose and passively rotating the head in yaw, either slowly at low acceleration, the Doll's Manoeuver, or by quicker high acceleration movements by the Halmagyi 'Head Impulse' or 'Head Thrust' Test (Halmagyi and Curthoys, 1988). The head impulse test involves low amplitude unpredictable fast head rotations. Source: Reproduced from Bronstein, A.M., and Lempert, T. 2006. *Dizziness: A Practical Approach to Diagnosis and Management*. Cambridge, Cambridge University Press.

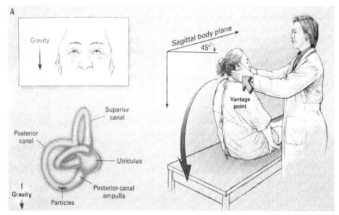

Figure 18.4 The Hallpike Manoeuvre

Source: Reproduced with permission: Furman J.M. and Cass S.P. 1999. Benign Paroxysmal Positional Vertigo. *New England Journal of Medicine*, 1999, 341, 1590–1596.

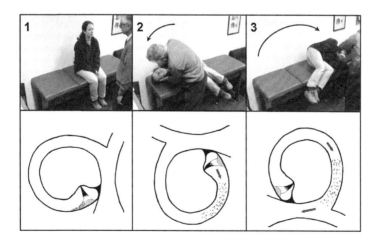

Figure 18.6 The positional manoeuvre and treatment (Semont Manoeuvre)

Source: Reproduced from Bronstein, A.M., and Lempert, T. 2006. *Dizziness: A Practical Approach to Diagnosis and Management*. Cambridge, Cambridge University Press.

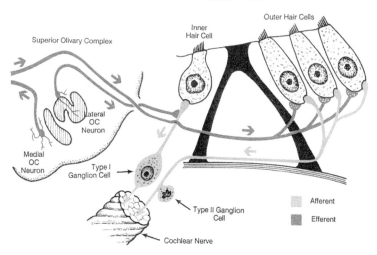

Figure 19.4 Diagram to illustrate efferent supply to inner and outer hair cells from medial and lateral olivocochlear bundles

The exact function of the efferent auditory system remains poorly understood, but it is thought that there is an auto-regulatory feedback mechanism that is mainly inhibitory, but may also be excitatory at different levels, and thus adjust and improve the processing of the auditory signal (Suga *et al.*, 2000) . The efferent fibres leave the brainstem in the superior division of the vestibular nerve. The reader is referred to the detailed description of cochlear physiology and mechanics by Pickles (2007). (Schuknecht, H.F. 1993. *Pathology of the Ear*. Philadelphia, Lea & Febiger, p. 67)

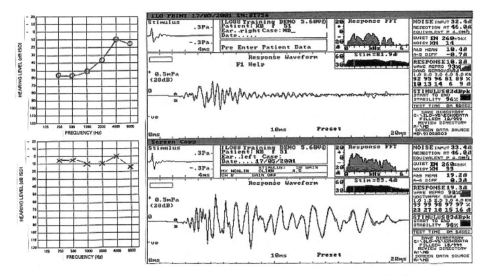

Figure 19.8 Otoacoustic emissions recorded from each ear in a normal subject

Otoacoustic emissions represent weak signals generated by the contractile properties of the outer hair cells in the cochlea in response to acoustic stimuli are time locked and averaged using computer analysis. These responses are measured in the external auditory canal, and provide direct objective information about the integrity of the outer hair cells.

Chapter 11

EXCESSIVE DAYTIME SLEEPINESS: CLINICAL CONSIDERATIONS

Thomas C. Britton, Andrew R. C. Cummin and Anthony N. Nicholson

Many disorders of the sleep–wake continuum lead to impaired daytime wakefulness with the possibility that cognition may be prejudiced. These disorders have particular relevance to the practice of aviation medicine in the selection of aircrew during young adulthood or if unwanted daytime sleepiness develops in middle age. In the clinical approach to excessive daytime sleepiness it is important for the practitioner to distinguish between sleepiness and fatigue – difficult though that can sometimes be – and to appreciate that they may coexist, as in obstructive sleep apnoea. Indeed, individuals often refer to both as tiredness. Due attention must be given to that possibility as subjective scales may assume that the subject can differentiate between sleepiness and fatigue. The complaint of fatigue is outside the scope of this text. There is a wide variety of scales and questionnaires concerned with its assessment, and the reader is referred to the review by Shen, Barbera and Shapiro (2006).

Sleepiness is not easy to define or to measure, but it is important to appreciate that the ability or the tendency to fall asleep quickly (sleep propensity) is not necessarily an indication of an undue generalized sleepiness that could impair the day-to-day life of the individual and imply sleep pathology. Falling asleep in well-defined circumstances (as in the measurement of sleep latencies) is a process that is distinct from a stable underlying and ongoing state of sleepiness. It may be related to experience or circumstances operant at that time. The separate phenomena of falling asleep quickly and underlying sleepiness are reflected in sleepiness scales and sleep latencies, and so it is essential to ensure that the scales and latencies are correctly interpreted. It is the approach of the aeromedical practitioner to excessive daytime sleepiness that is dealt with in this chapter, with emphasis on the measurements related to sleep, the differential diagnoses and the implications of each diagnosis to aircrew.

Sleepiness

Subjective assessments are well established in the investigation of the sleep–wake continuum (Chapter 10: Investigation of Sleep and Wakefulness in Aircrew). The most widely used are the Stanford (Hoddes *et al.*, 1973), the Karolinska (Akerstedt and Gilberg, 1990) and the Epworth (Johns, 1994) Sleepiness Scales. Visual analogue scales may also be used. They provide longitudinal data and are used mainly in research protocols concerned with evaluating the effects of drugs that modulate sleep and wakefulness.

Sleepiness Scales

The Stanford Sleepiness Scale (SSS) incorporates questions dealing with activity, alertness, cognition and sleepiness. It is concerned with feelings. It records the perceived level of sleepiness at the time of the assessment, but does not attempt to measure the general ongoing background level of daytime sleepiness. The Karolinska Sleepiness Scale (KSS) is similar. The scale provides an assessment of perceived alertness and sleepiness at the time of the assessment. Both of these scales are useful when there is the need to measure sleepiness at a particular time. They are sensitive to sleep deprivation and time of day, and may be repeated at short intervals of time. However, though the information obtained from both scales may suggest to the physician that the individual could have ongoing undue daytime sleepiness, they do not provide direct evidence for 'excessive daytime sleepiness' with its implication of sleep pathology.

The Epworth Sleepiness Scale (Johns, 1991, 1994, 1998, 2000; Chervin, 2003; Chervin and Aldrich, 1999) is an increasingly used instrument in the clinical setting. It is concerned with the chance of falling asleep in various situations encountered during day-to-day life. It is, therefore, independent of short-term variations. The subjects are required to assess their chance of falling asleep or dozing during various activities that range from lying down and resting in the afternoon to sitting and talking. Unlike the Stanford and Karolinska Scales, the Epworth Scale does not attempt to provide an indication of the severity of sleepiness at the time of the assessment. It indicates, in general terms, whether the individual is likely to have an undue level of background sleepiness, though the likelihood may be underestimated. The Epworth Scale is dependent on the estimates of the individual and, traditionally, a score above 10 is used to indicate unusual sleepiness. However, in a study of a randomly sampled community population (Sanford *et al.*, 2006) this score was exceeded by nearly one-third. That would indicate that, despite the usefulness of the Epworth Scale, caution must be exercised in assigning the significance to the calculated value if that is being used to indicate an unusual degree of sleepiness. On the other hand, there is always the possibility that if employment may be at stake, subjective assessments may err towards an underestimate of the degree of sleepiness.

Latencies to Daytime Sleep

The multiple sleep latency test (Carskadon and Dement, 1977; Carskadon *et al.*, 1986; Richardson *et al.*, 1978) measures the time taken to fall asleep. It is concerned with the tendency at particular times of the day and in particular circumstances to doze off or fall asleep, and so enter drowsy sleep. The test consists of four to six naps taken at two-hourly intervals from around an hour and a half after awakening. The subjects are encouraged to fall asleep in a darkened room, and the electroencephalogram and electro-oculogram are used to determine the latency to the first epoch of sleep observed on each occasion. The sleep latencies are sensitive to the time of day. They have a characteristic pattern. During the morning, latencies reduce, and that is presumably linked to the decreasing influence of the previous nocturnal sleep. During the afternoon, latencies increase and that is presumably linked to the underlying circadian rhythm of increasing alertness. If appropriate, recordings can be continued beyond sleep onset to detect sleep-onset rapid eye movements that could be relevant to the diagnosis of narcolepsy.

In the analysis of the data the latencies are often averaged over the day to provide an overall indication of sleep propensity – an averaged tendency to sleep. However, there is uncertainty concerning the clinical significance of such averaged values, and values of the individual points on the curve should be noted. Unfortunately, it has been widely assumed that the individual who is sleepy will fall asleep more quickly than one who is not sleepy. However, though the latencies are sensitive to the time of day, sleep deprivation and the effects of drugs that modulate alertness, it cannot be assumed that short latencies indicate an ongoing day-to-day state of undue sleepiness with the potential 'diagnosis' of pathological sleepiness. Indeed, Johns (2000) calculated from published studies that the normal range was from 3.2 to 20.0 minutes based on two standard deviations of the mean value.

As far as the potential clinical significance of the individual latencies is concerned, it must be borne in mind that short latencies are often observed in healthy adults (Levine et al., 1988;

Manni et al., 1991), and that sleepiness does not mean being able to fall asleep rapidly in conducive circumstances (Lavie and Zvuluni, 1992; Harrison and Horne, 1996). Further, in a study on sleep latencies recorded over a period of 30 hours in healthy subjects, it was not possible to establish correlations between sleep latency and the waking electroencephalogram, performance or arousal indices, and it was concluded that caution is necessary in the use of latencies alone to indicate daytime function (Nicholson et al., 1989). Similar concerns were raised by Johnson et al. (1990) from a study on daytime sleepiness in healthy young adults, and Johns (1998, 2000) has raised doubts as to whether the test can be used as an indicant of excessive daytime sleepiness.

Maintenance of Wakefulness

Maintenance of Wakefulness Test

This test is concerned with the ability to maintain wakefulness at the time of the assessment (Mittler et al., 1982). Subjects, at two-hourly intervals, sit upright in a darkened room and remain awake as long as they can. The assessment takes place within a specified period of time, say 20 or 40 minutes, and the time to the first epoch of any stage of sleep is recorded. The normative study carried out by Doghramji et al. (1997) indicated that the lower limits for the time to fall asleep (taken as two standard deviations below the mean) were 10.9 minutes with the 20-minute test and 19.4 minutes with the 40-minute test. The maintenance of wakefulness test, as with the multiple sleep latency test, measures sleep latencies, though in different circumstances, and does not necessarily indicate a pervasive ongoing excessive sleepiness. It is useful when there are concerns about the ability to stay awake and so to sustain attention, though that is not being directly measured.

Oxford Sleep Resistance (OSLER) Test

The maintenance of wakefulness and multiple sleep latency tests require electroencephalographic recordings, and so present logistic problems in routine clinical practice. In that context, the Oxford Sleep Resistance (OSLER) Test was developed, in which subjects are required to operate a switch in response to a light that is illuminated for a second in every three seconds. When the subject fails to respond for 21 seconds, sleep is considered to have occurred. In the initial evaluation, the usefulness of the test was compared with that of the maintenance of wakefulness test in patients with symptomatic sleepiness. It was concluded that the test discriminated as well as the maintenance of wakefulness test between healthy individuals and patients with obstructive sleep apnoea (Bennett *et al.*, 1997). In a subsequent study using the OSLER Test (Priest *et al.*, 2001), micro-sleeps recorded electroencephalographically were observed in sleep-deprived subjects particularly when consecutive stimuli were missed. It was concluded that the test was a reliable and useful method to assess daytime somnolence.

Correlations: Scales and Latencies

It is evident that subjective assessments of sleepiness and measures of sleep latency reflect different phenomena (Sangal *et al.*, 1992; Chervin *et al.*, 1995). They may assess sleepiness at a particular time in a particular circumstance or they may indicate the underlying sleepiness of the individual (Cludyts *et al.*, 2002).

The Stanford and Karolinska Scales seek information concerning perceived sleepiness at a particular time (state sleepiness); the Epworth Scale seeks information concerning the perception of background sleepiness (global or trait sleepiness). Multiple sleep latencies record how rapidly the individual falls asleep in circumstances that encourage sleep (sleep drive) and so may be useful when there is the need to know whether alertness is impaired. Benbadis *et al.* (1999) have studied the association between the Epworth scale and the multiple sleep latency test. Maintenance of wakefulness records how long the individual can stay awake (wake drive) and may be useful when there is the need to know whether the ability to stay awake is impaired. The limited statistical correlations that exist between these measures are of little help in clinical practice.

Interpretation

Tests that involve the measurement of sleep latencies and the maintenance of wakefulness measure aspects of sleep propensity. Sleep latencies measure the ability to fall asleep, and the maintenance of wakefulness measures ability to stay awake. Although it might indicate sleepiness related to underlying pathology, the ability to fall asleep quickly when required is not necessarily pathological and for aircrew moving across time zones or sleeping on board might well even have benefits. Furthermore, an individual wishing to perform well on a sleep latency test could easily alter the outcome by striving to stay awake. The test would then become a measure of whether the patient could stay awake if required to do so, which is a quite different measure and is in fact the focus of the maintenance of wakefulness test. On the face of it, a test that measures the ability to stay awake might be a more appropriate test, but there is a paucity of data on normal values, and a 'normal' value is no guarantee that the individual will be able to stay awake in the workplace. Similarly, normal subjects who are unable to stay awake in the circumstances of the maintenance of wakefulness test may be able to stay awake in the more rousing environment of work, operating machinery or when driving a motor vehicle or flying an aircraft.

Circadian Disorders

The nature of circadian rhythmicity is dealt with in Chapter 2 (Circadian System and Diurnal Activity). Normally, the endogenous rhythms (as well as the alternation of wake and sleep) are synchronized to the day and night of the environment, but in some individuals these relations no longer hold (Sack *et al.*, 2007). The possibility of disorders of the circadian system should be considered during the medical screening of aircrew as disorders of the circadian system may be associated with impaired wakefulness or even excessive daytime sleepiness.

The most common disorder of the circadian system is the delayed sleep phase syndrome described initially by Weitzman *et al.* (1981). There is a tendency to fall asleep late at night or in the very early hours of the morning (up to six hours later than normal), with difficulty in rising in the morning with adequate alertness to meet the usual demands of work. If undisturbed, sleep is of the normal length of time and is free of pathology. There are less common disorders, but these are less likely to be encountered in aeromedical practice. The advanced sleep phase syndrome is where the sleep period is advanced with

early sleep onset and early awakening in the day. A sleep–wake rhythm that is free-running is often seen in the blind, while complete irregularity of the sleep–wake rhythm may accompany a concomitant disorder of the central nervous system.

Disorders of the circadian system may present as excessive daytime sleepiness at inconvenient times of the day. In that context, it must be borne in mind that aircrew may need to work early mornings and late nights as in short-haul operations or cope with irregularity of rest and activity after transmeridian flights with the inevitable displacement of the sleep–wake pattern from the ongoing day and night. It is, therefore, important that the aeromedical practitioner is able to identify a circadian rhythm disorder in prospective aircrew and to discriminate between the effects of the working environment and a circadian rhythm disorder on the alertness of aircrew.

The initial investigation of a potential disorder of the circadian system involves recording, preferably over several weeks, the sleep–wake pattern in a diary, together with wrist movement (continuously over each 24 hours) by an actigraph (Ancoli-Israel *et al.*, 2003). With phase disorders the diaries and actigraphy usually reveal over weekends and during holidays (when the individual is no longer constrained by the conventional hours of work) a delay or advance of the sleep period, respectively. In the free-running disorder they reveal the irregularity of the sleep–wake pattern. The endogenous melatonin profile has also been used as a marker for the circadian position (Lewy *et al.*, 1999).

The syndrome that involves a phase-delay disorder may well be encountered in young adult aircrew. An attempt can be made to realign the rhythm by delaying bedtime by three hours a day every two days until the desired rest and activity pattern is achieved. To be successful, it is important to adhere rigidly to the new regime. An attempt to induce a phase advance can also be made by exposing the individual to bright light for periods up to 60 minutes in the morning, and a parallel technique has been used with the advanced syndrome. In this context, short wavelength light has been studied (Lockley *et al.*, 2003). However, both chronotherapy and phototherapy have their limitations. Melatonin taken in the evening when the phase is delayed or in the morning when the phase is advanced is another approach. Its effectiveness is probably related to its sedative activity and lowering of body temperature.

It has to be accepted that these approaches may fail to prove to be sufficiently robust to ensure that an individual with a circadian disorder could cope with an irregular pattern of work arising from the need for air operations to be scheduled around the clock and with time-zone changes, and maintain critical levels of alertness. The disengagement of the sleep–wake pattern from the day–night alternation may persist, and it is for that reason that the aeromedical practitioner needs to consider carefully whether an individual with a circadian disorder would be suitable for training as aircrew. With a diagnosis later in life, the question would still remain whether the condition is compatible with continued employment in circumstances that inevitably lead to sleep disturbance during rest periods and demand work free of impaired wakefulness at all hours round the clock

Narcolepsy and the Narcoleptic Syndrome

In the younger patient with excessive daytime sleepiness, the aeromedical practitioner will need to consider the possibility of an underlying neurological condition such as narcolepsy or idiopathic hypersomnia. The main differential diagnosis will be circadian rhythm disorders, especially in those individuals who are subject to frequent transmeridian travel. On the other hand, older individuals who develop excessive daytime sleepiness for the first time may have disturbed night-time sleep due to neurological or respiratory disorders. Neurological disorders that will need to be considered include narcolepsy, restless legs syndrome, neurodegenerative diseases and insidiously developing neuromuscular respiratory failure.

The narcoleptic syndrome is a chronic neurological condition that most commonly develops in the second or third decades of life (Zeman *et al.*, 2004). Its prevalence is estimated to be about 3 to 5 per 10,000 in the European population, making it approximately four times less common than multiple sclerosis. However, many patients are undiagnosed, and even for those patients who are diagnosed correctly, the delay to diagnosis is often around ten years from their first symptoms. Approximately 50 per cent of adults with the disorder retrospectively report symptoms beginning in their teenage years. Both sexes are equally affected. Rare familial cases are described. The narcoleptic syndrome refers to the tetrad of symptoms that includes narcolepsy (sudden attacks of sleep), cataplexy (sudden loss of muscle tone often triggered by emotion), sleep paralysis (awakening from sleep still paralyzed) and hypnogogic/ hypnopompic hallucinations. The importance of cataplexy within this tetrad has long been recognized, and, recently, has been linked to the absence of the neuropeptide, hypocretin/orexin, within the cerebrospinal fluid (Baumann and Bassetti, 2005). Narcolepsy is often divided into narcolepsy with cataplexy and narcolepsy without cataplexy.

Clinical Features

The first symptom of narcolepsy is usually excessive daytime sleepiness, with patients often falling asleep at times and in situations that are inappropriate (Zeman *et al.*, 2004). Patients, who are often at school or college when the symptoms begin, typically fall asleep in class or lectures and are then accused of being lazy or of not going to bed early enough. The urge to fall asleep can be overwhelming, but the duration of sleep is usually relatively short, lasting from 5 to 20 minutes, and most will describe the nap as being refreshing. In contrast, those with idiopathic hypersomnia, the chronic fatigue syndrome or depression generally report longer non-refreshing daytime naps lasting up to an hour or more.

Cataplexy is the sudden loss of muscle tone often triggered by emotion. It may result in complete loss of posture and falls with consequent injuries, but may only manifest itself as a slight loss of neck posture or drop in tone of the facial musculature. Cataplexy appears to have significance in relation to the presence of certain neuroendocrine changes within the hypothalamus. Hypnogogic hallucinations are characteristic visual images that the patient may report on going off to sleep. Such hallucinations are often described as vivid dream-like experiences or frightening elementary shapes and forms moving towards them as they fall asleep. Similar experiences may be reported on waking – hypnopompic hallucinations.

Sleep paralysis occurs when the patient wakes from sleep, but discovers that they are unable to move. Often they will report a sense of pressure on the chest. Occasional episodes of sleep paralysis are common in the general population, but patients with narcolepsy may have frequent attacks, typically occurring as they fall asleep, whereas idiopathic sleep paralysis is more likely to occur in the middle to latter part of the night. In addition to the cardinal features of the condition, patients often describe poor nocturnal sleep with frequent awakenings, together with behavioural abnormalities that include sleepwalking and behavioural disorders associated with rapid eye movement sleep (Bonakis *et al.*, 2009).

Pathophysiology

The symptoms of narcolepsy can be regarded as a disorder of the control of rapid eye movement (REM) sleep, whereby components of the REM sleep state intrude into wakefulness or orthodox (non-REM) sleep. Cataplexy can be viewed as REM-sleep atonia, with the active inhibition of muscle tone that normally accompanies REM sleep intruding into wakefulness, while hallucinations can be viewed as an intrusion of REM-sleep mentation (or dreams) into wakefulness. In sleep paralysis, patients may awaken without the normal reversal of the motor inhibition that occurs during REM-sleep. Whether all of the abnormalities seen in narcolepsy can be explained on the basis of a loss of REM-sleep regulation remains uncertain.

Animal studies have identified several brainstem structures that are important for the control of REM sleep, mainly within the pons and midbrain, although hypothalamic and forebrain mechanisms may also be involved (Jones, 2008). REM-on cells, which fire selectively during REM sleep periods, appear to be cholinergic, while REM-off cells are generally noradrenergic or serotonergic. The lower brainstem relay for motor inhibition in REM sleep appears to lie in the ventromedial medulla and contains glutaminergic cells which project to inhibitory spinal interneurons. The exact neurochemical basis underlying narcolepsy remains unknown, but may involve increased cholinergic activity within midbrain and pontine nuclei.

Ninety per cent of patients with narcolepsy with cataplexy have absent or low concentrations of hypocretin (orexin) in the cerebrospinal fluid (Bourgin *et al.*, 2008). Hypocretin is a neuropeptide produced in the posterolateral hypothalamus that has been shown to play a part in arousal, muscle tone and locomotion, the regulation of feeding behaviour and autonomic functions. Its role in the control of REM sleep remains controversial, but it probably acts as a sleep–wake stabilizer, preventing sudden and inappropriate transitions between REM and orthodox sleep. Those with narcolepsy with cataplexy appear to have a selective loss of the hypocretin-producing cells within the posterolateral hypothalamus.

The loss of cells that produce hypocretin within the hypothalamus (in those with narcolepsy with cataplexy) may have an autoimmune basis. In support of an autoimmune basis is the finding that almost all patients with narcolepsy with cataplexy have the human leucocyte antigen (HLA) type DQB1*0602 that is closely linked to an increased susceptibility to autoimmune disease. However, HLA-type DQB1*0602 does not predict the disease as it is present in approximately 25 per cent of the Caucasian population. Furthermore, there is little other evidence to support an autoimmune basis and patients do not generally have oligoclonal bands within the cerebrospinal fluid or an excess of other autoantibodies.

Absent or low levels of hypocretin have been described in a number of other conditions including head trauma, encephalitis, inflammatory neuropathies and diencephalic tumours. Narcolepsy-like sleep disturbances have been described in some of these cases, but not all. The exact nature of the link between deficiency of hypocretin and sleep disorders remains uncertain. Patients with narcolepsy without cataplexy have normal levels of hypocretin levels. Further, the relationship of narcolepsy without cataplexy to narcolepsy with cataplexy and to idiopathic hypersomnia remains unclear (Bourgin *et al.*, 2008).

Differential Diagnosis

Individuals with excessive daytime sleepiness associated with typical cataplexy should not pose a diagnostic problem. Some may initially present just with cataplexy, although this is rare since excessive daytime sleepiness almost always precedes the development of cataplexy. Indeed, the onset of excessive daytime sleepiness can precede the onset of cataplexy by many years, so patients initially presenting with just excessive daytime sleepiness will be the more common situation. For the rare patient who presents initially with just cataplexy, a clear and accurate history is paramount because the fact that they do not lose awareness during their attacks is often missed. Cataplexy is probably most often mistaken for an epileptic process, especially if there is irregular twitching of the limbs or face during the attack. Cataplexy can also be confused with faints or vasovagal attacks, since both are characteristically triggered by strong emotions; the retention of awareness during the attack is again the most important diagnostic feature pointing towards cataplexy. Other less common conditions that may enter the differential diagnosis of cataplectic attacks include startle epilepsy, hyperekplexia and gelastic epilepsy.

A diagnosis of narcolepsy would be of serious import to those seeking employment in aviation and to those already employed as it would permanently disqualify them from a licence. However, the aeromedical practitioner must bear in mind that the differential diagnosis for excessive daytime sleepiness is very wide and includes, amongst many other conditions, insufficient sleep, obstructive sleep apnoea and circadian rhythm disorders. Idiopathic hypersomnia is clinically difficult to differentiate from narcolepsy, although polysomnography can be helpful. Secondary causes of narcolepsy are rare, but well described, and include hypothalamic tumours, head injuries and a number of congenital syndromes.

Investigation

Investigation of a patient with suspected narcolepsy will vary depending on the circumstances and the certainty of the clinical diagnosis. A patient with narcolepsy and typical cataplexy may need no additional tests. Others with excessive daytime sleepiness will require investigations to exclude alternative diagnoses and, where possible, to provide evidence to support the diagnosis of narcolepsy. However, no single definitive test for narcolepsy is as yet available. Tomography and imaging are generally normal in those with narcolepsy, though sometimes requested to exclude the rare secondary causes of narcolepsy due to diencephalic lesions and tumours.

Most with suspected narcolepsy will have undergone polysomnography followed by recordings of daytime sleep latencies. Ideally, they should complete a sleep diary for two weeks prior to the overnight polysomnography to exclude a significant circadian rhythm disorder as a cause for their excessive daytime sleepiness. Polysomnography should identify patients with other causes of excessive daytime sleepiness, including restless legs syndrome, periodic limb movements during sleep or obstructive sleep apnoea. Polysomnography will also provide objective evidence of the quality and quantity of night-time sleep prior to a multiple sleep latency test.

The analysis of daytime sleep latencies provides an average value (Littner et al., 2005; Aldrich et al., 1997). Normal individuals will have an average latency of more than ten minutes. A sleep latency of less than five minutes is generally considered abnormal and consistent with an increased daytime sleepiness. Sleep-onset REM episodes on two or more of the naps is considered supportive of a diagnosis of narcolepsy. Whilst the multiple sleep latency test can be used to support a diagnosis of narcolepsy, it cannot be used to exclude the diagnosis, as not all with narcolepsy have reduced sleep latencies and the test is very dependent on the cooperation from the patient in trying to fall asleep. Thus one would need to exercise caution in using the test to assess an individual who has been reported falling asleep by their work colleagues.

The maintenance of wakefulness test is not commonly used in clinical practice to assess patients with narcolepsy, since it is of limited diagnostic value (Littner et al., 2005). However, it might be considered when trying to assess the functional impact of excessive daytime sleepiness or where there is concern about the ability to remain awake. Patients with untreated narcolepsy usually have a latency to sleep of about ten minutes compared with 18 minutes in healthy subjects.

In the past, HLA typing was often carried out since it was the first biological marker of narcolepsy to be identified. Almost all with narcolepsy with cataplexy will be HLA DQB1*0602 positive, though the rate varies a little with ethnicity. However, the specificity of HLA typing is low, since about 25 per cent of the Caucasian population are carriers – for every HLA DQB1*0602 positive individual with narcolepsy, there will be about 600 similarly positive individuals who do not have narcolepsy. The test is now rarely required. Absence of HLA DQB1*0602 in an individual with excessive daytime sleepiness would, however, be a strong pointer against the diagnosis of narcolepsy.

Measurements of hypocretin in the cerebrospinal fluid are a reliable way of confirming a diagnosis of narcolepsy with cataplexy, a level below 110 pg mL^{-1} being indicative of the diagnosis (Bourgin et al., 2008). However, hypocretin levels are not commonly measured in clinical practice because the diagnosis is rarely in doubt when the patient has narcolepsy with typical cataplexy. Patients with narcolepsy without cataplexy, where the clinical diagnosis is often less certain, usually have normal levels of hypocretin, and the test is, therefore, of little practical value.

The primary duty of the aeromedical practitioner is to ensure that an adequate assessment has been carried out as the diagnosis of narcolepsy permanently disqualifies the individual from a licence.

Idiopathic Hypersomnia

Some people who have an increased propensity to fall asleep during the day do not seemingly have narcolepsy and do not have any other obvious cause for their symptoms, such as insufficient sleep. Such individuals are now usually labelled as having idiopathic hypersomnia. However, the distinction between normal long sleepers at one end of the spectrum and individuals with narcolepsy without cataplexy at the other end is often difficult (Billiard, 2007). Idiopathic hypersomnia usually appears between the ages of 15 and 30 years, with males and females being equally affected (Ohayon, 2008). There are no reliable data on the prevalence of idiopathic hypersomnia, but it is considered to be rare, with a prevalence in the region of 0.3 per cent.

Clinical Features

Idiopathic hypersomnia presents as excessive daytime sleepiness with frequent daytime naps. In contrast with narcolepsy, the daytime naps are often of relatively long duration (one to two hours) and are rarely reported to be refreshing. They are not associated with dreaming. Night-time sleep is of normal or longer than normal duration, but is characteristically reported to be unrefreshing. Patients sleep deeply and are difficult to rouse, and they are liable to confusional arousals. The criteria for the diagnosis of idiopathic hypersomnia (American Academy of Sleep Medicine, 2005) require that the condition has been present for at least six months and that there has been no significant head injury during the preceding 18 months. In addition, there must be an absence of any medical or psychiatric disorders that could account for the excessive daytime sleepiness. Based on the duration of night-time sleep, idiopathic hypersomnia is now divided into two categories – idiopathic hypersomnia with long sleep time of more than ten hours and idiopathic hypersomnia without long sleep time, more than six but less than ten hours.

The pathophysiological basis of idiopathic hypersomnia is unknown. There is no association with the human leucocyte antigen DQB1*0602, and the levels of hypocretin in the cerebrospinal fluid are normal (Mignot, 2008). The main differential diagnosis will be between normal long sleepers and those with narcolepsy without cataplexy. Between 3 and 10 per cent of the population will report 'sleeping too much', and self-reported sleep duration is longer than eight and a half hours in about 10 per cent of the population (Van Dongen *et al.*, 2005). However, normal long sleepers do not report excessive daytime sleepiness. Distinguishing between idiopathic hypersomnia and narcolepsy without cataplexy is more problematic and will depend on the history and an analysis of daytime sleeps. Overnight polysomnography will be required to exclude other causes of excessive daytime sleepiness, with sleep latencies carried out the next day. The average sleep latency should be less than eight minutes, and there should be less than two episodes with sleep-onset REM sleep. Idiopathic hypersomnia with long sleep time is associated with more than ten hours of nocturnal sleep. The maintenance of wakefulness test may be of value in assessing the impact on daytime alertness (Grossman *et al.*, 2004).

Individuals with idiopathic hypersomnia should be careful to avoid any circumstances that might exacerbate the excessive sleepiness. Ideally, they should keep to a good sleep routine, although this may not be easy to achieve in aviation personnel. The judicious use of caffeine is often helpful. Modafinil is effective (Banerjee *et al.*, 2004), but some require amphetamine-based medications. A diagnosis of idiopathic hypersomnia will generally be associated with a degree of uncertainty, and distinguishing this disorder from normal longer sleepers or from narcolepsy without cataplexy is often problematic. The employment or continued employment of aviation personnel with a diagnosis of idiopathic hypersomnia demands careful consideration and rests on a case-by-case basis.

Incipient Neurodegenerative Diseases

Most neurodegenerative conditions, such as the Parkinsonian disorders or the dementias, are associated, at least in their later stages, with significant sleep problems including excessive daytime sleepiness, loss of the normal circadian rhythm and disturbed nocturnal sleep. Such sleep problems will not be an issue for the aeromedical physician who is looking after otherwise fit personnel. However, the onset of sleep problems in an otherwise fit individual can occasionally presage the development of more significant neurological disease, sometimes by many years or decades. In such circumstances, there is the need for a high index of suspicion for neurological disease after the more common causes of sleep problems have been excluded. Parkinson's disease and other Parkinsonian disorders, such as multiple system atrophy and Lewy-body dementias, appear especially likely to present with excessive daytime sleepiness, unexplained sleep attacks or behavioural disorders associated with REM sleep.

Parkinson's disease is frequently associated with excessive daytime sleepiness, with 40 per cent of patients with active Parkinson's disease having an Epworth Sleepiness score of more than 10, compared with 19 per cent in controls (Brodsky *et al.*, 2003). Patients with Parkinson's disease are also liable to sudden onset sleep attacks similar to narcolepsy and report falling asleep while driving more frequently (21 per cent) than controls (6 per cent). The excessive daytime sleepiness that occurs in Parkinson's disease may be due partly to medication and partly to fragmentation of night-time sleep and insomnia – often as a result of stiffness, restless legs, nocturnal cramps or urinary symptoms. However, some of the excessive daytime sleepiness appears to be an intrinsic part of the condition itself.

A REM sleep behaviour disorder (RBD) can predate the motor manifestations of Parkinsonism by many years or decades (Postuma *et al.*, 2009). It is characterized by loss of the normal muscle atonia that accompanies REM sleep. As a consequence, patients may 'act out their dreams', often falling out of bed, inadvertently hitting or punching their bed partner or shouting instructions. Patients may be unaware of the condition unless they injure themselves, the relevant history being provided by the bed partner. Patients diagnosed with RBD are at risk of developing Parkinson's disease and other Parkinsonian disorders – the risk being about 50 per cent at ten years. Whether all patients with RBD eventually develop Parkinsonism is unknown. Aviation personnel who are found to have RBD will need careful screening to ensure that they do not have the beginnings of Parkinson's disease.

Recent developments in our understanding of Parkinsonism have led to the view that the neurodegenerative process is not restricted to the nigrostriatal tract, as was once believed, but instead begins in the medulla and dorsal brainstem nuclei before spreading up through the brainstem (Braak *et al.*, 2003). On this basis, it is easy to appreciate how brainstem structures involved in sleep regulation, such as the medullary and pontine nuclei, can become affected before the substantia nigra within the midbrain. A diagnosis of Parkinson's disease, by virtue of its progressive nature, would generally disqualify an individual from holding a licence, while individuals with the REM sleep behavioural disorder would need to be considered on a case-by-case basis.

Periodic Limb Movements and the Restless Legs Syndrome

Periodic limb movements in sleep (PLMS) and the restless legs syndrome (RLS) are closely related conditions that can cause insomnia and excessive daytime sleepiness. In both conditions, the cause of the excessive daytime sleepiness appears to be disruption of sleep by frequent limb movements. Patients who have more than 15 periodic limb movements per hour of sleep associated with complaints of insomnia or excessive daytime sleepiness are defined within the International Classification of Sleep Disorders as having the periodic limb movement disorder. The population prevalence of PLMS is about 5 per cent, the condition being more common in Caucasians than African Americans (Scofield *et al.*, 2008). In the general population, PLMS is closely linked to complaints of insomnia. Although caffeine consumption is held to exacerbate the condition, the overall consumption of caffeine by such patients is not significantly different from controls.

The restless legs syndrome affects an estimated 7 to 10 per cent of the population, the condition being more common in Caucasians than African Americans, and those from the Far

East having the lowest prevalence (Montplaisir *et al.*, 2006). The syndrome becomes more common with increasing age and is associated with iron deficiency, pregnancy and end-stage renal disease, as well as neuropathies. More than 60 per cent of cases are thought to be familial and several genetic loci have been identified. Approximately 80 to 90 per cent have periodic leg movements. The limb movements are usually brief and rather jerky, lasting one to two seconds each and occurring repetitively in clusters of approximately every 15 to 90 seconds, generally during light (drowsy and stage 2) sleep. Both legs are usually affected, but not always symmetrically. Typically, the movements consist of extension of the big toes with dorsiflexion of the ankle and flexion of the knee and hip, similar to the Babinski withdrawal response, although other movement patterns are frequently seen (de Weerd *et al.*, 2004). Each movement is associated with a brief arousal, reflected in the electroencephalogram, an arousal being more likely with larger movements. Whether the limb movement causes the arousal or the arousal leads to the limb movement remains uncertain.

Patients are sometimes aware of their leg movements as they are falling asleep, or they may awaken with an urge to move their feet or hang their legs outside the bed. Such symptoms are similar to those experienced by patients with the restless legs syndrome, but those with periodic leg movements who are aware of their leg movements are sometimes labelled as having periodic limb movements during wakefulness (PLMW) in recognition of the fact that the movements do not strictly occur when they are asleep. Such observations also reinforce the view that periodic leg movements and the restless legs syndrome are really part of a continuum rather than distinct diseases.

Correctly identifying leg movements as the cause of excessive daytime sleepiness may be difficult if patients are unaware of their limb movements and if there is no history from a bed partner. In most cases, polysomnography throughout the night will be required to establish the diagnosis and exclude other causes of excessive daytime sleepiness. Management should initially be directed towards identifying and avoiding factors that might be exacerbating the condition. Irregular sleep routines, caffeine consumption, use of hypnotics or tricyclic antidepressants and stress can all worsen the condition and should be avoided where possible. Medications that are used in the restless legs syndrome are also helpful in those with periodic movements, and include the non-ergot dopamine agonists, levodopa and clonazepam. Iron deficiency should be corrected (Trenkwalder *et al.*, 2005). Patients with mild disturbances may wish to manage their symptoms without pharmacological therapy. Although such patients may have some insomnia, this probably does not affect cognitive function (Gamaldo *et al.*, 2008). More severe symptoms can affect daytime functioning, and aviation crew will need to be assessed on a case-by-case basis.

Neuromuscular Respiratory Failure

Isolated neuromuscular respiratory failure can occur in a number of conditions, including motor neuron disease, acid maltase deficiency, myotonic dystrophy and myasthenia gravis. In general, such conditions will produce excessive daytime sleepiness as a result of nocturnal hypoventilation and sleep fragmentation. They may also produce exertional dyspnoea. Sleep studies with appropriate respiratory recordings should identify the cause of the excessive daytime sleepiness as being due to neuromuscular respiratory failure, which typically manifests first during REM sleep. However, careful analysis will be required to ensure that such patients are correctly separated from the more common sleep-disordered breathing, obstructive sleep apnoea. Most causes of isolated neuromuscular respiratory failure are chronic and progressive, and would therefore disqualify an individual from an aircrew licence. Myasthenia gravis is also a lifelong condition, but it is not progressive and is treatable. Specialist advice would need to be taken about management and the risks of sudden incapacity arising in the future.

Obstructive Sleep Apnoea Syndrome

It is remarkable that obstructive sleep apnoea syndrome was not recognized as a major clinical problem until towards the end of the twentieth century, though descriptions of the condition date back to ancient times. As recently as 1981 it was claimed that obstructive sleep apnoea syndrome was uncommon in Britain (Shapiro *et al.*, 1981). We now know that the prevalence of obstructive sleep apnoea is especially high (perhaps as high as 4 per cent) in middle-aged men (Young *et al.*, 1993), and it is this demographic group that forms a large proportion of those working as experienced aircrew.

Pathophysiology

The pathogenesis of obstructive sleep apnoea syndrome is not fully understood, but the problem arises from recurrent obstruction or narrowing of the pharynx during sleep. Anatomical and functional factors, some genetically determined, combine to cause a loss of pharyngeal patency, perhaps because of craniofacial differences or, especially in the obese, the deposition of fat. The functional element is critical (White, 2005). Patency is maintained during wakefulness as a result of the activity of the pharyngeal dilator muscles, but in sleep, especially rapid eye movement sleep, the normal reduction muscular tone which includes the pharyngeal muscles, in susceptible individuals, causes the pharynx to narrow or become occluded.

Mild narrowing of the pharynx during sleep may just result in snoring as air passing through the narrowing sets up vibrations. If the pharynx becomes occluded, the patient is unable to breathe. Following increasing efforts to breathe against the obstruction, dilator muscle activity is eventually restored, the airway opens and breathing starts again, often with a snort. During this process there may be an arousal. The duration of the obstruction varies from a few seconds to over a minute and, depending on the duration and other factors such as lung volume, may be accompanied by marked but transient arterial oxygen desaturation. Some patients are aware of some of these episodes and may wake choking or gasping, but more often apnoeas pass unnoticed.

If recurrent arousals fragment and disrupt sleep, the patient may wake in the morning feeling unrefreshed and may be sleepy during the day. Sleep fragmentation and the resulting poor sleep quality may cause other symptoms such as poor concentration or grumpiness. Some patients may have drenching night sweats, presumably as a result of the sympathetic response to the apnoeas. Nocturia can also be a feature but may have a different mechanism

(Lin *et al.*, 1993). There is good evidence that obstructive sleep apnoea causes an elevation of systemic blood pressure especially during sleep.

Investigation

A full assessment of the patient with obstructive sleep apnoea involves polysomnography in which both sleep and breathing are recorded (Bulow, 1963). In addition to a limited montage for sleep staging, it is necessary to have measures of airflow at the nose/mouth and an estimate of movements of the thorax and abdomen. Various sensors can be used and may vary between sleep centres. Careful inspection of the data enables measures such as the frequency of apnoeas, hypopnoeas and arousals. Whether the apnoeas are central or obstructive can be determined from the thoracoabdominal movements.

Classification

Obstructive sleep apnoea is arbitrarily classified as mild, moderate or severe depending on the number of apnoeas and hypopnoeas per hour – the apnoea/hypopnoea index. However, the index is poorly correlated with daytime somnolence. Patients with obstructive apnoeas are not necessarily symptomatic and, since sleepiness is common in the general population, obstructive sleep apnoea is not necessarily the cause of an individual patient's sleepiness. Sometimes apnoeas only occur in the supine position when gravity tends to contribute to airway occlusion, or in rapid eye movement sleep when there is atonia of the pharyngeal dilators and other muscles.

At the mild end of the spectrum is simple snoring. Snoring occurs when the upper airway is narrow enough for the passage of air to cause vibrations, but sufficient patency is maintained to allow the flow of air. In simple snoring there is no significant airway occlusion and the apnoea/hypopnoea index is usually less than five events per hour; arousals do not occur and problems are largely confined to the bed partner. Some individuals may have arousals as a result of the effort to breathe against increased upper airway resistance rather than a complete pharyngeal occlusion, but the existence of this so-called upper airway resistance syndrome has been disputed (Douglas, 2000).

Functional Impairment

The apnoeic events that occur during sleep in individuals with obstructive sleep apnoea may lead to electroencephalographic arousals with impaired sleep continuity and to intermittent hypoxaemia. The functional consequences can be severe. It is well established that obstructive sleep apnoea leads to cognitive impairment as well as excessive daytime sleepiness, though the parts played by the impaired sleep and the intermittent hypoxaemia in the genesis of the observed deficits have been under discussion for many years (Findley *et al.*, 1986; Telekivi *et al.*, 1988). Broad-ranging neuropsychological deficits have been reported. Studies have been carried out with patients across many decades of life with sleep apnoea of varying severity, and a wide variety of tests has been used with differing designs. Cognitive impairment may involve intellectual and executive functions, performance on simulators, vigilance, attention and memory (Bédard *et al.*, 1991; Decary *et al.*, 2000; Naëgelé *et al.*, 1998; Engelman *et al.*, 2000: Fulda and Schultz, 2001; Aloia *et al.*, 2004; Mazza *et al.*, 2005; Saunamäki and Jehkonen, 2007; Lis *et al.*, 2008).

However, the relevance of the deficits to the day-to-day function of a particular individual is difficult to predict. Nevertheless, it is recognized that drivers with obstructive sleep apnoea are more likely than healthy individuals to be involved in collisions, and the risk increases with the severity of their condition. Performance decrements on driving simulators and sustained attention tasks are comparable with those of mild intoxication. While the various performance deficits may be reversed by effective treatment, questions remain as to their cause. Nocturnal hypoxaemia may be more associated with decrements in tests of global cognitive functioning, and sleep fragmentation more with decrements in tests of attention and vigilance (Aloia *et al.*, 2004).

To complicate matters, it would appear that even relatively mild degrees of respiratory disturbance in subjects without either marked hypoxaemia or sleepiness and free of comorbidity may be associated with cognitive deficits. There is evidence that vigilance and working memory may be impaired in such patients, though the ability to compensate with tasks that are stimulating is retained. One cannot discount the possibility that mild sleep-disordered breathing might cause an increased vulnerability to accidents or to mistakes during occupational tasks (Redline *et al.*, 1997).

Cerebral Pathology

In animal models of obstructive sleep apnoea, intermittent hypoxia causes brain injury, but standard magnetic resonance imaging of the brain of patients with obstructive sleep apnoea does not show obvious cerebral damage (Davies *et al.*, 2001). In the research setting, sophisticated imaging techniques have shown structural changes most consistently in the limbic system, but these do not fully explain the functional abnormalities. Studies using magnetic resonance imaging have shown that deficits may be associated with morphological changes. Macey *et al.* (2002) observed loss of grey matter in multiple areas, though it was uncertain whether these changes were pre-existing abnormalities that could have contributed to the genesis or maintenance of the disorder or whether they were a consequence of apnoea.

Lower concentrations of grey matter have also been reported within the left hippocampus (Morrell *et al.*, 2003, 2004). Axonal loss and impaired myelin have been found in the frontal periventricular matter (Alchanatis *et al.*, 2004), and, using functional magnetic resonance imaging, Thomas *et al.*(2005) reported loss of prefrontal activation in patients performing a working memory task. However, uncertainties remain in the alignment of neuropsychological impairments with the morphological changes. Morphological changes can be observed in the absence of unequivocal behavioural impairments, suggesting that imaging techniques may be particularly sensitive in detecting the central effects of sleep apnoea.

A study that involved cognitive assessments and brain imaging (Yaouhi *et al.*, 2009) raised the possibility that morphological changes may be present many years before there is clinical evidence of sleep apnoea, with the severity of the neurobehavioural manifestations becoming apparent only slowly. White matter may be extensively affected, and it has been suggested that this may represent injury that has accumulated over time (Macey *et al.*, 2008).

Clinical Management

Not all patients with obstructive apnoeas during sleep have excessive somnolence. The reason for this is not understood. It is possible that obstructive apnoeas disrupt the sleep of some but not others, perhaps related to different arousal thresholds. Perhaps, in some patients, the airway may reopen without sleep becoming fragmented, and this may be why neither the apnoea/hypopnoea index nor the number of arousals demonstrated electroencephalographically can be used clinically as a reliable predictor of functional impairment or daytime sleepiness. A further problem is that some arousals may not be detected by standard scoring criteria of electrical events.

Symptomatic cases require treatment. In principle, any treatment that prevents recurrent obstruction of the upper airway during sleep and restores sleep quality should be effective. Sometimes, usually in mild cases, obstructive apnoeas are confined to the supine position, and postural measures to prevent the patient sleeping on their back may be all that is required. While not usually the treatment of choice, devices that advance the mandible can be effective. Worn at night, they pull the lower jaw forward, making more space in the pharynx.

Tonsillectomy and adenoidectomy are often effective in children, and the occasional, usually young, adult with large tonsils may also benefit. Orthognathic surgery is a promising approach for those with micrognathia or retrognathia, but, on the whole, surgery in adults is disappointing, though there may still be a role in very severe cases for tracheostomy. Uvulopalatopharyngoplasty and laser-assisted uvulopalatoplasty are not generally recommended.

Continuous Positive Airway Pressure

Continuous positive airway pressure (CPAP) is the mainstay of treatment for obstructive sleep apnoea syndrome. It can be very effective for patients with symptoms and has a firm evidence base. It is self-evident that patients without symptoms cannot be made to feel better. On the other hand, sleep apnoea can be associated with a number of cardiovascular diseases, and there is a small but significant improvement in hypertension after treatment. Whether airway pressure reduces cardiovascular complications is not known. Currently, treatment is offered to improve symptoms and performance, but for treatment to be effective the patient must be able to use the machine sufficiently and effectively.

Effective treatment abolishes obstructive apnoeas, improves sleep quality, lessens unwanted sleepiness and restores alertness. The response to treatment may be rapid, but those in critical employments are generally required to be on effective treatment for six weeks before returning to duty. Difficulties may arise if there are problems with mask leaks or usage is inadequate. Some individuals find themselves removing the mask during sleep and temporary difficulties may arise during episodes of coryza or allergic rhinitis. Modern machines record usage, residual apnoeas and mask leaks, and machine downloads can be invaluable in determining whether or not those in safety-critical jobs are receiving sufficient effective treatment.

A particular problem is that patients in safety-critical occupations may make light of their degree of sleepiness.

The inevitable effects of shift work and frequent time-zone changes on somnolence complicate matters further. Furthermore, residual sleepiness following treatment is a well-recognized problem, and, with increasing evidence of structural brain changes possibly accumulating over years, the aeromedical practitioner should bear in mind the possibility of residual cognitive impairment in those with treated sleep apnoea (Bédard *et al.*, 1991, 1993) and make an informed decision as to whether cognitive testing might be useful in assessing a particular individual.

Approach to Aircrew

In the investigation of impaired wakefulness or undue sleepiness in aircrew, the initial assessment by the aeromedical practitioner is critical. It involves considerations of the pattern of their rest and activity and of the possibility of sleep pathology. The issues that arise directly from their irregularity of work and rest have been dealt with in Chapter 3 (Aircrew and Alertness). If the problem of undue sleepiness is not related to the work schedules, the aeromedical practitioner needs to assess the severity of the complaint and, together with the clinical data, decide whether to seek the advice of a physician with experience in sleep disorders. In the assessment of the severity of the complaint of undue sleepiness, it is important that careful thought is given to the use of scales of sleepiness and to recordings of sleep latencies. It would be inappropriate to influence the clinical picture by sleepiness scales and by sleep latencies that were not of direct relevance.

The Stanford and Karolinska Sleepiness Scales, daytime sleep latencies and the maintenance of wakefulness test relate to the actual time of the assessments and to the circumstances prevailing at that time. Such information may be useful, but is of limited value in deciding whether there is an excessive and pervasive sleepiness affecting daily life. Further, though falling asleep rapidly (as indicated by sleep latencies) occurs in individuals with excessive daytime sleepiness, an increased sleep propensity is not necessarily an invariable indicant of undue and day-to-day pervasive sleepiness (Johnson *et al.*, 1990; Johns, 2000). Neither is falling asleep rapidly essential for the diagnosis of a sleep disorder (Harrison and Horne, 1996). It is important that latencies to sleep are placed in their correct setting. Falling asleep rapidly has been encountered in operating aircrew *without* the complaint of undue sleepiness and in aircrew *with* the complaint of undue sleepiness.

Indeed, in a study of the nocturnal sleep and daytime alertness of aircrew operating a transatlantic schedule (Nicholson *et al.*, 1986), falling asleep rapidly was encountered in several of the aircrew without any clinical evidence of undue sleepiness. Daytime sleep latencies were recorded after an overnight rest period – though not within the schedule. Indeed, in that study, the rapidity with which some aircrew fell asleep would easily have been within the range that is often quoted as being 'pathologically sleepy', with the further implication of an underlying sleep disorder. However, in the absence of clinical evidence of undue sleepiness, such short latencies were considered to be an indication of a relative ease that aircrew may have in falling asleep – possibly a learned behaviour concerned with the need to cope with irregularity of their work and rest and sleeping in unfamiliar surroundings over many years. The existence of low sleep latencies is an important consideration in the assessment of aircrew, but needs to be placed in perspective.

Case Histories

Case histories in the aeromedical literature concerning the clinical investigation of aircrew with the complaint of excessive daytime sleepiness have highlighted the uncertainty engendered by scales and latencies in coming to a definitive decision as to whether the individual has undue sleepiness incompatible with their duties.

In one report (Smart and Singh, 2006) subjective evidence of underlying sleepiness was provided by the Epworth Sleepiness Scale (score of 13). Nocturnal sleep onset latencies varied between 12.5 and 24.0 minutes and the daytime sleep latencies were between 4.0 and 6.0 minutes. The mean wakeful time of the maintenance of wakefulness test with a 40-minute protocol was 10.25 minutes. In this trainee pilot, the Epworth scale and the maintenance test indicated an undue degree of underlying perceived sleepiness and difficulty in staying awake, respectively. However, an interpretation of undue sleepiness from the daytime latencies would have been an assumption as these latencies are indicants of the rate of falling asleep. The crucial investigations were the Epworth Scale and maintenance of wakefulness test. They provided little help in coming to a specific clinical diagnosis, but they were useful in the subsequent aeromedical management.

In other reports, formal subjective assessments of the perceived underlying sleepiness have not been made. One report involved two pilots – one complaining of undue sleepiness and the other falling asleep during a flight (Grossman *et al.*, 2004). Nocturnal sleep-onset latencies were 7 and 9 minutes respectively,

and the average of the daytime sleep latencies indicated that they fell asleep rapidly during the day (3 and 8 minutes respectively). However, the maintenance of wakefulness in both pilots, each with a 40-minute protocol, demonstrated clearly that their ability to stay awake was not, to any degree, compromised. There was little evidence of an impairment of wakefulness that would be incompatible with duties demanding a high degree of alertness. In both cases, it would appear that the short daytime sleep latencies were related solely to the ability of the aircrew to fall asleep quickly and did not indicate any underlying sleep pathology. That conclusion would be in accord with the absence of the onset of sleep after 40 minutes within the maintenance of wakefulness test. A diagnosis of sleep pathology could only have been made on the clinical picture.

In another case, a crew member was referred with undue sleepiness that was noted during ground and flight operations (Withers *et al.*, 1999). An assessment of the perceived underlying sleepiness using a scale was not included in the report. The nocturnal sleep latency was 4 minutes and the average of the daytime sleep latencies (4.25 minutes) indicated that the subject fell asleep rapidly in such circumstances. A diagnosis of sleep pathology was made on clinical grounds, though such a diagnosis could not have been inferred from the daytime sleep latencies. In the discussion of the case, the authors referred to the usefulness of the maintenance of wakefulness test (with a protocol of 40 minutes) in assessing the ability to stay awake, though it would appear that the test was not part of the clinical investigation.

The Way Ahead

The case histories cited in this chapter involved operational aircrew without complaints of undue sleepiness and aircrew complaining of undue sleepiness, and were from aeromedical centres worldwide that often consulted physicians with expertise in sleep disorders in the assessment of the individual concerned. The histories indicated that caution is necessary in the interpretation of sleepiness scales and sleep latencies. Nevertheless, in the approach to aircrew, it is useful, early on, to have some idea whether there is any likelihood of undue sleepiness. In that context, the Epworth Scale may be helpful. The averaged scale indicates the perceived likelihood of an ongoing day-to-day pervasive background of sleepiness. The assessment would have been based on experience garnered over several weeks and in a variety of circumstances – though it would be important to ensure that the perceived tendencies to fall asleep were not overly influenced by any specific experience related to an operational schedule. It must also be borne in mind that there is the possibility that with subjective scales the severity of the complaint may be underestimated.

A careful clinical history supported by the Epworth Sleepiness Scale would enable the aeromedical practitioner to decide whether there is any likelihood of a sleep disorder and whether there is undue sleepiness that needs further investigation. It is the clinical picture and informed clinical judgement that are the keys to the diagnosis and management of sleep disorders in aircrew. The expertise of the respiratory physician or the neurologist, each versed in sleep medicine, together with the experience of the aeromedical practitioner, are the means by which adequate decisions concerning the diagnosis, management and employability of aircrew with sleep disorders can be made.

References

Akerstedt, T. and Gilberg, M. 1990. Subjective and objective sleepiness in the active individual. *International Journal of Neuroscience*, 52, 29–37.

Alchanatis, M., Deligiorgis, N., Zias, N., Amfilochiou, A., Gotsis, E., Karaktsani, A. *et al.* 2004. Frontal brain lobe impairment in obstructive sleep apnoea: A proton MR spectroscopy study. *European Respiratory Journal*, 24, 980–86.

Aldrich, M.S., Chervin, R.D. and Malow, B.A. 1997. Value of the multiple sleep latency test (MSLT) for the diagnosis of narcolepsy. *Sleep*, 20, 620–29.

Aloia, M.S., Arnedt, J.T., Davis, J.D., Riggs, R.L. and Byrd, D. 2004. Neuropsychological sequelae of obstructive sleep apnea-hypopnea syndrome: A critical review. *Journal of the International Neuropsychological Society*, 10, 772–85.

American Academy of Sleep Medicine. 2005. *International Classification of Sleep Disorders: Diagnostic and Coding Manual – Second Edition*. Westchester, IL: American Academy of Sleep Medicine.

Ancoli-Israel, S., Cole, R., Alessi, C., Chambers, M., Moorcroft, W. and Pollak, C.P. 2003. The role of actigraphy in the study of sleep and circadian rhythms. *Sleep*, 26, 342–92.

Banerjee, D., Vitiello, M. and Grunstein, R. 2004. Pharmacotherapy for excessive daytime sleepiness. *Sleep Medicine Reviews*, 8, 339–54.

Baumann, C.R. and Bassetti, C.L. 2005. Hypocretins (orexins) and sleep-wake disorders. *Lancet Neurology*, 4, 673–82.

Bédard, M.A., Montplaisir, J., Richer, F., Rouleau, I. and Malo, J. 1991. Obstructive sleep apnea syndrome: Pathogenesis of neuropsychological deficits. *Journal of*

Clinical and Experimental Neuropsychology, 13, 950–64.

Bédard, M.A., Montplaisir, J., Malo, J., Richer, F. and Rouleau, I. 1993. Persistent neuropsychological deficits and vigilance impairment in sleep apnea syndrome after treatment with continuous positive airways pressure (CPAP). *Journal of Clinical and Experimental Neuropsychology*, 15, 330–41.

Benbadis, S.R., Mascha, E. and Perry, M. 1999. Association between Epworth sleepiness scale and the multiple sleep latency in a clinical population. *Annals of Internal Medicine*, 130, 289–92.

Bennett, L.S., Stradling, J.R. and Davies, R.J.O. 1997. A behavioural test to assess daytime sleepiness in obstructive sleep apnoea. *Journal of Sleep Research*, 6, 142–5.

Billiard, M. 2007. Diagnosis of narcolepsy and idiopathic hypersomnia: An update based on the International Classification of Sleep Disorders: Second Edition. *Sleep Medicine Reviews*, 11, 377–88.

Bonakis, A., Howard, R.S., Ebrahim, I.O., Merritt, S. and Williams, A. 2009. REM sleep behaviour disorder (RBD) and its associations in young patients. *Sleep Medicine*, 10, 641–5.

Bourgin, P., Zeitzer, J.M. and Mignot, E. 2008. CSF hypocretin-1 assessment in sleep and neurological disorders. *Lancet Neurology*, 7, 649–62.

Braak, H., Rüb, U., Gai, W.P. and Del Tredici, K. 2003. Idiopathic Parkinson's disease: Possible routes by which vulnerable neuronal types may be subject to neuroinvasion by an unknown pathogen. *Journal of Neural Transmission*, 110, 517–36.

Brodsky, M.A., Godbold, J., Roth, T. and Olanow, C.W. 2003. Sleepiness in Parkinson's disease: A controlled study. *Movement Disorders*, 18, 668–72.

Bulow, K. 1963. Respiration and wakefulness in man. *Acta Physiologica Scandinavica: Supplement*, 209, 1–110.

Carskadon, M.A. and Dement, W.C. 1977. Sleep tendency: An objective measure of sleep loss. *Sleep Research*, 6, 200.

Carskadon, M.A. and Dement, W.C. 1982. The multiple sleep latency test: What does it measure? *Sleep*, 5, S67–72.

Carskadon, M.A., Dement, W.C., Mittler, M.M., Roth, T., Westbrook, P.R. and Keenan, S. 1986. Guidelines for the multiple sleep latency test (MLST): A standard measure of sleepiness. *Sleep*, 9, 519–24.

Chervin, R.D. 2003. Epworth Sleepiness Scale? *Sleep Medicine*, 4, 175–6.

Chervin, R.D. and Aldrich, M.S. 1999. The Epworth Sleepiness Scale may not reflect objective measures of sleepiness or sleep apnoea. *Neurology*, 52, 125–31.

Chervin, R.D., Kraemer, H.C. and Guilleminault, C. 1995. Correlates of sleep latency on the multiple latency test in a clinical population. *Electroencephalography and Clinical Neurophysiology*, 95, 147–53.

Cluydts, R., de Valck, E., Verstraeten, E. and Theys, P. 2002. Daytime sleepiness and its evaluation. *Sleep Medicine Reviews*, 6, 83–96.

Davies, C.W., Crosby, J.H., Mullins, R.L., Traill, Z.C., Anslow, P., Davies, R.L. and Stradling, J.R. 2001. Case control study of cerebrovascular damage defined by magnetic resonance imaging in patients with OSA and normal matched control subjects. *Sleep*, 24, 715–20.

Decary, A., Rouleau, I. and Montplaisir, J. 2000. Cognitive deficits associated with sleep apnea syndrome: A proposed neuropsychological test battery. *Sleep*, 23, 1–13.

Doghramji, K., Mittler, M.M., Sangal, R.B., Shapiro, C., Taylor, S., Walseben, J. *et al.* 1997. A normative study of the maintenance of wakefulness test (MWT). *Electroencephalography and Clinical Neurophysiology*, 103, 554–62.

Douglas, N.J. 2000. Upper airway resistance is not a distinct syndrome. *American*

Journal of Respiratory and Critical Care Medicine, 161, 1413–6.

Engleman, H.M., Kingshott, R.N., Martin, S.E. and Douglas, N.J. 2000. Cognitive function in the sleep apnea/hypopnea syndrome (SAHS). *Sleep*, 23, S102–8.

Findley, I.J., Barth, J.T., Powers, D.C., Wilhoit, S.C., Boyd, D.G. and Suratt, P.M. 1986. Cognitive impairment in patients with obstructive sleep apnoea and associated hypoxaemia. *Chest*, 90, 686–90.

Fulda, S. and Schultz, H. 2001. Cognitive dysfunction in sleep disorders. *Sleep Medicine Reviews*, 5, 423–45.

Gamaldo, C.E., Benbrook, A.R., Allen, R.P., Oguntimein, O. and Earley, C.J. 2008. A further evaluation of the cognitive deficits associated with restless legs syndrome (RLS). *Sleep Medicine*, 9, 500–505.

Grossman, A., Barenboim, E., Azaria, B., Sherer, Y. and Goldstein, L. 2004. The maintenance of wakefulness test as a predictor of alertness in aircrew members with idiopathic hypersomnia. *Aviation, Space, and Environmental Medicine*, 75, 281–3.

Harrison, Y. and Horne, J.A. 1996. 'High sleepability without sleepiness'. The ability to fall asleep rapidly without other signs of sleepiness. *Clinical Neurophysiology*, 26, 15–20.

Hoddes, E., Zarcone, V., Smythe, H., Phillips, R. and Dement, W.C. 1973. Quantification of sleepiness: A new approach. *Psychophysiology*, 10, 431–6.

Johns, M.W. 1991. A new method for measuring daytime sleepiness: The Epworth sleepiness scale. *Sleep*, 14, 540–45.

Johns, M.W. 1994. Sleepiness in different situations measured by the Epworth Sleepiness Scale. *Sleep*, 17, 703–10.

Johns, M. 1998. Rethinking the assessment of sleepiness. *Sleep Medicine Reviews*, 2, 3–15.

Johns, M.W. 2000. Sensitivity and specificity of the multiple latency test (MLST), the maintenance of wakefulness test and the Epworth sleepiness scale: Failure of the MLST as a gold standard. *Journal of Sleep Research*, 9, 5–11.

Johnson, L.C., Spinweber, C.L., Gomez, S.A. and Matteson, L.T. 1990. Daytime sleepiness, performance, mood, nocturnal sleep: The effect of benzodiazepine and caffeine on their relationship. *Sleep*, 13, 121–35.

Jones, B.E. 2008. Modulation of cortical activation and behavioral arousal by cholinergic and orexinergic systems. *Annals of the New York Academy of Sciences*, 1129, 26–34.

Lavie, P. and Zvuluni, A. 1992. The 24-hour sleep propensity function: Experimental bases for somnotypology. *Psychophysiology*, 29, 566–75.

Levine, B., Roehrs, T., Zorick, F. and Roth, T. 1988. Daytime sleepiness in young adults. *Sleep*, 11, 39–46.

Lewy, A.J., Cutler, N.L. and Sack, R.L. 1999. The endogenous melatonin profile as a marker for circadian position. *Journal of Biological Rhythms*, 14, 227–36.

Lin, C.C., Tsan, K.W. and Lin, C.Y. 1993. Plasma levels of atrial natriuretic factor in moderate to severe obstructive sleep apnea syndrome. *Sleep*, 16, 37–9.

Lis, S., Krieger, S., Hennig, D., Roder, C., Kirsch, P., Seeger, W. *et al.* 2008. Executive functions and cognitive sub-processes in patients with obstructive sleep apnoea. *Journal of Sleep Research*, 17, 271–80.

Littner, M.R., Kushida, C., Wise, M., Davila, D.G., Morgenthaler, T., Lee-Chiong, T. *et al.* 2005. Practice parameters for clinical use of the multiple sleep latency test and the maintenance of wakefulness test. Standards of Practice Committee of the American Academy of Sleep Medicine. *Sleep*, 28, 113–21.

Lockley, S.W., Brainard, G.C. and Czeisler, C.A. 2003. High sensitivity of the human circadian melatonin rhythm to resetting by short wavelength light. *Journal of Clinical Endocrinology and Metabolism*, 88, 4502–5.

Macey, P.M., Henderson, L.A., Macey, K.E., Alger, J.R., Frysinger, R.C., Woo, M.A. *et al.* 2002. Brain morphology associated with obstructive sleep apnea. *American Journal of Respiration and Critical Care Medicine*, 166, 1382–7.

Macey, P.M., Kumar, R., Woo, M.A., Valladares, E.M., Yan-Go, F.L. and Harper, R.M. 2008. Brain structural changes in obstructive sleep apnea. *Sleep*, 31, 967–77.

Manni, R., Ratti, M.T., Barzaghi, N., Galimberti, C.A., Zucca, C., Perucca, E. *et al.* 1991. Daytime sleepiness in healthy, university students: A multiparametric study. *Italian Journal of Neurological Sciences*, 12, 203–9.

Mazza, N.S., Pepin, J.L., Naëgelé, B., Plante, J., Deschaux, C. and Levy, P. 2005. Most obstructive sleep apnoea patients exhibit vigilance and attention deficits on an extended battery of tests. *European Respiratory Journal*, 25, 75–80.

Mignot, E. 2008. Excessive daytime sleepiness: Population and etiology versus nosology. *Sleep Medicine Reviews*, 12, 87–94.

Mittler, M.M., Gujavarty, K.S. and Browman, C.P. 1982. Maintenance of wakefulness test: A polysomnographic technique for evaluating treatment of efficacy in patients with excessive somnolence. *Electroencephalography and Clinical Neurophysiology*, 53, 658–61.

Montplaisir, J., Michaud, M. and Petit, D. 2006. New trends in restless legs syndrome research. *Sleep Medicine Reviews*, 10, 147–51.

Morrell, M.J., Giassie, R., Simonds, A., Murphy, K., McRobbie, D.W. and Corfield, D.R. 2004. Obstructive sleep apnea is associated with changes in brain morphology in the hippocampus and para-hippocampus. *European Respiratory Journal*, 24, S446.

Morrell, M.J., McRobbie, D.W., Quest, R.A., Cummin, A.R., Ghiassi, R. and Corfield, D.R. 2003. Changes in brain morphology associated with obstructive sleep apnea. *Sleep Medicine*, 4, 451–4.

Naëgelé, B., Pépin, J.L., Lévy, P., Bonnet, C., Pellet, J. and Feuerstein, C. 1998. Cognitive executive dysfunction in patients with obstructive sleep apnoea syndrome (OSAS) after CPAP treatment. *Sleep*, 21, 392–7.

Nicholson, A.N., Pascoe, P.A., Spencer, M.B., Stone, B.M. and Green, R.L. 1986. Nocturnal sleep and daytime alertness of aircrew after transmeridian flights. *Aviation, Space, and Environmental Medicine*, Suppl., 57, B42–52.

Nicholson, A.N., Stone, B.M., Wright, N.A. and Belyavin, A.J. 1989. Daytime sleep latencies: Relationships with the electroencephalogram and with performance. *Journal of Psychophysiology*, 3, 387–95.

Ohayon, M. 2008. From wakefulness to excessive sleepiness: What we know and still need to know. *Sleep Medicine Reviews*, 12, 129–41.

Postuma, R.B., Gagnon, J.F., Vendette, M., Fantini, M.L., Massicotte-Marquez, J. and Montplaisir, J. 2009. Quantifying the risk of neurodegenerative disease in idiopathic REM sleep behaviour disorder. *Neurology*, 72, 1296–300.

Priest, B., Brichard, C., Aubert, G., Liistro, G. and Rodenstein, D.O. 2001. Microsleep during a simplified maintenance of wakefulness test: A validation study of the OSLER Test. *American Journal of Respiration and Critical Care Medicine*, 163, 1619–25.

Redline, S., Strauss, M.E., Adams, N., Winters, M., Roebuck, T., Spry, K. *et al.* 1997. Neuropsychological function in mild sleep-disordered breathing. *Sleep*, 20, 160–67.

Richardson, G.S., Carskadon, M.A., Flagg, W., van den Hoed, J., Dement, W.C. and Mittler, M.M. 1978. Excessive daytime sleepiness in man: Multiple sleep latency measures in narcoleptic and control subjects. *Electroencephalography and Clinical Neurophysiology*, 45, 621–7.

Sack, R.L., Auckley, D., Auger, R., Carskadon, M., Wright, K.P., Vitello, M.V. and Zhdanova, I.V. 2007. Circadian rhythm sleep disorders: Part II, Advanced sleep phase disorder, delayed sleep phase disorder, free-running disorder, and irregular sleep-wake rhythm: An American Academy of Sleep Medicine review. *Sleep*, 30, 1484–501.

Sanford, S.D., Lichstein, K.L., Durrence, H.H., Riedel, B.W., Taylor, D.J. and Bush, A.J. 2006. The influence of age, gender, ethnicity, and insomnia on Epworth sleepiness scores: A normative US population. *Sleep Medicine*, 7, 319–26.

Sangal, R.B., Thomas, L. and Mittler, M.M. 1992. Maintenance of wakefulness test and multiple sleep latency test: Measurement of different abilities in patients with sleep disorders. *Chest*, 101, 898–902.

Saunamäki, T. and Jehkonen, M. 2007. A review of executive functions in obstructive sleep apnea syndrome. *Acta Neurologica Scandinavica*, 115, 1–11.

Scofield, H., Roth, T. and Drake, C. 2008. Periodic limb movements during sleep: Population prevalence, clinical correlates, and racial differences. *Sleep*, 31, 1221–7.

Shapiro, C.M., Catterall, J.R., Oswald, I. and Flenley, D.C. 1981. Where are the British sleep apnoea patients? *Lancet*, 2, 523.

Shen, J., Barbera, J. and Shapiro, C.M. 2006. Distinguishing sleepiness and fatigue: Focus on definition and measurement. *Sleep Medicine Reviews*, 10, 63–76.

Smart, L.T. and Singh, B. 2006. Excessive daytime sleepiness in a trainee military pilot. *Aviation, Space, and Environmental Medicine*, 77, 753–7.

Telekivi, T., Kajaste, S., Partinen, I., Koskenvuo, M., Salmi, T. and Kaprio, J. 1988. Cognitive function in middle-aged snorers and controls: Role of excessive daytime somnolence and sleep-related hypoxic events. *Sleep*, 11, 454–62.

Thomas, R.J., Rosen, B.R., Stern, C.E., Weiss, J.W. and Kwong, K.K. 2005. Functional imaging of working memory in obstructive sleep-disordered breathing. *Journal of Applied Physiology*, 98, 2226–34.

Trenkwalder, C., Paulus, W. and Walters, A.S. 2005. The restless legs syndrome. *Lancet Neurology*, 4, 465–75.

Van Dongen, H.P., Vitellaro, K.M. and Dinges, D.F. 2005. Individual differences in adult human sleep and wakefulness: Leitmotif for a research agenda. *Sleep*, 28, 479–96.

de Weerd, A.W., Rijsman, R. and Brinkley, A. 2004. Activity patterns of leg muscles in periodic limb movement disorder. *Journal of Neurology Neurosurgery and Psychiatry*, 75, 317–9.

Weitzman, E.D., Czeisler, C.A., Coleman, R.M., Spielman, A.J., Zimmerman, J.C. and Dement, W.C. 1981. Delayed sleep phase syndrome: A chronobiological disorder with sleep-onset insomnia. *Archives of General Psychiatry*, 38, 737–46.

White, D.P. 2005. Pathogenesis of obstructive and central sleep apnoea, 2005. *American Journal of Respiratory and Critical Care Medicine*, 172, 1363–70.

Withers, B.G., Loube, D.I. and Husak. J.P. 1999. Idiopathic hypersomnia in an aircrew member. *Aviation, Space, and Environmental Medicine*, 70, 797–801.

Yaouhi, K., Bertran, F., Clochon, P., Mezenge, F., Denise, P., Foret, J. *et al.* 2009. A combined neuropsychological and brain imaging study of obstructive sleep apnea. *Journal of Sleep Research*, 18, 36–48.

Young, T., Palta, M., Dempsey, J., Skatrud, J., Weber, S. and Badr, S. 1993. The occurrence of sleep-disordered breathing among middle-aged adults. *New England Journal of Medicine*, 328, 1230–35.

Zeman, A., Britton, T., Douglas, N., Hansen, A., Hicks, J., Howard, R. *et al.* 2004. Narcolepsy and excessive daytime sleepiness. *British Medical Journal*, 329, 724–8.

Chapter 12

THE DIAGNOSIS OF EPILEPSY

Matthew C. Walker

The recognition of epilepsy as a distinct disorder has a long history. More than 3,000 years ago, epilepsy was described in a Babylonian cuneiform, making it one of the earliest documented conditions (Wilson and Reynolds, 1990). Five hundred years later, there are references to epilepsy in Greek texts; the word 'epilepsy' is derived from the ancient Greek, meaning to possess or to seize.

An epileptic seizure is a transient, excessive discharge of neurons in the cerebral cortex causing an event which is clinically discernible by the person experiencing the seizure and/or by an observer. The clinical manifestations of a seizure are determined by where in the cortex the seizure begins and the speed and extent of its spread. Epileptic seizures have a sudden onset, spread within minutes and usually cease spontaneously. A characteristic feature of seizures is that, within an individual, they are consistent both in the brain area in which they begin and in their pattern of spread. Frequently, seizures are followed by a period of drowsiness and confusion termed the post-ictal period. Seizure types can be divided into partial seizures, arising from one part of the brain, and generalized seizures, arising simultaneously throughout the cortex; respectively, these constitute approximately 40 per cent and 50 per cent of seizures in newly diagnosed epilepsy (10 per cent of seizures in this group are unclassifiable) (Sander *et al.*, 1990).

Seizures can be acutely precipitated by drugs, alcohol, head trauma, stroke or other factors. These are termed acute precipitated or acute symptomatic seizures. Such seizures need to be distinguished from recurrent unprovoked seizures, which have a much higher chance of recurrence (see below). Epilepsy is the propensity (chance) to have seizures, and this can result from a number of underlying aetiologies. Epilepsy is one of the most common serious neurological conditions, affecting approximately 0.5 per cent of the population at any point in time (Figure 12.1) (Wallace *et al.*, 1998). In developed countries, there may be as many as 80,000 to 100,000 new cases of treated epilepsy per year. In adults, the incidence is highest before the age of 25 years and then again in the elderly (> 75 years) (Wallace *et al.*, 1998). The incidence is lowest between the ages of 25 and 60 years. The lifetime chance of having epilepsy is approximately 3 per cent.

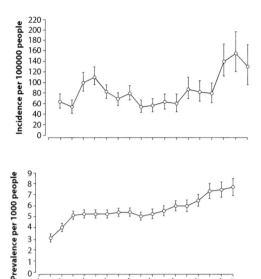

Figure 12.1 Incidence and prevalence of epilepsy in the United Kingdom (from Wallace et al., 1998)

Mechanisms and Aetiology

The brain consists of networks of excitatory and inhibitory neurons, and early views on the mechanisms underlying seizures considered that seizures were generated by a disruption of the normal balance between excitation and inhibition in the brain. This view is now considered oversimplified, as the generation of physiological oscillations, and probably seizures, depends upon an interplay between excitatory and inhibitory neurons (Duncan et al., 2006). The occurrence of epileptic activity is an emergent property of networks. The transition from normal to epileptiform behaviour probably results from greater spread and neuronal recruitment secondary to a combination of enhanced connectivity, enhanced excitatory transmission, a failure of inhibitory mechanisms and changes in intrinsic neuronal properties. An acute

precipitant can alter these, resulting in a seizure. However, epilepsy is secondary to chronic changes in network and neuronal properties that lead to an increased propensity for having spontaneous seizures.

Generalized epilepsies result in seizures occurring throughout the cortex because of a lowering of seizure threshold, and are usually genetically determined. Such seizures often involve the recruitment of thalamocortical networks that rapidly generalize the seizure activity. Partial seizures are due to focal disruption of normal network activity, and partial epilepsies can be genetically determined or secondary to local pathology. The probable aetiology depends on the age of the patient and the type of seizures. The commonest acquired causes in young infants are hypoxia or birth asphyxia, perinatal intracranial trauma, metabolic disturbances, congenital malformations of the brain, and infection. In young children and adolescents, idiopathic epilepsies (genetically determined) account for the majority of seizure disorders, although trauma and infection also play a role.

The range of causes of the onset of epilepsy in young adults is broad. Idiopathic epilepsy, epilepsy due to birth trauma and epilepsy due to abnormal cortical development (cortical dysgenesis) can begin in early adulthood. Other important causes of seizures in adulthood are infection, trauma and alcohol abuse, and, in older age groups, brain tumours and cerebrovascular disease (Sander et al., 1990). Brain tumours are responsible for the development of epilepsy in approximately 20 per cent of cases between the ages of 50 and 60 years (Sander et al., 1990). Over the age of 60 years, cerebrovascular disease is the commonest cause of epilepsy and is present in approximately a half of the patients.

Classification of Seizures

The International Seizure Classification Scheme is the most widely used scheme and it is based on the clinical and electroencephalographic manifestations of the individual seizure (Commission on Classification and Terminology of the International League Against Epilepsy, 1985, 1989). It divides epileptic seizures into two main groups according to the source of the primary epileptic discharge: those originating from localized cortical areas, the epileptic focus or foci (partial seizures), and those characterized by synchronous discharges over both hemispheres (generalized seizures). There is a group of seizures that are deemed 'unclassifiable' even after extensive investigation, such as may occur in patients with infrequent and unwitnessed seizures.

Partial Seizures

Partial or focal seizures arise from an epileptic focus. The clinical manifestations of a partial seizure depend on the area of cerebral cortex involved and the extent and manner of spread. Importantly, seizures spread rapidly in a matter of minutes, differentiating them from other phenomena such as migrainous aura. The most common sites of origin of epileptic seizures are the temporal lobes. Approximately 60 per cent of complex partial seizures have their origin in the temporal lobe; the rest (extra-temporal seizures) usually arise from the frontal lobe. Seizures originating in the parietal or occipital regions are relatively rare. The partial nature of the seizure and the location and lateralization of the focus can often be identified from the clinical signs present either during or after the seizure (post-ictally). Partial seizures are subdivided into three groups: simple partial, complex partial and secondary generalized seizures.

Simple partial seizures

Simple partial seizures are the result of localized epileptic activity during which consciousness is fully preserved. The symptoms depend upon the localization of the seizure activity, but characteristically the symptoms are distinct and stereotypical. Typical simple partial seizures include focal motor (often occurring as a Jacksonian march evolving, as predicted, by spread along the motor cortex), autonomic symptoms (vomiting, pallor, flushing, sweating), somatosensory or special sensory symptoms (seeing flashing lights, experiencing unpleasant odours or tastes, vertigo, parasthesia, pain), and psychic/dysmnestic symptoms (strong feelings of *déjà vu*, depersonalization, fear, illusions, hallucinations). Probably the commonest aura in temporal lobe epilepsy is a rising epigastric feeling. Occasionally (especially with frontal lobe epilepsy), people have problems describing their aura, but will recognize the feeling as distinct and stereotypical.

Simple partial seizures usually start suddenly, evolve over a matter of minutes (less than five minutes) and are brief, unless progression occurs. It is rare for simple partial seizures to be the sole manifestation of epilepsy, although this observation may be confounded by under-diagnosis of simple partial seizures in the population. Certain of the phenomenon detailed above, in particular the psychic symptoms, are experienced frequently in the general population as a non-epileptic symptom. This is particularly so for *déjà vu* which may be experienced by anything up to 90 per cent of the population (Warren-Gash and Zeman, 2003) and is especially common in people with psychiatric problems (anxiety, depression). Epileptic *déjà vu* cannot be differentiated from *déjà vu* of other causes by semiology alone. Epileptic *déjà vu* is usually frequent, prolonged, more intense and associated with other symptoms such as fear or rising epigastric aura. The occurrence of complex partial seizures or secondary generalized seizures will usually clinch the diagnosis, but isolated frequent *déjà vu* does occur and can be a diagnostic challenge. In such instances, further investigations such as neuroimaging and electroencephalography can be helpful (see below).

Complex partial seizures

Complex partial seizures involve an impairment of consciousness, which can sometimes be mild or unrecognized by the person having the seizure. Complex partial seizures can evolve from a simple partial seizure (the 'aura') or there can be an alteration of consciousness from the onset. Initially, there is often motor arrest and a blank stare and then the seizure progresses to altered or 'automatic' behaviour. If the seizure consists only of a blank stare, then it is important to differentiate this from absence seizures (in which there is immediate and rapid recovery) and non-epileptic episodes of loss of concentration (which the person can be 'snapped out of').

The automatisms associated with complex partial seizures depend upon the location of the seizure. In temporal lobe seizures, the automatisms usually involve distal movements such as plucking at clothing and fiddling with various objects. Lip smacking or chewing movements, grimacing, undressing, the carrying out of purposeless activities or of aimless wandering may all occur on their own or in different combinations. Sometimes those with a complex partial seizure are able to carry on with a simple task with very few outward signs of a seizure; on occasion more complex tasks such as driving may be performed. These seizures usually last a matter of minutes. There is amnesia for the event and post-ictal confusion that can last up to 20 minutes. Temporal lobe seizures contrast with frontal lobe seizures in which there are often bilateral posturing and hypermotor automatisms with large gestural components (such as pushing), running, cycling of legs and scissoring of legs. These seizures are usually brief with rapid recovery and have to be distinguished from psychogenic non-epileptic seizures (see below).

Secondarily generalized seizures

Secondarily generalized attacks are partial seizures, either simple or complex, in which the epileptic activity spreads to both cerebral hemispheres, so that a generalized seizure, usually a tonic-clonic convulsion, ensues. The patient may have an aura, but this is not always the case. The spread of the discharge can occur so quickly that no features of the localized onset are apparent to the patient or to an observer. On rare occasions, a secondarily generalized seizure may take the form of a tonic, atonic or unilateral tonic-clonic seizure.

Generalized Seizures

Generalized seizures are characterized by the simultaneous involvement of the whole cortex at the onset of the seizure. This can usually be demonstrated by electroencephalography. Patients experiencing generalized seizures lose consciousness at the beginning of the seizure, so that there is no warning. There are various types of generalized seizures: generalized tonic-clonic seizures, absence seizures, myoclonic, tonic and atonic seizures.

Generalized tonic-clonic seizures

Generalized tonic-clonic convulsions, or convulsive seizures, are common. In this type of seizure, there is no aura, but the patient may experience a prodrome, sometimes lasting hours, of general malaise. At the onset of the seizure (the tonic phase), the patient becomes stiff, often crying out. The tongue may also be bitten during this phase, usually on the sides. Apnoea occurs, and the patient becomes cyanosed. The patient falls, and clonic movements occur, usually involving all four limbs, but often predominantly affecting the arms. The clonic movements are usually quite regular and then slow and become less regular towards the end of the seizure. Incontinence commonly occurs at the end of the clonic phase. The convulsion rarely lasts longer than a minute or two and then is followed by a post-ictal phase of drowsiness, and confusion, lasting up to 20 minutes. Tonic-clonic seizures at night can be recognized in the morning from tongue biting with blood on the pillow, aching limbs, headache and feeling unwell. Incontinence alone is rarely the result of a nocturnal seizure.

Absence seizures

Typical absence attacks start almost exclusively in childhood and early adolescence, but can continue into adulthood. The individual has motor arrest, and stares; there may be fluttering of the eyelids and swallowing. The attacks usually last only a few seconds and often pass unrecognized. Absence seizures are associated with a characteristic electroencephalographic pattern with anterior predominant 3-per-second generalized spike-and-wave discharges. They may be precipitated by hyperventilation, which is a useful diagnostic manoeuvre, and by missing sleep. Atypical absences are usually associated with more severe epilepsy syndromes, such as the Lennox–Gastaut syndrome. The electroencephalogram (EEG) of atypical absences is less homogenous and more irregular. The onset and cessation of the seizure is not as abrupt as with typical absence seizures, and additional features are usually pronounced. The presence of photosensitivity depends upon the epilepsy syndrome, ranging from 20 to 40 per cent of individuals with absence seizures.

Myoclonic seizures

Myoclonus seizures are abrupt, brief, involuntary jerks which can involve the whole body, or just part of it, such as the arms or the head. Myoclonus is not necessarily epileptic and can occur from brainstem and spinal pathology. In addition, physiological myoclonic phenomena also occur in healthy people, particularly when they are just going off to sleep (hypnic jerk). Myoclonus also occurs in the context of a seizure disorder. In primary generalized epilepsy, myoclonic jerks occur most commonly in the morning, shortly after waking. They vary in severity from barely perceptible jerks to falls. They also occur in devastating epilepsies (such as the progressive myoclonic epilepsies) with associated cognitive decline and other neurological symptoms.

Atonic and tonic seizures

These types of generalized attacks are rare, accounting for fewer than 1 per cent of epileptic seizures in the general population. Atonic seizures (drop attacks) involve a sudden loss of tone in the postural muscles, and the patient falls to the ground. There are no convulsive movements. Recovery is rapid, with no perceptible post-ictal symptomatology. Atonic seizures usually occur in people with severe epilepsy, learning difficulties and multiple seizure types, often starting in early childhood – those with the syndrome described by Lennox (1884–1960) and Gastaut (1915–1995). If such attacks are occurring in someone of normal intelligence, then other possibilities, such as cardiac or psychogenic attacks, need to be considered. Tonic seizures result in a sudden increase in the muscle tone of the body, usually resulting in a fall backwards on to the ground. Recovery is generally rapid. Tonic seizures, similar to atonic seizures, are also associated with severe epilepsies, but can also occur in frontal lobe epilepsy syndromes.

The Diagnosis

The diagnosis of epilepsy depends upon a careful history and witnessed account. In particular, the semiology of the events should be carefully documented, including the extent to which the events are stereotypical. The seizure description should include premonitory symptoms,

	Epilepsy	Syncope	Psychogenic non-epileptic seizure
Circumstance	Unpredictable Sleep or awake	Upright	Audience
Precipitant	Occasional	Occasional	Occasional
Aura and prodrome	Stereotypical Brief Evolve	Presyncope Can be prolonged	Dissociative Aura Autonomic Aura
Event	Stereotypical Brief Evolve	Pallor Variable semiology	Slumping Waxing and waning Eyes shut Variable semiology Arched back/ thrashing Directed violence Long
After event	Marked confusion	Unwell Confusion (None or brief)	Tearfulness

the circumstance in which the event took place (including possible precipitants), aura, description and duration of seizure (usually from witness), and lastly post-ictal symptoms. The temporal aspects of events (when in a day, how often, how long) are also important in differentiating epileptic seizures from other paroxysmal events. Other important aspects in the history are: antecedent events such as a history of febrile seizures, head injuries, encephalitis or meningitis; family history of epilepsy; drug use, including illicit drug use; alcohol use; and past medical history, including cardiac history. Clinical examination should include not only a full neurological examination but also a cardiovascular examination, recognizing that syncopal attacks can present as seizure-like events. In considering the differential diagnosis, there are four common areas of misdiagnosis in adults: syncope, migraine, psychogenic non-epileptic attacks and parasomnias (Crompton and Berkovic, 2009). Features of three of these are given below. Overall, about a fifth of patients referred to tertiary centres for refractory epilepsy do not have epilepsy (Duncan *et al.*, 2006).

Syncope

Syncopal attacks can be differentiated from epileptic seizures in that they usually occur whilst upright (sitting or standing) and are associated with a presyncopal aura (nausea, sweating, greying of vision, feeling hot and cold). However, cardiac arrhythmias can occur whilst lying, and sudden cardiac arrhythmias can present with collapse without warning. It is not uncommon for small amplitude, non-rhythmical jerking (of probable brainstem origin) to occur and this is often misreported as clonic jerks. After the attack, people are rarely

confused for long, but can continue to complain of autonomic symptoms such as nausea. It is worth also recognizing that in some circumstances a syncopal attack can result in a brief seizure-like event especially in children (termed a reflex anoxic seizure), and, rarely, a period of anoxia can result in an epileptic seizure (this is an acute precipitated anoxic seizure). The diagnosis of syncope is also dealt with in Chapter 13 (Syncope: Physiology, Pathophysiology and Aeromedical Implications).

Migraine

Migrainous aura can sometimes be confused with epileptic aura, especially when they are not followed by a headache (acephalgic migraine). Migrainous aura, however, usually spread over a longer period (> 5 minutes) and there are often differences in the quality of the aura. Visual aura in migraine are usually simple shapes and are black or white, whilst in seizures the visual aura can be complex and are often coloured. Furthermore, seizure aura will always start on the same side, whilst migrainous aura start on either side. Isolated episodes of olfactory hallucinations can also be secondary to migrainous phenomena (Fuller and Guiloff, 1987). Migraines rarely result in loss of consciousness, and, if this occurs, it is usually as a result of brainstem involvement such as in basilar migraine accompanied by other brainstem symptoms and signs.

Psychogenic Non-Epileptic Seizures

Psychogenic non-epileptic seizures (also termed non-epileptic attack disorder, dissociative seizures and pseudoseizures) are commonly misdiagnosed as epileptic seizures (Reuber and Elger, 2003). They occur more commonly in women and are associated with prior physical and sexual abuse. Although associated with other psychiatric conditions, such as depression and anxiety disorders, they can occur in isolation. The semiology falls into two specific categories (Meierkord *et al.*, 1991). In one category, there are motor events with pelvic thrusting, head turning from side to side, waxing and waning of motor activity and eyes held shut. In the other, there are collapse attacks with eyes shut and no motor activity (a 'swoon'). The attacks often occur in specific circumstances, there may be an aura of a dissociative feeling ('out of body' feeling) and, although the attacks may share specific features, they are rarely identical. The attacks are often prolonged and can be confused with status epilepticus. Tongue biting can occur, but this usually involves the tip rather than the side of the tongue (as is usual in epileptic seizures). Other injuries also occur, with carpet burns to the face being a specific sign of psychogenic non-epileptic seizures. After the attacks, there is no confusion, but there may be tearfulness. Such attacks are involuntary and are not malingering.

Parasomnia

Parasomnia occur either in rapid eye movement (REM) sleep (REM parasomnia) or in non-REM sleep, usually in slow-wave sleep (non-REM parasomnia). Seizures occur predominantly in non-REM sleep and occur in both light and deep sleep. In view of this, parasomnia and seizures exhibit different patterns of occurrence during the night. REM parasomnia occur predominantly in the second part of the night, non-REM parasomnias occur predominantly during the first third of the night, and seizures occur throughout the night. These events differ in frequency, with parasomnia one to three times a night and seizures many times per night. The semiology also differs. REM parasomnia involve dream phenomena such as nightmares and acting out of dreams (the REM behavioural disorder). Non-REM parasomnia have an indistinct offset and consist of sleepwalking, night terrors and confusional arousals. These lack the stereotypy, complexity and posturing apparent with seizures. Non-REM parasomnia often last for much longer than seizures and lack a distinct offset. It can, however, sometimes be difficult to differentiate parasomnia from seizures, and a sleep study with video-EEG telemetry may be necessary.

Risks of Further Seizures

After the First Seizure

Epilepsy is the propensity to have seizures; thus, following a first seizure, the probability of having further seizures is of paramount importance in deciding whether to label a person as having epilepsy (having the propensity) and in deciding whether to treat. Early studies suggested that after one seizure only 30 to 60 per cent have a recurrence within two years (Berg and Shinnar, 1991). Overall, approximately 90 per cent of the risk of having further seizures occurs in two years. These studies, however, had an inherent selection bias. They were hospital studies and therefore first seizure cases were ascertained some time after the first seizure (those with a high chance of early recurrence were therefore indirectly excluded). In an unselected community-based study (Hart *et al.*, 1990), the seizure recurrence rate following a first seizure was much higher – 67 per cent within 12 months, and 78 per cent within 36 months.

Certain factors had a large effect on recurrence rates so that seizures associated with a neurological deficit present at birth had a 100 per cent relapse within the first 12 months, whilst seizures occurring within the context of an acute insult or precipitant had only a 40 per cent relapse over the same time period. The difference in the risk of recurrent seizures between acute symptomatic (defined as a seizure in close temporal association with a transient central nervous system insult, taken as within one week of the insult) and unprovoked seizures in the context of similar insults (traumatic brain injury, stroke or infection involving the central nervous system) has recently been addressed (Hesdorffer et al., 2009). The first unprovoked seizure group had a significantly higher risk of subsequent unprovoked seizure within ten years (65 per cent) compared with the first acute symptomatic seizure group (19 per cent), regardless of aetiology, and, as in most studies, most of this risk was within the first one to two years.

The electroencephalogram (EEG) can also have a predictive value, although this varies from study to study perhaps due to interpretation (see below) (Gilbert et al., 2003). More recently, a pragmatic study of patients presenting with seizures was used to assess prognostic factors. This study was similarly confounded by delay from seizure to presentation, but nevertheless it permitted the determination of prognostic factors. A score was assessed: 0 for one seizure prior to presentation, 1 for two to three seizures prior to presentation and 2 for four or more seizures prior to presentation. Then 1 was added to the score if there was a neurological disorder, deficit, learning disability or developmental delay, and

1 for an abnormal EEG (this included the presence of abnormal slow and/or epileptiform abnormalities). A total score of 0 was low risk, 1 was medium risk and 2–4 was high risk. The probability of a seizure by one, three and five years in different risk groups with delayed (until a further seizure) treatment is given below (after Kim et al., 2006):

	Seizure by 1 year	Seizure by 3 years	Seizure by 5 years
Low risk	0.19	0.28	0.3
Medium risk	0.35	0.5	0.56
High risk	0.59	0.67	0.73

After Specific Insults

Certain acquired insults significantly increase the risk of seizures – in particular, infection of the central nervous system, cerebrovascular events and head injury. These can result in acute seizures (within one week of the insult) or later unprovoked seizures (see above). It is this latter risk that is considered here. The risks associated with infection depend upon the nature of the infection. Cysticercosis is one of the major causes of epilepsy worldwide; most infected people do not develop epilepsy, but seizures are the commonest presenting symptom of neurocysticercosis, occurring in up to 90 per cent with 40 per cent having a further unprovoked seizure within two years (Carpio and Hauser, 2002). Brain abscesses are also associated with a high seizure risk, with up to 70 per cent developing epilepsy (Legg et al., 1973). Following viral encephalitis the risk of epilepsy (if no acute seizures) is 10 per cent after 20 years, with most of the risk in the first four years, and after bacterial meningitis the risk of epilepsy (if no acute seizures) after 20 years is 2.4 per cent, which is marginally greater than the risk for the general population. Aseptic meningitis carried no increased risk of seizures, and early acute symptomatic seizures doubled the above risks.

Post-stroke seizures are not uncommon (Burn *et al.*, 1997) and depend on the nature and position of the stroke (anterior circulation strokes, not surprisingly, have the greatest risk of post-stroke epilepsy). The probability of having a post-stroke seizure was 6 per cent within the first year; the risk then increased by about 1.5 per cent a year, so that by five years the cumulative risk was approximately 12 per cent (Burn *et al.*, 1997). This five-year risk was very much greater for intracerebral haemorrhage (26 per cent) and subarachnoid haemorrhage (34 per cent). Importantly, those who were alive and independent at six months had a five-year risk of 2.7 per cent (Burn *et al.*, 1997).

Traumatic brain injury has been long associated with epilepsy. Penetrating injuries such as gunshot wounds have the highest risk, with over 50 per cent developing epilepsy (Salazar *et al.*, 1995). Population based studies with non-penetrating head injuries have lower incidences, and the incidences are related to severity of head injury (Christensen *et al.*, 2009; Annegers *et al.*, 1998). In the largest study to date (Christensen *et al.*, 2009), head injury was divided into mild brain injury, severe brain injury and skull fracture. Mild brain injury was defined as loss of consciousness (less than 30 minutes), amnesia, confusion/disorientation or as temporary focal neurological deficit and a Glasgow Coma Scale (Teasdale and Jennett, 1974) of 14 or more after 30 minutes and post-traumatic amnesia less than 24 hours. Severe brain injury included those with brain contusion or intracranial haemorrhage.

Overall, the risk of epilepsy was twice as high after mild brain injury or skull fracture, and seven times higher after severe brain injury than those without head injury. Importantly, the risk was still higher than the general population more than ten years following head injury for all subtypes, but for the mild and severe head injury groups the risks were substantially greater in the first six months. Overall, however, the risks were small, with a risk following mild head injury of approximately 0.7 per cent in the first year and a ten-year cumulative risk of 1.3 per cent, and for severe head injury 3.1 per cent in the first year and a ten-year cumulative risk of 4.7 per cent. In the other study (Annegers *et al.*, 1998), the figures for severe head injury are larger, which may be due to some of the less severe head injuries being included in a separate group of moderate head injury, and also the population being studied dating back to 1935 when medical care may have been inferior. When does the increased risk for head injury cease? This is difficult to determine, but, certainly in one study (Annegers *et al.*, 1998), the increased risk from 20 to 30 years is marginal, indicating that after 20 years the risk of epilepsy is probably not much different from that of the general population.

The Investigation

In the investigation of seizures or potential seizures, full blood counts and analysis of blood glucose and electrolytes (in particular sodium) should be carried out, although there are few data to support routine use of these tests. Lumbar puncture and toxicology screens should also be considered (Krumholz *et al.*, 2007). All people with a putative seizure should have an electrocardiogram to exclude causes such as the prolonged QT syndrome

(Petkar *et al.*, 2006). In those in whom the diagnosis is uncertain, 24-hour Holter monitoring and tilt-table testing may also be necessary (Petkar *et al.*, 2006). In all adults with an unprovoked seizure, electroencephalography and neuroimaging are necessary.

Electroencephalography

Epileptiform abnormalities and normal variants

Since the 1940s, the electroencephalogram has played a pivotal role in epilepsy, not only for the diagnosis of epilepsy but also for determining the epilepsy syndrome and the risk of seizures. Activation procedures (hyperventilation and photic stimulation) should also be performed unless contraindicated (Mendez and Brenner, 2006). Hyperventilation is usually carried out for three to five minutes, and is probably most effective at inducing epileptiform abnormalities in idiopathic generalized epilepsy in which up to 80 per cent will have 3Hz spike and wave activity. Photic stimulation can be carried out in a variety of fashions but usually consists of stimulation from 1 to 30Hz. A typical protocol is flashes delivered in trains of 10 seconds for each frequency, with intervals of 7 seconds between starting at 1 Hz and progressing to 20 Hz, and then decreasing from 60 Hz to 25 Hz (Kasteleijn-Nolst Trenité *et al.*, 1999).

The features that are most important are spikes (defined as discharges that have a duration of less than 70 milliseconds) and sharp waves (defined as discharges that last 70 to 200 milliseconds). Although these do not have different pathological or aetiological significance (both being considered 'epileptiform abnormalities'), spikes are more easily distinguished from the background EEG, whilst fluctuations of sharpened background rhythms can be mistaken as sharp waves. This error most commonly occurs when alpha activity extends to temporal regions and is fragmented, such as occurs during drowsiness. In addition, when there are intermixed frequencies such as theta and faster beta rhythms, a sharply contoured EEG can be mistaken as sharp waves. To avoid these misinterpretations, only 'sharp waves' that are of high amplitude and stand out from the background activity and are followed by a slow wave should be defined as 'epileptiform'. Another, not uncommon, error is to mistake the combination of fast activity and delta induced by hyperventilation as generalized spike/wave discharges. In a study of misinterpreted EEGs, it was fluctuations in background activity leading to transients with a sharpened morphology that were most often misinterpreted as pathological (Gilbert *et al.*, 2003). However, in addition to these errors of interpretation, there are a number of physiological variants that can be and are misinterpreted as epileptiform, but which are entirely benign (Tatum *et al.*, 2006). These can be divided into benign rhythmic activity and benign spike/sharp wave activity.

Benign rhythmic activity

Alpha rhythm variants can on occasions cause some confusion, but it is usually rhythmic or semi-rhythmic theta that is most often misinterpreted as being pathological. Bursts of rhythmic temporal theta occurring in drowsiness (also known as psychomotor variant) can occur in up to 2 per cent of EEGs, bilaterally or independently over either temporal region (often with a left temporal bias); this pattern is benign. Similarly, rhythmic, unresponsive midline theta over the vertex (occasionally termed a Ciganek rhythm) is of no clinical significance. More problematic are bursts of generalized 6 Hz spike and wave which are usually a benign phenomenon (Figure 12.2a). This pattern falls into one of two groups – WHAM (wake, high amplitude, anterior and male) and FOLD (female, occipital, low amplitude and drowsiness). Nevertheless, this pattern can sometimes be difficult to distinguish from pathological patterns. Features that would indicate a pathological spike/wave pattern are high-amplitude spikes, anterior emphasis, frequency less than 6 Hz and presence during deep sleep.

Therefore, in cases of uncertainly, a sleep EEG can be helpful. Lastly, a pattern termed sub-clinical rhythmic electrographic discharge in adults (SREDA) (usually over 50 years of age) can last up to a minute in the temporal/parietal region. Again, this is of no known pathological significance but can be misinterpreted as sub-clinical seizure activity. The pattern does not show the evolution typical of seizures and is not followed by slow-wave activity.

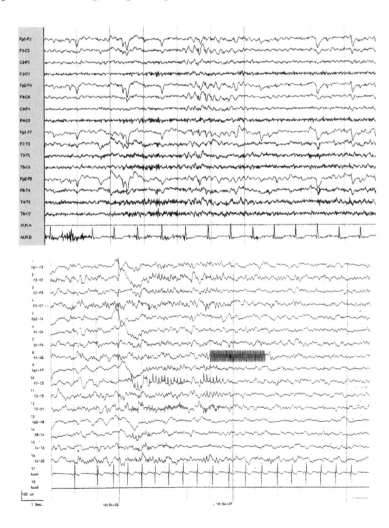

Figure 12.2 Examples of benign EEG patterns a) 6 Hz spike-wave burst and b) 14 and 6 Hz positive bursts

Source: From Tatum *et al.*, 2006. Reproduced with permission (American Electroencephalographic Society: Lippincott Williams & Wilkins).

Benign spike/sharp wave activity

As already discussed, sharpened background activity can be mistaken as sharp waves. However, there are also a number of physiological variants that are benign and are therefore important to recognize. Posterior occipital sharp transients of sleep (POSTs) and Lamda waves, which are also sharp posterior transients, can be mistaken for posterior sharp waves. POSTs are usually easily recognized, and Lamda occurs in young adults (or children) when reading or scanning a text. Three other patterns are important to recognize – wicket spikes, 14 Hz and 6 Hz positive spikes (Figure 12.2b) and small sharp spikes of sleep (sometimes referred to as benign epileptiform transients of sleep). Wicket spikes occur in older adults (> 30 years) in the temporal region (bilaterally or independently) during drowsiness or light sleep. They are usually of alpha frequency and are not associated with a slow wave. Fourteen Hz and 6 Hz positive spikes are bursts of spindle-like discharges over the posterior region, lasting up to a second and occurring in adolescence or young adults. Lastly, small sharp spikes of sleep are small and brief spikes that occur usually over the mid-temporal region during light sleep.

Epileptiform abnormalities without seizures

Having identified EEG abnormalities that can confidently be considered pathological, it is necessary to determine the risk of epilepsy associated with abnormalities in those free of seizures. This should be considered in two separate situations: screening of the general population and making the diagnosis in someone with a blackout. First of all, the use of the EEG as a screening tool in the general population without prior risk factors. Many of the early studies in this area are confounded by inclusion of non-epileptic EEG patterns (see above). These patterns are common in the general population. In a sleep EEG study of 100 male volunteer active-duty soldiers, 14 Hz and 6 Hz positive spikes occurred in 12 per cent, small sharp spikes in 11 per cent and 6 Hz spike and wave in 1 per cent (Jabbari *et al.*, 2000). Indeed, in this study none had true epileptiform activity. Furthermore, population EEG studies are usually not unselected populations and are usually carried out on patients. Thus, one of the classic papers on this issue (Zivin and Ajmone-Marsan, 1968) considered the records of 6,497 non-epileptic patients of whom 142 (2.2 per cent) had 'epileptiform' abnormalities. On closer inspection, 15 of the EEGs demonstrated 6 Hz spike and wave, and moreover most patients had concomitant disease (such as brain infections, mental retardation, psychosis, neoplasms). Indeed, only 142 could be considered 'normal', of which none had an abnormal EEG. This is in keeping with large studies in fit young adults in which a reasonable estimate of the incidence of epileptiform abnormalities is approximately 0.5 per cent (Gregory *et al.*, 1993; Richter *et al.*, 1971; Oberholtz *et al.*, 1975) or less (0.1 per cent) (LeTourneau and Merren, 1973).

If such people do have an epileptiform abnormality on the EEG, what is the subsequent risk of developing epilepsy? This is again a contentious area. In community studies, where most epileptiform discharges are in patients with acute or progressive cerebral lesions, a high percentage may go on to have seizures; these are, however, usually acutely provoked seizures (Sam and So, 2001) and are secondary to the underlying pathology. In fit young adults, the risks are substantially less, with most follow-up studies giving an estimate of incidence of epilepsy in those with epileptiform abnormalities of 2.5 per cent (Gregory *et al.*, 1993). In most of these studies, the mean follow-up is not given, but assuming a ten-year follow-up and a population incidence of 60 per 100,000 person-years in this age group (Wallace *et al.*, 1998), then this risk represents approximately five times the population risk.

This may, however, misrepresent the risk as it is likely that most of the risk of an abnormal EEG will be acute (soon after the EEG) and that the risk will diminish with time. The specificity of an epileptiform abnormality is therefore low. What about sensitivity of epileptiform abnormalities, as with the chance of finding an epileptiform abnormality in someone with epilepsy? A single EEG recording of someone with epilepsy has a 55 per cent chance of revealing an epileptiform abnormality (Fowle and Binnie, 2002), while combining a wake and sleep record can increase this to 80 per cent (Fowle and Binnie, 2002). Mitchell and Schenk (2003) have estimated the costs of screening EEG to prevent accidents. On the basis of an annual risk of seizures of 0.05 per cent and taking 10,000 aircrew, five would develop seizures in a year. Given an average in-flight time of 500 hours per year (that is, 1/20 of a year), the chance of an in-flight seizure would be 0.25 per year. If there is a chance of detecting epileptiform abnormalities in half the patients who have or will develop epilepsy (this may be an overestimate), then it would be possible to exclude 0.125 in-flight seizures per year or a seizure every eight years. Given an estimate of 1/1000 risk that an in-flight incapacitation will result in an accident, this would prevent an accident once every 8,000 years in 10,000 pilots. If each EEG costs 300 Euro, then screening 10,000 aircrew every year for

8,000 years would cost 2.4 billion Euro to prevent one accident.

Given these data and arguments, the EEG would not appear to be a particularly economic screening test to identify those likely to have seizures. There is, however, a separate argument that even interictal EEG abnormalities can be of relevance (Binnie, 2003). The observation that 'interictal' generalized spike/wave in the setting of someone with absence epilepsy can transiently disturb cognitive and motor performance is well established (Aarts *et al.*, 1984). Even brief bursts of spike/wave (< 3 seconds) can significantly slow reaction times 50 per cent of the time. However, this effect is not confined to generalized spike/wave as focal spikes can disrupt cognitive performance and this effect may last for up to two seconds (Binnie, 2003). Often, the disruption is subtle and can only be established with careful testing.

Perhaps of more relevance are the effects of these discharges on performance in everyday life, and such a study has been carried out on driving performance (Kasteleijn-Nolst Trenité *et al.*, 1987). In this study, interictal discharges had a significant effect on three out of six people, impairing both their ability to maintain course and abilities on an attentional task. It could be argued that these effects are small, and that since interictal discharges are less frequent during attentional tasks, they are likely to be rare. Nevertheless, these findings have been used to justify EEG recordings in both air traffic controllers and pilots. Further, evidence of the potential role of interictal EEG abnormalities is from data from the Royal Danish Air Force during the early 1950s, in which EEGs were recorded on applicants but not used to exclude from training (Lennox-Buchthal *et al.*, 1959). Follow-up indicated that those with marked (defined as > 10 per cent of frequencies below 6 Hz) or paroxysmal (spikes or sharp waves) abnormalities were three times more likely than those without abnormalities to have a crash due to pilot error. The reasons for these crashes (seizures, inattention during interictal discharges or some other condition) are not clear.

Bayesian Inference

The use of the EEG to diagnose epilepsy in someone with a blackout is best considered using Bayesian inference – that is, we should create a prior assessment of the chances of the blackout being epileptic and then see how the EEG will modify the probability (Figure 12.3). Given a prior probability of epilepsy (P), a probability of epileptiform abnormalities (EA) in fit adults without epilepsy of 0.005 and a probability of having an epileptiform abnormality on a standard EEG of 0.5 if the person has epilepsy, the probability of someone having epilepsy if an EA is found on the EEG is

P (epilepsy given an EA on EEG) = P x (probability of EA if epilepsy) / (probability of EA)
Probability of EA = (1-P) x 0.005 + P × 0.5 = 0.495P + 0.005
so P (epilepsy given an EA on EEG) = 0.5P / (0.495P + 0.005)

If it is considered that there is a 10 per cent chance that an event was a seizure, then finding an epileptiform abnormality will change the chances of the person having epilepsy to over 90 per cent.

Conversely, the value of using the EEG to confirm that someone does not have epilepsy (using a lack of EEG abnormalities to change the probability of our estimate that someone does not have epilepsy) can be estimated (Figure

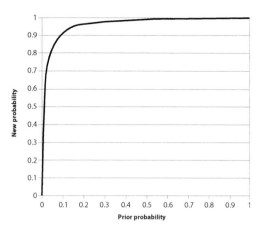

Figure 12.3 Probability of epilepsy given prior probability after epileptiform abnormality on EEG. Demonstrates that the EEG recording has a large effect on probability

12.4). There is a prior probability of P that someone does not have epilepsy. The probability of someone in the fit adult population having no epileptiform abnormalities is 0.995 (1 − 0.05). The probability of someone with epilepsy not having epileptiform abnormalities is 0.5 (1 − 0.5).

P (no epilepsy given no EA) = P × (probability of no EA if no epilepsy) / (probability of no EA)
Probability of EA = (1-P) x 0.5 + P × 0.995 = 0.495P + 0.5
P (no epilepsy given no EA) = 0.995P / (0.495P + 0.5)

In this situation, the EEG has only a small effect on modifying the prior probability (Figure 12.4).

From these calculations it can be seen that the EEG is useful to change confidence that someone in whom epilepsy is suspected has epilepsy, but it is not so useful in confirming that someone does not have epilepsy. For this reason, EEG should perhaps be

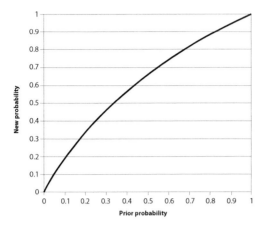

Figure 12.4 Probability of no epilepsy given prior probability and how probability is modified by no epileptiform abnormality on EEG. Demonstrates minimal effect of EEG recording on modifying prior probability

recorded in all people in whom epilepsy is suspected, but it is unnecessary when there is confidence that someone does not have epilepsy. It is important to recognize that these estimates are based on previously fit young adults. In people with neurological disease, in which there is a higher probability of epileptiform abnormalities, these probabilities are altered. Indeed, the probability of epileptiform abnormalities following intracranial operations or cerebral palsy increases to 0.1 (10 per cent). In these situations, a prior probability of 10 per cent would only be increased to 36 per cent by an epileptiform abnormality, and a prior probability of 60 per cent would be increased to approximately 90 per cent by an epileptiform abnormality.

Neuroimaging

Ideally, almost all patients with epilepsy should have neuroimaging,

and this is certainly true for those with partial epilepsy or with drug-resistant epilepsy of any type. Neuroimaging is recommended in all adults presenting with a first unprovoked seizure in recent guidelines from the American Academy of Neurology as the yield is likely to be at least 10 per cent (Krumholz *et al.*, 2007). Magnetic resonance imaging is preferable to a computerized tomography scan as the yield is much greater – CT scans may miss over two-thirds of the abnormalities detected by MR imaging (Bronen *et al.*, 1996). Imaging, however, cannot be used to make the diagnosis of epilepsy as 10 per cent of those with psychogenic non-epileptic seizures have abnormalities, including abnormalities strongly associated with epilepsy such as hippocampal sclerosis (Reuber *et al.*, 2002). Other imaging methods are mainly used in research or in pre-surgical assessment, including positron emission tomography (PET) which uses short-lived positron-emitting isotopes of biologically active tracers to determine regional blood flow, oxygen metabolism, glucose metabolism and receptor binding. Ictal single-photon emission computed tomography (SPECT) using a tracer to monitor blood flow has not only been used in pre-surgical assessment of patients to identify the ictal onset zone, but has also been used in the diagnosis of epilepsy to differentiate non-epileptic from epileptic attacks in challenging cases.

Implications to Aircrew

It is evident that many issues have to be taken into consideration when dealing with the possibility of epilepsy in both potential and operating aircrew. In the former the possibility of epilepsy may arise during the screening process, and with the latter the possibility may arise for clinical or other reasons. Essentially, epilepsy is the propensity to have seizures. Seizures are a common event that can occur at any age, but, in the first place, they need to be differentiated from other paroxysmal events, including syncope, psychogenic non-epileptic seizures, migraine and parasomnia. The issues have been dealt with in this chapter in relation to the diagnosis of epilepsy, and the reader is also referred to later chapters dealing with these disorders in a wider context.

As far as potential aircrew are concerned, if there is the possibility of epilepsy based on the history or the clinical examination alone, it may be unwise to permit the applicant to proceed further, particularly if there is clear evidence of a previous single seizure. The impact that a single seizure will have on the propensity to have further seizures depends upon the aetiology of that seizure and the time since that seizure occurred. The risk of further seizures diminishes greatly after two years, but depending upon aetiology and EEG, the risk may remain raised for beyond ten years. The aeromedical practitioner is confronted with a difficult situation when having to make the decision as to whether an apparently fit individual, but with so-called 'abnormalities' in the EEG, seeks employment as aircrew. It is important that less familiar and benign EEG patterns do not unduly influence the assessment. Nevertheless, it is only for those where there is unequivocal evidence that the EEG recordings are benign, as discussed above, that a career as aircrew would be a possibility.

In the event of a single seizure in operating aircrew, it is necessary to assess carefully the risk of further seizures. The risk depends upon whether the seizures were provoked or unprovoked, and is also dependent upon the EEG findings and the presence of neurological deficit.

The EEG can be used to determine seizure risk in those without seizures. It is true that the yield of a screening EEG is small (< 0.5 per cent), but in those with epileptiform abnormalities the risk of unprovoked seizures may be increased fivefold. Nevertheless, the economics of yearly EEG screening have been brought into question. This has, however, to be balanced against the observation that certain interictal EEG patterns such as generalized spike and wave may lead to transient cognitive impairment. Further, certain insults (such as infection, traumatic brain injury and stroke) may increase the risk of seizures, and this increased risk can persist for years. In such individuals, a very cautious approach should be adopted with respect to the possibility of continued flying.

References

Aarts, J.H., Binnie, C.D., Smit, A.M. and Wilkins, A.J. 1984. Selective cognitive impairment during focal and generalized epileptiform EEG activity. *Brain*, 107, 293–308.

Annegers, J.F., Hauser, W.A., Coan, S.P. and Rocca, W.A. 1998. A population-based study of seizures after traumatic brain injuries. *New England Journal of Medicine*, 338, 20–24.

Berg, A.T. and Shinnar, S. 1991. The risk of seizure recurrence following a first unprovoked seizure: A quantitative review. *Neurology*, 41, 965–72.

Binnie, C.D. 2003. Cognitive impairment during epileptiform discharges: Is it ever justifiable to treat the EEG? *Lancet Neurology*, 2, 725–30.

Bronen, R.A., Fulbright, R.K., Spencer, D.D., Spencer, S.S., Kim, J.H. *et al.* 1996. Refractory epilepsy: Comparison of MR imaging, CT, and histopathologic findings in 117 patients. *Radiology*, 201, 97–105.

Burn, J., Dennis, M., Bamford, J., Sandercock, P., Wade, D. and Warlow, C. 1997. Epileptic seizures after a first stroke: The Oxfordshire Community Stroke Project. *British Medical Journal*, 315, 1582–7.

Carpio, A. and Hauser, W.A. 2002. Prognosis for seizure recurrence in patients with newly diagnosed neurocysticercosis. *Neurology*, 59, 1730–34.

Christensen, J., Pedersen, M.G., Pedersen, C.B., Sidenius, P., Olsen, J. and Vestergaard, M. 2009. Long-term risk of epilepsy after traumatic brain injury in children and young adults: A population-based cohort study. *Lancet*, 373, 1105–10.

Commission on Classification and Terminology of the International League Against Epilepsy. 1985. Proposal for classification of epilepsies and epileptic syndromes. *Epilepsia*, 26, 268–78.

Commission on Classification and Terminology of the International League Against Epilepsy. 1989. Proposal for revised classification of epilepsies and epileptic syndromes. *Epilepsia*, 30, 389–99.

Crompton, D.E. and Berkovic, S.F. 2009. The borderland of epilepsy: Clinical and molecular features of phenomena that mimic epileptic seizures. *Lancet Neurology*, 8, 370–81.

Duncan, J.S., Sander, J.W., Sisodiya, S.M. and Walker, M.C. 2006. Adult epilepsy. *Lancet*, 367, 1087–100.

Fowle, A.J. and Binnie, C.D. 2000. Uses and abuses of the EEG in epilepsy. *Epilepsia*, 41, Suppl. 3, 10–18.

Fuller, G.N. and Guiloff, R.J. 1987. Migrainous olfactory hallucinations. *Journal of Neurology, Neurosurgery and Psychiatry*, 50, 1688–90.

Gilbert, D.L., Sethuraman, G., Kotagal, U. and Buncher, C.R. 2003. Meta-analysis of EEG test performance shows wide variation among studies. *Neurology*, 60, 564–70.

Gregory, R.P., Oates, T. and Merry, R.T. 1993. Electroencephalogram epileptiform abnormalities in candidates for aircrew training. *Electroencephalography and Clinical Neurophysiology*, 86, 75–7.

Hart, Y.M., Sander, J.W., Johnson, A.L. and Shorvon, S.D. 1990. National General Practice Study of Epilepsy: Recurrence after a first seizure. *Lancet*, 336, 1271–4.

Hesdorffer, D.C., Benn, E.K., Cascino, G.D. and Hauser, W.A. 2009. Is a first acute symptomatic seizure epilepsy? Mortality and risk for recurrent seizure. *Epilepsia*, 50, 1102–8.

Jabbari, B., Russo, M.B. and Russo, M.L. 2000. Electroencephalogram of asymptomatic adult subjects. *Clinical Neurophysiology*, 111, 102–5.

Kasteleijn-Nolst Trenité, D.G., Binnie, C.D., Harding, G.F. and Wilkins, A. 1999. Photic stimulation: Standardization of screening methods. *Epilepsia*, 40, Suppl. 4, 5–9.

Kasteleijn-Nolst Trenité, D.G., Riemersma, J.B.J., Binnie, C.D., Smit, A.M. and Meinardi, H. 1987. The influence of subclinical epileptiform EEG discharges on driving behaviour. *Electroencephalography and Clinical Neurophysiology*, 67, 167–70.

Kim, L.G., Johnson, T.L., Marson, A.G. and Chadwick, D.W. (MRC MESS Study group). 2006. Prediction of risk of seizure recurrence after a single seizure and early epilepsy: Further results from the MESS trial. *Lancet Neurology*, 5, 317–22.

Krumholz, A., Wiebe, S., Gronseth, G., Shinnar, S., Levisohn, P., Ting, T. *et al.* (Quality Standards Subcommittee of the American Academy of Neurology and the American Epilepsy Society). 2007. Practice parameter: Evaluating an apparent unprovoked first seizure in adults (an evidence-based review): Report of the Quality Standards Subcommittee of the American Academy of Neurology and the American Epilepsy Society. *Neurology*, 69, 1996–2007.

Legg, N.J., Gupta, P.C. and Scott, D.F. 1973. Epilepsy following cerebral abscess: A clinical and EEG study of 70 patients. *Brain*, 96, 259–68.

Lennox-Buchthal, M., Buchthal, F. and Rosenfalck, P. 1959. Correlation of electroencephalographic findings with crash rate of military jet pilots. *Epilepsia*, 1, 366–72.

LeTourneau, D.J. and Merren, M.D. 1973. Experience with electroencephalography in student naval aviation personnel, 1961–1971: A preliminary report. *Aerospace Medicine*, 44, 1302–4.

Meierkord, H., Will, B., Fish, D. and Shorvon, S. 1991. The clinical features and prognosis of pseudoseizures diagnosed using video-EEG telemetry. *Neurology*, 41, 1643–6.

Mendez, O.E. and Brenner, R.P. 2006. Increasing the yield of EEG. *Journal of Clinical Neurophysiology*, 23, 282–93.

Mitchell, S.J. and Schenk, C.P. 2003. The value of screening tests in applicants for professional pilot medical certification. *Occupational Medicine*, 53, 15–18.

Oberholtz, H., Kugler, J. and Jessberger, W. 1975. EEG criteria for flying fitness applied by the German Air Force Institute of Aviation Medicine. *Aviation, Space, and Environmental Medicine*, 46, 194–7.

Petkar, S., Cooper, P. and Fitzpatrick, A.P. 2006. How to avoid a misdiagnosis in patients presenting with transient loss of consciousness. *Postgraduate Medical Journal*, 82, 630–41.

Reuber, M. and Elger, C.E. 2003. Psychogenic nonepileptic seizures: Review and update. *Epilepsy and Behavior*, 4, 205–16.

Reuber, M., Fernández, G., Helmstaedter, C., Qurishi, A. and Elger, C.E. 2002. Evidence of brain abnormality in patients with psychogenic nonepileptic seizures. *Epilepsy and Behavior*, 3, 249–54.

Richter, P.L., Zimmerman, E.A., Raichle, M.E. and Liske, E. 1971. Electroencephalograms of 2,947 United States Air Force Academy Cadets (1965–1969). *Aerospace Medicine*, 42, 1011–4.

Salazar, A.M., Jabbari, B., Vance, S.C., Grafman, J., Amin D. and Dillon, J.D. 1985. Epilepsy after penetrating head injury. I. Clinical correlates: A report of the Vietnam Head Injury Study. *Neurology*, 35, 1406–14.

Sam, M.C. and So, E.L. 2001. Significance of epileptiform discharges in patients without epilepsy in the community. *Epilepsia*, 42, 1273–8.

Sander, J.W., Hart, Y.M., Johnson, A.L. and Shorvon, S.D. 1990. National General Practice Study of Epilepsy: Newly diagnosed epileptic seizures in a general population. *Lancet*, 336, 1267–71.

Tatum, W.O. IV, Husain, A.M., Benbadis, S.R. and Kaplan, P.W. 2006. Normal adult EEG and patterns of uncertain significance. *Journal of Clinical Neurophysiology*, 23, 194–207.

Teasdale, G. and Jennett, B. 1974. Assessment of coma and impaired consciousness: A practical scale. *Lancet*, 2, 81–4.

Wallace, H., Shorvon, S. and Tallis, R. 1998. Age-specific incidence and prevalence rates of treated epilepsy in an unselected population of 2,052,922 and age-specific fertility rates of women with epilepsy. *Lancet*, 352, 1970–73.

Warren-Gash, C. and Zeman, A. 2003. Déjà vu. *Practical Neurology*, 3,106–9.

Wilson, J.V. and Reynolds, E.H. 1990. Texts and documents: Translation and analysis of a cuneiform text forming part of a Babylonian treatise on epilepsy. *Medical History*, 34, 185–98.

Zivin, L. and Ajmone-Marsan, C. 1968. Incidence and prognostic significance of epileptiform activity in the EEG of nonepileptlc subjects. *Brain*, 91, 751–77.

Chapter 13

SYNCOPE: PHYSIOLOGY, PATHOPHYSIOLOGY AND AEROMEDICAL IMPLICATIONS

David A. Low and Christopher J. Mathias

❖

Syncope (or fainting) is defined as a transient loss of postural tone and/or consciousness due to transient global cerebral hypoperfusion (Moya *et al.*, 2009). The regulation of blood pressure and thus maintenance of cerebral blood flow within normal limits are critical in preserving adequate cerebral oxygenation and ensuring consciousness (van Lieshout *et al.*, 2003). Neural and non-neural mechanisms must ensure effective and rapid return of blood to the heart and continued delivery to the brain, particularly in the upright posture, where the anatomical positions of the brain and the heart and the hydrostatic gradient imposed by gravitational stress result in about 70 per cent of the body's blood volume being located below the heart (Rowell, 1993). A precipitous decrease in blood pressure may lead to inadequate cerebral perfusion, potentially causing reduced physical and/or mental capacity and syncope. Moreover, a syncopal episode may lead to injury through loss of postural tone and to seizures as a result of cerebral hypoxia. Furthermore, if the syncopal attack and the cerebral hypoperfusion continue to be unresolved, irreversible damage can occur. The cardiovascular system has to monitor and regulate blood pressure continuously through the autonomic modulation of the heart and circulation that plays a key role in determining and integrating haemodynamic adjustments.

Autonomic Control of the Circulation

The autonomic nervous system has a central role in the regulation of blood pressure. Normal physiologic feedback mechanisms work through craniosacral parasympathetic and thoracolumbar sympathetic neural pathways to maintain blood pressure, and thus adequate cerebral perfusion (Figure 13.1).

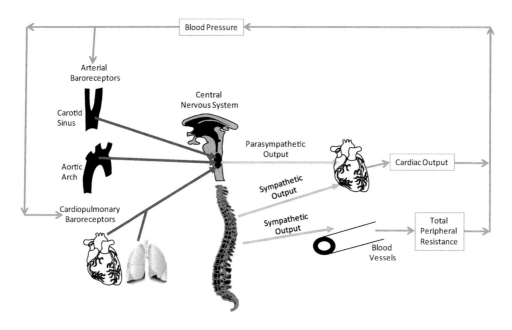

Figure 13.1 Scheme outlining autonomic neural pathways that control arterial blood pressure (see colour section)

There are specific neurotransmitters in each pathway that influence ganglionic and post-ganglionic activity (Figure 13.2). Acetylcholine is the pre-ganglionic neurotransmitter for both the parasympathetic and sympathetic pathways, and is also the post-ganglionic neurotransmitter of parasympathetic neurons that stimulate muscarinic receptors. In contrast, sympathetic post-ganglionic neurons release noradrenaline, along with other co-transmitters, such as adenosine triphosphate, that act on alpha- or beta-adrenergic receptors. One exception is at the adrenal cortex where there is no post-synaptic neuron, though the presynaptic neuron releases acetylcholine to act on nicotinic receptors which stimulates the release of adrenaline and noradrenaline into the circulation as hormones that can also act on the adrenergic receptors.

Reflex compensatory changes occur within the autonomic nervous system in response to alterations in blood pressure as part of the cardiopulmonary and arterial baroreflexes that participate continuously in the regulation of cardiovascular function to produce alterations in efferent sympathetic adrenergic and parasympathetic neural activity and subsequent haemodynamic adjustments (Figure 13.1). Arterial and cardiopulmonary baroreceptors respond to mechanical deformation via local changes in blood pressure and volume to correct alterations in blood pressure via changes in cardiac output and/or total peripheral resistance. There are two types of arterial baroreceptors: carotid baroreceptors, located in the internal carotid artery, and aortic baroreceptors, located in the aorta arch. Cardiopulmonary baroreceptors are mechanically sensitive receptors located in the four chambers of the heart that respond to changes in cardiac and pulmonary filling volumes (Ray and Saito, 2000). Afferent information from these baroreceptors is relayed

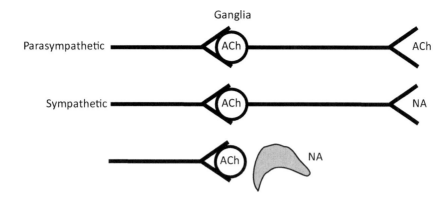

Figure 13.2 Outline of the major transmitters at autonomic ganglia and post-ganglionic sites supplied by the sympathetic and parasympathetic efferent pathways

to the cardiovascular centre in the brainstem. Efferent information via the parasympathetic and sympathetic neural pathways is then provided to effector organs, for example the heart and regional vascular beds, to correct the change in blood pressure and complete the baroreflex. The heart is under the dual control of the parasympathetic and sympathetic neural pathways, an increase in parasympathetic neural activity causing a reduction in heart rate. In contrast, increases in sympathetic nerve activity result in elevations in heart rate and vascular resistance of various regional vascular beds. In addition, increased sympathetic nerve activity is also directed to the adrenal gland, which stimulates the release of noradrenaline.

Orthostasis

Due to the hydrostatic gradient imposed by gravity on the cardiovascular system, syncope is most likely to occur in the upright posture due to arterial blood pressure at the brain being less than that at the heart and the pooling of blood below the heart. Thus, the effect of orthostatic stress on the cardiovascular system must be considered. Upon assumption of the upright posture, between 300 and 800 millilitres of blood is translocated to the lower limbs. The rise in pressure in the capillaries of the lower limbs also causes the movement of fluid from the blood to the tissues, resulting in plasma volume loss (Brown and Hainsworth, 1999). As a consequence of blood pooling and the superimposed decline in plasma volume, the return of venous blood to the heart is reduced and central blood volume falls (van Lieshout *et al.*, 2003). Reductions in filling of the right ventricle lead to a reduction in stroke volume and a fall in cardiac output, despite an elevation of the heart rate (Harms *et al.*, 1999), but blood pressure is preserved by compensatory vasoconstriction of resistance and capacitance vessels in the splanchnic, musculoskeletal, cutaneous and renal vascular beds (Rowell, 1984) (Figure 13.3).

During prolonged orthostatic stress, additional adjustments are mediated by the humoral limb of the neuroendocrine system. In response to decreases in effective blood volume, increases in activity of the vasopressin and renin-angiotensin-aldosterone systems occur that further augment sympathetic nerve activity and preserve effective blood volume (Rowell, 1993). Other non-neural mechanisms that assist with the maintenance of blood pressure during orthostatic stress are the skeletal muscle pump (such as during muscular contraction) and the thoracoabdominal respiratory pump (for example, the lowering and raising of the ribcage and diaphragm). These mechanisms serve to increase venous return to the heart and attenuate pooling in the dependent veins.

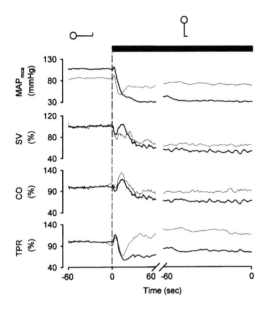

Figure 13.3 Average cardiovascular responses to standing in healthy aged matched control subjects and in patients with significant autonomic dysfunction during the first and the last 60 seconds of five minutes of standing (black bar)

Blood pressure (MAP) was measured non-invasively from a digital artery and stroke volume (SV), cardiac output (CO) and total peripheral resistance (TPR) were calculated according to the Modeflow technique and are presented as percentage changes from the supine position. Although not shown, heart rate increased from 66 to 81 and from 60 to 81 beats.min-1 in the patient and healthy control groups, respectively, by the end of standing. Bold lines are data from patients and grey lines represent healthy controls. From Harms *et al.*, (2000) with permission.

The haemodynamic adjustments to an upright posture are analogous to those produced during headwards accelerations experienced by a pilot. Intuitively, it would be assumed that footwards accelerations, which produce the movement of blood towards the central circulation and the head, would not threaten the effective maintenance of blood pressure, but this is not necessarily so. Footwards accelerations ($-G_z$) initially increase blood pressure and cerebral blood flow, but secondary baroreflex-mediated responses induce bradycardia alongside arteriolar dilatation, which can reduce arterial pressure and cerebral blood flow to syncopal levels if the acceleration is prolonged and uncorrected.

Cerebral Perfusion

Blood flow to the brain is controlled via adjustments in systemic haemodynamics – the perfusion pressure (Ogoh *et al.*, 2005; Ogoh *et al.*, 2008; van Lieshout *et al.*, 2003) – and also through local vascular regulation (Panerai, 2008; Paulson *et al.*, 1990). The brain is able to maintain its blood flow in the face of a wide range of arterial blood pressures – a process termed cerebral autoregulation (CA) that has both fast- and slow-acting regulatory components. Fast (or dynamic CA) refers to the ability to restore cerebral blood flow in the face of blood pressure changes within seconds and reflects the latency of the cerebral vasoregulatory system, whereas static CA reflects the overall 'steady-state' efficiency of the system (Panerai, 2008; Tiecks *et al.*, 1995; van Beek *et al.*, 2008). Cerebral blood flow is also locally adjusted to changes in the metabolic activity of the brain (alterations in carbon dioxide, oxygen and glucose content), myogenic and humoral factors and autonomic neural activity (Panerai, 2008; Paulson *et al.*, 1990). Although there is some variation, syncope typically ensues when cerebral perfusion has decreased by ~ 50 per cent, when mental confusion becomes prominent and cerebral oxygenation becomes affected (Madsen *et al.*, 1998; van Lieshout *et al.*, 2003) (Figure 13.4).

Classification of Syncope

A syncopal attack is characterized by rapid onset, short duration and by a spontaneous and complete recovery (Moya *et al.*, 2009). It can have many causes, and so classifications vary. The classification below is adapted from (Moya *et al.*, 2009) and (Mathias, 2009)

O Autonomic (neurally) mediated syncope
  – Vasovagal
  – Situational
  – Carotid sinus
O Orthostatic hypotension
  – Neurogenic causes
    • Disease, especially autonomic failure syndromes
  – Non-neurogenic causes
    • Blood/plasma loss – haemorrhage, burns, sweating
    • Fluid/electrolyte – fluid loss (vomiting, diarrhoea) renal/endocrine (salt losing nephropathy, adrenal insufficiency)
    • Drug-induced
    • Alcohol
    • Physical deconditioning
O Cardiac syncope
  – Arrhythmia
  – Structural disorders – myocarditis, pericarditis, aortic stenosis

Autonomic (neurally or reflex) mediated syncope is the most frequent cause of syncope. Autonomic (neurally) mediated syncope traditionally refers to a heterogeneous group of conditions in which the cardiovascular reflexes that are normally useful in controlling the circulation become intermittently inappropriate, in response to a trigger, resulting in vasodilatation through sympathetic nerve activity withdrawal and/or bradycardia via increased vagal

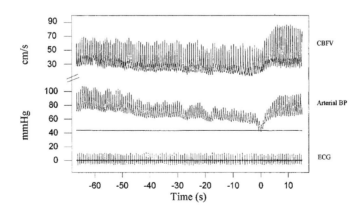

Figure 13.4 Continuous and non-invasive beat-to-beat tracings of blood pressure and middle cerebral artery blood velocity (CBFV) prior to and during a syncopal episode in a subject during 60 degrees head-up tilt. Also, notice the widening of the ECG (e.g., bradycardia) just prior to time 0. From Carey *et al.*, (2001) with permission.

activity and thereby a fall in arterial blood pressure and global cerebral perfusion. There are three major forms of autonomic (neurally) mediated syncope: vasovagal syncope, carotid sinus hypersensitivity and situational syncope. Vasovagal syncope is the most common form and is also referred to as common faints or emotional syncope as provoking factors include fear, pain and psychological factors. Nausea and other gastrointestinal upsets, probably through activation of visceral afferents, may also be causative.

Carotid sinus hypersensitivity syncope is rare in younger individuals but more common after the age of 50 (Humm and Mathias, 2006) and occurs when there is a disproportionate efferent response to mechanical manipulation of the carotid sinuses and the carotid baroreceptors, for example whilst turning the head or buttoning the collar. In situational syncope, various, but specific, factors and conditions predispose the individual to syncope. These include induction of a Valsalva manoeuvre (as in defecation), hyperventilation during heavy resistance exercise, the playing of musical instruments and following paroxysms of coughing. There may be situations in which autonomic syncope occurs with uncertain or even apparently absent triggers. In some this may be due to pseudo-syncope, which can be difficult to diagnose (Mathias *et al.*, 2000). When the cause is uncertain, or even if the condition is in doubt, the term 'atypical syncope' has been used (Moya *et al.*, 2009). Evaluation of syncope may need the facilities of a dedicated autonomic laboratory as a wide range of investigations is sometimes needed (Mathias and Bannister, 2002).

For pilots and other air personnel, the most relevant major group of syncope to consider is autonomic (neurally) mediated syncope, previously referred to by a variety of names, including reflex and neurocardiogenic. The other two major groups of syncope, cardiac and orthostatic hypotension (with neurogenic or non-neurogenic causes), are less likely in young and usually physically fit individuals, as their incidence increases with age and comorbidity. Individuals with autonomic failure syndromes (such as multiple system atrophy and pure autonomic failure) regularly experience orthostatic hypotension (see Figure 13.5a) and at times syncope due to

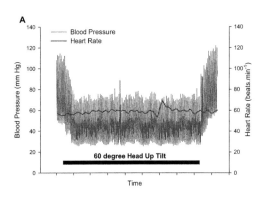
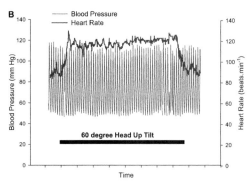

Figure 13.5 Continuous blood pressure and heart rate tracings of orthostatic hypotension in an autonomic failure patient (A) and postural tachycardia in a PoTS patient (B) during 60 degree head up tilt tests. From Mathias (2009) (see colour section)

their inability to increasing sympathetic nerve activity when needed, as a result of central or peripheral autonomic damage. Cardiac syncope is associated with an arrhythmia or structural disease and is characterized by the suddenness of its onset and the lack of warning symptoms of cerebral hypoperfusion. An exception is the volume depletion subtype of orthostatic hypotension syncope, where excessive dehydration through sweating and/or blood loss, for example, could provoke a syncopal event in a pilot.

Clinical Picture

There are number of symptoms that occur before syncope given that it is a neurally mediated event. These may include sweating, pallor, hyperventilation, nausea and feelings of 'dizziness'. These may be in addition to the symptoms mainly resulting from a fall in blood pressure and diminsihed organ perfusion, as described below in patients with ortostatic hypotension (Figure 13.7).

○ Cerebral hypoperfusion
  - Dizziness
  - Visual disturbances
    • Blurred – tunnel
    • Scotoma (partially diminished visual acuity)
    • Greying/blacking out
    • Colour defects
  - Cognitive deficits
○ Muscle hypoperfusion
  - Paracervical and suboccipital ('coat-hanger') ache
  - Lower back/buttock ache
○ Subclavian steal-like syndrome
○ Renal hypoperfusion
  - Oliguria (decreased urine output)
○ Spinal cord hypoperfusion

○ Non-specific
  - Weakness, lethargy, fatigue

Hyperventilation is often a result of the psychological stress that can accompany or even provoke syncope and results in a reduction of arterial blood carbon dioxide concentration (for example, hypocapnia), which has two implications for the maintenance of blood pressure and cerebral blood flow. A decrease in arterial blood carbon dioxide concentration will cause a reduction in cerebral blood flow, thus further threatening cerebral perfusion, but, conversely, also causes vasodilation in other vascular beds and consequently lowers vascular resistance (Norcliffe-Kaufmann *et al.*, 2008). Despite these two differing effects of hypocapnia, such responses will overall further predispose an individual to a syncopal event. Furthermore, relative hypoperfusion of other vascular beds above the heart can occur and produce symptoms. For example, collapse of retinal perfusion becomes manifest before the loss of consciousness, thus resulting in sensations of 'greying' or 'blacking' out (van Lieshout *et al.*, 2003) prior to and/or during a syncopal event. Using the arm muscles, especially when upright, can increase symptoms of cerebral hypoperfusion by a subclavian steal-like mechanism, further reducing brain blood flow. These symptoms can be used as warning signs of an imminent syncopal attack and prompt manoeuvres to help prevent such an occurrence. For a pilot, however, such simple but very effective interventions, such as lying flat, are practically not feasible and therefore could have critical consequences for the individual.

In autonomic (neurally) mediated syncope, the function of the autonomic nerves serving the baroreflex is essentially normal, except when there is an intermittent 'abnormality', and it is usually subclassified on the causative mechanisms of the efferent neural pathway that predominates. In the 'vasodepressor' type, hypotension is the result of a loss of sympathetic nerve activity and vasoconstrictor tone that causes excessive vasodilatation (Figure 13.6a). In the 'cardio-inhibitory' type, bradycardia or asystole predominates via increased vagal nerve activity (Figure 13.6b). In the 'mixed' type, both mechanisms are operative (Figure 13.6c). The subtype of syncope does not always depend on the nature of the trigger and can vary within the same individual.

Another haemodynamic response that can occur, but not in all individuals, in the immediate presyncopal phase is a reduction and abrupt cessation of sympathetic nerve activity (Iwase et al., 2002) (Figure 13.7).

Conversely, large increases in adrenaline can occur, which contributes to a reduced total vascular resistance through vasodilatation prior to syncope (Goldstein et al., 2003). Furthermore, during steady-state orthostatic stress the baroreflexes function normally, and are even improved; however, immediately before the onset of syncope, baroreflex control of sympathetic nerve activity and heart rate is significantly impaired (Ichinose et al., 2006; Ogoh et al., 2004). Finally, evidence for impaired dynamic cerebral autoregulation prior to the onset of syncope is equivocal (Carey et al., 2001; Schondorf et al., 2001; Zhang et al., 1998), which likely relates to the differences in analysis techniques and approaches. Although the different pathways and types of syncope have been well described, the specific trigger(s) for the initiation of the cascade of events that occur in individual attacks is less well understood.

Autonomic (neurally) mediated syncope is regarded as the most common cause of intermittent and

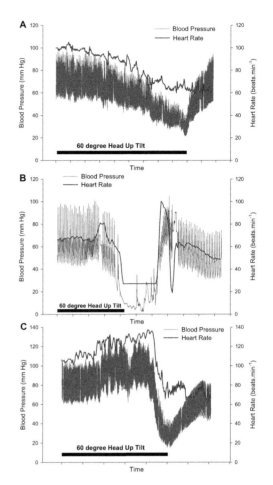

Figure 13.6 Continuous blood pressure and heart rate tracings during the predominantly vasodepressor (A), cardio-inhibitory (B) and mixed (cardio-inhibitory and vasodepressor, C) forms of vasovagal syncope during 60 degree head up tilt tests. From Mathias (2009) (see colour section)

usually extremely short-lived autonomic cardiovascular dysfunction. Another cause of intermittent autonomic dysfunction, mainly associated with postural change and exercise, which only recently has been recognized, is the postural tachycardia syndrome (PoTS) (Schondorf and Low, 1993). This

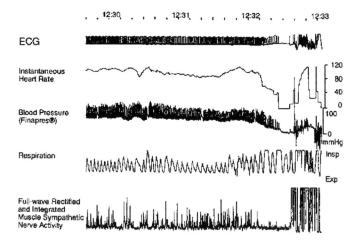

Figure 13.7 Continuous recordings of the electrocardiogram, heart rate, blood pressure, respiration and muscle sympathetic nerve activity prior to and during a syncopal event

Notice the withdrawal of sympathetic nerve activity just prior to syncope. Muscle sympathetic nerve activity was recorded from the peroneal nerve using the microneurography technique. From Iwase *et al.*, (2002) with permission.

syndrome is characterized by a substantial rise in heart rate ($\geq$ 30 beats.min^{-1}) and orthostatic intolerance symptoms attributed to cerebral hypoperfusion and sympathetic over-activation (palpitations, tremulousness and sweating) but without orthostatic hypotension (Figure 13.6b) (Mathias, 2009). In our experience, syncope also occurs in a third of such patients investigated, although symptoms in the presyncopal phase, especially palpitations, enable them to take preventive action. It predominantly affects women below the age of 50 years and may be preceded by a viral illness. Fatigue occurs in some, and prolonged physical inactivity (for example, deconditioning) and hyperventilation may be contributory. The most common associated disorder, in our experience, is the joint hypermobility syndrome (Ehlers–Danlos III).

There is a range of non-pharmacological measures that can help prevent precipitous reductions in blood pressure. Pre-emptive action should be taken; thus, ensuring an adequate fluid intake during flight is essential in the aeromedical environment to counter dehydration. Ingestion of water has also been shown to have a moderate pressor effect in middle-aged to older individuals and to improve orthostatic tolerance (Mathias, 2000) (Figure 13.8).

Physical manoeuvres such as muscle tensing and abdominal compression, as well as devices such as lower limb elastic stockings and abdominal binders, can decrease venous pooling by activation of the calf muscle pump and increasing sympathetic nerve activity and reduce orthostatic hypotension (Krediet *et al.*, 2007; Mathias, 2003; Smit *et al.*, 2004) (Figure 13.9).

These strategies have been implemented in the use of muscle tensing, short-term Valsalva manoeuvres that increase intrathoracic and intra-abdominal pressures by expiring against a closed glottis, and anti-G suits in pilots, which are effective in abating syncope. In situational syncope, management should be directed towards the underlying cause and pathophysiological basis.

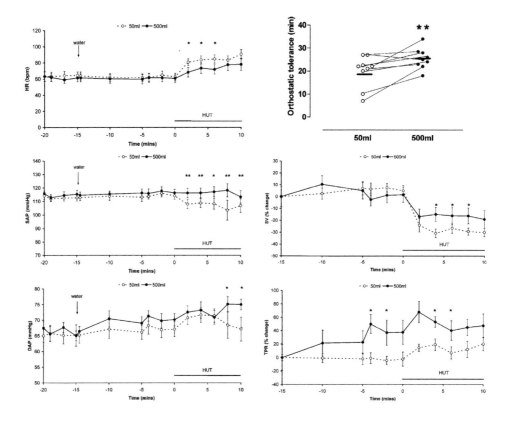

Figure 13.8 Orthostatic tolerance and hemodynamic responses during supine rest and 60° head up tilt (HUT) after ingestion of 50 or 500 mL distilled water in nine healthy participants who were experiencing attacks of syncope of unknown cause (mean age, 36.8 ± 4.2 years; four males)

After 20 minutes of HUT, increasing levels of lower body negative pressure (LBNP) were applied (while still tilted) until syncopal symptoms. Orthostatic tolerance was measured as the time to the onset of syncopal symptoms during either HUT or HUT+LBNP. Blood pressure was measured non-invasively from a digital artery and stroke volume and total peripheral resistance were calculated according to the Modeflow technique. HR=heart rate, SAP=systolic blood pressure, DAP=diastolic blood pressure, SV=stroke volume, TPR=total peripheral resistance. *P<0.05 and **P<0.01 compared with 50 mL of water. There was a significant increase in orthostatic tolerance (e.g., syncope was delayed) of 5.6±1.9 minutes after 500 mL of water (top right panel), which was mediated by increases in DAP (lower left panel) and TPR (lower right panel) in the supine position, SAP (middle left panel), DAP and TPR during tilting and an attenuation in the reduction in SV (middle right panel) during HUT. An improvement in the control of cerebral perfusion was also recorded (data not shown). Reproduced with permission, from Claydon *et al.*, (2006)

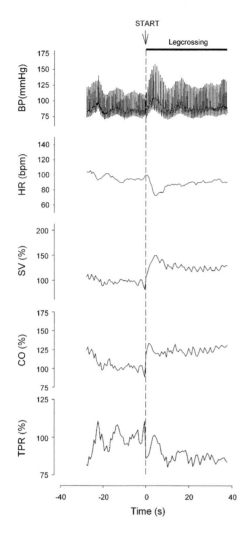

Figure 13.9 Typical haemodynamic responses during leg crossing and isometric contractions of the lower limbs and abdomen during standing in an individual subject

Blood pressure (BP) was non-invasively measured from a digital artery and stroke volume (SV), cardiac output (CO) and total peripheral resistance (TPR) were calculated according to the Modeflow technique and are presented as percentage changes from their starting values during standing. Notice the increase in blood and pulse pressure. From van Dijk *et al.*, (2005) with permission.

Furthermore, cognitive behavioural psychotherapy is helpful if there is coexisting phobia, panic attack or anxiety disorder.

The Aviation Domain

The environment that a pilot encounters during flight can present significant challenges to the maintenance of blood pressure, which have implications if they are unsuccessfully met. The cognitive changes demonstrated in a human deficit clinical model – pure autonomic failure, where there is no central involvement – suggest that a low blood pressure may decrease cognitive function, and this may occur even in normal healthy individuals (Heims *et al.*, 2006). Furthermore, cognitive function may also be transiently affected when symptoms of syncope occur, such as dizziness or lightheadedness, unsteadiness and blurred or impaired vision. The consequences of one or a combination of these events, as well as a syncopal episode, could have grave repercussions for a pilot (Burton and Whinnery, 1985; Kobayashi and Miyamoto, 2000; van Dijk *et al.*, 2003; Yilmaz *et al.*, 1999). Although the orthostatic stress of a seated position is less severe than the upright posture, the pilot is faced with a number of challenges that could threaten the effective regulation of blood pressure within normal limits during flight. Orthostasis in the seated position for a prolonged duration and/or the long duration of acceleration forces (headwards $+G_Z$ or footwards $-G_Z$) imposed by various manoeuvres during flight can alter the hydrostatic gradient of the pilot and predispose them to syncope if unchecked. Prolonged orthostasis also results in plasma volume loss from the blood to the surrounding tissues, which can also reduce tolerance to orthostatic stress (el-Sayed *et al.*, 1995).

The reduced partial pressure of oxygen of the cabin environment that occurs with ascent to altitude could also increase the risk of syncope. The hyperventilation response to hypoxia decreases the body's partial pressure of carbon dioxide which reduces cerebral perfusion (Lennox and Gibbs, 1932) and thus could hasten the occurrence of syncope. However, there would appear to be a general lack of effect of hypoxia on tolerance to orthostatic stress and cardiovascular function, except for individuals who display large increases in adrenaline during such exposure (Rowell and Blackmon, 1987; Rowell and Blackmon, 1989; Rowell and Seals, 1990). In contrast, rapid changes in partial pressure of oxygen within the aircraft, such as those that occur with rapid decompression/depressurization, can result in severe hypoxia and would reduce tolerance to acceleration $(+G_Z)$ forces (Macmillan, 1999).

Pilots can also be exposed to heat stress prior to and during flight. The thermal load from the avionics, aerodynamic friction, solar radiation and protective clothing of pilots, which can retard heat loss/exchange, as well as low-flying manoeuvres and anti-G straining manoeuvres, which increase metabolic rate, can promote heat storage (Maidment, 1999). Subsequent rises in body temperature and increases in cutaneous vasodilatation and sweating and associated dehydration worsen orthostatic hypotension and tolerance to $+G_Z$ (Lind et al., 1968; Wilson et al., 2006).

Aeromedical Considerations

In the assessment of an aviator presenting with a history of a syncopal episode, it is, of course, important to take into consideration the varied stresses of the aviation domain, including those particular situations away from home if the aviator is operating worldwide. As well as hypotension, hypoxia and dehydration, dealt with above, the aeromedical practitioner needs to consider a day-to-day lifestyle that may involve a host of possibly precipitating factors that include fatigue arising from the need to cope with sleep disturbance, environmental factors that may be encountered in foreign climes and the possibility of adverse operating situations with high workload and uncertainty (Clint, 2008).

However, though syncope in an aviator may occur in response to varied stresses, it may equally involve disease of the cardiovascular and nervous systems, even though the individual will have been screened regularly. It is, therefore, important that assessments of aircrew reporting a syncopal episode are carried out carefully and in detail. Subsequent to the episode, the physical examination is often normal and thus the history is especially important; sometimes witness accounts are useful. Antecedent events, contributing albeit rarely to syncope, such as personal psychological trauma, may result in autonomic (neurally) mediated syncope. It is likely that the history will prove to be of overriding relevance in deciding on the cause, on the prognosis and on the implications of the event to future employment.

Syncope or Seizure

The differentiation of epilepsy from syncope can present a problem to the medical practitioner, and the inability to exclude even the likelihood of epilepsy can be detrimental to the career of an aviator. For a detailed treatment of the differential diagnosis, the reader is referred to Sheldon et al. (2002). Briefly, syncope occurs in the upright position, usually with prodromal symptoms that include nausea, yawning and deep breathing, and there may be visual symptoms. There is a sudden collapse and a brief period of unconsciousness, but there may be a rapid recovery afterwards with little or no apparent confusion. In some episodes of syncope there may be brief convulsive movements such as twitching of the hands and face, tonic postures and myoclonic jerks, but not usually a generalized tonic–clonic seizure. These movements are more likely to occur if the individual is kept upright. Urinary incontinence may occur in syncope, though that would increase the suspicion of an epileptic event if in combination with tongue biting, seizure and a post-ictal confusional state.

Lightheadedness, sweating and cardiac symptoms such as palpitations also suggest syncope, whereas events related to the nervous system such as *déjà vu*, aphasia, an aura and post-event delirium suggest epilepsy. Witness accounts of aphasia, delirium, automatism and posturing as well as a description of the convulsion may point to epilepsy. If there is any uncertainty in the mind of the aeromedical practitioner with regard to the differential diagnosis between syncope and epilepsy, referral to a neurologist with expertise of cardiovascular autonomic disorders, and with facilities for detailed autonomic investigation, is desirable and sometimes essential.

Syncope and Cardiac Arrhythmias

Cardiac arrhythmias are often a major cause of syncope, but usually below 20 years where there may be an underlying genetic disorder (such as the Brugada syndrome) or over the age of 55 years where ischemic heart disease, amongst other factors, may be contributory. In aviators between the ages of 20 and 55 years who have been cleared as previously being fit, this may still need to be considered (Gould, 2010). Referral to a cardiologist, especially to one specializing in arrhythmias, is recommended. Investigations may include 24-hour, or longer, periods of electroencephalographic recording. Whether implanted loop recorders, such as the Reveal device, have a role in the aviator setting remains to be debated.

Syncope of Unknown Origin

Determining the cause of syncope in an aviator, and also the pathophysiological mechanisms responsible, is an essential aim. Despite intensive investigation, definitive diagnosis may not be achieved in up to a third of such individuals, as based on the experience in large centres dealing with different age groups and a wide range of disorders. In those with normal evaluations (which typically include tilt-table studies, with or without drugs), an absence of history of cardiovascular disease and a normal electrocardiogram, it is more likely that the risk is low and that the individual would have a good prognosis. It may be that provocative factors need to be considered as part of the workup, and, if necessary, investigations which are well established in autonomic centres and laboratories considered. These include food challenge, cervical and neck movements and even carotid sinus massage. Assessing the risk of recurrence may be difficult when the aetiology cannot be established with certainly. Identifying possible precipitating factors is of particular value in management.

Summary

Syncope, when it occurs in an aviator, is often benign, but it warrants careful and individual consideration. The setting in which the event occurred needs to be carefully considered, and the combination of clinical history, investigations and, in particular cases, specific provocation tests (as used in autonomic departments) are needed to determine the underlying diagnosis and the pathophysiological mechanisms responsible. This is of crucial importance as this determines prognosis, and thus the likelihood of continued employment. It is also of relevance to management, which usually would consist of non-pharmacological measures. These would focus on preventing episodes that predispose subjects, even in extreme situations, to syncope. Rarely, support is needed because of extreme psychological trauma, often highly specific, and thus excluding situations which otherwise would not impair the aviator's performance. In the aviation setting, it would be most unlikely to consider medication, as used widely in clinical practice, such as the use of mineralocorticoids (fludrocortisone), vasoconstrictors (midodrine), beta-adrenergic blockers and even scopolamine. These usually are given to subjects with recurrent presyncope or syncope who are not responsive to non-pharmacological measures, but this would most likely to jeopardize the flight status of an aviator.

References

van Beek, A.H., Claassen, J.A., Rikkert, M.G. and Jansen, R.W. 2008. Cerebral autoregulation: An overview of current concepts and methodology with special focus on the elderly. *Journal of Cerebral Blood Flow Metabolism*, 28, 1071–85.

Brown, C.M. and Hainsworth, R. 1999. Assessment of capillary fluid shifts during orthostatic stress in normal subjects and subjects with orthostatic intolerance. *Clinical Autonomic Research*, 9, 69–73.

Burton, R.R. and Whinnery, J.E. 1985. Operational G-induced loss of consciousness: Something old; something new. *Aviation, Space, and Environmental Medicine*, 56, 812–7.

Carey, B.J., Manktelow, B.N., Panerai, R.B. and Potter, J.F. 2001. Cerebral autoregulatory responses to head-up tilt in normal subjects and patients with recurrent vasovagal syncope. *Circulation*, 104, 898–902.

Clint, D. 2008. You're the flight surgeon. *Aviation, Space, and Environmental Medicine*, 79, 714–5.

Critchley, H.D and Mathias, C.J. 2003. Blood pressure, attention and cognition: Drivers and air traffic controllers. *Clinical Autonomic Research*, 13, 399–401.

van Dijk, N., Colman, N., Dambrink, J.H. and Wieling, W. 2003. Pilots with vasovagal syncope: Fit to fly? *Aviation, Space, and Environmental Medicine*, 74, 571–4.

Goldstein, D.S., Holmes, C., Frank, S.M., Naqibuddin, M., Dendi, R., Snader, S. and Calkins, H. 2003. Sympathoadrenal imbalance before neurocardiogenic syncope. *American Journal of Cardiology*, 91, 53–8.

Gould, R.K. 2010. Syncope as the first sign of complete heart block in a military aviator. *Aviation, Space, and Environmental Medicine*, 81, 431–2.

Harms, M.P., Wesseling, K.H., Pott, F., Jenstrup, M., van Goudoever, J., Secher, N.H. and van Lieshout, J.J. 1999. Continuous stroke volume monitoring by modelling flow from non-invasive measurement of arterial pressure in humans under orthostatic stress. *Clinical Science (London)*, 97, 291–301.

Heims, H.C., Critchley, H.D., Martin, N.H., Jager, H.R., Mathias, C.J. and Cipolotti, L. 2006. Cognitive functioning in orthostatic hypotension due to pure autonomic failure. *Clinical Autonomic Research*, 16, 113–20.

Humm, A.M. and Mathias, C.J. 2006. Unexplained syncope – Is screening for carotid sinus hypersensitivity indicated in all patients aged > 40 years? *Journal of Neurology, Neurosurgery and Psychiatry*, 77, 1267–70.

Ichinose, M., Saito, M., Fujii, N., Kondo, N. and Nishiyasu, T. 2006. Modulation of the control of muscle sympathetic nerve activity during severe orthostatic stress. *Journal of Physiology*, 576, 947–58.

Iwase, S., Mano, T., Kamiya, A., Niimi, Y., Fu, Q. and Suzumura, A. 2002. Syncopal attack alters the burst properties of muscle sympathetic nerve activity in humans. *Autonomic Neuroscience*, 95, 141–5.

Kobayashi, A. and Miyamoto, Y. 2000. In-flight cerebral oxygen status: Continuous monitoring by near-infrared spectroscopy. *Aviation, Space, and Environmental Medicine*, 71, 177–83.

Krediet, C.T., Go-Schon, I.K., Kim, Y.S., Linzer, M., van Lieshout, J.J. and Wieling, W. 2007. Management of initial orthostatic hypotension: Lower body muscle tensing attenuates the transient arterial blood pressure decrease upon standing from squatting. *Clinical Science (London)*, 113, 401–7.

Lennox, W.G. and Gibbs, E.L. 1932. The blood flow in the brain and the leg of man, and the changes induced by alteration of blood gases. *Journal of Clinical Investigation*, 11, 1155–77.

van Lieshout, J.J., Wieling, W., Karemaker, J.M. and Secher, N.H. 2003. Syncope, cerebral perfusion, and oxygenation. *Journal of Applied Physiology*, 94, 833–48.

Lind, A.R., Leithead, C.S. and McNicol, G.W. 1968. Cardiovascular changes during syncope induced by tilting men in the heat. *Journal of Applied Physiology*, 25, 268–76.

Macmillan, A.J.F. 1999. The Pressure Cabin. In: J. Ernsting, A.N. Nicholson and D.J. Rainford (eds) *Aviation Medicine*. Oxford: Butterworth Heinemann, 112–27.

Madsen, P., Pott, F., Olsen, S.B., Nielsen, H.B., Burcev, I. and Secher, N.H. 1998. Near-infrared spectrophotometry determined brain oxygenation during fainting. *Acta Physiologica Scandinavica*, 162, 501–7.

Maidment, G. 1999. Thermal Stress and Survival. In: J. Ernsting, A.N. Nicholson and D.J. Rainford (eds) *Aviation Medicine*. Oxford: Butterworth Heinemann, 556–7.

Mathias, C.J. 1998. Cardiovascular autonomic function in parkinsonian patients. *Clinical Neuroscience*, 5, 153–66.

Mathias, C.J. 2000. A 21st century water cure. *Lancet*, 356, 1046–8.

Mathias, C.J. 2003. Autonomic diseases: Management. *Journal of Neurology, Neurosurgery and Psychiatry*, 74, Suppl. 3, iii, 42–7.

Mathias, C.J. 2009. Autonomic Dysfunction. In: C. Clarke, R. Howard, M. Rossor and S. Shorvon (eds) *Neurology: A Queen Square Textbook*. Oxford: Wiley-Blackwell, 871–92.

Mathias, C.J. and Bannister, R. 2002. Investigation of Autonomic Disorders. In: C.J. Mathias and R. Bannister (eds) *Autonomic Failure: A Textbook of Clinical Disorders of the Autonomic Nervous System*. New York, NY: Oxford University Press, 169–95.

Mathias, C.J., Deguchi, K., Bleasdale-Barr, K. and Smith, S. 2000. Familial vasovagal syncope and pseudosyncope: Observations in a case with both natural and adopted siblings. *Clinical Autonomic Research*, 10, 43–5.

Moya, A., Sutton, R., Ammirati, F., Blanc, J.J., Brignole, M., Dahm, J.B. *et al.* 2009. Guidelines for the diagnosis and management of syncope (version 2009): The Task Force for the Diagnosis and Management of Syncope of the European Society of Cardiology (ESC). *European Heart Journal*, 30, 2631–71.

Norcliffe-Kaufmann, L., Kaufmann, H. and Hainsworth, R. 2008. Enhanced vascular responses to hypocapnia in neurally mediated syncope. *Annals of Neurology*, 63, 288–94.

Ogoh, S., Brothers, R.M., Barnes, Q., Eubank, W.L., Hawkins, M.N., Purkayastha, S. *et al.* 2005. The effect of changes in cardiac output on middle cerebral artery mean blood velocity at rest and during exercise. *Journal of Physiology*, 569, 697–704.

Ogoh, S., Brothers, R.M., Eubank, W.L. and Raven, P.B. 2008. Autonomic neural control of the cerebral vasculature: Acute hypotension. *Stroke*, 39, 1979–87.

Ogoh, S., Volianitis, S., Raven, P.B. and Secher, N.H. 2004. Carotid baroreflex function ceases during vasovagal syncope. *Clinical Autonomic Research*, 14, 30–33.

Panerai, R.B. 2008. Cerebral autoregulation: From models to clinical applications. *Cardiovascular Engineering*, 8, 42–59.

Paulson, O.B., Strandgaard, S. and Edvinsson, L. 1990. Cerebral autoregulation. *Cerebrovascular and Brain Metabolism Reviews*, 2, 161–92.

Ray, C.A. and Saito, M. 2000. The Cardiopulmonary Reflex. In: B. Saltin, R. Boushel, N.H. Secher and J.H. Mitchell (eds) *Exercise and Circulation in Health and Disease*. Champaign, IL: Human Kinetics, 43–52.

Rowell, L.B. 1984. Reflex control of regional circulations in humans. *Journal of the Autonomic Nervous System*, 11, 101–14.

Rowell, L.B. 1993. *Human Cardiovascular Control*. New York, NY: Oxford University Press.

Rowell, L.B. and Blackmon, J.R. 1987. Human cardiovascular adjustments to acute hypoxaemia. *Clinical Physiology*, 7, 349–76.

Rowell, L.B. and Blackmon, J.R. 1989. Hypotension induced by central hypovolaemia and hypoxaemia. *Clinical Physiology*, 9, 269–77.

Rowell, L.B. and Seals, D.R. 1990. Sympathetic activity during graded central hypovolemia in hypoxemic humans. *American Journal of Physiology*, 259, H1197–206.

el-Sayed, H., Goodall, S.R. and Hainsworth, R. 1995. Re-evaluation of Evans blue dye dilution method of plasma volume measurement. *Clinical and Laboratory Haematology*, 17, 189–94.

Schondorf, R., Benoit, J. and Stein, R. 2001. Cerebral autoregulation in orthostatic intolerance. *Annals of the New York Academy of Sciences*, 940, 514–26.

Schondorf, R. and Low, P.A. 1993. Idiopathic postural orthostatic tachycardia syndrome: An attenuated form of acute pandysautonomia? *Neurology*, 43, 132–7.

Sheldon, R., Rose, S., Ritchie, D., Connolly, S.J., Koshman, M.L., Lee, M.A. *et al.* 2002. Historical criteria that distinguish syncope from seizures. *Journal of the American College of Cardiology*, 40, 142–8.

Smit, A.A., Wieling, W., Fujimura, J., Denq, J.C., Opfer-Gehrking, T.L., Akarriou, M. *et al.* (2004). Use of lower abdominal compression to combat orthostatic hypotension in patients with autonomic dysfunction. *Clinical Autonomic Research*, 14, 167–75.

Tiecks, F.P., Lam, A.M., Aaslid, R. and Newell, D.W. 1995. Comparison of static and dynamic cerebral autoregulation measurements. *Stroke*, 26, 1014–9.

Wilson, T.E., Cui, J., Zhang, R. and Crandall, C.G. 2006. Heat stress reduces cerebral blood velocity and markedly impairs orthostatic tolerance in humans. *American Journal of Physiology – Regulatory, Integrative and Comparative Physiology*, 291, R1443–8.

Yilmaz, U., Cetinguc, M. and Akin, A. 1999. Visual symptoms and G-LOC in the operational environment and during centrifuge training of Turkish jet pilots. *Aviation, Space, and Environmental Medicine*, 70, 709–12.

Zhang, R., Zuckerman, J.H. and Levine, B.D. 1998. Deterioration of cerebral autoregulation during orthostatic stress: Insights from the frequency domain. *Journal of Applied Physiology*, 85, 1113–22.

Chapter 14

HYPOGLYCAEMIA AND HYPOGLYCAEMIA AWARENESS

Simon R. Heller

Cerebral tissue is uniquely sensitive to the effects of glucose deprivation that can lead to profound defects in cognitive ability, loss of consciousness and permanent cerebral damage. For this reason most countries bar individuals with insulin-treated diabetes from holding amateur and professional pilot licences. Yet, as with the regulations applied to drivers of automobiles and larger vehicles, the law is inconsistent across and even within countries. Many countries permit flying in individuals taking sulphonylureas (which can cause profound hypoglycaemia and cerebral dysfunction) and in other countries aircrew taking insulin are allowed to fly combat missions.

In this chapter the pathophysiology of hypoglycaemia is reviewed, describing the physiological mechanisms that virtually prevent hypoglycaemia in the non-diabetic and explaining how these defences are compromised in diabetes. These acquired defects can lead to the syndrome of 'hypoglycaemia unawareness', a situation in which insulin-treated patients can develop severe acute cognitive impairment without warning. These observations are relevant to anyone undertaking vulnerable and potentially hazardous occupations. They apply particularly to those who supervise participants in these activities, and, within the context of this book, those who advise aircrew.

Part 1: GLUCOSE METABOLISM

The specialized function of the mammalian brain is reflected in its high metabolic rate and its dependence on glucose as a source of fuel (McCall, 2004). The brain makes up 2 per cent of body weight, but accounts for 20 per cent of oxygen consumption (Clarke and Sokoloff, 1999). The pressing energy demands are derived largely from oxidative metabolism of glucose and explain why cerebral tissue is generally an obligate user of glucose. However, in certain circumstances, other fuels such as lactate and ketones may play a role. Dependence of the nervous system on glucose is reflected in the speed at which cerebral dysfunction develops if there is diminished supply, as in hypoglycaemic states. Clinical observations suggest that normal function is dependent largely upon a continuous supply of glucose and that there is little storage capacity either in the form of glucose or glycogen.

Glucose reaches the neurons and glial cells of the nervous system by a process of facilitated diffusion involving specialized carrier proteins, the glucose transporters (McCall, 2004). When positioned in the cell membrane, they allow glucose to move down a concentration gradient. The glucose transporter-1 (GLUT-1) permits transfer of glucose across the endothelial cells of the blood–brain barrier which then enter the cell bodies of neurons and adjacent glial cells. Neuronal glucose uptake is dependent on the glucose transporter-3 (GLUT-3) and presumably provides the main route of entry for glucose to support cerebral metabolic activity. The role of glial cells in supporting neuronal function has been the subject of recent research. The GLUT-1 glucose transporter is also expressed in glial cells, and it has been assumed that glucose entry is mediated by this mechanism. However, the insulin-sensitive glucose transporter-4 is also expressed, and evidence is emerging that glial cells may store glycogen under the influence of insulin (Brown, 2004). As glucose enters glial cells, it is phosphorylated and it may be stored as glycogen or metabolized to lactate. The latter can then be transported by neurons through the action of monocarboxylate transporters.

Neuronal activity may be supported both by the metabolism of glucose that enters directly and also through lactate provided by adjacent glial cells. It has been suggested that glycogenolysis might fulfil a physiological role, whereby additional energy is supplied by the transfer of lactate derived from glycogen during periods of intense neuronal activity. In vitro studies have confirmed the ability of lactate to support neuronal metabolism (Brown et al., 2001), and there are also studies in humans that have demonstrated that systemic delivery of lactate during experimental hypoglycaemia (Maran et al., 1994) can preserve cognitive function. However, the precise role of glycogen remains to be defined. Results are awaited from experiments using methodologies such as nuclear magnetic resonance spectroscopy which allows sequential measurements of glycogen under different experimental conditions (Choi et al., 2003). It remains to be seen whether these data will lead to advances in the preventative treatment of hypoglycaemia.

Clinical Considerations

The physiological mechanisms that prevent hypoglycaemia are so effective that, even under extreme physiological conditions, circulating glucose concentrations are prevented from falling to levels in which brain function is compromised. Nevertheless, since it is obviously difficult to explore the effects of hypoglycaemia on cerebral function in animal models, studies involving non-diabetic humans have defined the effects of glucose-lowering medication, such as insulin, and have established how the effects of hypoglycaemia differ in individuals with diabetes.

Clinical experience illustrates vividly that severe hypoglycaemia leads to profound deterioration in cognitive ability. What is more relevant, particularly for those who regulate high-risk occupations and activities, is the glucose level at which deterioration begins and whether this is consistent within and between individuals. It is also important to identify any factors that might influence this threshold such as the individual's age and the type and duration of diabetes or treatment. Although some animal models can provide a crude representation of cognitive impairment in humans, useful research in this area has been largely confined to human investigation. Most of the work has been undertaken within the last 20 years, having had to await the development of appropriate methods of inducing hypoglycaemia in the laboratory and reliable measures of cognitive function. An appreciation of the different methods used both to induce experimental hypoglycaemia and to measure different aspects of cognitive function is important to understanding the data obtained from different studies and their clinical relevance.

Models and Methodology

Early human studies used boluses of intravenous insulin to induce hypoglycaemia (Fisher *et al.*, 1988). While this provided a potent stimulus for hormonal and cardiovascular responses to a major stress, it proved largely unhelpful in establishing the consequences of hypoglycaemia on cerebral function. Such experiments resulted in a rapidly induced, short-lived period of profound hypoglycaemia totally inappropriate to measure subtle deterioration in cognitive function or define the glucose thresholds at which changes develop. Furthermore, measurements were made on the background of initially high followed by rapidly falling insulin concentrations that might themselves induce artefactual changes in cerebral function. The earliest studies used slow infusions of insulin. This limited the rapid changes in blood glucose, and it proved possible to match the insulin infusion to balance the effects of counter-regulatory hormones which could produce relatively stable blood glucose levels. It was the application of an automated device that delivered both glucose and insulin based on continuous measurement of intravenous glucose (Biostator) and then the glucose clamp technique that allowed precise measurements of cognitive function and defined blood glucose thresholds at which brain function began to deteriorate.

The glucose clamp was originally developed to measure insulin resistance (De Fronzo *et al.*, 1979). It consists of a generally fixed infusion rate of intravenous insulin following initial priming, together with an intravenous infusion of 20 per cent glucose solution adjusted according to frequently measured (every five minutes) blood or plasma glucose concentrations that maintain glucose concentrations at any desired level. The rate of glucose infusion is also an index of the strength of the counter-regulatory response at hypoglycaemic levels. The release of hormones such as glucagon and adrenaline reduce the need for exogenous glucose to maintain glucose levels since they raise blood glucose by stimulating hepatic glucose release and impairing peripheral glucose uptake. Initial studies involved clamping glucose at normal concentrations followed by measurements at one or two hypoglycaemic plateaus (Heller *et al.*, 1987a). This approach has subsequently been refined into a 'slow-fall technique' where blood glucose is lowered sequentially through four or five plateaus (Amiel *et al.*, 1988). This approach allows the precise definition of a glucose threshold for the activation of physiological defences and the onset of cognitive dysfunction.

Measuring Cognitive Dysfunction

Hypoglycaemia has the potential to impair a range of cognitive functions. Batteries of different tests have been used in the hope of identifying those aspects of cognitive function that are particularly affected by hypoglycaemia and at what blood glucose concentration this occurs. A number of tests have emerged that are particularly suited to measuring different components of brain function, but investigators and clinicians must be aware of methodological limitations when interpreting the results of this work (Heller and Macdonald, 1996). These include the need to use methods of measuring performance that can be performed repeatedly within the laboratory by individuals who are receiving intravenous insulin and glucose infusions. This clearly imposes practical constraints on the type of test.

There are also potential artefactual influences and other limitations imposed by delivering a test battery (Herbert, 1978). Applying a test battery may reduce the sensitivity of psychomotor testing since each test is regarded by the subject as a fresh challenge. There is the need to allow for practice effects since improving performance may mask deterioration at hypoglycaemic levels. Furthermore, tests undertaken at the start of a hypoglycaemic plateau may vary from those undertaken at the end as the effects of hypoglycaemia become manifest. Some of these problems can be overcome by the use of a euglycaemic control arm, but this and many of the other desirable features of an experimental protocol are sometimes avoided due to the extra complexity and expense.

Another relevant factor is that, while some tests purport to be measuring specific areas of cognitive dysfunction, they often involve a number of different areas of the brain (Deary, 1993). However, despite these limitations, it is possible to group the different tests according to the area of cognition they are assessing. It would clearly be difficult to devise a test that measured purely motor function, but it is the main component of a number of tests including the peg-board and finger tapping (Stevens et al., 1989). The striking observation in studies involving these tests is that performance is essentially unaffected in both diabetic and non-diabetic subjects, even down to glucose levels as low as 2.0 mmol/l (Pramming et al., 1986; Stevens et al., 1989; Holmes et al., 1986; Hoffman et al., 1989).

Vigilance

Tests of vigilance measure performance with different forms of reaction time. These range from merely responding to a visual or auditory stimulus by pressing a button to a test where the subject is required to choose a series of responses according to the stimulus. The test now most widely used in the latter category is the 'four-choice' test, in which subjects select one of four buttons matching the position of one of four lights illuminated in random order (Wilkinson and Houghton, 1975). Trail-making is a traditional test of vigilance, in which subjects are timed while connecting numbered and labelled points sequentially. However, results from studies that have incorporated this test have revealed considerable inconsistency. Impairment was detected at a glucose level of 3.4 mmol/l in one study involving non-diabetic subjects, while in another, at a glucose level of 2.5 mmol/l, there was no deterioration in performance. Similar inconsistencies have been observed in diabetic subjects, and the observations may be explained by the relative simplicity of the task.

Reaction Time

Simple reaction time (RT) has been reported to deteriorate in non-diabetic subjects at glucose levels between 2.0 and 2.7 mmol/l (Herold *et al.*, 1985; Mitrakou *et al.*, 1991; Wirsen *et al.*, 1992) but is unaffected at higher levels (Stevens *et al.*, 1989). Simple RT is generally reported to deteriorate in diabetic subjects below 2.8 mmol/l (Herold *et al.*, 1985; Wirsen *et al.*, 1992), though no deterioration was found by Holmes *et al.* (1983) even at low glucose levels. By contrast, impairment in four-choice RT appears to occur at all levels below 3.2 mmol/l in both diabetic (Heller *et al.*, 1987a; Holmes *et al.*, 1986; Wirsen *et al.*, 1992) and non-diabetic (Heller *et al.*, 1987a; Blackman *et al.*, 1990; Snorgaard *et al.*, 1991) subjects. The data suggest, perhaps unsurprisingly, that more complex tasks are more sensitive to hypoglycaemia. They indicate that performance begins to deteriorate, at least in most individuals, at an arterialized glucose concentration of between 3.5 and 3.0 mmol/l.

Stroop and Symbol Substitution

Observations with the Stroop colour–word interference and digit symbol substitution (Ryan, 1994) tests during experimental hypoglycaemia are not totally consistent, but studies have reported deterioration in performance below a glucose concentration of around 3.3 mmol/l in diabetic subjects with either test (Holmes *et al.*, 1984; Stevens *et al.*, 1989). Most of the vigilance tests that have been used during experimental hypoglycaemia measure more complex behaviour and test a number of components of cognition. The data are not entirely consistent, and this may relate in part to methodological differences between studies in the way in which hypoglycaemia is induced and tests are administered. It probably also reflects inter-individual variability in both non-diabetic and diabetic subjects. Overall, the data indicate that performance as measured by tests of vigilance deteriorates at a glucose concentration below 3.3 mmol/l.

Memory

An important component of cognitive performance is memory. Early studies used tests of short-term memory such as word and story recall (Holmes *et al.*, 1986; Wirsen *et al.*, 1992). Recently, more sophisticated tests of verbal, visual and working memory have been incorporated (Sommerfield *et al.*, 2003a, 2003b). Interestingly, all the studies have demonstrated impairment in all aspects of memory in both diabetic and non-diabetic individuals, but only below a glucose value of 2.7 mmol/l. This observation is limited to some degree as the more recent experiments have largely measured memory at a single glucose plateau of 2.5 mmol/l rather than explored the threshold at which memory begins to deteriorate. However, the data suggest that, at mild hypoglycaemic levels, aspects of memory may be relatively preserved.

Global Activity

The tests described above have been used to test different components of cognitive ability. However, perhaps more relevant to clinical practice, in particular the ability of patients with diabetes to manage more complex tasks, are tests of global activity. This was highlighted by McAulay and colleagues when reporting studies measuring deterioration in attention and problem-solving ability during experimental hypoglycaemia (McAulay *et al.*, 2001, 2006). Their data are limited to the extent that they measure performance at one level of hypoglycaemia rather than establishing glycaemic thresholds. Nevertheless, they have been able to show that both measures of attention and problem solving were impaired during moderate hypoglycaemia (2.5 mmol/l) in non-diabetic and diabetic individuals.

Simulation

Arguably, the most relevant studies that can inform the issues surrounding flying and risk due to cognitive impairment are those that measure driving performance during experimental hypoglycaemia. It is clearly impossible for ethical and practical reasons to observe performance during clinical hypoglycaemia while driving on the road, but a number of investigators have tried to solve these problems using driving simulators. Such an approach has potential limitations. The use of driving simulators as fairground entertainment highlights their novelty value, and there is a potential danger that subjects' enjoyment and interest is increased, thus reducing the sensitivity of the test. Practice effects may be particularly important as participants become increasingly used to the device and gradually overcome the technical challenges. Thus, to add value, driving simulators need to be sufficiently sophisticated to represent accurately a realistic impression of a driving situation. Investigators also need to be able to manipulate glucose concentrations reliably and consistently, and include the appropriate euglycaemic control arms.

The need to develop a robust approach is exemplified by a recent study which came to the doubtful conclusion that driving ability is unaffected in either patients with Type 1 or Type 2 diabetes at glucose levels as low as 2.7 mmol/l (Stork *et al.*, 2007).

In contrast, Cox and colleagues developed a reliable device in the early 1990s in collaboration with the computer manufacturer Atari. The simulator was relatively simple, but the instrument represented the driving situation with appropriate audio and visual simulation reasonably accurately, and measured limited aspects of driving performance. The group then went on to develop a more sophisticated machine that could measure additional aspects of performance and extended the duration of the driving task. These investigators have undertaken a series of useful studies, generally using a 'Biostator' device to control blood glucose. They have provided important additional information linking the experimental work exploring cognitive dysfunction, the ability of individuals to recognize that their performance is impaired and decisions they take about taking charge of a vehicle despite objective evidence of cognitive impairment.

In an early study using an uncomplicated simulator, they demonstrated in individuals with Type 1 diabetes that driving was generally unimpaired at a glucose concentration of 3.6 mmol/l, but deteriorated at a concentration of 2.6 mmol/l, with impairment in a number of performance measures including swerving and time off the road (Cox *et al.*, 1993). Importantly, of the third who exhibited global deterioration in driving performance, only 50 per cent recognized that they were unfit to drive. In a more recent study, also involving patients with Type 1 diabetes, they identified impaired aspects of driving performance at glucose concentrations of around 3.6 mmol/1 (Cox *et al.*, 2000) and at every glucose value below. There was widespread variability, with severe impairment observed in 38 per cent of the participants. More worrying is that there was little relationship between impaired driving performance and the ability to recognize this and decide not to drive. Although most recognized that their driving performance had deteriorated, only 30 per cent of those took corrective action in terms of stopping and taking treatment to raise their blood glucose. The authors concluded that patients should not drive if their blood glucose was below 5.0 mmol/l.

Glycaemic Thresholds

A summary of the blood/plasma levels (mmol/1 or mg/dl) for the glycaemic thresholds linked to cognitive impairment in non-diabetics and diabetics is useful at this stage.

Part 2:
COUNTER-REGULATION

Humans have evolved effective systems that preserve blood glucose even under extreme physiological circumstances (such as prolonged starvation) such that hypoglycaemia and resulting impaired cognition due to central glucose deprivation is extremely uncommon (Cryer, 2001). Glucose enters the bloodstream by ingestion and intestinal absorption, by the breakdown of hepatic and renal glycogen stores (glycogenolysis) and by gluconeogenesis, in which glucose is generated from lactate plus three carbon precursors derived from the breakdown of skeletal muscle and adipose tissue. Glycogenolysis and gluconeogenesis occur in both the liver and kidney since only these tissues contain the necessary enzymes to drive the processes. Quantitatively, the liver is the major organ controlling glucose concentrations, storing glucose as glycogen during feeding and releasing

| | Blood/Plasma level mmol/l (mg/dl) | | Source |
	Non-diabetic	Diabetic	
Motor	< 2.0 (35)	< 2.0 (35)	Holmes et al., 1986
			Hoffman et al. 1989
			Pramming et al., 1986
Vigilance	< 3.3 (55)	< 3.3 (55)	Blackman et al., 1990
			Heller et al., 1987a
			Holmes et al., 1984, 1986
			Snorgaard et al., 1991
			Stevens et al., 1989
Memory	< 2.7 (45)	< 2.7 (45)	Holmes et al., 1986
			McAulay et al., 2001. 2006
			Sommerfield et al., 2003a, 2003b
			Wirsen et al., 1992
Driving		< 3.6 (60)	Cox et al., 2000

glucose through glycogenolysis and gluconeogenesis during the fasting state.

The physiological processes that maintain blood glucose, described above, are under hormonal control. Insulin is the main regulatory hormone secreted from the β-cells of the pancreatic islets (Rizza *et al.*, 1981). Activation of insulin receptors in skeletal muscle and adipose tissue increases peripheral glucose uptake and storage. Insulin also suppresses glycogenolysis and gluconeogenesis, promoting hepatic and renal storage of glucose as glycogen. Conversely, falling insulin concentrations lead to a release of hepatic glucose and diminished peripheral glucose uptake. Glucose concentrations are also controlled by the actions of additional 'counter-regulatory hormones'. The regulatory and glucose-lowering effects of insulin are opposed by the counter-regulatory hormones, glucagon, adrenaline, cortisol and growth hormone, as well as by activation of the sympathoadrenal system. Glucagon, released from the α-cells of the islet as glucose concentrations fall, stimulates hepatic glycogenolysis and so increases hepatic glucose uptake. It also stimulates hepatic gluconeogenesis, although, because it does not mobilize gluconeogenic precursors from peripheral tissue, the effect is somewhat limited.

The prevailing glucose concentration has a direct effect both on glucagon release from the pancreatic α-cells and βislet cell secretion with the portal insulin/glucagon ratio controlling hepatic gluconeogenesis and glycogenolysis and determining overall hepatic glucose output. Normally, insulin concentrations of 30 µIU/mL are sufficient to suppress hepatic glucose release completely. Insulin increases peripheral glucose uptake indirectly by suppressing lipolysis at relatively low concentrations, but direct stimulation of peripheral glucose uptake in skeletal and cardiac muscle and adipose tissue occurs only at substantially higher concentrations, above 30–40 µIU/mL. However, since under basal conditions most glucose uptake is into insulin-independent tissues such as brain and red blood cells, insulin normally has little effect on peripheral glucose uptake.

Catecholamines, as circulating adrenaline and noradrenaline released from post-ganglionic sympathetic neurons, have a direct effect on hepatic glycogenolysis and gluconeogenesis. Other effects are indirect. Increased lipolysis and rising non-esterified fatty acid levels reduce peripheral glucose uptake and increase glycerol delivery to the liver. Glucagon release is stimulated through an α-adrenergic effect and, importantly, insulin release is inhibited through a β-effect. Cortisol stimulates hepatic gluconeogenesis directly, as well as increasing hepatic delivery of the gluconeogenic substrates, alanine and lactate, through effects on skeletal muscle and adipose tissue. Growth hormone also increases lipolysis and directly stimulates hepatic gluconeogenesis, and other hormones such as vasopressin and angiotensin II may also play a role. Finally, glucose itself can regulate carbohydrate metabolism by directly stimulating peripheral glucose uptake and inhibiting hepatic glucose output.

Physiological Mechanisms

Two physiological mechanisms specifically prevent hypoglycaemia in non-diabetic individuals and correct hypoglycaemia in diabetic humans. They are the inhibition of insulin secretion and counter-regulatory responses. Experimental studies in humans have demonstrated that insulin secretion is inhibited at a plasma glucose level of around 4.5 mmol/l (Schwartz *et al.*, 1987; Fanelli *et al.*, 1994) in non-diabetic individuals. The resulting increase in hepatic glucose output due to the reduction of the portal insulin/glucagon ratio delivered to hepatocytes is sufficient to stabilize blood glucose. In diabetic humans who have insufficient or absent endogenous insulin, and who are relying on either injected insulin or sulphonylurea-stimulated insulin secretion, the additional hormonal counter-regulatory mechanisms are crucial in preventing or reversing hypoglycaemia. In summary, the physiological defences to hypoglycaemia are:

○ Inhibition of insulin secretion
○ Counter-regulatory hormone release
  – Glucagon
  – Adrenaline
  – Growth hormone
  – Cortisol
○ Sympathoadrenal activation
○ Symptoms
  – Autonomic
  – Neuroglycopenic.

In the early 1980s, Cryer, Gerich and colleagues carried out a series of studies that established the components of the endocrine defence to hypoglycaemia (Rizza *et al.*, 1979; Cryer and Gerich, 1983). They showed that hypoglycaemia elicited increases in glucagon and adrenaline, leading to hepatic glucose release, initially from glycogenolysis with an increasing proportion due to gluconeogenesis. In addition, peripheral glucose uptake was progressively inhibited, partly directly, but also secondarily, to increases in circulating non-esterified fatty acids following adrenaline stimulated lipolysis. These investigators demonstrated that inhibiting glucagon release pharmacologically impaired glucose recovered by around 40

per cent, but that if both glucagon and adrenaline were blocked, then glucose recovery from acute hypoglycaemia was totally inhibited. Release of other hormones, including growth hormone and cortisol, also raised blood glucose by stimulating gluconeogenesis, and during severe hypoglycaemia (Cryer and Gerich, 1983) the liver released glucose independent of hormonal control – hepatic autoregulation (Bolli *et al.*, 1985). However, the failure of glucose recovery from experimental hypoglycaemia when both glucagon and sympathoadrenal responses were blocked suggested that other mechanisms do not have a major physiological role to play following acute hypoglycaemia.

The threshold for the release of glucagon occurs at a circulating plasma glucose level of around 3.5 mmol/l. The mechanism underlying the glucagon response to hypoglycaemia is somewhat controversial. Data derived from animal models indicate that activation of the autonomic nervous system after central activation drives the release of glucagon (Taborsky *et al.*, 1998). In humans, the release of glucagon during hypoglycaemia may be more dependent on a local paracrine effect. Local release of insulin from the β-cells within the pancreatic islets tonically inhibits glucagon release from adjacent α-cells (Unger, 1983). Studies in humans have demonstrated that the induction of hypoglycaemia by boosting endogenous insulin provokes a much smaller glucagon response than when induced by exogenous insulin (Peacey *et al.*, 1997; Raju and Cryer, 2005). These and other data suggest that glucagon secretion during hypoglycaemia occurs as endogenous insulin secretion shuts off when the blood glucose level drops below normal. This is particularly relevant to individuals with diabetes since a failure of endogenous insulin secretion may disrupt this mechanism and so interfere with a major protective response.

Release of adrenaline and activation of the sympathoadrenal system occurs at around 3.5 mmol/l and is mediated by central activation of the autonomic nervous system (Schwartz et al., 1987). In non-diabetic humans, the ability of the β-cell to suppress insulin secretion as glucose values approach the lower limit of the normal range means that these additional protective mechanisms rarely operate. In contrast, patients with diabetes who are taking exogenous insulin or therapeutic agents that boost endogenous insulin are regularly exposed to situations where insulin levels are inappropriately high at glucose concentrations below normal. Under these circumstances, integrity of the physiological defences will determine whether glucose concentrations are maintained and severe hypoglycaemia prevented. As studies in normal subjects have demonstrated, the array of physiological defences can prevent a fall in blood glucose in the presence of substantially raised insulin concentrations (Heller and Cryer, 1991a). Ironically, a number of mechanisms conspire to compromise those with diabetes, which makes them vulnerable to hypoglycaemia and the resulting impairment in cognitive function.

Glucose Sensing

There are a number of sites throughout the body where specialized cells respond to either a rise or fall in circulating glucose levels by initiating physiological responses largely designed to restore homeostasis. The most obvious example is the islet β-cells that respond to a rise in glucose by secreting insulin. Other areas that sense glucose include the portal vein and intestine and, in particular, the brain, which is largely responsible for initiating the physiological defence to a falling blood glucose. Studies undertaken predominantly in animals have, in the last few years, begun to provide a clearer picture of how a falling glucose is detected and initiates a coordinated physiological response designed to raise blood glucose towards normal (McCrimmon, 2008). A better understanding of the mechanisms that underlie these responses and their impairment in those with diabetes may lead to therapeutic interventions to mitigate the problems of hypoglycaemia induced by treatment.

There are critical areas within the brain responsible for initiating protective physiological responses to hypoglycaemia. Lesions within the ventromedial hypothalamus result in diminished physiological responses to hypoglycaemia (Borg et al., 1994). Induction of local hypoglycaemia using targeted infusions of 2-deoxyglucose within this area leads to rises in counter-regulatory hormones (Borg et al., 1995). The relevance of this area of the hypothalamus may relate to its unique status within the brain, since at this site the blood–brain barrier breaks down, allowing specialized cells to access blood glucose concentrations directly.

The precise way in which hypoglycaemia is sensed is being elucidated. Potential mechanisms include the generation of adenosine triphosphate (ATP) following phosphorylation by glucokinase, and the activation of adenosine monophosphate kinase and chloride channels involving neurons that are activated by either high or low glucose concentrations. Synaptic pathways projecting across the brain from these highly specialized cells lead to a coordinated response with activation of the autonomic nervous system and release of counter-regulatory hormones, including adrenaline and noradrenaline at post-ganglionic sympathetic neurons. Impairments in these responses that develop in those with diabetes may be due to acquired defects in the release of different neurotransmitters. At present, the precise mechanisms remain unclear, but are the subject of experimental work in animal models.

Part 3:
HYPOGLYCAEMIA

The difficulty in agreeing a common definition of hypoglycaemia hampered the early collection of reliable data assessing the risk of hypoglycaemia, particularly severe episodes. These are now generally defined as episodes requiring the help of another person for recovery, although some centres only report episodes resulting in coma or seizure – an end-point that is easier to identity. Comparing the frequency of mild episodes is far more difficult since symptoms are often non-specific and are rarely confirmed with a simultaneous measurement of blood glucose level. It is also apparent from studies of overnight glucose monitoring (Gale and Tattersall, 1979; Matyka *et al.*, 1996) and from continuous glucose monitoring that even prolonged periods of hypoglycaemia remain unnoticed, particularly at night (Kaufman *et al.*, 2002).

Reported rates of hypoglycaemia vary, depending upon whether they are recorded during clinical trials in selected populations or gathered from population-based surveys obtained during 'real-life' therapy. The 'risk' of hypoglycaemia is usually reported either as the percentage of individuals affected by at least one episode or as the number of episodes per patient, or even '100 patient-years'. Both methods obscure the important observation that

even among those populations where rates of hypoglycaemia are high, most individuals experience few if any events and frequent episodes are confined to a small minority.

In an early population based study in Denmark involving 411 individuals with Type 1 diabetes receiving the standard therapy of the time, severe hypoglycaemia occurred at a mean rate of 1.6 attacks per patient year (Pramming *et al.*, 1991). Importantly, a survey undertaken 15 years later among a similar population found no decrease in rates of hypoglycaemia despite advances in therapy such as insulin analogues in the interim (Pedersen-Bjergaard *et al.*, 2004). A risk of a severe hypoglycaemic episode (defined as coma, seizure or needing the assistance of another person) of around 10 per cent in a year was reported for participants in a clinical trial that established the benefits of tight control (Diabetes Control and Complications Trial Research Group, 1993). These patients were in the control arm of the trial, were taking one or two injections of insulin a day and had a mean Hb_{A1c} of 9.5 per cent. Rates of severe episodes increased threefold in those assigned to intensive therapy and who had a mean Hb_{A1c} of 7.5 per cent. There was also a striking inverse relationship between the risk of severe hypoglycaemia and the level of glycaemic control achieved as expressed by Hb_{A1c} (Diabetes Control and Complications Trial Research Group, 1997).

Patients with Type 2 diabetes can experience hypoglycaemia whether treated with insulin or sulphonylureas, and severe and occasionally fatal outcomes have been recorded for both treatments. Reported rates of hypoglycaemia in clinical trials may underestimate hypoglycaemic risk. In the United Kingdom Prospective Diabetes Study (1998b), a trial of intensive therapy among patients with Type 2 diabetes, the proportion of patients suffering a major hypoglycaemic event per year was 0.4 per cent for those taking chlorpropamide, 0.6 per cent for glibenclamide and 2.3 per cent for insulin. Median Hb_{A1c} values were comparable with studies of intensive insulin therapy in Type 1 diabetes, suggesting that the risks of hypoglycaemia are less in those with Type 2 diabetes, but higher during insulin treatment. Population-based studies suggest severe hypoglycaemia may be more common. Akram *et al.* (2006) reported a frequency of 0.44 episodes each year, around a third of those reported for individuals with Type 1 diabetes, a rate confirmed in a British population (Donnelly *et al.*, 2005). Since the prevalence of Type 2 diabetes is far greater, these data indicate that severe hypoglycaemia is the greater overall problem in individuals with Type 2 diabetes.

Symptomatic episodes are a universal experience for virtually everyone with Type 1 diabetes, and common in those with Type 2 diabetes who are treated with either insulin or sulphonylureas. The frequency of symptomatic episodes has been calculated in a population-based study to be around 4,300 per 100 patient-years for those with Type 1 diabetes and 1,600 in insulin-treated Type 2 diabetes. The studies reported have generally failed to take into account the duration of diabetes, and few have compared rates of severe hypoglycaemia in both types of diabetes within the same study. There is evidence in both types of diabetes that the duration of the disease has a major influence on the risk of severe hypoglycaemic episodes. This hypothesis was specifically tested in a population-based multicentre study undertaken in individuals attending specialist clinics (United Kingdom Hypoglycaemia Study Group, 2007).

The Group found a rate of severe hypoglycemia of 110 episodes per 100 patient-years in patients with Type 1 diabetes diagnosed for less than five years. In patients with a long duration of diabetes, greater than 15 years, rates of severe hypoglycaemia were three times as high. Individuals with Type 2 diabetes, treated with insulin for less than two years, had rates of severe hypoglycaemia of 10 per 100 patient-years compared with 70 episodes per 100 patient-years in those with a duration of insulin treatment greater than five years, and these were experienced by 7 and 25 per cent of the respective populations over nine to 12 months (Figure 14.1).

These and other data demonstrate that the risk of severe episodes increases with increasing duration of insulin treatment and in either type of diabetes. Indeed, the risks of severe hypoglycaemia are comparable in patients treated with sulphonylureas and in those with Type 2 diabetes recently started on insulin. In patients with Type 2 diabetes with a long duration of insulin treatment, rates of hypoglycaemia are low during the first years following insulin initiation and rise progressively and eventually approach those of Type 1 diabetes. As discussed below, this appears to be due to a failure of protective physiological mechanisms, a loss of functioning β-cells and endogenous insulin secretion. Indeed, in other studies reduced endogenous insulin secretion is a major independent predictor of severe hypoglycaemia (Bott *et al.*, 1997).

Intensive Insulin Therapy

Trials of intensive therapy described above confirmed the importance of tight glycaemic control in reducing the rate of onset of complications, although these benefits were gained at the expense of

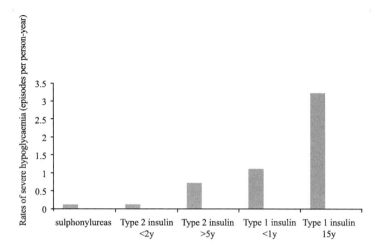

Figure 14.1 Rates of severe hypoglycaemia in different types of diabetes
Rates are similar in patients with Type 2 diabetes taking sulphonylureas and in those that have recently started on insulin, but are much higher with longstanding Type 1 diabetes. Data from United Kingdom Hypoglycaemia Study Group (2007).

an increased risk of hypoglycaemia. The studies demonstrated a clear relationship between the level of glycaemic control as measured by HbA_{1c} and the rate of severe hypoglycaemic episodes. Many clinicians (and patients) believe that attempting to keep blood glucose close to normal brings with it an inevitable high risk of severe hypoglycaemia, particularly as tight control leads to impaired counter-regulatory and symptomatic defences to hypoglycaemia.

However, these views have been challenged by Mühlhauser and Berger (1993) with suggestions that outcomes are more a consequence of inexpert delivery of intensive insulin therapy rather than pathophysiological inevitability. They and others have shown that delivering high-quality training to patients before they embark on intensive therapy can improve glycaemic control without a rise in rates of severe hypoglycaemia (Pieber *et al.*, 1995). In one observational study involving over 600 patients with Type 1 diabetes who undertook the training, levels of glycaemic control as reported by the Diabetes Control and Complications Trial Research Group (1993) were achieved, yet the number of severe hypoglycaemic episodes (defined as coma or seizure) fell from 0.28 to 0.17 cases per patient per year (Bott *et al.*, 1997). A more recent study has demonstrated no relationship between Hb_{A1c} and risk of severe hypoglycaemia (Sämann *et al.*, 2005).

In summary, there are different views regarding the risk of severe hypoglycaemia associated with intensive insulin therapy. The conventional view has been that, in those with Type 1 diabetes, aiming for near normoglycaemia brings with it a high risk of severe hypoglycaemic episodes. This is thought to be a consequence of repeated hypoglycaemia leading to a vicious circle of impaired counter-regulatory and symptomatic responses, with resulting hypoglycaemia unawareness leading to increased vulnerability to further episodes. Others believe that severe episodes are not necessarily inevitable with intensive insulin therapy and that high-quality training that specifically targets ways of reducing hypoglycaemic risk and encouraging patient independence produces no increase in rates of severe hypoglycaemia. Further research is needed.

Symptomatology

Activation of the autonomic nervous system in response to impending hypoglycaemia leads to the release of counter-regulatory hormones which, by inhibiting peripheral glucose uptake and increasing hepatic glucose output, resist the glucose-lowering effects of insulin. The autonomic nervous system, particularly the sympathoadrenal component, also plays an important part in generating symptoms that alert patients to a falling glucose level. The recognition of impending hypoglycaemia is essential for patients to take action by ingesting refined carbohydrate before a severe episode supervenes. Most individuals treated with insulin or sulphonylurea experience mild hypoglycaemia, and the presence and intensity of different symptoms varies between and within the same individual. Some patients develop sweating during nocturnal hypoglycaemic episodes, but never during the day, while others rely on subtle changes in the ability to reason or altered vision to alert them to an impending episode. Most learn to recognize a pattern of symptoms that they then depend upon to alert them to an impending attack.

Factor analysis has been applied to descriptions by patients of their individual symptoms. The identification of symptom clusters indicates groups of symptoms generated by similar physiological responses (Hepburn and Deary, 1991). Adults with Type 1 diabetes generally reported three groups of symptoms. They were 1) autonomic (corresponding to those caused by sympathoadrenal activation),

2) neuroglycopenic (corresponding to symptoms generated by cerebral dysfunction such as loss of concentration and confusion) and 3) malaise that included nausea and headache. Reported symptoms appear to vary according to age and type of diabetes. Older patients with Type 2 diabetes reported non-specific neurological symptoms (Jaap et al., 1998), suggesting effects of hypoglycaemia on vulnerable areas of the elderly brain, while children reported autonomic and neuroglycopenic symptoms, plus those due to change in behaviour and emotion (McCrimmon et al., 1995). Different distributions of symptoms may reflect differences in pathophysiology.

The symptoms of hypoglycaemia (grouped by factor analysis after questioning of 295 patients) with Type 1 diabetes are given below (Hepburn and Deary, 1991):

❍ Autonomic
  – Sweating
  – Palpitations
  – Shaking
  – Hunger
❍ Neuroglycopenic
  – Confusion
  – Drowsiness
  – Odd behaviour
  – Speech difficulty
  – Incoordination
❍ General malaise
  – Headache
  – Nausea.

Hypoglycaemia and Awareness

A large body of experimental work has identified both the components of the pathophysiological response to hypoglycaemia and the glucose thresholds at which they are activated. Key to understanding how patients are alerted to hypoglycaemia and the development of hypoglycaemia unawareness is an understanding of the relationship between the various components. Although there is some inter-individual variation, in non-diabetic adults the first response is activation of glucagon release that occurs at a plasma glucose of around 3.6 mmol/l (Schwartz *et al.*, 1987). Activation of the autonomic nervous system, manifest by an increase in plasma adrenaline, occurs at glucose concentrations just below this level at 3.6 mmol/l (Schwartz *et al.*, 1987). Since autonomic symptoms result from activation of the sympathoadrenal system, tremor, palpitations and sweating develop at similar circulating glucose levels – around 3.3 mmol/l (Heller *et al.*, 1987a). Symptom scores that reflect both neuroglycopenic and autonomic symptoms increase at similar glucose levels (Mitrakou *et al.*, 1991). Cerebral function, as measured by a variety of cognitive function tests, begins to deteriorate at just under 3.3 mmol/l, and becomes progressively more impaired as the level of blood glucose falls (Heller *et al.*, 1987a; Heller and Macdonald, 1996). Thus, symptoms are generated at a glucose concentration slightly above those for significant cognitive dysfunction.

The proximity of the thresholds for the activation of protective responses (increase in counter-regulatory hormones and generation of symptoms) to those for impaired cognition shows how potentially vulnerable patients with diabetes are to developing problems in recognizing the onset of hypoglycaemia. Nevertheless, since symptoms occur at a blood glucose level before major deterioration in cognitive function occurs, the data suggest that individuals with Type 1 diabetes will be alerted to hypoglycaemia before they have developed serious cognitive decline. That would give them time to take action

by ingesting refined carbohydrate such as a glucose drink. However, if these thresholds changed such that activation of a sympathoadrenal response now occurred at lower glucose levels, then this would place those individuals at far greater risk (Figure 14.2a and b). In these circumstances, by the time that peripheral responses were generated they could have developed severe cerebral dysfunction and so be incapable of responding appropriately. As described below, this is a situation that could explain why some patients fail to recognize impending hypoglycaemia and are prone to repeated severe episodes.

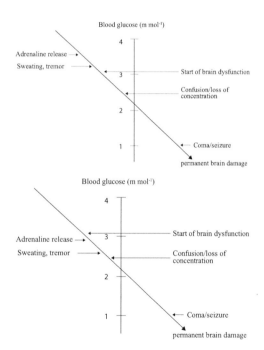

Figure 14.2 a) Glucose thresholds for the physiological responses to hypoglycaemia in non-diabetic subjects and in diabetic patients with normal awareness and b) Glucose thresholds for the responses to hypoglycaemia in patients with hypoglycaemia unawareness

Protection against Hypoglycaemia

The major factor contributing to hypoglycaemia in insulin-treated diabetes is inappropriately high insulin levels. In the non-diabetic physiological state, systemic insulin profiles consist of stable basal concentrations in the fasting or post-absorptive state and sharp peaks of insulin concentration during feeding. Since insulin is secreted into the portal vein, around 50 per cent is removed during its passage through the liver, which limits systemic insulin concentrations even during feeding. Furthermore, as glucose concentrations fall below 4 mmol/l, insulin secretion is rapidly and completely inhibited, a response that explains why hypoglycaemia is so rare in the non-diabetic individual.

In contrast, a subcutaneous bolus of insulin will raise circulating insulin levels that remain raised whatever the blood glucose concentration until that depot is totally absorbed. These observations explain why patients with diabetes are so vulnerable to hypoglycaemia. This is particularly the case in the post-absorptive state, in between meals and at night when the actions of insulin are not resisted following the ingestion of food. In this situation, the additional physiological protection, described in detail above in the form of counter-regulatory hormone release, together with the onset of symptoms, is essential in protecting patients from severe hypoglycaemic episodes.

Endocrine responses to hypoglycaemia are comparable with non-diabetic individuals at diagnosis (Bolli *et al.*, 1983), but as the duration of the disease increases, individuals develop defects in their counter-regulatory defences. The glucagon rise in response to hypoglycaemia becomes impaired in most patients with Type 1 diabetes

within two to three years of diagnosis. One study found defective responses in a patient with a duration of diabetes as short as two weeks (Gerich *et al.*, 1973). Impairment is progressive, and after ten years the failure of glucagon secretion during hypoglycaemia is virtually universal (Bolli *et al.*, 1983). The α-cell can respond normally to other secretagogues such as arginine (Gerich *et al.*, 1973); the defect is a specific failure to respond to hypoglycaemia. Of the hypotheses that have been proposed to explain this observation, progressive autoimmune destruction of pancreatic β-cells interfering with local paracrine crosstalk appears the most convincing.

At diagnosis, increases in adrenaline during hypoglycaemia are normal but, like glucagon responses, become progressively impaired with increased duration (Bolli *et al.*, 1983). As with glucagon, the defect is afferent: increases in adrenaline during exercise and other stressors are normal, but there is a failure of secretion in response to hypoglycaemia (Hirsch and Shamoon, 1987). The integrity of the sympathoadrenal counter-regulatory response is variable and diminishes at different rates between individuals. The defect progresses more slowly than the impaired glucagon response, although many patients demonstrate impaired responses. One review estimated that around 40 per cent of those with Type 1 diabetes with a duration of diabetes of over 15 years had impaired responses (Gerich and Bolli, 1993). The precise mechanism remains unclear. There appears to be a failure of the nervous system to activate the sympathoadrenal system until glucose levels fall well below those seen in studies involving non-diabetic subjects; that is, adrenaline concentrations begin to rise at glucose concentrations of around 2.5 mmol/l, as opposed to 3.5 mmol/l. However, the reason why glucose sensors fail to activate the appropriate pathways is currently unknown.

Experimental studies have suggested that suppression of both glucagon and adrenaline largely prevents any rise in blood glucose from hypoglycaemic levels until insulin concentrations have waned. Clinical studies confirmed the major consequences of a bilateral defect. In one study (White *et al.*, 1983) patients with defective increases of both adrenaline and glucagon, when tested in the laboratory, had a ninefold increase in rates of severe hypoglycaemia during the ensuing year of standard treatment. These risks were due in part to the failure of the release of hormones that resist the glucose-lowering effects of insulin.

However, the activation of the autonomic nervous system produces peripheral responses that the patient (and family) learn to recognize as symptoms and signs. Thus, the increased frequency of severe episodes is also related to failure to recognize and treat impending hypoglycaemia before it results in severe cognitive impairment (hypoglycaemia unawareness). Clearly, counter-regulatory failure and hypoglycaemia unawareness are related syndromes, and both reflect different aspects of defective physiological defences to hypoglycaemia in individuals with Type 1 diabetes. Defects in the autonomic response to hypoglycaemia may not only be confined to impaired secretion. There is evidence of altered β-adrenergic sensitivity in some patients with Type 1 diabetes, although to what extent these changes contribute to hypoglycaemia unawareness and susceptibility to severe hypoglycaemia is not clear (Trovik *et al.*, 1994; Fritsche *et al.*, 1998).

Hypoglycaemia Unawareness

The observation that some individuals are unable to recognize the onset of hypoglycaemia was reported over 50 years ago (Lawrence, 1941; Balodimos and Root, 1959), but systematic studies have had to await sophisticated methods of inducing experimental hypoglycaemia and measuring physiological responses. The problem of unawareness has probably become more common as patients have been encouraged to maintain tighter levels of glycaemic control to prevent diabetic complications. It has been difficult to obtain reliable estimates of the incidence and prevalence of hypoglycaemia unawareness or compare rates between populations due to the lack of an agreed definition, and because the condition is, at least in part, reversible. It appears that unawareness that develops in the early years after diagnosis is often temporary, due in part to tightened glycaemic control or conditions such as pregnancy or ingestion of alcohol. In longstanding Type 1 diabetes, a reduced ability to identify impending hypoglycaemia is common and less reversible, perhaps indicating a different pathogenic mechanism.

One of the first systematic surveys of a secondary care population reported some degree of hypoglycaemia unawareness in around 20 per cent of patients with Type 1 diabetes (Pramming *et al.*, 1991). In a more recent observational study, involving patients attending secondary care clinics in the United Kingdom and Denmark, reduced awareness of hypoglycaemia was present in 40 per cent of those with a duration of diabetes of less than ten years, and in those with a duration of diabetes between 20 and 30 years the incidences were 10 and 50 per cent respectively (Pedersen-Bjergaard *et al.*, 2004). Since the syndrome of hypoglycaemia unawareness identifies those with impaired counter-regulatory responses to hypoglycaemia, such patients would be expected to be at greater risk of severe hypoglycaemia. Prospective studies have confirmed this, reporting a six- to sevenfold increased risk of severe hypoglycaemia during standard insulin therapy in those with partial or complete hypoglycaemia unawareness (Gold *et al.*, 1994).

As discussed above, and as others have pointed out, the syndromes of counter-regulatory failure and hypoglycaemia unawareness are related. Both represent a failure of central mechanisms to respond to a falling glucose level by activating the autonomic nervous system and place patients at high risk of severe episodes. Cryer (1994) has proposed the term 'hypoglycaemia-associated autonomic failure' (HAAF) to describe this syndrome which develops so commonly in Type 1 diabetes.

Part 4:
IMPAIRED COUNTER-REGULATION

Multiple factors contribute to defective physiological protection resisting a falling glucose level, some of which offer therapeutic opportunities to reduce the risk of hypoglycaemia. As discussed above, there is overwhelming evidence that glucose counter-regulation and symptomatic awareness are intact at diagnosis, but become progressively impaired with increased diabetes duration. This explains why duration of Type 1 diabetes is a powerful independent risk factor predicting severe hypoglycaemia in retrospective (Pedersen-Bjergaard *et al.*, 2004) and prospective surveys. (United Kingdom Hypoglycaemia Study Group, 2007). The mechanisms that underlie these observations are less clear. There is good evidence to attribute the

progressive failure of glucagon secretion directly to the disease process in Type 1 diabetes – that is, the loss of pancreatic β-cell cells through autoimmune destruction (Peacey *et al.*, 1997; Raju and Cryer, 2005). However, the cause of the central defect leading to impaired sympathoadrenal activation and the onset of autonomic symptoms remains unknown. One plausible explanation is that repeated episodes of hypoglycaemia lead to progressive destruction of the glucose-sensing neurons that mediate the counter-regulatory response. Whatever the mechanism, it is important to recognize the greater vulnerability of those with longstanding diabetes to severe hypoglycaemia.

In summary, the possible mechanisms associated with hypoglycaemia unawareness, linked to clinical situations such as the duration of the disease, metabolic control and alcohol ingestion, are:

o Long duration:
   – Unknown, perhaps repeated hypoglycaemic damage to gluco-sensitive neurons
o Tight metabolic control:
   – Antecedent hypoglycaemia possibly leading to impaired neurotransmission in key neural pathways
   – Altered catecholamine sensitivity
o Alcohol ingestion
   – Suppression of autonomic peripheral responses (tremor)
   – Impaired cognition.

Clinicians had initially speculated that tight glycaemic control might protect physiological defences to hypoglycaemia, but studies in the 1980s reported that patients who intensified their glycaemic control developed impaired glucose counter-regulation and symptomatic responses (Simonson *et al.*, 1985; Amiel *et al.*, 1987). There appeared to be a resetting of glycaemic thresholds, with increases in adrenaline developing at glucose concentrations of around 2.5 mmol/l rather than the normal 3.5 mmol/l (Amiel *et al.*, 1988). The possibility that hypoglycaemia itself might contribute to impaired counter-regulatory responses had been raised by an earlier observation involving non-diabetic patients undergoing insulin shock treatment for schizophrenia that had demonstrated progressively diminished sympathoadrenal responses with repeated hypoglycaemic treatments (Goldfien *et al.*, 1961). However, it was not until the early 1990s that a series of studies established that repeated episodes of hypoglycaemia in both non-diabetic (Heller and Cryer, 1991b; Widom and Simonson, 1992) and diabetic individuals (Dagogo-Jack *et al.*, 1993) led to diminished sympathoadrenal and symptomatic responses to hypoglycaemia, an effect that could last for at least a week (George *et al.*, 1995). It seems likely that this pathogenetic mechanism makes an important contribution to counter-regulatory failure and reduced

symptoms and increases the risk of severe hypoglycaemia during intensive insulin therapy (Figure 14.3).

Autonomic Neuropathy

The use of the term 'hypoglycaemia-associated autonomic failure' (HAAF) to describe the combined syndromes of counter-regulatory failure and hypoglycaemia unawareness highlights the involvement of the autonomic nervous system. It is important to distinguish this type of 'autonomic failure' from classical autonomic neuropathy that develops in some individuals with diabetes as part of the spectrum of microvascular complications. In early reports of hypoglycaemia unawareness, the syndrome was attributed to autonomic neuropathy (Campbell *et al.*, 1977; Hoeldtke *et al.*, 1982), yet many individuals with impaired sympathoadrenal hypoglycaemic responses have normal autonomic function (Heller *et al.*, 1987a; Ryder *et al.*, 1990). The selective nature of the autonomic defect and the ability of those with counter-regulatory failure to generate normal adrenergic responses

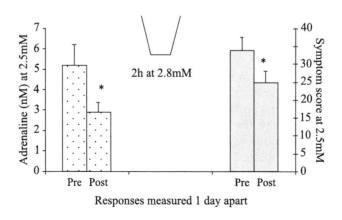

Figure 14.3 **Effect of '1' episode of antecedent hypoglycaemia in non-diabetic subjects. Adrenaline concentrations and symptom scores are significantly impaired after a single episode of hypoglycaemia. Data from Heller and Cryer (1991)**

to other stimuli, such as exercise, suggest that the efferent pathway of the autonomic nervous system is unaffected. Furthermore, some patients with established autonomic neuropathy exhibit normal sympathoadrenal responses to hypoglycaemia (Hepburn et al., 1993). However, recent work has indicated that some patients with autonomic neuropathy exhibit diminished sympathoadrenal responses to hypoglycaemia (Bottini et al., 1997; Lee et al., 2004), but this may relate more to a long duration of diabetes. On balance, the available evidence indicates that defective physiological responses to hypoglycaemia are not directly caused by classical autonomic neuropathy.

Alcohol

Excess and prolonged alcohol intake may cause secondary diabetes due to chronic pancreatitis. Such individuals usually require insulin treatment but, due to loss of glucagon secreting α-cells, are highly insulin-sensitive and prone to hypoglycaemic episodes (Sjoberg and Kidd, 1989). Alcohol also has acute effects that can increase the risk of severe hypoglycaemia. Alcohol inhibits some sympathoadrenal responses to hypoglycaemia such as tremor, leading to a reduction in symptomatic awareness. Acute alcohol ingestion inhibits gluconeogenesis in part secondary to a fall in circulating fatty acids (Avogaro et al., 1993), and this may prolong an established episode. Finally, the features of intoxication may be indistinguishable from those caused by impaired cerebral function such as confusion, disinhibition or a diminished conscious level. The consequences of leaving an individual to 'sleep off' what is actually severe hypoglycaemia may be disastrous. Alcohol can transform an episode of

moderate hypoglycaemia into something much more severe, even leading in some circumstances to irreversible brain damage or death. Anecdotal reports (Luthra and Donaldson, 1997) and clinical experience indicate that alcohol is an important cause of severe hypoglycaemia.

Pathophysiology of Unawareness

As has been presented elsewhere in this review, there is evidence that activation of the sympathoadrenal system and the onset of symptoms during hypoglycaemia develop at glucose thresholds that may vary according to the influence of factors such as duration of the disease, glycaemic control and antecedent hypoglycaemia. The extent to which glycaemic thresholds for the onset of cognitive dysfunction can vary is less clear, as the data from various studies and their interpretation are somewhat contradictory. There is disagreement between those who believe that the glycaemic threshold at which cerebral function begins to deteriorate is fixed at around 3.2 mmol/l, and others citing evidence that the threshold is flexible and alters in response to other factors such as antecedent hypoglycaemia. Resolution of these opinions would be important since the relationship between the different effects of hypoglycaemia explains why some patients fail to recognize that their blood glucose is low.

Activation of the Sympathoadrenal System

It has been proposed that unawareness of hypoglycaemia in those with impaired autonomic responses develops due to an alteration of the glycaemic threshold for the activation of the sympathoadrenal system and related symptoms that develop at glucose concentrations of around 2.5 mmol/l (Heller and Macdonald, 1996; Amiel, 1998). In contrast, the threshold for impaired cognition is relatively fixed at around 3.0 mmol/l, and cognitive ability deteriorates as neurons are progressively deprived of an essential substrate as glucose levels fall further. Those affected are incapacitated due to cerebral dysfunction by the time they begin to generate peripheral responses due to autonomic activation, and are unable to take the appropriate actions to raise their blood glucose. Unless assisted by others, their blood glucose will continue to fall until the sympathoadrenal response is sufficiently powerful to balance the glucose-lowering effect of injected insulin. The duration of coma or incapacity will depend upon the dissipation of injected insulin that then allows blood glucose to rise. Even in those prone to these types of hypoglycaemic episodes, death from hypoglycaemic brain damage is rare. It appears the sympathoadrenal system is eventually activated, albeit at low glucose concentrations, and that this is sufficient to stabilize blood glucose in the presence of insulin concentrations produced during everyday treatment.

Counter-Regulatory Failure

Based on early animal work that demonstrated the ability of the brain to respond to chronic hypoglycaemia by up-regulating glucose transport, a model has been proposed of 'maladaptation'. It was argued that, in response to hypoglycaemia, cerebral tissue extracted more glucose from the bloodstream, and that glucose had to fall to a lower hypoglycaemic level to activate a counter-regulatory response. Studies in rats have convincingly demonstrated that chronic hypoglycaemia leads to an increase in the expression of glucose transporters with increased cerebral glucose uptake, possibly due to increased expression of glucose transporters (McCall et al., 1986; Kumagai et al., 1995). Such pathogenic mechanisms have been supported by human studies that reported increased cerebral glucose uptake in non-diabetic humans subjected to mild experimental hypoglycaemia for many hours (Boyle et al., 1994) and preserved glucose uptake during hypoglycaemia in patients with Type 1 diabetes with tight glycaemic control (Boyle et al., 1995). However, there are a number of problems with this model. Perhaps the most important is that these changes apparently require periods of hypoglycaemia of a few days to produce changes in glucose transport, whereas functional changes can be demonstrated in humans (and animals) after periods of mild hypoglycaemia lasting just a few hours.

If cerebral tissue can extract greater amounts of glucose after prolonged or repeated hypoglycaemia, then this might be expected to preserve cognitive function during hypoglycaemia, whereas those with diminished counter-regulatory responses appear to be at greater risk of severe hypoglycaemia. It is, however, noteworthy that recent studies involving diabetic individuals have failed to find any change in cerebral glucose uptake (Segel et al., 2001). A plausible alternative explanation has invoked increases in cortisol concentrations. Rises in cortisol can produce comparable impairments in counter-regulatory and symptomatic responses with those observed after antecedent hypoglycaemia (Davis et al., 1996). Quite how cortisol might suppress subsequent activation of the autonomic nervous system is not entirely clear. Further experiments have suggested that the level of cortisol observed during experimental hypoglycaemia is insufficient to generate impairments in the counter-regulatory response (Raju *et al.*, 2003).

It is possible that activation of glucocorticoid receptors is responsible for deficient defences to hypoglycaemia and unawareness in different ways. Sherwin and colleagues have undertaken a series of studies using a rat model of hypoglycaemia to demonstrate opposing effects on the counter-regulatory response through stimulation by the cortisol-releasing hormone (CRH) and urocortin of CRH-R1 and CRH-R2 receptors respectively within the ventromedial hypothalamus (McCrimmon *et al.*, 2006; Cheng *et al.*, 2007; Sherwin, 2008). They hypothesize that repeated periods of hypoglycaemia may upregulate CRH-R2 receptors, leading to a deficient counter-regulatory response. However, more experimental work needs to be done. It will be a major challenge to confirm these pathways and relate the findings to humans since current experimental techniques do not permit detailed exploration of the pathways.

The observation that periods of mild hypoglycaemia lasting for a few hours inhibit physiological responses to subsequent episodes highlights a mechanism whereby one hypoglycaemic episode leads to diminished counter-regulatory defences to further hypoglycaemia and subsequent vulnerability to further episodes (Figure 14.4). It also indicates that such defects are functional and so may be reversible. A number of clinical studies have confirmed that even prolonged hypoglycaemia unawareness can be reversed, at least in part (Fanelli *et al.*, 1993; Cranston *et al.*, 1994), although counter-regulatory hormone responses were not restored to normal (Dagogo-Jack *et al.*, 1994). Not only did strict avoidance of all episodes

of hypoglycaemia lead to restoration of symptoms, but two studies demonstrated alteration of glycaemic thresholds for the onset of symptoms and adrenaline increase to a level higher than that which initially provoked cerebral dysfunction (Fanelli *et al.*, 1993: Cranston *et al.*, 1994) (Figure 14.5). No study has observed that glucagon responses were restored.

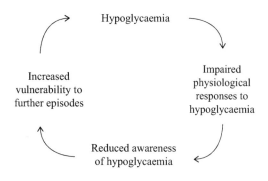

Figure 14.4 The vicious circle of repeated hypoglycaemia

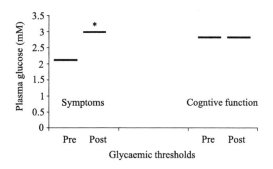

Figure 14.5 Reversing hypoglycaemia unawareness. Effect of a hypoglycaemia avoidance programme that involved 12 males with unawareness and three weeks absence of hypoglycaemia. After 'reversal', thresholds for the release of adrenaline rise to blood glucose concentrations above those for cognitive impairment. Data from Cranston *et al.* (1994)

Practical Approach to Hypoglycaemia

These studies may offer a practical approach to dealing with individuals with problems with hypoglycaemia, but success is by no means guaranteed. The critical steps appear to involve increased blood glucose monitoring, acceptance by the patient that glucose targets may be loosened (although it is possible to reverse unawareness without drastic deterioration in glycaemic control) and frequent contact with specialist nurses. Although the period of hypoglycaemia avoidance necessary to reset glycaemic thresholds may be as short as two to three weeks, establishing this behaviour in an affected individual may take many months and some patients are unable to change their approach (Heller, 2001). A detailed review of approaches to preventing the development of hypoglycaemia unawareness and avoiding severe hypoglycaemia during everyday therapy is beyond the scope of this chapter and the reader is directed to a recent account (Heller, 2008). In summary, the development of new insulin analogues, more sophisticated glucose monitoring devices and insulin infusion pumps have led to only modest reductions in the risk of hypoglycaemia during treatment. The most cost-effective approaches involve the delivery of structured skills training and equipping patients with the knowledge and ability to implement intensive insulin therapy safely. There is also evidence that training to become more aware of the blood glucose level through external clues (blood glucose awareness training) can reduce the risk of severe episodes (Schachinger et al., 2005).

Current Issues

The publication of the United Kingdom Prospective Diabetes Study Group (1998a) increased the pressure to intensify therapy in individuals with Type 2 diabetes. However, the potential risk of severe hypoglycaemia, together with other side effects of treatment such as weight gain, prevented patients from achieving tight glycaemic targets. The ACCORD study (Action to Control Cardiovascular Risk in Diabetes), designed to test the benefits of very low glucose targets in individuals with Type 2 diabetes, was terminated early due to unexpected increases in sudden death (Gerstein et al., 2008), although whether this was due to the increased risk of hypoglycaemia is still unclear.

Many studies have explored whether Type 2 diabetes modifies physiological defences to hypoglycaemia and whether these differ from the situation in Type 1 diabetes. Early reports indicated that glucagon responses were relatively intact, in contrast with those with Type 1 diabetes (Boden et al., 1983; Heller et al., 1987b), but more recent work has demonstrated that patients with insulin-treated Type 2 diabetes and diminished endogenous insulin secretion exhibit reduced glucagon responses when compared with patients on oral agents or non-diabetic controls (Segel et al., 2002). This reflects data from recent epidemiological studies demonstrating that the risk of hypoglycaemia increases with increasing duration of diabetes (United Kingdom Hypoglycaemia Study Group, 2007). As in Type 1 diabetes, progressive β-cell damage is associated with impaired counter-regulatory responses to hypoglycaemia – in particular, impaired glucagon secretion (Segel et al., 2002).

Studies have also explored the effects of repeated episodes of hypoglycaemia among patients with Type 2 diabetes, one reporting unchanged adrenaline and symptomatic responses after a single hypoglycaemic episode (Peacey *et al.*, 1996) and another demonstrating equivalent reductions in adrenaline and symptomatic responses following antecedent hypoglycaemia as those seen in Type 1 diabetes (Davis *et al.*, 1999). Other work has reported that glycaemic thresholds for physiological defences to hypoglycaemia can vary in those with Type 2 diabetes, as previously demonstrated in Type 1 diabetes. This ranges from observations that patients with tight glycaemic control exhibit thresholds for counter-regulatory hormone and symptom increases below normal (Korzon-Burakowska *et al.*, 1998) to reports of autonomic responses being initiated at glucose concentrations above 4 mmol/l (Spyer *et al.*, 2000). Thus, the same factors that influence impaired responses in Type 1 diabetes may also contribute to defects in patients with Type 2 diabetes. The low risk of hypoglycaemia during the first few years of treatment is related to relative preservation of β-cell function. Those with long-duration Type 2 diabetes may eventually be just as vulnerable to the failure of physiological defences to hypoglycaemia as patients with Type 1 diabetes (Cryer, 2008).

Part 5:
IMPLICATIONS FOR THE PRACTICE OF AVIATION MEDICINE

Like others responsible for regulating medical practice in potentially hazardous occupations, those involved in the licensing of aircrew need to balance the risks to the public and the individuals themselves against the wish to minimize the possibility of aircrew losing their operating licence. This applies particularly to ingested medication, and considerable work has been undertaken to identify and ensure the use of medication that has minimal side effects and does not impair operational performance. However, uncertainty surrounding the risks of hypoglycaemia as a result of taking medication (both sulphonylureas and insulin) in different types of diabetes has led to a lack of consistency in regulations surrounding the licensing of aircrew. The International Civil Aviation Organization (2008) considers that those with insulin-treated diabetes are unfit, while elsewhere in their manual it is acknowledged that some member states permit insulin-treated individuals to fly. The Federal Aviation Authority grants Special Issuance Medical certification to aircrew taking oral anti-diabetic medication including sulphonylureas, a dispensation extended to some aircrew using insulin (Orford and Silberman, 2008). Prospective aircrew have to provide evidence supported by a physician of the absence of a history of severe hypoglycaemia, and they have to undertake regular blood glucose monitoring and show that they know the correct actions to be taken if they develop hypoglycaemia.

Type 1 Diabetes

Relaxation of previously stringent regulations even extends to military aircrew. Recent communications claim unimpaired operational capability of aircrew with Type 1 diabetes in such circumstances (Grossman *et al.*, 2005: Carter *et al.*, 2005). The authors acknowledge that the critical issue is the risk of impaired cognitive function. They institute a careful approach, with insistence on regular glucose monitoring, 'aggressive treatment' and a high degree of cooperation from aircrew with a short duration of diabetes. Some aircrew participate in blood glucose awareness training, in which individuals learn to recognize at an early stage the symptoms of hypoglycaemia. Some individuals also used a hypoglycaemic clamp to familiarize themselves with their particular hypoglycaemic symptoms.

However, it is conceivable that symptoms induced by using a clamp may be different from those experienced during a clinical episode. The concentration of circulating insulin, the rate of change of the blood glucose level (Mitrakou *et al.*, 1993) and the state of arousal (Heller and Macdonald, 1991) may all modify hypoglycaemic symptoms. Of more concern is that symptoms may vary within the same individual and that patients often overestimate their ability to recognize a falling blood glucose level (Heller *et al.*, 1995). The careful approach described will reduce the likelihood of a severe hypoglycaemic episode, but would not eliminate such an event. It is noteworthy that only individuals with short-duration diabetes were permitted to fly. This was an important safeguard since it is patients of long duration who are more vulnerable to sudden cognitive impairment without warning induced by hypoglycaemia.

The duration of any cognitive impairment induced by hypoglycaemia must also be considered. Even if patients can rely on a powerful symptomatic response to alert them to a falling glucose level, by the time they take action their performance may have deteriorated due to an acute cognitive decline. In addition, and of considerable significance, is that recovery of cognitive performance is often delayed after hypoglycaemia for at least an hour (Zammitt *et al.*, 2008). Performance and recovery may also be compromised by environmental challenges. For example, with transport

aircrew, it is conceivable that the relative hypoxia of the aircraft cabin and a limited degree of hypoglycaemia could have a synergistic adverse effect, and the altitude of the destination airport may be above that to which they are normally accustomed. In summary, despite good symptomatic awareness and an immediate response to symptoms, those with Type 1 diabetes are at risk of an acute and lengthy decline in performance after even mild hypoglycaemia (Heller and Nicholson, 2006). Although blood glucose monitoring can give advance warning of impending hypoglycaemia, frequent measurements are often impractical in flight.

It is also a challenge to devise insulin regimens that can cope with flying duties which can extend to any time of the day and night, involve multiple time-zone changes and varying flight duty periods. The inevitable disruption of sleep patterns might increase susceptibility to a decline in performance during an episode of hypoglycaemia. Other factors to be considered include the need to accommodate the storage of insulin to different and changing climatic conditions, and the responsibility placed on the healthy pilot particularly during critical periods of the flight. There will also be the burden on the healthy pilot during the recovery of cognition after a hypoglycaemic episode, and this could be significant in the event of combat.

Type 2 Diabetes

The situation among those with a relatively short duration of Type 2 diabetes is certainly different and merits careful consideration. The recent findings of the United Kingdom Hypoglycaemia Study Group (2007) clearly showed that although both patients treated with sulphonylurea or insulin were prone to occasional hypoglycaemic episodes, the risk in those with Type 2 diabetes was around tenfold less than those with Type 1 diabetes. There is certainly a case for scrutinizing such cases more sympathetically, although each one must be considered carefully and on its own merits.

Conclusion

Insulin-induced hypoglycaemia has the potential to cause widespread and major pathophysiological effects, particularly within the central nervous system. Any individual who takes insulin or sulphonylureas is vulnerable, but those with longstanding diabetes whose defences to resist hypoglycaemia are often severely compromised are at greatest risk. Since hypoglycaemia unawareness is rarely all or nothing, and even those who recognize the onset of hypoglycaemia are likely to exhibit some impairment of performance, permitting such patients to undertake flying duties seems unwise. However, those with Type 2 diabetes who are taking sulphonylureas or who have a short history of insulin treatment might be capable of safely undertaking a flying role, if there is no history of severe hypoglycaemia, they can reliably recognize the onset of symptoms and they are prepared to measure their blood glucose both before and during a flight.

References

Akram, K., Pedersen-Bjergaard, U., Carstensen, B., Borch-Johnsen, K. and Thorsteinsson, B. 2006. Frequency and risk factors of severe hypoglycaemia in insulin-treated Type 2 diabetes: A cross-sectional survey. *Diabetic Medicine*, 23, 750–56.

Amiel, S.A. 1998. Cognitive function testing in studies of acute hypoglycaemia: Rights and wrongs? *Diabetologia*, 4, 713–9.

Amiel, S.A., Sherwin, R.S., Simonson, D.C. and Tamborlane, W.V. 1988. Effect of intensive insulin therapy on glycemic thresholds for counter-regulatory hormone release. *Diabetes*, 37, 901–7.

Amiel, S.A., Tamborlane, W.V., Simonson, D.C. and Sherwin, R.S. 1987. Defective glucose counter-regulation after strict glycemic control of insulin-dependent diabetes mellitus. *New England Journal of Medicine*, 316, 1376–83.

Avogaro, A., Belttramellom, P., Gnudt, L., Moran, A., Valerio, A., Miola, M. *et al.* 1993. Alcohol intake impairs glucose counter-regulation during acute insulin-induced hypoglycemia in IDDM patients: Evidence for a critical role of free fatty acids. *Diabetes*, 42, 1626–34.

Balodimos, M.C. and Root, H.E. 1959. Hypoglycaemic insulin reactions without warning symptoms. *Journal of the American Medical Association*, 171, 101–7.

Blackman, J.D., Towle, V.L., Lewis, G.F., Spire, J.P. and Polonsky, K.S. 1990. Hypoglycemic thresholds for cognitive dysfunction in humans. *Diabetes*, 39, 828–35.

Boden, G., Soriano, M., Hoeldtke, R.D. and Owen, O.E. 1983. Counter-regulatory hormone release and glucose recovery after hypoglycemia in non-insulin-dependent diabetic patients. *Diabetes*, 32, 1055–9.

Bolli, G., De Feo, P., Compagnucci, P., Cartechini, M.G., Angeletti, G., Santeusanio, F. *et al.* 1983. Abnormal glucose counter-regulation in IDDM: Interaction of anti-insulin antibodies and impaired glucagon and epinephrine secretion. *Diabetes*, 32, 134–41.

Bolli, G., De Feo, P., Perriello, G., De Cosmo, S., Ventura, M., Campbell, P. *et al.* 1985. Role of hepatic autoregulation in defence against hypoglycaemia in humans. *Journal of Clinical Investigation*, 75, 1623–31.

Borg, W.P., During, M.J., Sherwin, R.S., Borg, M.A., Brines, M.L. and Shulman, G.I. 1994. Ventromedial hypothalamic lesions in rats suppress counter-regulatory responses to hypoglycemia. *Journal of Clinical Investigation*, 93, 1677–82.

Borg, W.P., Sherwin, R.S., During, M.J., Borg, M.A. and Shulman, G.I. 1995. Local ventromedial hypothalamus glucopenia triggers counter-regulatory hormone release. *Diabetes*, 44, 180–84.

Bott, S., Bott, U., Berger, M. and Mühlhauser, I. 1997. Intensified insulin therapy and the risk of severe hypoglycaemia. *Diabetologia*, 40, 926–32.

Bottini, P., Boschetti, E., Pampanelli, S., Ciofetta, M., Del Sindaco, P., Scionti, L. *et al.* 1997. Contribution of autonomic neuropathy to reduced plasma adrenaline responses to hypoglycaemia in IDDM. *Diabetes*, 46, 814–23.

Boyle, P.J., Kempers, S.F., O'Connor, A.M. and Nagy, R.J. 1995. Brain glucose uptake and unawareness of hypoglycemia in patients with insulin-dependent diabetes mellitus. *New England Journal of Medicine*, 28, 1726–31.

Boyle, P.J., Nagy, R.J., O'Connor, A.M., Kempers, S.F., Yeo, R.A. and Qualls, C. 1994. Adaptation in brain glucose uptake following recurrent hypoglycemia. *Proceedings of the National Academy of Sciences of the United States of America*, 91, 9352–6.

Brown, A.M. 2004. Brain glycogen re-awakened. *Journal of Neurochemistry*, 89, 537–52.

Campbell, L.V., Kraegen, E.W. and Lazarus, L. 1977. Defective blood glucose counter-regulation in diabetics is a selective form of autonomic neuropathy. *British Medical Journal*, 2, 1527–9.

Brown, A.M., Wender, R. and Ransom, R. 2001. Metabolic substrates other than glucose support axon function in central white matter. *Journal of Neuroscience Research*, 66, 839–43.

Carter, D., Azaria, B. and Goldstein, L. 2005. Diabetes mellitus Type 1 in five military aviators: Flying with insulin. *Aviation, Space, and Environmental Medicine*, 76, 861–2.

Cheng, H., Zhou, L., Zhu, W., Wang, A., Tang, C., Chan, O. *et al.* 2007. Type 1 corticotropin-releasing factor receptors in the ventromedial hypothalamus promote hypoglycemia-induced hormonal counter-regulation. *American Journal of Physiology: Endocrinology and Metabolism*, 293, E705–12.

Choi, I.Y., Seaquist, E.R. and Gruetter, R. 2003. Effect of hypoglycemia on brain glycogen metabolism in vivo. *Journal of Neuroscience Research*, 72, 25–32.

Clarke, D.D. and Sokoloff, L. 1999. Circulation and Energy Metabolism of the Brain. In: G.J. Siegel, B.W. Agranoff, R.W. Albers, S.K. Molinoff, P.B. Fisher and M.D. Uhler (eds) *Basic Neurochemistry*. Philadelphia, PA: Lippincott-Raven, 637–69.

Cox, D.J., Gonder-Frederick, L. and Clarke, W. 1993. Driving decrements in Type I diabetes during moderate hypoglycemia. *Diabetes*, 42, 239–43.

Cox, D.J., Gonder-Frederick, L., Kovatcher, B.P., Julian, C.M. and Clarke, W.L. 2000. Progressive hypoglycemia's impact on driving simulation performance: Occurrence, awareness and correction. *Diabetes Care*, 23, 163–70.

Cranston, I., Lomas, J., Maran, A., MacDonald, I. and Amiel, S.A. 1994. Restoration of hypoglycaemia unawareness in patients with long-duration insulin-dependent diabetes. *Lancet*, 344, 283–7.

Cryer, P.E. 1994. Hypoglycemia unawareness in IDDM. *Diabetes Care*, 16, 40–47.

Cryer, P.E. 2001. The Prevention and Correction of Hypoglycemia. In: L.S. Jefferson and A.D. Cherrington (eds) *Handbook of Physiology. Section 7: The Endocrine System. Volume II: The Endocrine Pancreas and Regulation of Metabolism*. New

York, NY: Oxford University Press, 1057–92.

Cryer, P.E. 2008. Hypoglycemia: Still the limiting factor in the glycemic management of diabetes. *Endocrine Practice*, 14, 750–56.

Cryer, P.E. and Gerich, J.E. 1983. Relevance of glucose counter-regulatory systems to patients with diabetes: Critical roles of glucagon and epinephrine. *Diabetes Care*, 6, 95–9.

Dagogo-Jack, S.E., Croft, S. and Cryer, P.E. 1993. Hypoglycemia-associated autonomic failure in insulin-dependent diabetes mellitus. *Journal of Clinical Investigation*, 91, 819–28.

Dagogo-Jack, S., Rattarasam, C. and Cryer, P.E. 1994. Reversal of hypoglycemia unawareness, but not defective glucose counter-regulation, in IDDM. *Diabetes*, 43, 1426–34.

Davis, S.N., Mann, S., Tate, D., Brown, J., Ping, L. and Costa, F. 1999. Effects of antecedent hypoglycemia (AH) on counter-regulatory response to subsequent hypoglycemia in patients with Type 2 diabetes. *Diabetes*, 48, 1590.

Davis, S.N., Shavers, C., Costa, F. and Mosqueda-Garcia, R. 1996. Role of cortisol in the pathogenesis of deficient counter-regulation after antecedent hypoglycemia in normal humans. *Journal of Clinical Investigation*, 98, 680–89.

De Fronzo, R., Tobin, J.D. and Andres, R. 1979. Glucose clamp technique: A method for quantifying insulin secretion and resistance. *American Journal of Physiology*, 237, E214–23.

Deary, I.J. 1993. Effects of Hypoglycaemia on Cognitive Function. In: B.M. Frier and B.M. Fisher (eds) *Hypoglycaemia and Diabetes*. London: Edward Arnold, 80–92.

Diabetes Control and Complications Trial Research Group. 1993. The effect of intensive treatment of diabetes on the development and progression of long-term complications in insulin-dependent

diabetes mellitus. *New England Journal of Medicine*, 329, 683–9.

Diabetes Control and Complications Trial Research Group, 1997. Hypoglycemia in the Diabetes Control and Complications Trial. *Diabetes*, 46, 271–86.

Donnelly, L.A., Morris, A.D., Frier, B.M., Ellis, J.D., Donnan, P.T., Durrant, R. *et al.* 2005. Frequency and predictors of hypoglycaemia in Type 1 and insulin-treated Type 2 diabetes: A population-based study. *Diabetic Medicine*, 22, 749–55.

Fanelli, C.G., Epifano, L., Rambotti, A.M., Pampanelli, S., Vincenzo, A., Modarelli, F. *et al.* 1993. Meticulous prevention of hypoglycemia normalizes the glycemic thresholds of most of neuroendocrine responses to, symptoms of, and cognitive function during hypoglycemia in intensively treated patients with short-term IDDM. *Diabetes*, 42, 1683–9.

Fanelli, C., Pampanelli, S., Epifano, L., Rambotti, A.M., Ciofetta, M., Modarelli, F. *et al.* 1994. Relative roles of insulin and hypoglycaemia on induction of neuroendocrine responses to, symptoms of, and deterioration of cognitive function in hypoglycaemia in male and female humans. *Diabetologia*, 37, 797–807.

Fisher, B.M., Gray, C.E., Beastall, G.H. and Frier, B.M. 1988. Responses to acute insulin-induced hypoglycaemia in diabetic patients: A comparison of short-acting human and porcine insulins. *Diabetic Research*, 8, 1–8.

Fritsche, A., Stumvoll, M., Grub, M., Sieslack, S., Renn, W. and Schmülling, R.M. 1998. Effect of hypoglycemia on beta-adrenergic sensitivity in normal and Type 1 diabetic subjects. *Diabetes Care*, 21, 1505–10.

Gale, E.A.M. and Tattersall, R.B. 1979. Unrecognised nocturnal hypoglycaemia in insulin dependent diabetics. *Lancet*, 1, 1049–52.

George, E., Harris, N., Bedford, C., Macdonald, I.A., Hardisty, C.A. and Heller, S.R. 1995. Prolonged but partial impairment of the hypoglycaemic physiological response following short-term hypoglycaemia in normal subjects. *Diabetologia*, 38, 1183–90.

Gerich, J.E., Langlois, M., Noacco, C., Karam, J.H. and Forsham, P.H. 1973. Lack of glucagon response to hypoglycaemia in diabetes: Evidence for an intrinsic pancreatic alpha cell defect. *Science*, 182, 171–3.

Gerich, J.E. and Bolli, G.B. 1993. Counter-Regulatory Failure. In: B.M. Fisher and B.M. Frier (eds) *Hypoglycaemia and Diabetes: Clinical and Physiological Aspects*. London: Edward Arnold, 253–67.

Gerstein, H.C., Miller, M.E., Byington, R.P., Goff, D.C. Jr, Bigger, J.T., Buse, J.B. *et al.* 2008. Effects of intensive glucose lowering in Type 2 diabetes. *New England Journal of Medicine*, 358, 2545–59.

Gold, A.E., MacLeod, K.M. and Frier, B.M. 1994. Frequency of severe hypoglycemia in patients with Type I (insulin dependent) diabetes with impaired awareness of hypoglycemia. *Diabetes Care*, 17, 697–703.

Goldfien, A., Moore, R., Zileli, S., Havens, L.L., Boliong, L. and Thorn, G.W. 1961. Plasma epinephrine and norepinephrine levels during insulin-induced hypoglycaemia in man. *Journal of Clinical Endocrinology and Metabolism*, 21, 296–303.

Grossman, A., Barenboim, E., Azaria, B., Goldstein, L. and Cohen, O. 2005. Blood glucose awareness training helps return insulin-treated aviators to the cockpit. *Aviation, Space, and Environmental Medicine*, 76, 586–8.

Heller, S.R. 2001. How Should Hypoglycaemia Unawareness Be Managed? In: G. Gill, G. Williams and J. Pickup (eds) *Difficult Diabetes*. Oxford: Blackwell, 168–87.

Heller, S.R. 2008. Minimizing hypoglycemia while maintaining glycemic control in diabetes. *Diabetes*, 57, 3177–83.

Heller, S.R., Chapman, J., McCloud, J. and Ward, J. 1995. Unreliability of reports of hypoglycaemia by diabetic patients. *British Medical Journal*, 310, 440.

Heller, S.R. and Cryer, P.E. 1991a. Hypoinsulinemia is not critical to glucose recovery from hypoglycemia in humans. *American Journal of Physiology*, 261, E41–8.

Heller, S.R. and Cryer, P.E. 1991b. Reduced neuroendocrine and symptomatic responses to subsequent hypoglycemia after one episode of hypoglycemia in non-diabetic humans. *Diabetes*, 40, 223–6.

Heller, S.R. and Macdonald, I.A. 1991. Physiological disturbances in hypoglycaemia: Effect on subjective awareness. *Clinical Science*, 81, 1–9.

Heller, S.R. and Macdonald, I.A. 1996. The measurement of cognitive function during acute hypoglycaemia: Experimental limitations and their effect on the study of hypoglycaemia unawareness. *Diabetic Medicine*, 13, 607–15.

Heller, S.R., MacDonald, I.A., Herbert, M. and Tattersall, R.B. 1987a. Influence of sympathetic nervous system on hypoglycaemic warning symptoms. *Lancet*, 2, 359–63.

Heller, S.R., MacDonald, I.A. and Tattersall, R.B. 1987b. Counter-regulation in Type 2 (non-insulin-dependent) diabetes mellitus: Normal endocrine and glycaemic responses, up to ten years after diagnosis. *Diabetologia*, 30, 924–9.

Heller, S.R. and Nicholson, A.N. 2006. Aircrew and Type 1 diabetes mellitus. *Aviation, Space, and Environmental Medicine*, 77, 456–8.

Hepburn, D.A. and Deary, I.J. 1991. Symptoms of acute hypoglycaemia in humans with and without IDDM (Factor analysis approach). *Diabetes Care*, 14, 949–57.

Hepburn, D.A., Macleod, K.M. and Frier, B.M. 1993. Physiological, symptomatic and hormonal responses to acute hypoglycaemia in Type 1 diabetic patients with autonomic neuropathy. *Diabetic Medicine*, 10, 940–49.

Herbert, M. 1978. Assessment of performance in studies of anaesthetic agents. *British Journal of Anaesthesia*, 50, 33–8.

Herold, K.C., Polonsky, K.S., Cohen, R.M., Levy, J. and Douglas, F. 1985. Variable deterioration in cortical function during insulin-induced hypoglycemia. *Diabetes*, 34, 677–85.

Hirsch, B.R. and Shamoon, H. 1987. Defective epinephrine and growth hormone responses in Type 1 diabetes are stimulus specific. *Diabetes*, 36, 20–26.

Hoeldtke, R.D., Boden, G., Shuman, C.R. and Owen, O.E. 1982. Reduced epinephrine secretion and hypoglycemia unawareness in diabetic autonomic neuropathy. *Annals of Internal Medicine*, 96, 459–62.

Hoffman, R.G., Sleelman, D.J., Hinnen, D.A., Conley, K.L., Guthrie, R.A. and Knapp, R.K. 1989. Changes in cortical functioning with acute hypoglycemia and hyperglycemia in Type 1 diabetes. *Diabetes Care*, 12, 193–7.

Holmes, C.S., Hayford, J.T., Gonzalez, J.L. and Weydert, J.A. 1983. A survey of cognitive functioning at different glucose levels in diabetic persons. *Diabetes Care*, 6, 180–85.

Holmes, C.S., Koepke, K.M. and Thompson, R.G. (1986). Simple versus complex impairments at three blood glucose levels. *Psychoneuroendocrinology*, 11, 353–7.

Holmes, C.S., Koepke, K.M., Thompson, R.G., Gyves, P.W. and Weydert, J.A. 1984. Verbal fluency and naming performance in Type 1 diabetes at different blood glucose concentrations. *Diabetes Care*, 7, 454–9.

International Civil Aviation Organization. 2008. Metabolic, Nutritional and Endocrine Diseases. In: *Manual of Civil Aviation Medicine – Preliminary Edition*. Montreal: International Civil Aviation Organization, III, 4–14.

Jaap, A.J., Jones, G.C., McCrimmon, R.J., Deary, I.J. and Frier, B.M. 1998. Perceived symptoms of hypoglycaemia in elderly Type 2 diabetic patients treated with insulin. *Diabetic Medicine*, 15, 398–401.

Kaufman, F.R., Austin, J., Neinstein, A., Jeng, L., Halvorson M., Devoe, D.J. *et al.* 2002. Nocturnal hypoglycemia detected with the Continuous Glucose Monitoring System in pediatric patients with Type 1 diabetes. *Journal of Pediatrics*, 141, 625–30.

Korzon-Burakowska, A., Hopkins, D., Matyka, K., Lomas, J., Pernet, A., Macdonald, I. *et al.* 1998. Effects of glycemic control on protective responses against hypoglycemia in Type 2 diabetes. *Diabetes Care*, 21, 283–90.

Kumagai, A.K., Kang, Y.S., Boado, R.J. and Pardridge, W.M. 1995. Upregulation of blood-brain barrier GLUT1 glucose transporter protein and mRNA in experimental chronic hypoglycaemia. *Diabetes*, 44, 1399–404.

Lawrence, R.D. 1941. Insulin hypoglycaemia: Changes in nervous manifestations. *Lancet*, 2, 602.

Lee, S.P., Yeoh, L., Harris, N.D., Davis, C.M., Robinson, R.T., Leathard, A. *et al.* 2004. Influence of autonomic neuropathy on QTc interval lengthening during hypoglycemia in Type 1 diabetes. *Diabetes*, 53, 1535–42.

Luthra, Y.K. and Donaldson, D. 1997. Lessons to be learned: A case study approach. Severe hypoglycaemia in insulin-dependent diabetes mellitus (IDDM) – living to tell the tale. *Journal of the Royal Society of Health*, 117, 377–80.

McAulay, V., Deary, I.J., Ferguson, S.C. and Frier, B.M. 2001. Acute hypoglycemia in humans causes attentional dysfunction while nonverbal intelligence is preserved. *Diabetes Care*, 24, 1745–50.

McAulay, V., Deary, I.J., Sommerfield, A.J. and Frier, B.M. 2006. Attentional functioning is impaired during acute hypoglycaemia in people with Type 1 diabetes. *Diabetic Medicine*, 23, 26–31.

McCall, A.L. 2004. Cerebral glucose metabolism in diabetes mellitus. *European Journal of Pharmacology*, 490, 147–58.

McCall, A.L., Fixman, L.B., Fleming, N., Tornheim, K., Chick, W. and Rudeman, N.B. 1986. Chronic hypoglycemia increases brain glucose transport. *American Journal of Physiology*, 251, E442–7.

McCrimmon, R. 2008. The mechanisms that underlie glucose sensing during hypoglycaemia in diabetes. *Diabetic Medicine*, 25, 513–22.

McCrimmon, R.J., Gold, A.E., Deary, I.J., Kelner, C.J. and Frier, B.M. 1995. Symptoms of hypoglycemia in children with IDDM. *Diabetes Care*, 18, 858–61.

McCrimmon, R.J., Song, Z., Cheng, H., McNay, E.C., Weikart-Yeckel, C., Fan, X. *et al.* 2006. Corticotrophin-releasing factor receptors within the ventromedial hypothalamus regulate hypoglycemia-induced hormonal counter-regulation. *Journal of Clinical Investigation*, 116, 1723–30.

Maran, A., Cranston, I., Lomas, J., Macdonald, I. and Amiel, S.A. 1994. Protection by lactate of cerebral function during hypoglycaemia. *Lancet*, 343, 16–20.

Matyka, K., Watts, A.P., Stores, G. and Dunger, D.B. 1996. High prevalence of nocturnal hypoglycaemia in young children with insulin-dependent diabetes mellitus studied overnight at home. *Diabetic Medicine*, 13, Suppl. 3, S13.

Mitrakou, A., Ryan, C., Veneman, T., Mokan, M., Jenssen, T., Kiss, I. *et al.* 1991. Hierarchy of glycemic thresholds for counter-regulatory hormone secretion, symptoms and cerebral dysfunction. *American Journal of Physiology*, 260, E67–74.

Mitrakou, A., Mokan, M., Ryan, C., Venema, T., Cryer, P. and Gerich, J. 1993. Influence of plasma glucose rate of decrease on hierarchy of responses to hypoglycemia. *Journal of Clinical Endocrinology and Metabolism*, 76, 462–5.

Mühlhauser, I. and Berger, M. 1993. Diabetes education and insulin therapy: When will they ever learn? *Journal of Internal Medicine*, 233, 321–6.

Orford, R.R. and Silberman, W.S. 2008. Pilot Health and Aeromedical Certification. In: J.R. Davis, R. Johnson, J. Stepanek and J.A. Fogarty (eds) *Fundamentals of Aerospace Medicine – Fourth Edition*. Philadelphia, PA: Lippincott Williams and Wilkins, 318–48.

Peacey, S.R., Bedford, C., Marlow, S., Harris, N., MacDonald, I.A., Hardisty, C.A. and Heller, S.R. 1996. Antecedent hypoglycemia does not alter the physiological response to subsequent hypoglycemia in NIDDM. *Diabetes*, 45, 199.

Peacey, S.R., Rostami-Hodjegan, A., George, E., Tucker, G.T. and Heller, S.R. 1997. The use of tolbutamide-induced hypoglycemia to examine the intraislet role of insulin in mediating glucagon release in normal humans. *Journal of Clinical Endocrinology and Metabolism*, 82, 1458–61.

Pedersen-Bjergaard, U., Pramming, S., Heller, S.R., Wallace, T.M., Rasmussen, A.K., Jørgensen, H.V. *et al.* 2004. Severe hypoglycaemia in 1076 adult patients with Type 1 diabetes: Influence of risk markers and selection. *Diabetes/Metabolism Research and Reviews*, 20, 479–86.

Pieber, T.R., Brunner, G.A., Schnedl, W.J., Schattenberg, S., Kaufmann, P. and Krejs, G.J. 1995. Evaluation of a structured outpatient group education program for intensive insulin therapy. *Diabetes Care*, 18, 625–30.

Pramming, S., Thorsteinsson, B., Bendtson, I. and Binder, C. 1991. Symptomatic hypoglycaemia in 411 Type 1 diabetic patients. *Diabetic Medicine*, 8, 217–22.

Pramming, S., Thorsteinsson, B., Theilgaard, A., Pinner, E.M. and Binder, C. 1986. Cognitive function during hypoglycaemia in Type 1 diabetes mellitus. *British Medical Journal*, 292, 647–50.

Raju, B., McGregor, V.P. and Cryer, P.E. 2003. Cortisol elevations comparable to those that occur during hypoglycemia do not cause hypoglycemia-associated autonomic failure. *Diabetes*, 52, 2083–9.

Raju, B. and Cryer, P.E. 2005. Loss of the decrement in intraislet insulin plausibly explains loss of the glucagon response to hypoglycemia in insulin-deficient diabetes: Documentation of the intraislet insulin hypothesis in humans. *Diabetes*, 54, 757–64.

Rizza, R.A., McGregor, V.P, and Cryer, P.E. 1979. Role of glucagon, catecholamines, and growth hormone in human glucose counter-regulation: Effects of somatostatin and combined alpha- and beta-adrenergic blockade on plasma glucose recovery and glucose flux rates after insulin-induced hypoglycemia. *Journal of Clinical Investigation*, 64, 62–71.

Rizza, R.A., Mandarino, L.J. and Gerich, J.E. 1981. Dose-response characteristics for effects of insulin on production and utilization of glucose in man. *American Journal of Physiology*, 240, E630–39.

Ryan, C.M. 1994. Measures of Cognitive Function. In: C. Bradley (ed.) *Handbook of Psychology and Diabetes*. Chur, Switzerland: Harwood Academic Publishers, 191–222.

Ryder, R.E.J., Owens, D.R., Hayes, T.M., Ghatei, M.A. and Bloom, S.R. 1990. Unawareness of hypoglycaemia and inadequate hypoglycaemic counter-regulation: No causal relation with diabetic autonomic neuropathy. *British Medical Journal*, 301, 783–7.

Sämann, A., Mühlhauser, I., Bender, R., Kloos, Ch. and Müller, A. 2005. Glycaemic control and severe hypoglycaemia following training in flexible, intensive insulin therapy to enable dietary freedom in people with Type 1 diabetes: A prospective implementation study. *Diabetologia*, 48, 1965–70.

Schachinger, H., Hegar, K., Hermanns, N., Straumann, M., Keller, U., Fehm-

Wolfsdorf, G. *et al*. 2005. Randomized controlled clinical trial of Blood Glucose Awareness Training (BGAT III) in Switzerland and Germany. *Journal of Behavioral Medicine*, 28, 587–94.

Schwartz, N.S., Clutter, W.E., Shah, S.D. and Cryer, P.E. 1987. Glycemic thresholds for activation of glucose counter-regulatory systems are higher than the threshold for symptoms. *Journal of Clinical Investigation*, 79, 777–81.

Segel, S.A., Fanelli, C.G., Dence, C.S., Markham, J., Videen, T.O., Paramore, D.S. *et al*. 2001. Blood-to-brain glucose transport, cerebral glucose metabolism, and cerebral blood flow are not increased after hypoglycemia. *Diabetes*, 50, 1911–7.

Segel, S.A., Paramore, D.S. and Cryer, P.E. 2002. Hypoglycemia associated autonomic failure in advanced Type 2 diabetes. *Diabetes*, 51, 724–33.

Sherwin, R.S. 2008. Bringing light to the dark side of insulin: A journey across the blood-brain barrier. *Diabetes*, 57, 2259–68.

Simonson, D.C., Tamborlane, W.V., De Fronzo, R.A. and Sherwin, R.S. 1985. Intensive insulin therapy reduces counter-regulatory hormone responses to hypoglycaemia inpatients with Type 1 diabetes. *Annals of Internal Medicine*, 103, 184–90.

Sjoberg, R.J. and Kidd, G.S. 1989. Pancreatic diabetes mellitus. *Diabetes Care*, 12, 715–24.

Snorgaard, O., Lassen, L.H., Rosenfalck, A.M. and Binder, C. 1991. Glycaemic thresholds for hypoglycaemic symptoms, impairment of cognitive function, and release of counter-regulatory hormones in subjects with functional hypoglycaemia. *Journal of Internal Medicine*, 229, 343–50.

Sommerfield, A.J., Deary, I.J., McAulay, V. and Frier, B.M. 2003a. Short-term, delayed, and working memory are impaired during hypoglycemia in individuals with Type 1 diabetes. *Diabetes Care*, 26, 390–96.

Sommerfield, A.J., Deary, I.J., McAulay, V. and Frier, B.M. 2003b. Moderate hypoglycemia impairs multiple memory functions in healthy adults. *Neuropsychology*, 17, 125–32.

Spyer, G., Hattersley, A.T., MacDonald, I.A., Amiel, S. and MacLeod, K.M. 2000. Hypoglycaemic counter-regulation at normal blood glucose concentrations in patients with well controlled Type 2 diabetes. *Lancet*, 356, 1970–74

Stevens, A.B., McKane, W.R., Bell, P.M., Bell, P., King, D.J. and Hayes, J.R. 1989. Psychomotor performance and counter-regulatory responses during mild hypoglycemia in healthy volunteers. *Diabetes Care*, 12, 12–17.

Stork, A.D., van Haeften, T.W. and Veneman, T.F. 2007. The decision not to drive during hypoglycemia in patients with Type 1 and Type 2 diabetes according to hypoglycemia awareness. *Diabetes Care*, 30, 2822–6.

Taborsky, G.J. Jr, Ahrén, B. and Havel, P.J. 1998. Autonomic mediation of glucagon secretion during hypoglycemia: Implications for impaired alpha-cell responses in Type 1 diabetes. *Diabetes*, 47, 995–1005.

Trovik, T.S., Jaeger, R., Jorde, R. and Sager, G. 1994. Reduced sensitivity to beta-adrenoceptor stimulation and blockade in insulin dependent diabetic patients with hypoglycaemia unawareness. *British Journal of Clinical Pharmacology*, 38, 427–32.

Unger, R.H. 1983. Insulin-glucagon relationships in the defense against hypoglycemia. *Diabetes*, 32, 575–83.

United Kingdom Prospective Diabetes Study Group. 1998a. Effect of intensive blood-glucose control with metformin on complications in overweight patients with Type 2 diabetes. *Lancet*, 352, 854–65.

United Kingdom Prospective Diabetes Study Group. 1998b. Intensive blood-glucose control with sulphonylureas or insulin compared with conventional treatment and risk of complications in patients with Type 2 diabetes. *Lancet*, 352, 837–53.

United Kingdom Hypoglycaemia Study Group. 2007. Risk of hypoglycaemia in Types 1 and 2 diabetes: Effects of treatment modalities and their duration. *Diabetologia*, 50, 1140–47.

White, N.H., Skor, D.A., Cryer P.E., Levandoski, L.A., Bier, D.M. and Santiago, J.V. 1983. Identification of Type 1 diabetic patients at increased risk for hypoglycemia during intensive therapy. *New England Journal of Medicine*, 308, 485–91.

Widom, B. and Simonson, D.C. 1992. Intermittent hypoglycemia impairs glucose counter-regulation. *Diabetes*, 41, 1597–602.

Wilkinson, R.T. and Houghton, D. 1975. Portable four-choice reaction time test with magnetic tape memory. *Behavioral Research Methods and Instrumentation*, 7, 441–6.

Wirsen, A., Tallroth, G., Lindgren, M. and Agardh, C.D. 1992. Neuropsychological performance differs between Type 1 diabetic and normal men during insulin-induced hypoglycaemia. *Diabetic Medicine*, 9, 156–65.

Zammitt, N.N., Warren, R.E., Deary, I.J. and Frier, B.M. 2008. Delayed recovery of cognitive function following hypoglycemia in adults with Type 1 diabetes: Effect of impaired awareness of hypoglycemia. *Diabetes*, 57, 732–6.

Chapter 15

HEADACHE

Thomas C. Britton

Headache is one of the more common neurological symptoms presenting to the practitioner of aviation medicine, and correct diagnosis and management are crucial to the livelihood and welfare of aircrew, as well as the safety of others. Headache as the only symptom of a brain tumour is rare (Wang *et al.*, 2001), but even migraine and tension-type headache can be a cause of significant disability and functional impairment (Lipton *et al.*, 2001; Steiner *et al.*, 2003) and they require careful assessment. Distinguishing primary headaches from secondary (or symptomatic) headaches and more serious underlying causes is not always straightforward. The history and the neurological examination remain the cornerstone of clinical diagnosis, but magnetic resonance imaging (MRI) and computerized tomography (CT) are increasingly carried out to 'exclude' more serious pathology. While such investigations will almost invariably exclude the pathology being considered, incidental abnormalities may be revealed. An understanding of the significance of such findings is needed, particularly in the context of occupational medicine.

Migraine and tension-type headache are likely to be the most frequent reasons for referral to the aeromedical practitioner. Chronic daily headache and the overuse of medication, although commonly seen in neurological practice, are less likely to be issues. Chronic daily headache is defined as headaches with the features of episodic migraine or tension-type headache occurring on more than 15 days per month for at least three consecutive months, while headache due to the overuse of medication should be considered in patients taking analgesic medications on more than ten days a month (International Headache Society, 2004). Both chronic daily headache and headache due to the overuse of medication disqualify candidates applying for an aviation licence and will not be discussed further.

Individuals with cluster (migrainous neuralgia) and thunderclap headaches present from time to time and need to be investigated and treated. Certain secondary causes of headache, including giant cell arteritis (temporal arteritis) and trigeminal neuralgia, also warrant consideration. Other secondary causes of headache (trauma, vascular disease, structural lesions, infection, metabolic disturbances, drugs, disorders affecting the ear, nose and throat, psychiatric disorders, cranial neuralgias and facial pain) are either dealt with in other chapters or are outside the scope of this book.

Migraine

Migraine remains a clinical diagnosis as no specific laboratory or imaging findings are associated with the condition. The criteria of the International Headache Society (2004) separate migraine with aura (classical migraine) from migraine without aura (common migraine), and these are given below:

○ Common migraine (without an aura) involves headaches lasting between four hours and three days with
  – at least two characteristics (unilateral, pulsating, moderate or severe intensity and aggravated by movement), and
  – associated with either nausea and/or vomiting as well as photophobia and phonophobia, and
  – is not attributable to another cause.
○ Classical migraine (with aura) involves
  – reversible focal dysfunction that develops slowly over more than four minutes and lasts less than an hour followed by
  – migraine headache within an hour.

Chronic migraine and other rarer forms of migraine such as familial hemiplegic migraine are also recognized entities. These are unlikely to be encountered in aircrew and would require specialist investigation. Migraine is more common in women, and a family history is found in up to 90 per cent of patients. The prevalence of migraine in Europe and in the United States is about 18 per cent in women and 6 per cent in men (Lipton *et al.*, 2001). Although migraine is usually separated into those attacks preceded by aura and

those that are unaccompanied by aura, both types may occur within the same individual. Indeed, in clinical practice it is common to encounter patients who have their first attack of migraine with aura in their 20s and 30s and who give a history of occasional headaches over many years which in retrospect is likely to have represented common migraine. There is a tendency for the headache associated with migraine to become less severe with age, while the aura may become more troublesome or noticeable. Some older patients can present with a typical migrainous aura without headache.

Clinical Features

Classical migraine (migraine with aura) may be preceded by a prodrome occurring up to a day before the onset of headache, in which the observant patient may be aware of a change in mood, often reporting feeling uncommonly well with increased appetite.

Auras

The migraine aura is characteristically a positive visual phenomenon evolving over 20 minutes. The patient is usually first aware of a small patch of blurred or distorted vision, sometimes with scintillating, kaleidoscopic colours – termed teichopsia – just a short distance away from central vision. The disturbance then spreads across the visual field to affect a quadrant, half or even the entire visual field.

From the clinical perspective, it is important to note that the patient is aware of (or can 'see') a visual disturbance – that is, they report a positive symptom. In contrast, patients who have had a stroke affecting their visual pathways usually have negative symptoms, only being aware of a hemianopia if they try to read and notice that the words on one or other side 'are not there', or if they bump into an object in their hemianopic field. Focal seizures may of course produce positive symptoms, including poorly defined elemental visual forms and paraesthesiae, but the evolution (or 'march') of such symptoms is generally much faster than the evolution of a migrainous aura.

A typical visual aura characteristically interferes with vision, and patients report that part of their vision is obscured such that they may have difficulty reading or seeing the whole of an object. However, patients rarely report being completely 'blind', usually noting that they can 'see around' the visual disturbance. Static visual field testing in patients with migraine with aura rarely identifies a specific abnormality, although subtle abnormalities can be detected with more sophisticated neurophysiological tests of the visual system (Schoenen, 2006).

Typical visual auras are often associated with sensory symptoms in the limbs or around the face, usually in the form of paraesthesiae which, like the visual aura, evolve over 15 to 20 minutes. Some patients will report difficulty with speech in association with their classical visual aura. Other types of transient neurological disturbance have also be labelled as migrainous aura, including more complex visual disturbances, ataxia, vertigo, dysarthria and impairment of consciousness, although usually only after thorough neurological assessment and always with a degree of caution. Mild unilateral limb weakness occurring with the aura is also reported, but hemiplegic migraine (often familial) is now classified separately. The motor weakness of the latter condition characteristically develops with the headache and lasts for the duration of the attack.

Headache

The headache of migraine usually begins 20 to 40 minutes after the end of the aura, the headache building up in intensity over one to two hours. The headache is typically pulsating and unilateral, and characteristically contralateral to the preceding sensory aura. However, the pain is sometimes more constant and generalized, and may affect the face or, not uncommonly, the back of the head and neck. The severity of headache can be variable. Although the criteria of the International Headache Society (2004) require the headache to be of 'moderate to severe' intensity, some patients with unequivocal migraine (with preceding typical visual aura) may report just a mild 'heaviness' of the head; indeed, it is quite common to encounter patients in the clinic who report having had severe migrainous headaches with nausea and vomiting when younger and who in later years have typical migrainous visual auras that are followed by no (or just a minor) headache.

With the onset of headache, patients usually develop nausea and may vomit – most commonly occurring about an hour after the headache has begun. Other symptoms of heightened 'sensitivity' include photophobia and phonophobia. Patients may also report the dislike of strong odours (osmophobia), but this symptom needs to be distinguished from strong smells that can be a trigger for some auras (see below) and from the occasional patient who has temporal lobe epilepsy associated with olfactory hallucinations followed by a headache. The patient with migraine generally prefers to lie down in a darkened room until the headache has settled (usually getting into bed rather than lying on top of it), and they will often become irritable if unnecessarily stimulated.

However, some patients with migraine may be able to continue to function (for example, if at work), albeit at a reduced level. Patients usually look pale and will report that movement aggravates their symptoms. The headache of migraine usually settles after sleep, but may last up to two to three days. After the headache has disappeared, many patients will still feel lethargic and 'not with it' for several further days.

Triggers

Although chocolate and cheese (and other tyramine-rich foodstuffs) are often incriminated, there is little hard evidence that specific dietary factors are important in triggering headaches or migraines. Monosodium glutamate, found in many prepared foods, may trigger headaches in some susceptible individuals, but it is difficult to avoid the additive completely in a present-day diet. Radical exclusion diets are rarely effective. Drugs such as certain calcium channel blockers (nifedipine) and nitrate medications not uncommonly cause headaches, and it is always prudent to review the medication chart. Whether such drugs 'trigger' typical migraine is uncertain, although glyceryl trinitrate and alcohol have been used in research as a means of triggering cluster headache.

Lifestyle

Most authorities would agree that lifestyle issues play a significant role in triggering migraine. Prolonged fasts and irregular meal times are often associated with headaches. The patient who misses breakfast often develops migraine mid-morning, while the busy office worker who misses lunch may develop a headache in the mid-afternoon. An irregular sleeping habit is also a common trigger for migraine,

and potentially a significant problem for aviation personnel who may be coping with time-zone changes, as with crews operating intercontinental schedules, or who may have early mornings and late nights, as with crews involved in short-haul flying. For the office-based worker, lack of sleep on weekdays or (perhaps more commonly) sleeping in at the weekend are commonly associated with headaches. For patients who develop their headaches after sleeping in at the weekend, successful management should be directed towards ensuring adequate sleep during the week (to avoid building up a sleep debt) rather than just rising at the same time at the weekend. Stress and periods following intense stress are also commonly associated with a higher risk of developing a migraine, although advising a patient to avoid stress and to relax is usually unhelpful. Regular structured exercise (not the exertion of simply walking to work) may be useful.

Pathophysiology

The cause of migraine remains unknown. It is not now thought to be simply 'vascular' in aetiology. The vascular theory was based upon the notion that vasoconstriction of cerebral blood vessels was the cause of the migrainous aura, and that subsequent vasodilatation of extracranial vessels resulted in the headache. In support of the vascular theory, cerebral blood flow studies revealed reduced flow associated with the aura, while dilatation of scalp vessels occurred with the headache phase. However, migraine auras rarely respect vascular territories, making it unlikely that vasospasm of individual arteries could be responsible for the aura. Furthermore, flow studies revealed a period of hyperaemia prior to the period of reduced flow (Olesen *et al.*,

1981) which the vascular theory did not predict. Additional shortcomings with the theory were identified when it was noted that the headache phase could begin prior to the vasodilatation of extracranial vessels (Cutrer *et al.*, 1998).

Most evidence now points towards the aura of migraine having a neurogenic basis (Moskowitz, 2007). The typical visual aura takes about 20 minutes to spread across the visual field, which is consistent with a disturbance of cortical function. The rate of spread is similar to that observed in the phenomenon of spreading electrical depression as first described by Leão (1944). Leão, who was studying the mechanisms underlying epilepsy, prodded the exposed brains of rats with a small rod and recorded a slow wave of electrical depression spreading out across the cortex at a rate of about 3 millimetres a minute. The depression has been shown to consist initially of a wave of increased electrical and metabolic activity, followed by a period of electrical (and metabolic) silence. Although spreading depression would appear to have many of the temporal characteristics required for a migraine aura and it is not constrained by vascular boundaries, it should be emphasized that, at this time, it has not been directly recorded during a migraine aura in humans.

What accounts for the headache phase of migraine with aura remains uncertain. Cortical spreading depression, which is thought to be the basis of the aura, is known to be associated with the release of various excitatory neurotransmitters as well as significant metabolic changes. However, brain tissue is itself insensitive. Pain-sensitive structures within the cranial cavity include the meninges and the proximal arteries and dural sinuses. This apparent dilemma led to the neurovascular theory of migraine. In this theory, the constituents released from the brain by cortical spreading depression are believed to activate the trigeminal innervation of the meninges. Activation of the trigeminal system then leads to vasodilation of blood vessels and headache (Moskowitz, 2007).

Functional imaging and tomography

These investigations (functional magnetic resonance imaging and positive and single photon emission tomography) have confirmed the vascular changes that occur with migraine, but more recently there has been interest in changes in brainstem activity. Interestingly, there appears to be increased activity within the upper brainstem. It is not simply due to the perception of pain (related to the trigeminal nerve nuclei) as there is still increased activity even after the headache is successfully treated with sumatriptan (Bahra *et al.*, 2001). It is possible that the primary 'generator' of migraine lies within the brainstem, with the migrainous auras resulting from changes in cortical excitability due to modulation by brainstem nuclei.

Genetic considerations

Although no structural brain differences have been identified in patients with migraine, there is some neurophysiological evidence to suggest neuronal hyperexcitability even between attacks (Ambrosini *et al.*, 2003). The rare genetic causes of migraine also provide support for the view that neuronal excitability lies at the heart of condition (Montagna, 2004), with both the calcium channel gene mutation (familial hemiplegic migraine type 1) and the sodium-potassium adenosine triphosphatase mutations (familial hemiplegic migraine type 2) being predicted to increase glutamate release at the nerve terminal (Moskowitz, 2007).

However, the exact relationship of these rare genetic conditions to the more common forms of migraine remains uncertain and, in particular, the currently identified mutations responsible for familial hemiplegic migraine do not appear to play a direct role in the more common types of migraine.

Summary

Patients with migraine appear to have an inherent susceptibility to attacks, which clearly separates them from the norm. The increased susceptibility may be the result of neuronal hyperexcitability. Migrainous auras are believed to be associated with cortical spreading depression. The headache results either directly from brainstem structures or via activation of the trigeminal nerve, which is also responsible for the vascular changes seen in association with migraine (the trigeminovascular or neurovascular theory of migraine).

Investigation

The diagnosis of migraine is clinical and no specific laboratory or imaging investigations are required. However, tests are often sought, including brain imaging and a routine blood screen, probably to reassure the practitioner as much as the patient. Although computed tomography of the brain will usually identify major structural intracranial lesions, magnetic resonance imaging is much more sensitive and avoids the use of ionizing radiation. Imaging is generally normal in patients with migraine, although there is a higher incidence of non-specific white matter hyperintensities (Kruit et al, 2004). The significance of these abnormalities of the white matter is uncertain. There is no evidence that they are linked to

neurological deficits, although long-term follow-up studies have not yet been completed. More recently, a possible link between migraine, non-specific white matter lesions on imaging and patency of the foramen ovale has been suggested, although the evidence is still weak (Schwedt *et al.*, 2008).

Distinguishing the non-specific white matter abnormalities seen with typical migraine from more significant intracranial lesions depends on careful and accurate reporting of the scan. Ideally, all imaging should be reported by a neuroradiologist or a radiologist with a special interest in neurological imaging. The non-specific white matter abnormalities with migraine may be mistaken for patches of demyelination or vasculitis, leading to considerable anxiety and unnecessary investigations. On the other hand, there are some rare neurological disorders that can produce migraine-like attacks and progressive neurological disease, such as CADASIL (cerebral autosomal dominant arteriopathy with subcortical infarcts and leukoencephalopathy), which would be important to identify. Research concerned with cerebral blood flow has shown that the aura of migraine is associated with a reduction in cerebral blood flow over the occipital cortex, while the headache phase may be associated with increased cerebral blood flow contralaterally. Functional imaging has revealed increased activity with brainstem structures during the headache phase (May, 2004). These studies are clearly of interest in understanding the pathophysiology of migraine, but none is currently of value in the investigation of an individual patient.

Management

When a diagnosis of migraine is made, the nature of the condition should be explained to the patient, noting that it is a generally benign, albeit painful, disorder. There is no cure for migraine, and successful management should initially be directed toward identifying and avoiding triggering factors, if present. For patients with only infrequent and mild attacks which settle with rest, no further treatment may be necessary. Lifestyle issues are important in reducing the frequency of attacks, and patients should be advised to eat regular meals (but not more) and ensure that their sleeping habits are regular (if possible). Regular exercise tends to improve the sleep–wake cycle – as well as having general health benefits. Most patients will voluntarily take themselves off to a quiet place to sit or lie down as soon as their headache begins. Those who try to continue working when their headache begins are probably best advised to sit or lie down quietly. Those who do not experience severe vomiting early in the course of their migraine may find it helpful to take a small snack (a milk drink and a sandwich) along with their analgesic medication.

Therapeutics

Medication that might be triggering or aggravating the tendency to migraine should be discontinued or substituted, if possible. Use of oral contraceptives may be associated with a worsening of migraine, although this is not invariable. Some find that oral contraceptives actually improve their migraine, perhaps more often in those with migraine occurring around the time of menstruation – menstrual or catamenial migraine. The use of the combined oral contraceptive does give cause for concern because of the risk of ischaemic stroke. Migraine is associated with a small, but significant, increase in stroke (odds ratio

3.5) (Tzourio *et al.*, 1995), the risk being greater in women with migraine with aura (odds ratio 6.2). The risk is further increased by using the combined oral contraceptive pill (odds ratio 13.9). Use of the combined oral contraceptive in migraine with aura is not recommended, but the progesterone-only variety (not associated with the risk of ischaemic stroke) or the low-dose combined contraceptive may be considered. In giving advice, it should be borne in mind that that the absolute risk of a stroke in women aged 20–40 is low – around 7 per 100,000 per year.

Many drugs have been shown to reduce the severity or duration of migraine headaches. They include aspirin, paracetamol, ibuprofen, codeine, ergotamine-containing preparations and triptans. Such medications are often given in combination with an anti-emetic such as prochlorperazine or metoclopramide, with or without caffeine. Numerous over-the-counter preparations are available. The timing of ingestion is important. Delaying the administration until after the headache has become established significantly lessens its efficacy. For patients who have an aura, treatment as soon as the aura begins may even abort the attack prior to the onset of the headache phase, or at least significantly ameliorate its severity. For those with migraine without aura, medication should be taken as soon as possible after the onset of headache. Most patients use oral medication, but there are advantages to using other routes of administration. Subcutaneous injections or medications absorbed buccally may enter the bloodstream more rapidly and more reliably, while suppositories may be useful in those whose headaches are accompanied by severe vomiting.

Treatment with the newer anti-migraine drugs, including the so-called 'triptans' which have strong $5HT_{1B}$ and $5HT_{1D}$ agonist activity, appears to be particularly effective. Up to 50 per cent should expect to be pain-free (or have only a mild headache) by two hours, while the majority (80 per cent) should be helped within four hours. A sumatriptan-naproxen combination, taken within an hour of the onset of headache, will render half free within two hours compared with 15 to 20 per cent given a placebo (Silberstein *et al.*, 2008). Rebound headaches can be problematic with the 'triptans' and may require a further dose within the next 24 hours. Common side effects of 'triptans' include tingling, flushing and a feeling of fullness in the neck or chest.

While the majority of patients with migraine manage their attacks successfully using simple analgesics on an occasional basis (and often without ever having consulted a doctor), there are some patients who experience frequent and disabling attacks and for whom regular prophylactic medication may be considered. The decision as to when to start such medication will depend on individual circumstances. Weekly or more frequent attacks almost always require prophylactic medication, while less frequent attacks (once a month or less) may also be considered, especially if the attacks are severe and disabling. Prophylactic medications that are commonly used include propranolol, amitriptyline, pizotifen, valproate and topiramate. Not all of these, such as low-dose amitriptyline and valproate, are licensed for such use, and only the newer drugs have been subject to formal randomized, placebo-controlled trials. Medication is usually given for a period of three to six months, starting at a low dose and building up slowly until the migraines are satisfactorily controlled.

○ Propranolol, a beta-adrenergic blocker, is usually prescribed at an initial dose of 10 mg three times a day. Although often successful in controlling migraine, side effects and contraindications limit its use. They include the potential to exacerbate asthma and peripheral vascular disease, including the phenomenon described by Raynaud (1834–1881). Some may also experience unpleasant and vivid dreams, a side effect that may be less evident with the less lipophyllic beta blockers. Metoprolol, nadolol and timolol are reported to be effective, with intrinsic sympathomimetic activity seemingly being important for efficacy.

○ Pizotifen is an antihistamine and serotonin antagonist. It is given initially at a dose of 0.5 mg, with the dose being increased in weekly intervals (or longer) to 1.5 mg in the evening. Weight gain and increased appetite are common side effects and can limit its use. Sedation, dry mouth and drowsiness may sometimes be troublesome.

○ Low-dose amitriptyline was shown to be an effective prophylactic 20 years ago (Ziegler *et al.*, 1987), although the drug is not licensed for such use in the United Kingdom. It is usually given at a dose of 10 mg in the evening, the dose being increased every two weeks (or longer) to 20 to 30 mg. The original trials suggested that doses up to 60 or 70 mg could be beneficial. Improved quality of sleep is often reported, probably because of its tendency to suppress rapid eye movement sleep, although excess sedation and a hangover effect can occasionally be problematic. Weight gain is a potentially troublesome side effect. Other tricyclic anti-depressant drugs including imipramine and nortriptyline can be used instead of amitriptyline, but the serotonin re-uptake inhibitors do not appear to have a role in migraine prophylaxis.

○ Valproate was shown to be beneficial in the early 1990s. The drug should be started at a low dose to minimize the risk of side effects. The maintenance dose can be up to 500–1000 mg a day taken in two divided doses. Weight gain, dizziness and sedation often limit its use, and caution is necessary when considering its use in women of child-bearing age because of its teratogenic potential.

○ Topiramate is another anti-epileptic medication which has been shown to be useful (Brandes *et al.*, 2004). It is believed to have effects on both γ-amino-butyric acid (GABA) receptors, as an agonist, and glutamate receptors, as an antagonist, as well as having carbonic anhydrase activity. A starting dose of 25 mg at night for one week can be increased by 25 mg steps up to 50 mg twice a day. Side effects can be a limiting factor, particularly paraesthesiae, although weight loss is often seen as a beneficial side effect.

Cluster Headache

Cluster headache (migrainous neuralgia) is much less common than common migraine, but those with the condition are more likely to seek advice as the pain is invariably severe. The prevalence of cluster headache probably lies between 0.05 and 0.4 per cent of the population, compared with a prevalence for migraine of between 6 and 18 per cent. In contrast with migraine, most patients are male,

and the usual age at presentation is in the second to fourth decades.

Clinical Features

An attack of cluster headache generally lasts about 45 minutes, with the pain being felt in or around one or other eye. The pain is intense and will characteristically wake the patient from sleep. When awake, patients can rarely sit or lie still, preferring to pace around the room or press on their forehead. Some patients will describe an urge to hit their heads against the wall or on the floor to try to relieve the pain. Associated with the pain, the nose will feel congested and the patient may be aware of watering of the eye. The eyelid on the affected side may become oedematous and there may be a partial ptosis. An attack is therefore easy to distinguish from common migraine – the patient with a cluster headache appears agitated and restless in contrast with the patient with typical migraine who usually looks pale and lies quietly in a darkened room.

The name of the condition derives from the tendency for attacks to occur in clusters over a period of two to three months every year or so. A typical patient may describe attacks occurring every night (often at around 1 a.m.) for a period of six weeks or so, followed by spontaneous remission. During a cluster, attacks can occur more than once a day and can be triggered by alcohol or by the use of glyceryl trinitrate, the anti-anginal drug. Most patients quickly recognize the association with alcohol and will avoid alcohol for the duration of the cluster, although between clusters alcohol can usually be consumed without fear of triggering an attack. Recognizing the condition can be more problematic in those who present in their first bout, although a history of previous occasional isolated attacks can often be obtained. Bouts may recur more than once a year or only once every few years, but there is a tendency for attacks to be more common in springtime – at least in the northern hemisphere.

The headache usually remains on the same side for the duration of a cluster, but can switch sides in subsequent clusters. For some patients, attacks can occur outside of clusters, with some individuals experiencing a more chronic form of the condition – chronic cluster headaches as opposed to the more common episodic cluster headache. There is a paucity of literature on the long-term prognosis of cluster headache, but the available evidence suggests that it is a lifelong disorder in most people. In about 10 per cent, episodic cluster headache may develop into chronic cluster headache. However, a substantial proportion of people with cluster headache can expect to develop longer remission periods with increasing age.

The International Headache Society (2004) criteria for cluster headache requires a severe unilateral orbital or periorbital pain lasting between a quarter of an hour and three hours, occurring between every other day and up to eight times a day, that is not attributable to another cause, with, in addition, at least one of the following ipsilateral features:

❍   conjunctival   injection   and/or lachrymation
❍   nasal congestion and/or rhinorrhoea
❍   oedema of the eyelids
❍   sweating of the forehead and/or face
❍   miosis and/or ptosis
❍   a sense of restlessness.

Pathophysiology

The pain of an attack is thought to be linked to vasodilatation in the retro-orbital region. This causes compression on pain-sensitive structures and leads to autonomic dysfunction that accounts for the nasal congestion, lachrymation and partial ptosis. In support of this view is the tendency for attacks to occur at about 1 a.m. – a time when there is general vasodilatation. In addition, vasodilator agents such as alcohol and glyceryl trinitrate can reliably trigger attacks during a cluster. In contrast, treatments such as oxygen (which lead to vasoconstriction) are often useful in the acute management of an attack. Whether patients with cluster headache have some predisposing structural or vascular anomaly remains uncertain, although some investigators have noted that patients are more likely to have more coarse facial features with a more prominent nasolabial fold.

The recurrent clusters, often with a seasonal tendency, suggest an underlying chronobiological basis. Both structural and functional differences within the hypothalamus (a region known to be important in many aspects of chronobiology, including circadian rhythms) have been identified in those with cluster headache. Attacks of cluster headache triggered by glyceryl trinitrate are associated with increased activity within the hypothalamus on functional imaging. High-resolution imaging of the hypothalamus has also revealed differences in the size of the inferior posterior part of the hypothalamus (May et al., 1999). These changes appear to be specific for cluster headaches and are not seen with common migraine or migraine with aura.

Investigations

For a patient with established cluster headache, no further investigation is required. However, the situation is more difficult when the patient presents in their first bout – usually within the first few days of the bout, given the severity of the pain. Sometimes it is possible to obtain a previous history of a few short-lasting clusters, but, in those where there remains doubt as to the diagnosis, imaging of the brain and of the retro-orbital region is generally advised to exclude aneurysms or dissections of the carotid artery or, rarely, structural lesions such as a meningioma.

Management

Patients with cluster headache generally present early to their practitioner. Establishing the diagnosis and excluding other causes are important, but treatment should not be delayed as the pain of cluster headache can be severe enough for otherwise normal individuals even to contemplate suicide. Patients should be appropriately reassured that, although extremely painful, the condition will respond to treatment and should eventually spontaneously remit. Treatment can be divided into acute interventions and prophylactic treatment, although in practice they are generally initiated together; the pain is usually too severe and disruptive for attacks to be manageable using only acute interventions (May et al., 2006). Furthermore, given the rapid onset and short time to peak intensity of cluster headache, acute treatments are often of limited value.

No acute intervention can immediately abolish the pain of an acute attack of cluster headache, but many patients note that moving to an open window and taking deep breaths can be helpful. How and why hyperventilation helps remains uncertain, but vasoconstriction of the cranial arterial system may be important. For some, the administration of oxygen can abort an attack of cluster headache. A high flow rate (at least 8 litres per minute) with a tight-fitting mask is required, and patients are advised to sit upright. There are no contraindications for the use of oxygen. It is safe and without side effects. About 60 per cent of all patients with cluster headache respond to this treatment with a significant reduction in pain within half an hour. For those who benefit, oxygen therapy can be very effective, despite the logistical difficulties of arranging domiciliary oxygen.

Subcutaneous sumatriptan is the only licensed treatment for cluster headache, given at a dosage of 6 mg as soon as possible after the onset of pain. Approximately 75 per cent can expect to have relief of their symptoms within 15 minutes (Ekbom et al., 1993). Nasally administered sumatriptan may also be effective (van Vliet et al., 2003), but orally administered formulations are less helpful. Although the onset can often be predicted, sumatriptan is not effective if given in anticipation of an attack. Other parenterally administered 'triptan' medications may also be helpful but have not been examined in clinical trials. More recently, subcutaneous octreotide (100 µg) has been shown to be effective in the treatment of acute cluster headache attacks in a double-blind, placebo-controlled trial (Matharu et al., 2004).

Verapamil in dosages starting at 80 mg three times a day is probably the most commonly used prophylactic drug, although unlicensed. The dose may need to be increased to 960 mg per day, depending on response and side effects. It is thought to work predominantly via its calcium channel blocking properties, inhibiting calcium ion influx into the vascular smooth muscle cells and consequently blocking the sequence of events leading to muscle contraction. Cardiac side effects are potentially the most important; serial electrocardiograms are recommended during dose titration and may be needed in the longer term. Monitoring is concerned with changes suggestive of heart block, such as prolongation of PR interval, change in cardiac axis and/or broadening of QRS complex. A number of drugs interact with Verapamil and should be avoided, the most important being beta blockers and digoxin.

Corticosteroids are clearly effective in cluster headache, although there are no randomized, placebo-controlled trials to support their use. Open studies of steroids given under different regimens suggest that 70 to 80 per cent will respond to steroids. The usual initial daily dose of prednisolone is 60 to 100 mg for at least five days, then tapering the dose by 10 mg each day. Steroids can be used to obtain rapid control while the dosage of other prophylactic drugs, such as verapamil, is being increased. There are some patients who appear to require continuous administration of steroids, and intravenous steroids can occasionally be useful. Methysergide, lithium and topiramate are also commonly used as prophylactic agents, but their use in cluster headache is not licensed, and such patients should ideally be managed by a physician with a special interest in headache.

Tension-Type Headache

Like migraine, tension-type headache is a clinical diagnosis, and the International Headache Society (2004) has produced diagnostic criteria as follows:

○ Tension-type headaches are not associated with nausea or vomiting, photophobia or phonophobia and last between half an hour and seven days with at least two of the following features:
  – bilateral
  – pressing (not pulsating) quality
  – mild to moderate intensity
  – not aggravated by routine activities and
  – cannot be attributed to another cause.

Tension-type headache is common, with the population prevalence of an attack in the previous year being 63 per cent in men and 86 per cent in women (Rasmussen *et al.*, 1991). All ages are susceptible, but most are young adults. Fortunately, the headache is rarely severe and usually responds well to non-prescription drugs, and in most cases will not lead to seeking medical advice.

Clinical Features

Tension-type headache is typically of only mild to moderate severity, non-pulsating and bilateral, and often felt over the forehead or back of the neck. Patients frequently describe the pain as a feeling of tightness or squeezing. Compared with migraine, the pain is usually more gradual in onset and the duration more variable, lasting from half an hour to a week. A preceding sensory aura does not occur, and sensitivity to noise or light is less frequently reported. Tension-type headaches may occur acutely under emotional distress or intense worry and are often associated with insomnia and complaints of difficulty concentrating. Neurological examination should be normal, although there may be mild tenderness elicited over the scalp or neck. The temporal arteries should not be tender and there should be no nuchal rigidity.

Pathophysiology

The underlying pathophysiology of tension-type headache remains unknown. At one time, stress was thought to cause contraction of neck and scalp muscles, leading to pain as a result of sustained muscle contraction. However, there is no direct evidence to support this view, and the International Headache Society prefers the term 'tension-type headache' to 'tension headache' or 'muscle contraction headache'. Both muscular and psychogenic factors probably play a role.

Investigations

No specific investigations are required for tension-type headache, the diagnosis being made on clinical grounds alone. However, investigations are often requested to exclude other conditions. Whenever there is concern about a diagnosis of temporal arteritis, the sedimentation rate should be determined. For those with significant neck pain, radiographs or imaging of the cervical spine may be appropriate. Imaging of the brain, although often requested, is not required unless the headache is of recent onset in an older patient.

Management

Effective management of tension headache usually consists of simple, over-the-counter analgesics such as paracetamol, aspirin, ibuprofen and other non-steroidal anti-inflammatory agents, as well as massage, relaxation or even a hot bath. Patients with frequent tension-type headaches should be alerted to the risk of the overuse of medication. Some patients may benefit from low-dose amitriptyline, the drug being given in a similar way as when used as a prophylactic drug for migraine. Depression associated with tension-type headache should be treated appropriately.

Thunderclap Headache

An abrupt onset (that is, within seconds) of severe headache is always a cause for concern and requires further assessment, although often no specific underlying cause can be identified. Depending on the circumstances and the associated symptoms and signs, the patient needs to be evaluated for a possible subarachnoid haemorrhage with appropriate brain imaging and, if necessary, examination of the cerebrospinal fluid. Other causes are infections (including meningitis), cerebral venous sinus thrombosis, dissection of the carotid or vertebral arteries, and pituitary apoplexy, although there are usually other pointers to these diagnoses in the history or in the examination. A severe headache of sudden onset that occurs during sexual intercourse, beginning just before or at the time of climax and lasting less than half an hour, is likely to indicate benign coital headache. However, in many cases of thunderclap headache (benign thunderclap headache), there is no definite explanation despite careful investigation (Schwedt *et al.*, 2006).

Trigeminal Neuralgia

Trigeminal neuralgia is relatively uncommon, but its severity will almost invariably bring the patient to medical attention. The incidence of new cases varies between 4 and 20 per 100,000 of the population per year, the condition becoming more common with age. The incidence is similar to that of post-herpetic neuralgia. More women are affected than men, with a ratio of about 3:2, and the right side of the face is more frequently affected than the left for reasons that are not clear (Manzoni and Torelli, 2005).

Clinical Features

Trigeminal neuralgia is felt as a brief lancinating or shock-like facial pain, usually within the distribution of the mandibular division of the trigeminal nerve, and may at first be mistaken for dental pain. Occasionally, the pain is felt within the maxillary division, along the upper jaw or in the cheek. Trigeminal neuralgia within the ophthalmic division is much rarer and should prompt a search for other causes. Attacks of trigeminal neuralgia last only a few seconds, but the pain is so intense that patients will stop what they are doing, often cupping their hand around the affected jaw while they wait fearfully for the next attack. Repetitive bursts of attacks often occur over a few minutes. Between attacks (or bursts of attacks), some patients are aware of a more continuous dull ache within the same territory. Trigeminal neuralgia can be triggered by various factors, including cold air blowing over the face (especially on winter mornings), washing the face or cleaning the teeth. As a result of the pain, patients may stop brushing their teeth on the affected side, while males may shave only half of the face.

Pathophysiology

Trigeminal neuralgia arises as a result of irritation to the trigeminal nerve,

but in the majority of cases no specific structural lesion can be identified. In approximately 15 per cent, high-resolution imaging will identify a vascular loop in close proximity to the nerve near its root entry zone. The vascular loop is presumed to cause compression of the nerve, and it is on this basis that treatment with microvascular decompression is carried out.

In a small minority of patients, imaging will identify a structural abnormality other than a vascular loop. Such abnormalities can include demyelinating plaques (of multiple sclerosis) within the brainstem, tumours, intracranial aneurysms and abnormalities of the skull base. Those with an identifiable structural abnormality on imaging are labelled symptomatic trigeminal neuralgia, while those without any associated structural lesion (except for possible neurovascular contact) are labelled classic trigeminal neuralgia. Patients with classic trigeminal neuralgia should have no clinically evident neurological deficit.

Investigations

The diagnosis of trigeminal neuralgia is clinical and is based on the patient's description of the pain with its typical temporal and anatomical features. For those with classic trigeminal neuralgia, there should be no additional neurological findings and neurophysiological studies of the trigeminal nerve should be normal. Investigations are carried out to exclude secondary causes of trigeminal neuralgia and will generally include imaging of the brain and cerebellopontine angle, along with routine blood tests. These include a full blood count, erythrocyte sedimentation rate, electrolytes, glucose and liver enzyme levels. They are also useful prior to starting carbamazepine treatment. Angiography, examination of the cerebrospinal fluid and a search for metastatic disease depend on the individual case.

Management

The treatment of trigeminal neuralgia has been reviewed recently (Gronseth *et al.*, 2008) and is usefully considered from both the medical and surgical aspects.

Carbamazepine and oxcarbazepine are first-line therapies. Carbamazepine is probably more efficacious than oxcarbazepine but is associated with more side effects. The initial dose of carbamazepine is usually 100 mg twice daily, but the dose often needs to be escalated rapidly to control the pain. Unfortunately, rapid dose escalation of carbamazepine is associated with a greater risk of allergic reactions, and many patients require doses that produce side effects including nausea, ataxia and double vision. Oxcarbazepine is usually started at a dosage of 300 mg twice daily and increased to 900 mg twice daily. There is little evidence to guide the clinician when first-line medical therapy fails. Lamotrigine and baclofen are probably of benefit and commonly used. The efficacy of other drugs commonly used in neuropathic pain (gabapentin, pregabalin) is unknown. There are no published studies directly comparing polytherapy with monotherapy. Other drugs that have been used include valproate, clonazepam, phenytoin and topiramate.

Those with classic trigeminal neuralgia who do not respond to medical treatment or who develop unacceptable side effects on medical treatment should be considered for surgical management. Some with trigeminal neuralgia respond well to medical treatment initially, but their symptoms return once the dose of carbamazepine is reduced. In others,

medical treatment may have provided adequate benefit previously, but recurrent bouts of trigeminal neuralgia over the years may become less responsive to medication.

Several surgical techniques are used for trigeminal neuralgia. They include blocking or destruction of peripheral portions of the trigeminal nerve, trigeminal ganglion percutaneous procedures, posterior fossa microvascular decompression and gamma knife radiosurgery of the trigeminal root entry zone. None of these surgical techniques has been investigated in formal trials. Peripheral techniques involve blocking or destruction of portions of the trigeminal nerve distal to the trigeminal ganglion, usually within the cheek. Various methods and substances have been used, including streptomycin and lidocaine injections, cryotherapy, surgical extirpation (neurectomies), alcohol and phenol injections, peripheral acupuncture, and radiofrequency thermocoagulation. Few of these treatments have been subjected to clinical trials. Although there may be a good initial response, the recurrence of pain after a year is probably about 50 per cent. An advantage of these techniques, however, is their low morbidity.

Percutaneous procedures involving the trigeminal ganglion involve the insertion of a needle under radiographic control through the foramen ovale into the trigeminal cistern to make controlled lesions of the trigeminal ganglion or root. Various means are used, including radiofrequency thermocoagulation, chemical injection (glycerol) and mechanical compression by a balloon inflated into Meckel's Cave. The position of the needle and the size of the lesion can be controlled, to a certain extent, by waking the patient at the start of the procedure. There are no trials of any of these procedures, but uncontrolled case series suggest that 70 to 80 per cent can expect to be pain-free at one year, the proportion falling to about 50 per cent at three to five years. Sensory loss after these percutaneous procedures is present in almost half of patients, while about 5 per cent may develop troublesome dysaesthesias and 4 per cent develop anaesthesia dolorosa (severe spontaneous pain occurring in an anesthetized area). Corneal anaesthesia is a rare but potentially serious complication of treatment. Surgical mortality is extremely low and percutaneous procedures on the trigeminal ganglion can be carried out on patients who are in a relatively poor general medical condition.

Microvascular decompression is a major neurosurgical procedure, requiring a posterior fossa craniotomy to reach the trigeminal nerve and to separate it from any blood vessels. Patients need to be medically fit and accept the risks that include a mortality of 0.2 per cent. However, the results of microvascular decompression (at least from uncontrolled case series) suggest that 80 per cent will be pain-free at one year and 73 per cent at five years. Serious post-operative complications include leaks of the cerebrospinal fluid, haematomas, aseptic meningitis and hearing loss, but microvascular decompression probably offers the best prognosis for long-term control of what is otherwise a severely disabling condition.

Gamma knife surgery involves focused radiotherapy of the trigeminal root in the posterior fossa. Again, there are no trials of this technique, but case series suggest that 70 per cent may be free of pain at one year, the proportion falling to 50 per cent at three years. Although sensory symptoms and paraesthesiae are common side effects, anaesthesia dolorosa rarely occurs. Gamma knife surgery avoids the need for invasive surgery, and quality-of-life

studies suggest that the technique is successful for the majority of patients.

Giant Cell Arteritis

Giant cell arteritis (temporal arteritis) should always be considered in patients over the age of 50 years who present with a recent unilateral or temporal headache. The incidence of giant cell arteritis in populations of European origin is approximately 20 per 100,000 persons older than 50 years, the rates being higher in northern Europe than in Mediterranean countries. The incidence appears to be significantly less in Japan at 1 to 2 per 100,000 of the population over the age of 50 years. Women are affected two to three times more often than men. Some studies have reported seasonal variations, with an increase in incidence in late spring and early summer.

Clinical Features

Patients with giant cell arteritis are usually aged over 60 years and present with a mild to moderate unilateral headache, frequently in association with systemic symptoms of general malaise, anorexia and weight loss. Other characteristic features include scalp sensitivity (especially when brushing the hair) and jaw claudication when eating. Jaw claudication is a high predictor of giant cell arteritis but is not pathognomonic. Occasionally, intermittent claudication can affect the arms, tongue or the muscles involved in swallowing. It is not uncommon for these additional symptoms to have been present (in retrospect) for several weeks or months before the diagnosis is made. On examination, the superficial temporal arteries may be thickened and tender, and non-pulsatile. A mild pyrexia is common and may be the main clinical feature. Indeed, about 15 per cent of pyrexias of unknown origin in patients over 65 are eventually attributed to giant cell arteritis (Salvarani *et al.*, 2008).

Permanent, partial or complete loss of vision in one or both eyes is often an early manifestation of giant cell arteritis. The visual loss is painless, and once one eye is affected there is a high risk that the other eye will also become affected within one to two weeks unless adequate corticosteroid treatment is given. The arteritis can also affect the blood vessels arising from the aortic arch resulting in bruits, absent peripheral pulses, symptoms of claudication and, later, aneurysm formation. Neurologically, patients may develop neuropathies, transient ischaemic attacks and strokes. Scalp necrosis, ulceration or infarction of the tongue, pericardial and pleural effusions are occasionally encountered. Hunder *et al.* (1990) have prepared criteria for the diagnosis of giant cell arteritis as follows:

❍ 50 years or over
❍ localized pain in the head and of recent onset
❍ tenderness to palpation of temporal artery or decreased pulsation
❍ not related to arteriosclerosis of cervical arteries
❍ erythrocyte sedimentation rate greater than 50 mm per hour
❍ biopsy of artery with vasculitis characterized by mononuclear cell infiltration, granulomatous inflammation or multinucleated giant cells.

Pathophysiology

Giant cell arteritis affects the large and medium-sized arteries, especially the proximal aorta and its branches. These blood vessels are notable for their prominent internal elastic membrane and vasa vasorum, which may be relevant to the underlying pathophysiology. In contrast, the intracranial arteries, which are rarely directly affected by the condition, are thinner and do not have vasa vasorum. Histologically, the affected arteries show a granulomatous inflammatory infiltrate with lymphocytes, macrophages and multinucleated giant cells, the latter usually being located at the intima-media junction. The underlying cause of the arteritis remains unknown. The geographical and the apparent seasonal variation in the incidence of the disease suggest that both genetic and environmental factors are important. An infectious aetiology has been proposed, but as yet no specific virus has been identified as a trigger. There is some evidence for an association of giant cell arteritis with certain human leucocyte antigens.

Investigation

Once the diagnosis is considered, the sedimentation rate should be determined immediately. A markedly raised rate is strongly supportive of the diagnosis. However, a normal rate does not exclude the diagnosis, and if the condition is still suspected, then temporal artery biopsy should be undertaken. The long-term management of the condition is made easier if a definitive histological diagnosis can be obtained. Temporal artery biopsy is probably justified in all cases, even if the history is typical and the sedimentation rate is markedly raised. A temporal artery biopsy must not delay treatment but should ideally be undertaken within a few days of starting corticosteroids. Only about 50 per cent of routine biopsy samples show all the characteristic features of the condition and many biopsies will be non-diagnostic or even normal. However, a normal or non-diagnostic biopsy, as with a normal sedimentation rate, does not by itself exclude the diagnosis of giant cell arteritis, and the diagnosis should be made on the basis of all the clinical features.

Management

Treatment must be started immediately. High-dose steroids, such as prednisolone 60 mg daily, should be given, together with appropriate medication to reduce the risk of gastric ulceration and loss of bone density. Patients often report a sudden and dramatic improvement in their symptoms within a day. Even if the temporal artery biopsy is subsequently non-diagnostic, steroid treatment should be continued where there are strong clinical reasons for suspecting the diagnosis. Steroid treatment should be gradually reduced, but most patients will need to be on treatment for at least 18 months. The rate at which steroid treatment is reduced should be based on symptoms and the sedimentation rate. After an initial two- to four-week period of high-dose prednisolone, the dose can usually be lowered to around 40 mg per day. Thereafter, the dose should be reduced as the symptoms and the sedimentation rate allow, with a reduction of about 5 mg per day every four weeks down to 20 mg per day, and then in smaller steps of 1 to 2 mg per day every month. Even with gradual reduction of doses of steroids, clinical flares have been reported to occur in more than 50 per cent, particularly during the first year.

Steroid-related side effects are unfortunately very common, in part related to the age of the typical patient and in part to the high doses needed to control the symptoms adequately. In one population-based study, more than 80 per cent of patients with giant cell arteritis had adverse events, including bone fractures, avascular necrosis of the hip, diabetes mellitus, infections, gastrointestinal bleeding, cataract and hypertension. Calcium and vitamin D supplements, bisphosphonates and gastric protection should be considered in all patients, along with regular blood glucose estimations. Faced with increasingly problematic steroid-related side effects in a patient who is asymptomatic with respect to the original symptoms (and who may not be able to remember the initial headaches), a positive temporal artery biopsy obtained at the outset is always helpful. For those at particularly high risk of steroid-related side effects, methotrexate may be useful.

Headache and Aeromedical Practice

The complaint of headache by aircrew must always be taken seriously. Occasionally, headache may be the only presenting symptom of a brain tumour. However, even headaches that are not associated with structural intracranial lesions can often cause acute and unpredictable symptomatology that could compromise the safety of a flight. The decision as to whether an individual can be licensed to operate an aircraft, either commercial or private, rests finally with the aeromedical practitioner, but it is appropriate to consider the differential diagnoses and prognoses of the various conditions described in this chapter. In relation to migraine, it must be emphasized that attacks are often unpredictable and frequently associated with significant disability and functional impairment (Lipton et al., 2001; Steiner et al., 2003).

A diagnosis of migraine will, therefore, generally disqualify an applicant for a commercial licence, although the aeromedical practitioner might consider an individual with only occasional attacks as suitable for licensing as a private pilot. The diagnosis of migraine in an individual who already holds a commercial licence presents a difficult clinical decision but will likely result in some restriction to flying, depending on the nature and frequency of attacks. If the attacks are infrequent, they may be permitted to continue flying with a co-pilot, but the aeromedical practitioner must bear in mind that incapacitation associated with attacks of migraine can be prolonged, and due account would have to be taken of the operational implications of such an event.

Attacks of cluster headache are extremely disabling and would inevitably compromise the ability to operate an aircraft. Within a cluster, there would be the increased risk of further attacks that would not be predictable. Even when a cluster has been successfully treated, there would still be the risk of recurrence, and therefore, with a diagnosis of cluster headache, the practitioner would need to consider the advisability of a continued licence.

On the other hand, almost everyone suffers occasional tension-type headaches, and as long as the attacks remain infrequent and mild, they do not pose a significant problem for aircrew. However, again, the aeromedical practitioner may consider some restrictions to flying if the headaches interfere with normal activities, occur more than three times a year or require prescription medicines.

Thunderclap headache is generally considered a benign condition of unknown cause, provided a subarachnoid haemorrhage has been excluded. Follow-up of patients with thunderclap headache (Savitz *et al.*, 2009) who have undergone computed tomography and lumbar puncture suggests that the risk of a subsequent aneurysmal bleed is very low, and therefore, in uncomplicated cases, a diagnosis of isolated thunderclap headache should not have major implications for flight crew.

Trigeminal neuralgia is a disabling condition and would inevitably interfere with an individual's ability to continue flying. Treatment of the condition is not always satisfactory and there is also the risk that the pain will recur, even when initial medical or surgical treatment has been successful. When treated medically, patients also commonly experience side effects of medication. A diagnosis of trigeminal neuralgia should therefore inevitably lead to restriction of flying privileges. However, in the case of aircrew who have been successfully treated surgically, the aeromedical practitioner will need to consider the prognosis and the implications for flying on a case-by-case basis.

Giant cell arteritis can cause visual loss as well as strokes and neuropathies; however, with appropriate treatment over a period of time that is likely to be up to two years, the prognosis is good. During treatment, the aeromedical practitioner should take into account the side effects of treatment, including steroid-induced psychiatric disorders.

Acknowledgement

The author is grateful to Dr Sam Chong, Consultant Neurologist, King's College Hospital, London, for his helpful advice and suggestions.

References

Ambrosini, A., de Noordhout, A.M., Sandor, P.S. and Schoenen, J. 2003. Electrophysiological studies in migraine: A comprehensive review of their interest and limitations. *Cephalalgia* (Suppl.), 23, 13–31.

Bahra, A., Matharu, M.S., Buchel, C., Frackowiak, R.S. and Goadsby, P.J. 2001. Brainstem activation specific to migraine headache. *Lancet*, 357, 1016–7.

Brandes, J.L., Saper, J.R., Diamond, M., Couch, J.R., Lewis, D.W., Schmitt, J. *et al.* 2004. Topiramate for migraine prevention: A randomized controlled trial. *Journal of the American Medical Association*, 291, 965–73.

Cutrer, F.M., Sorensen, A.G., Weisskoff, R.M., Ostergaard, L., Sanchez del Rio, M., Lee, E.J. *et al.* 1998. Perfusion-weighted imaging defects during spontaneous migrainous aura. *Annals of Neurology*, 43, 25–31.

Ekbom, K., Monstad, I., Prusinski, A., Cole, J.A., Pilgrim, A.J. and Noronha, D. 1993. Subcutaneous sumatriptan in the acute treatment of cluster headache: A dose comparison study. The Sumatriptan Cluster Headache Study Group. *Acta Neurologica Scandinavica*, 88, 63–9.

Gronseth, G., Cruccu, G., Alksne, J., Argoff, C., Brainin, M., Burchiel, K. *et al.* 2008. Practice Parameter: The diagnostic evaluation and treatment of trigeminal neuralgia (an evidence-based review). Report of the Quality Standards Subcommittee of the American Academy of Neurology and the European Federation of Neurological Societies. *Neurology*, 71, 1183–90.

Hunder, G.G., Bloch, D.A., Michel, B.A., Stevens, M.B., Arend, W.P., Calabrese, L.H. *et al.* 1990. The American College of Rheumatology 1990 criteria for the classification of giant cell arteritis. *Arthritis and Rheumatism*, 33, 1122–8.

International Headache Society. 2004. The International Classification of Headache Disorders, Second Edition. *Cephalalgia* (Suppl.), 24, 1–160.

Kruit, M.C., van Buchem, M.A., Hofman, P.A.M., Bakkers, J.T., Terwindt, G.M., Ferrari, M.D. *et al.* 2004 Migraine is a risk factor for subclinical brain lesions. *Journal of the American Medical Association*, 291, 427–43.

Leão, A.A.P. 1944. Spreading depression of activity in the cerebral cortex. *Journal of Neurophysiology*, 7, 359–90.

Lipton, R.B., Stewart, W.F., Diamond, S., Diamond, M.L., Reed, M. *et al.* 2001. Prevalence and burden of migraine in the United States: Data from the American Migraine Study II. *Headache*, 41, 646–57.

Manzoni, G.C. and Torelli, P. 2005. Epidemiology of typical and atypical craniofacial neuralgias. *Neurological Sciences* (Suppl.), 26, 65–7.

Matharu, M.S., Levy, M.J., Meeran, K. and Goadsby, P.J. 2004. Subcutaneous octreotide in cluster headache: Randomized placebo-controlled double-blind crossover study. *Annals of Neurology*, 56, 488–94.

May, A. 2004. The contribution of functional neuroimaging to primary headaches. *Neurological Sciences*, 25, S85–8.

May, A.J., Ashburner, J., Büchel, C., McGonigle, D.J., Friston, K.J., Frackowiak, R.S.J. et al, 1999. Correlation between structural and functional changes in the brain in an idiopathic headache syndrome. *Nature Medicine*, 5, 836–8.

May, A., Leone, M., Afra, J., Linde, M., Sándor, P.S., Evers, S. *et al.* 2006. EFNS guidelines on the treatment of cluster headache and other trigeminal-autonomic cephalalgias. *European Journal of Neurology*, 13, 1066–77.

Montagna, P. 2004. The physiopathology of migraine: The contribution of genetics. *Neurological Sciences*, 25, S93–6.

Moskowitz, M.A. 2007. Pathophysiology of headache – past and present. *Headache* (Suppl.), 47, 58–63.

Olesen, J., Larsen, B. and Lauritzen, M. 1981. Focal hyperemia followed by spreading oligemia and impaired activation of rCBF in classic migraine. *Annals of Neurology*, 9, 344–52.

Rasmussen, B.K., Jensen, R., Schroll, M. and Olesen, J. 1991. Epidemiology of headache in a general population: A prevalence study. *Journal of Clinical Epidemiology*, 44, 1147–57.

Salvarani, C., Cantini, F. and Hunder, G.G. 2008. Polymyalgia rheumatica and giant-cell arteritis. *Lancet*, 372, 234–45.

Savitz, S.I., Levitana, E.B., Wearsa, R. and Edlow, J.A. 2009. Pooled analysis of patients with thunderclap headache evaluated by CT and LP: Is angiography necessary in patients with negative evaluations? *Journal of the Neurological Sciences*, 276, 123–5.

Schoenen, J. 2006. Neurophysiological features of the migrainous brain. *Neurological Sciences*, 27, 77–81.

Schwedt, T., Demaerschalk, B.M. and Dodick, D.W. 2008. Patent foramen ovale and migraine: A quantitative systematic review. *Cephalalgia*, 28, 531–40.

Schwedt, T.J., Matharu, M.S. and Dodick, D.W. 2006. Thunderclap headache. *Lancet Neurology*, 5, 621–31.

Silberstein, S.D., Mannix, L.K., Goldstein, J., Couch, J.R., Byrd, S.C. and Ames, M.H. 2008. Multimechanistic (sumatriptan-naproxen) early intervention for the acute treatment of migraine. *Neurology*, 71, 114–21.

Steiner, T.J., Scher, A.I., Stewart, W.F., Kolodner, K., Liberman, J. and Lipton, R.B. 2003. The prevalence and disability of adult migraine in England and their relationships to age, gender and ethnicity. *Cephalalgia*, 23, 519–27.

Tzourio, C., Tehindrazanarivelo, A., Iglésias, S., Alpérovitch, A., Chedru, F., d'Anglejan-Chatillon, J. *et al.* 1995. Case-control study of migraine and risk of ischaemic stroke in young women. *British Medical Journal*, 310, 830–33.

van Vliet, J.A., Bahra, A., Martin, V., Ramadan, N., Aurora, S.K., Mathew, N.T. *et al.* 2003. Intranasal sumatriptan in cluster headache: Randomized placebo-controlled double-blind study. *Neurology*, 60, 630–33.

Wang, H.Z., Simonson, T.M., Greco, W.R. and Yuh, W.T. 2001. Brain MR imaging in the evaluation of chronic headache in patients without other neurologic symptoms. *Academic Radiology*, 8, 405–8.

Ziegler, D.K., Hurwitz, A., Hassanein, R.S., Kodanaz, H.A., Preskorn, S.H. and Mason, J. 1987. Migraine prophylaxis: A comparison of propranolol and amitriptyline. *Archives of Neurology*, 44, 486–9.

.

Chapter 16

TRAUMATIC BRAIN INJURY
AND
AEROMEDICAL LICENSING

Garth S. Cruickshank

Traumatic brain injury represents a significant cause of neurological problems in those seeking aeromedical licensing. The initial injury can vary, at the mildest, from a short (less than 30-minute) period of loss of consciousness to severe injury with neurological deficit and evidence from a computer tomographic (CT) scan of intracranial bleeding or damage. Imaging has contributed much to the understanding of both the pathology of injury and its extent and, perhaps most usefully, to the prediction of outcome. For aeromedical licensing, the applicants will have recovered to a great extent and the assessor must weigh the factors that allow determination of the risk of disabling problems occurring in the future.

Guidance on civil aviation medicine, as with the publication from the International Civil Aviation Organization (2008), proposes that in-flight incapacitation should be estimated in terms of annual percentage risk. Whilst this has simplified the derivation of individual risk, new data and approaches have now brought into question the threshold levels used. The manual recommends a risk of disabling events at 'no greater than one per cent' per annum. This implies not only a detailed analysis of initial risk but also an understanding of the confidence limits for the profile with respect to time from injury. Whilst it is relatively easy for the assessor to be strict with the interpretation, more explicit and publicized description of risk thresholds will encourage the borderline applicant to test the robustness of the assessment process, especially where new evidence and its interpretation may be conditional issues.

In this chapter, acute care of traumatic brain injury is reviewed and followed by a detailed analysis of risk for post-traumatic epilepsy at the one per cent level. A review of the other sequelae focuses on the difficulties of assessing post-concussion, focal neurological deficits and cognitive problems. These issues retain the absolute need for clinical expertise in their interpretation for aeromedical licensing, where the evidence base is less than clear in describing risk related to an individual's performance.

Acute Care

In the United Kingdom, there are approximately a million reported head injuries per year. Of these, around 100,000 will need, at least, overnight observation in hospital, with around 10,000 triaged against standard criteria to require transfer or involvement of a specialist neurosurgical centre. This situation may change in favour of early direct referral to neurosurgical units if certain recommendations, for example those of the National Confidential Enquiry into Patient Outcome and Death (2007), become widely implemented. That would imply that, as well as taking patients requiring immediate neurosurgical interventions, all patients with a level of less than 14 on the Glasgow Coma Scale would be managed in neurosurgical units (London Trauma Office, 2010). It is important to realize that only a relatively small proportion, with more severe head injuries, apparently require intensive neurosurgical input, and as result the majority of head injuries are looked after by non-specialized medical personnel with limited training.

Concomitant with this is ability in history taking and clinical observation in a difficult acute area. It is increasingly clear that there is a need for neurotrauma expertise not only in acute care but also in the early risk assessment of head injuries. Indeed, there is increasing evidence from the ready availability of imaging that apparently mild to moderate head injuries may harbour structural damage (Schrader *et al.*, 2009). Furthermore, there is the lasting promise that a likely impact on future performance of

patients from apparently minor head injuries will remain a matter of concern to all who have the responsibility of advising both patients and regulators. It is, therefore, a challenge to the clinical assessor to recognize a pattern of risk to make the interpretation of future performance and current clinical need.

Severity of Head Injury

A key issue in the determination of possible sequelae from a head injury has traditionally and, indeed currently, depended upon the assessment of the severity of the injury. Clinical management hinges around the definition of conscious level by virtue of the Glasgow Coma Scale (Teasdale and Jennett, 1974; Jennett and Teasdale, 1977) and the presence or absence of skull fracturing as an additive factor to risk. In addition, the assessment of post-traumatic amnesia has been shown in numerous studies to support prediction of early discharge from hospital and late recovery outcome (Brown *et al.*, 2005). In the acute clinical situation, it is the level of the Glasgow Coma Scale that provides most useful insight into the risk of evolution of a primary head injury into secondary insults to the brain. Though invaluable in the acute situation, it also has significant bearing on the prediction of long-term sequelae. The Glasgow Coma Scale is given in an addendum to this chapter.

It has also to be remembered that in trying to assess the risks of delayed sequelae from brain trauma, population-based studies are very imprecise at determining specific risks. From an operational point of view, it is important to determine as precisely as possible over which time period the risk should be assessed. What would be the risk of developing a seizure (for example) in the next year? This is different from what the risk might be of having epilepsy after a head injury, which has no determined time frame. The first description is more useful for the assessor. Unfortunately, for those who have to carry out these assessments, the literature is sparse on classification into population groups by virtue of their subsequent profile – for example, the subsequent risk of developing a seizure at the end of one year after head injury, in the prospective year, with signs of contusion on the CT scan, but no alteration in the Glasgow Coma Scale.

In defining a particular risk, there are some limited data that help guide the definition of severity with respect to a particular head injury, but the assessor will need to use a degree of judgement as to where on a scale of risk severity a patient may sit. From a legislative point of view, regulatory authorities may use risk profiling in a pragmatic way, setting the risk of a disability event in the next year. One should note that this is quite a different assessment from saying what the risk of epilepsy or symptoms might be over a ten-year period.

Commonly, the severity of head injury is classified by the Glasgow Coma Scale at particular moments in time. It is frequently taught to medical students that the initial appraisal of the Glasgow Coma Scale arises from when the patient is first assessed after a head injury. Of course, this may be immediate or it may be after a delayed period. This primary assessment is made by whoever sees the patient initially and gives a description of whether the patient was moving, making sounds or opening their eyes. This can be readily reinterpreted in terms of the scale. Assuming there is at least some delay in transferring the patient from the site of injury to the accident and emergency department, the elapsed time means that a second assessment of

the scale at entry into the department allows for trajectory of the assessment to be determined and so facilitate early decisions about potential secondary risks and management. The delay in transferring patients from the site of injury to the department can, of course, vary enormously, but, from the point of view of the doctor in the department, this differential information is crucial.

What, then, was the level of the Glasgow Coma Scale at the time of the head injury? Often it is the assessment in the accident and emergency department rather than information at the site of injury, and it is important for the assessor to try to understand what may have occurred in the intervening period when they have to review the situation retrospectively. For example, it is often difficult to determine whether an episode of concussion has truly occurred in the hiatus that can surround trauma. Most experts in the area of brain injury now believe that any injury involving even a brief loss of consciousness must be considered as harbouring an area of brain injury, and that this must undoubtedly carry a risk of sequelae. Patients who are unconscious from the time of injury must be considered as having severe diffuse head injuries and likely to suffer the full spectrum of problems.

According to the International Civil Aviation Organization (2008), a mild closed head injury is defined as loss of, or alteration of, consciousness and/or post-traumatic amnesia of less than one hour. A moderate closed head injury is classified as sustaining an altered level of consciousness and/or post-traumatic amnesia of longer than one hour, but less than 24 hours. A severe closed head injury is classified as alteration in consciousness and/or post-traumatic amnesia of 24 hours or more. It is to be noted that these are essentially clinical classifications. The addition of information arising from early CT imaging may add to the capacity to define subsequent risks (Annegers *et al.*, 1998).

The classification used by the Children's Hospital at Westmead (Shores *et al.*, 1986) defines *mild* traumatic brain injury as a level on the Glasgow Coma Scale between 12 and 15 and a post-traumatic amnesia of less than 24 hours (Table 16.2), but that would be considered by the International Civil Aviation Organization to be a *moderate* injury (Table 16.1). Conversely, Annegers *et al.* (1998) classify mild traumatic brain injury as a brief loss of consciousness only and a post-traumatic amnesia of less than 30 minutes (Table 16.2). That would place an assessment for aeromedical seizure risk with a post-traumatic amnesia of more than 30 minutes, but less than one hour, into the *moderate* category, leading to a more restrictive interpretation. In practice, most publications in this area have adopted one of the classifications given in Table 16.1.

Clearly, it is important to ask and seek the actual clinical data on loss of consciousness and post-traumatic amnesia, rather than accept a reported definition of severity. Furthermore, where published outcome risk is available, the clinical information is more useful in individualizing risk than an undefined categorical assignment. Post-traumatic amnesia has been associated with cognitive, functional and behaviour recovery through several rigorous years of testing. More recent studies have revalidated post-traumatic amnesia in the post-scanning era. The duration of post-traumatic amnesia has been assessed in terms of a battery of outcome measures using recursive partitioning analysis, and was found to be the best predictor of

Table 16.1 Severity of traumatic brain injury

Traumatic Brain Injury	Clinical Observations	Cantu	American Academy of Neurology	Children's Hospital at Westmead	International Civil Aviation Organization
Mild	Glasgow Coma Scale Loss of consciousness Post-traumatic amnesia	15 None < 30 min	15 None: transient confusion symptoms resolve in 15 min	12–15 Loss < 24 hr	< 1 hr and/or < 1 hr
Moderate	Glasgow Coma Scale Loss of consciousness Post-traumatic amnesia	< 5 min > 30 min	As above: resolving in < 5 min Common	9–11 1–7 days	> 1 hr < 24 hr and/or > 1 hr < 24 hr
Severe	Glasgow Coma Scale Loss of consciousness Post-traumatic Amnesia	>/= 5 min >/= 24 hr	Any loss	3–9 1–4 weeks	> 24 hr and/ or > 24 hr
Very Severe	Glasgow Coma Scale Loss of consciousness Post Traumatic Amnesia			> 4 weeks	

Table 16.2 Classifications of severity of injury and ten-year risk of seizure

	LOC	Post Traumatic Amnesia >24hr	Focal Signs	Contusion (CT Scan)	Traumatic Intracranial Haemorrhage	Skull Fracture	Dural Tear	Early Epilepsy	Severity	10 Year TBI Risk of Seizure
Jennett (1988)		Present Absent Unknown	Present Absent Unknown				Present Absent Unknown	Present Absent Unknown	Presence, absence or unknown of these factors to give a 10-year risk of seizures (from 6 to 60%)	6–60%
		Present Absent Unknown	Present Absent Unknown		(Present)					(30%) 20% 13% 3%
	>24hr	>24hr		Present	Present				Severe: One or more of these features	13%
Annegers et al. (1998)	30min to 24hr						Present		Moderate: Either of these	2%
	<30min						Absent		Mild: Brief LOC only	1%
	? included in ICD	? included in ICD	? included in ICD	ICD 06.1–06.3	ICD 06.4–06.9	ICD 02.0–1.02.702.9			Severe: One or more of these features	~6%
Christensen et al. (2009)				Cerebral Contusions Lacerations Traumatic Oedema	Extradural Subdural Subarachnoid Cerebellar	Frontal Parietal Orbital Roof Skull base				
	Concussion S06.0								Mild: Brief LOC only	>1%

outcome for all end-points and elements of physical examination (Brown *et al.*, 2005). It is thus salutary to note that the use of post-traumatic amnesia in acute medicine (at least in the United Kingdom) is waning.

Referral and Initial Assessment

The situation under which head injuries occur may be obscure. Patients may self-refer after an incident which is apparently trivial, or they may discount it or even forget the incident. The latter is probably most common in those who develop a chronic subdural haematoma where information about the primary cause of the injury has either gone unnoticed or has been forgotten. A range of other mild to moderate head injuries are either self-referred or are referred by a supporting witness, resulting in a visit either to a medical practitioner or to an accident and emergency department. This is usually more common in situations in which there has been direct injury to the scalp or face manifest in bruising or laceration.

In the acute phase of traumatic brain injury, within the first few hours (four) after the injury, the essential issues for the clinician are to determine the general severity of the injury and, in particular, the level on the Glasgow Coma Scale, and whether there has been any skull fracturing. As discussed above, the Glasgow Coma Scale is usually taken at the time of the initial medical assessment, but it may be available from an earlier and immediately post-injury period. The presence or absence of fractures may be manifest through a bilateral periorbital haematoma, a subconjunctival haemorrhage, leakage of the cerebral spinal fluid or Battle's sign.[1] Leakage of the cerebral spinal fluid and Battle's sign are much later manifestations, with the former, perhaps, not occurring for several days and the latter not being present in the retroauricular region for four to eight hours. These obvious clinical signs confirm skull fracturing and are of enormous value in determining what the potential risk is in the acute situation and providing some insight into risks for long-term sequelae. An altered Glasgow Coma Scale, any level below 15, plus signs of a skull fracture as described above increase the risk of a secondary intracranial problem to around 25 per cent (Maas *et al.*, 2008). This forms the major paradigm for acute clinical management of a head injury where determining both conscious level and risk from skull fracturing provides immediate risk factors for the development of secondary brain injury (Figure 16.1).

Management

Initial assessment will involve a rapid review of the critical signs and injuries, together with an evaluation of the nature and severity of the injury. The assessment would include determination of the level on the Glasgow Coma Scale, details of post-traumatic amnesia, evaluation of scalp and skull damage for fracture or penetration, determination of pupil size and the function of the cranial nerves, and whether there are asymmetric responses to commands, speech or pain, together with a brief systemic check of all neurologic systems. The details should be recorded in the acute admission record, and they represent a valuable source of information on the primary status after the injury.

---

1   The sign refers to an ecchymosis of the post-auricular skin due to extravasation of blood along the path of the post-auricular artery. It is an external sign of a temporal bone fracture (Battle, 1890).

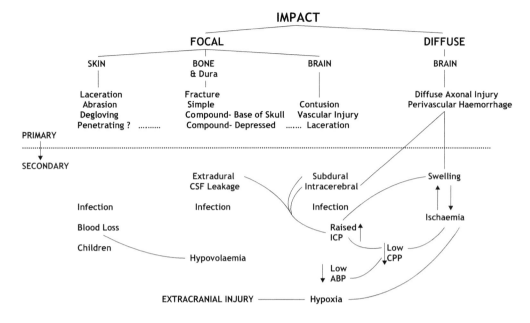

Figure 16.1 Paradigm for acute clinical management of a head injury

Conscious level and risk from skull fracturing provide immediate risk factors for the development of secondary brain injury. Flow diagram illustrates post traumatic events. The aim is to control the cerebral perfusion pressure (CPP) which is a function of mean arterial blood pressure (ABP), normally ~100 mmHg, less the intracranial pressure (ICP), normally <10 mmHg.

Patients who are unconscious from the time of injury will require acute neuromedical management, with the priorities being resuscitation and stabilization. These patients have almost certainly suffered severe diffuse axonal injury, and a low level on the Glasgow Coma Scale, at this time, indicates the likelihood of a poor outcome. One of the major problems for this group, and for others in whom injury to the brain itself occurs, is swelling or compression from bleeding. Both lead to a raised intracranial pressure of greater than 10 mm Hg. Raised intracranial pressure can overcome the cerebral perfusion pressure of the blood supply to the head, resulting in further ischaemia.

Most acute management under these conditions is directed at improving and maintaining the blood supply to the brain and even increasing the blood pressure to maintain cerebral perfusion against an elevated intracranial pressure. Where maintenance of the cerebral perfusion pressure to a level of at least 60 mm Hg cannot be achieved, decompression of the cranial cavity, either by clot removal or extensive decompressive craniectomy, is to be considered. The latter now forms a significantly increasing part of the armamentarium of managing head injuries and is analogous to managing a so-called compartment syndrome in other parts of the body (Pompucci *et al.*, 2007).

With the Glasgow Coma Scale assessed and the initial overview of the risk of skull fracturing completed, patients increasingly receive CT scans. It is at this point that one is able to determine the presence of intracranial injury in the form of contusion or haemorrhage within the parenchymal matter or the presence of extra-axial collections such as an extradural and/or a subdural haematoma. Additional information may arise from the visualization of subarachnoid blood and also from the presence of air within the intracranial cavity that is indicative of severe skull-based fracturing. Incipient or developing raised intracranial pressure, brain swelling, clot expansion or infarction can be detected on serial scans. Taken together with the clinical data, CT scans can help to establish the risk of further deterioration and/or the presence of brain swelling, particularly with reference to the visible subarachnoid spaces. For example, manifestly visible cerebrospinal fluid spaces around the midbrain basal cisterns indicate an intracranial pressure below 20 mm Hg. If these are not visible and are closed, the intracranial pressure is globally raised and likely to be above 20 mm Hg. Sustained elevated intracranial pressure impairs cerebral perfusion and compromises further brain function.

Outcome is much dependent upon the severity of the head injury and the capacity of the medical team to determine risks and manage a patient through the next (secondary) phase. It is well recognized that over the last 30 years, since the introduction of triaging criteria, there has been a 50 per cent reduction in patients who used to 'talk and die' (Dunn *et al.*, 2003). Early triage and transfer to immediate neurosurgical intervention, where required, has led to a substantial improvement in the number of patients who survive and, indeed, of those who make a good outcome. However, it is less certain for patients with apparent non-surgical lesions that acute neurosurgical care offers advantage over good-quality intensive care. Nevertheless, it has recently been suggested that there is an improvement of up to 12 per cent in outcome across the board for those managed in a neurosurgical environment (National Confidential Enquiry into Patient Outcome and Death, 2007).

However, it is important to realize that although subsequent problems that patients may have, if they survive their head injury, are likely to be due mainly to their primary injury, they may, in part, be due to secondary complications arising from the primary injury. The outcome may also be influenced by the timely use of interventions to control secondary problems. This may involve additional risks from monitoring intracranial pressure and the drainage procedures involving the ventricles, as well as those from the surgical trauma. There are a number of new interventions, such as oxygen measurement with microprobes and microdialysis, that involve parenchymal placement of probes. The introduction of these interventions has posed the question as to whether they lead to longer-term issues. The question is pertinent, as with assessment of risks, say, for driving, advisors to regulatory authorities have addressed the estimated additional risk. In general, the newer technologies have been used primarily in severe head injury, and consequently their contribution has been considered to be relatively minor in the context of an individual who has a major insult to the brain. However, it is pertinent to note that such interventions are now registered in regulatory publications such as *At a Glance Guide to the Current Medical Standards of Fitness to Drive* (Driver and Vehicle Licensing Agency: Drivers Medical Group, 2011).

Haematoma

Extradural

Classically, extradural haematoma is an injury of younger people in whom the dural attachment to the bone is less developed. A blow to the side of the head results in fracturing of the skull in the thinner temporal region. There is tearing of the middle meningeal artery and bleeding into the extradural space. The initial impact may be associated with a short concussive period, with loss of consciousness for less than 30 minutes, and there is the question whether this, in itself, may have resulted in some injury to the brain parenchyma. After this period there may be what is called 'a lucid interval' when, to all intents and purposes, the victim appears to be fully conscious. They may even be able to carry on participating in their activity or sport. However, as the clot accumulates in the extradural space, conscious level deteriorates, leading ultimately to impaired performance and, in some in cases, slipping into coma.

The level of consciousness after the initial concussive period may be impossible to separate from normality, and a recent high-profile celebrity case has lent weight to this.[2] Later, however, often after a prodromal period of severe headache and nausea with raised intracranial pressure, the level on the Glasgow Coma Scale drops and weakness develops in the contralateral limbs from local cortical pressure (focal symptoms). Later, the ipsilateral pupil will dilate and become unresponsive due to incipient tentorial (medial temporal) herniation against the oculomotor nerve. With adequate monitoring and early identification of deterioration, patients can usually be transferred to a facility where CT scans will confirm the extradural collection. Given the nature of the extradural haematoma, it is often difficult to see from the scan any sign of an underlying brain injury. Usually, there is little to see other than the clot, and most clinicians have taken this to imply that removal of the extradural

haematoma would not be associated with long-term neurological problems. Hence, very early evacuation of the clot is warranted in anyone who has signs of an extradural haemorrhage and a headache and, certainly, anyone who has an altered conscious level.

Patients with a less symptomatic extradural haematoma should be monitored in the neurosurgical environment to see whether the clot develops further. An unremitting headache or deterioration will require surgery. The chances of a good outcome and complete return to normality are excellent. Indeed, patients who have their extradural clot rapidly excised, despite acute focal deterioration, usually make a miraculous recovery, with low risk of sequelae. Contralateral deficits usually abate quickly, but one should be suspicious if a focal deficit takes a longer time to settle (weeks). This may indicate some contusional injury occurring either at the time of the impact or as a result of either the clot itself expanding or even the neurosurgical intervention. Magnetic resonance imaging would provide the most useful information and can be carried out later.

It is generally considered that the risk of sequelae from an extradural haematoma is relatively small and that these patients can return to driving after six months. There is no general requirement for any further investigation or imaging, although frequently they will have had post-operative scans to determine that the extradural haemorrhage has been completely excised. Those who do not make an immediate recovery often have a CT scan on the post-operative day, and this may or may not be useful in the assessment at a later date. Generally speaking, the better the immediate recovery, the less likely the need for further investigations. However, in the setting of a neurosurgical

---

2   Natasha Richardson, the English actress, sustained a head injury while taking a skiing lesson. The injury was followed by a lucid interval, but three hours later she complained of headache. She died two days after the accident, and the autopsy revealed an epidural (extradural) haematoma. There was much debate concerning the use of helmets while skiing and Richardson's refusal, immediately after the accident, to accept medical attention.

unit, subtle issues such as change in personality, symptoms of headache and memory dysfunction may not be easily determined where an extradural haematoma is part of a complex head injury. Twenty per cent of patients with an extradural haematoma on CT scan will have a small subdural haematoma at operation (or autopsy).

Subdural

Patients who sustain a subdural haematoma after head injury vary from the apparently unimpaired through to the fatally injured. In general, there appear to be two main issues. Have they been diagnosed by CT scanning? It seems likely that a number of patients who have received injuries that do not amount to any obvious impact on conscious level, particularly those who have alcohol-related injuries, may not undergo CT scanning. The mechanism of subdural haematoma under these conditions is most likely to be contusional and this may not always be easily recognized even on a CT scan where the major sites of impact are in the subtemporal and subfrontal areas adjacent to dense bone.

If diagnosed as having a subdural collection, then it is likely that the patient is flagged for at least a neurosurgical opinion and probably for some further assessment. In other words, they are identified as having had a head injury. In more severe collections with raised intracranial pressure and focal neurological performance, the next important decision would be whether the severity of these symptoms develop to the point at which neurosurgical intervention to remove the clot is indicated. This implies the risk that the intracranial pressure will rise or is, indeed, high. The brain has, as a result, not only suffered some primary insult

from the original head injury but is deteriorating further due to a secondary insult that surgery may control.

Older patients (and boxers who dehydrate to lose weight) are more likely to develop subdural haematomas from brain movement tearing polar and bridging veins between the cortical surface and the adjacent dura. These patients may have a similar presentation to those with extradural haematomas. Such isolated tears in the absence of cortical contusion can have a better than expected outcome if recognized and treated efficiently.

A small proportion may go on to have irremediable brain swelling and ultimately develop brainstem herniation and die, but a gratifyingly significant number are helped by surgical evacuation and make various levels of recovery. An increasing number will benefit from invasive monitoring such as intracranial pressure and microdialysis. It is unlikely that this group will survive without any deficit, though increasingly early intervention and care have opened the possibility that a few will be seeking not only to drive but to fly in the future. This is particularly true of younger patients. As a general rule, a high proportion of these patients will have significant injury to brain tissue.

Intracerebral

Patients who suffer an intracerebral haematoma usually derive this as a consequence of contusional cortical damage resulting in, for example, a burst temporal lobe or similar occurrence. In other words, the clot can be traced to the cortical surface. So-called 'isolated intracerebral haematoma from trauma' is relatively uncommon and begs the question as to whether the patient had some kind of spontaneous bleed outwith the immediate injury. Patients who are taking anticoagulant medication may fall into this category. Clearly, most of those with intraparenchymal injury have associated brain injury and as a result generally fall into the category of severe injury. They carry a high likelihood of survival sequelae.

Diffuse Axonal Injury

Patients with diffuse axonal injury tend to have widespread global damage to the brain, usually associated with the pathological description of shearing of axons between grey and white matter.

Co-located microvascular shearing is associated with petechial haemorrhages that may or may not be visible on CT scanning, but are increasingly being recognized on magnetic resonance scans as being more widespread than originally thought in the acute phase. Additionally, characteristic grey/white matter differentiation and loss of open basal cisterns are seen frequently. These patients tend to have a severely altered conscious level at presentation and will almost certainly have long-term problems if they survive.

Penetrating Injuries

Penetrating injuries to the skull associated with either implements or projectiles are not uncommon. The critical issue from the clinical point of view is to determine whether the lesion has actually penetrated through the skull, through the dura and into brain tissue. It is often surprisingly difficult to determine from history and/or examination as to whether this has occurred, particularly where the issue may involve fine instruments such as screwdrivers and the weapon has been removed. As a general rule, all scalp injuries could be potential sites for penetrating injury and this is where the history and a high level of suspicion from the clinician are required. Penetrating injuries to the brain carry a high risk of subsequent seizures which may be further exacerbated by resultant infection to an overall risk level greater than 50 per cent.

Associated with penetrating injuries will be skull fracturing, and the major determinant of the severity of this would be whether the fracture is linear or fragmented, and also whether the fragments are depressed beyond the inner table of the skull such that there may be risks to the dural membrane. Penetrating injuries are by definition compound fractures. Dural puncture is usually associated with cortical contusion, and penetrating injuries are always associated with a degree of brain contusion. Early recognition and CT scans, with or without magnetic resonance scans and vascular studies, may be indicated. Fragment removal may not always be immediately desirable in the context of existing brain swelling, but, usually, early debridement of the wound and closure of the skin is the primary objective. Again, these patients will always have post-injury sequelae, most of which would debar them from holding a pilot's licence in the future. However, as with all injuries, there is a spectrum of penetration, and, at the less serious end of the scale, assessors will be called upon to determine what the risk will be in the ensuing period with respect to future performance.

Intensive Care

Those more severely injured will require close observation in the acute admission and post-operative periods. Such care on specialist units affords moment-to-moment monitoring aimed at maintaining vital systems. Patients with brain swelling may need prolonged periods of ventilation until this settles. During this period, the primary target is to control the cerebral perfusion pressure (CPP) which is a function of mean arterial blood pressure, normally ~100 mm Hg, less the intracranial pressure, normally < 10 mm Hg (Figure 16.1). This is achieved by introduction of an intracranial pressure monitor and arterial lines. The critical cerebral perfusion pressure is around 60 mm Hg, and efforts are aimed at reducing the intracranial pressure and elevating mean arterial pressure to effect a cerebral perfusion pressure well above the critical level.

These processes are aided as cerebral vascular autoregulation is impaired, and, if the intracerebral pressure is stable, cerebral perfusion pressure becomes absolutely dependent on mean arterial pressure. Too low a perfusion pressure will result in ischaemia, brain swelling and aggregated damage to the local and global brain. This may worsen the original injury and lead to delayed ischaemic swelling and a prolonged stay in hospital or progressive deterioration. Too high a perfusion pressure, particularly with crystalloid infusion, can lead to hyperaemic brain swelling due to disturbed oncotic pressure balance. This inevitably leads, in turn, to brain swelling and ischaemia. Balanced control remains the crucial objective.

Hypoxic or ischaemic episodes involving changes in the perfusion pressure of as little as 10 mm Hg can result in aggregated worsening of injury (Miller *et al.*, 1998). Hypoxia associated with depressed blood pressure or concomitant respiratory pathology will add to existing injury in terms of severity and prolongation of hospital stay. Whether the nature of such

additional global hypoxic injury adds complexity to the risk of long-term problems, over that of severity alone, remains an issue in developing acute approaches to intensive care, as with, for example, neuroprotective agents. Medical assessors will see relatively few of these patients. However, early triage is likely to result in a greater percentage of patients with levels of better than 9 on the Glasgow Coma Scale being ventilated for their other injuries or to protect systems during transport. Many of these patients will be subject to the above constraints and increasing interventional monitoring.

Epilepsy

The risk of epilepsy is greater after head injury and increases after invasive neurosurgery. However, for practical purposes in survivors, the underlying brain injury from the trauma represents the most significant issue in assessing subsequent risk. For example, factors predisposing to late traumatic epilepsy include an intracranial haematoma that is surgically removed (35 per cent risk). However, when an intracerebral haematoma is seen on the CT scan, but surgical evacuation is not required, the risk of seizure is still high at 20 per cent. The diagnosis of seizure is not always easy, and for many who have made an apparently good recovery, there are significant personal incentives not to declare these. In most cases, however, there is not only the description of the patients or accompanying persons but also the documentation of the event from hospital records.

Regulatory bodies carry the responsibility for assessing the fitness to fly of commercial pilots. Criteria and guidelines are outlined in the *Manual of Civil Aviation Medicine: Preliminary Edition*

Part III published by the International Civil Aviation Organization (2008), and the particular level of acceptability, in terms of risk for holding a licence, is described conceptually in Volume One and categorically in Chapter Three. In Europe, regulations are issued to aeromedical examiners as the *Joint Aviation Requirements: Flight Crew Licensing 3 (Medical)* by the Joint Aviation Authorities (2006). Regulatory bodies usually provide an expert advisory service for complex or borderline cases, and the results are held in a secure database. However, there is the need to rationalize and standardize approaches to these cases, and, for the individual patient, their particular risk may not simply align with the described categories. For the assessor, as well as the onus of categorization from often incomplete information, there is the application of risk assessment criteria to individual applicants in a fair and robust way. In simple terms, for aeromedical licensing of those with a seizure risk of greater than 1 per cent per year, medical certification is not appropriate.

The level of risk of a seizure *in the next year* is determined by the time since the last seizure or initial head injury. If anti-epileptic medication is stopped or reduced, there is a period of increased risk over the next few months, but in the absence of recurrence during this period the risk follows a downward curve. For those who have a subsequent seizure and re-enter the 'at risk population', assessments of delayed risk of further seizures is complex. Nonetheless, in the situation of recurrent seizure risk in the non-traumatic brain injury group, a generally better prognostic group, recent data would suggest that a period of at least five years, with at least five years off anti-epileptic medication, would be required to establish a risk that might questionably approach 2 per

cent. This five-year period is likely to be more extended for injury with recurrent seizures, and unlikely to be approached where the criteria are set at 1 per cent (Bonnett *et al.*, 2010).

Attention is directed mainly at determining the risk of a first disabling event or seizure in post-injury patients at a time after their head injury that predicts their risk *in the next year* at less than 1 per cent for commercial crew. It is set at 2 per cent or 20 per cent for recreational licensing (see addendum). Importantly, the 1 per cent criterion specified for commercial aircrew is now (if these same approaches are applied) more accessible for a number of patients who have sustained a head injury, but the pragmatic application of safe and consistent rules demand expert critical appraisal.

Residual Risk versus Annual Risk

A further issue is the improving portfolio of evidence to support assessments of risk. The early approach taken by the pioneering work of Jennett and Teasdale (Jennett, 1988; Teasdale and Jennett, 1974, 1978) was an assessment of the apparent overall risk (10 years) of having a post-traumatic seizure and applying actuarial calculations to derive a table of initial risk against years for defining residual risk after a time period (Table 16.2). This approach allowed the aggregation of injury severity in terms of risk stratification. Hence, penetrating injury, post-traumatic amnesia and an intracranial haematoma could be used to assess the initial and, therefore, apparent later risk of seizures.

Subsequent population-based reports by Annegers *et al.* (1998) included imaging CT appearances in the definition of severe head injury (brain contusion together with the concept of risk in the subsequent year, rather than residual risk). They suggested that annual risk will lead to an acceptable level in a shorter time (Table 16.2; Figure 16.2). This is supported by more recent studies such as that by Christensen *et al.* (2009) which looked at a large Danish cohort of 1.5 million individuals from 1977 to 2002 (Table 16.2; Figure 16.2). This study reported that relative risks of epilepsy were raised twofold after mild head injury and sevenfold after severe head injury. The adjusted relative risk and confidence limits were calculated against the target population not having a seizure. In the mild head injury group, of 16,633 patients, 1.78/1,000 persons had a fit in the first to second year after head injury. The unadjusted risk in the second year was 0.178 per cent, with the adjusted relative risk being 2.26 (1.87–2.73). For severe head injuries, 17,354 patients, 6.06/1,000 had a seizure in the first to second year after head injury. Their annual unadjusted risk was around 0.6 per cent – below 1 per cent with a relative risk of 7.42 (4.68–11.9). The measure of interest is the probability of being seizure-free for the next year, having been seizure-free from the date of the injury to the time point in question. This requires the more subtle analysis of the data by Christensen *et al.* (2009), but based on this study (target population based), the risk remains above 1 per cent for only two years for even the severe group.

There are three sets of information that seem to set varying standards. The first is what a regulatory body may recommend using annual risk assessment rather than residual risk. The issue is best considered in an example. A male aged 41 has an extradural haematoma with perhaps a small subdural haematoma and some bleeding into the frontal lobe. He has a post-traumatic amnesia lasting two weeks. He has, by most definitions,

had a severe head injury. According to Jennett (1988), his seizure risk for the next ten years is 25 per cent. His *residual risk* falls to 9 per cent at two years, but does not fall below 2 per cent until eight years and below 1 per cent until ten years. However, his *annual risk* calculated from the difference in annual residual risk (Driver and Vehicle Licensing Agency, 2005) falls to 2 per cent by the end of the second year, to between 1 and 2 per cent from the third year onwards and to around 1 per cent after the seventh year (Figure 16.2).

This tends to suggest that there may be a continuing risk extending beyond the ten-year period. If the same patient data are used in the series published by Annegers *et al.* (1998), and categorized according to Table 16.2, the same patient has now a 13 per cent risk at ten years and his residual risk of seizures falls below 1 per cent after only eight years by interpolation, in agreement with Jennett (1998). However, the *annual risk* falls below 2 per cent after two years and 'not greater than 1 per cent' after five years, and remains below through ten years. It is important to note that, in comparison with the analysis carried out by Jennett (1998), the data from Annegers *et al.* (1998) are improved and modernized by the addition of CT data, even though the confidence limits for risk profiling within the three groups, particularly the severe group, are broad. This suggests that both sets of data are comparable even for severe traumatic brain injury.

The data from Annegers *et al.* (1998) would suggest earlier consideration of aeromedical licensing with some surety of annual risk lying consistently below 1 per cent after five years. However, the most recent data from Christensen *et al.* (2009) would appear to offer a clearer insight into the issues as it based on a large population of 78,572 individuals with traumatic brain injury. It explores

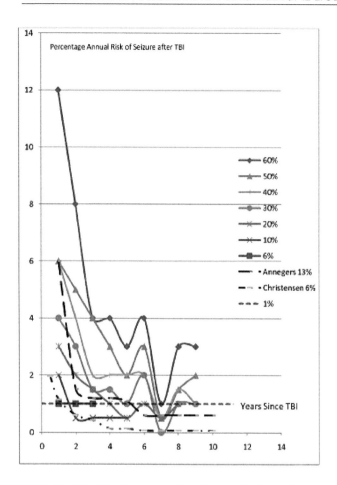

Figure 16.2 Percentage annual risk of seizure after traumatic brain injury
The data for Jennett (1988) is derived by calculating the difference in residual risk at ten years between successive years. Jennett (1998) expressed the ten year risk of seizures (severity: see 6–60 per cent plots) in terms of the aggregate of factors to give an overall beginning risk of developing a seizure. The plots for Annegers *et al.* (1989) and Christensen *et al.* (2009) relate to annual risk of epilepsy for individual classification of 'severe'.

the same or intending population for aeromedical licensing, and includes definition of intracranial pathology from CT scans. Jennett (1998) estimated that, overall, 5 per cent of head injuries will have epilepsy and this compares with the risk in this more recent study.

Using the above example of a severe head injury, with the data from Christensen *et al.* (1998), the residual risk of around 6 per cent falls to 1 per cent in the first year and below this after the third year (Table 16.2). The *annual risk* calculated directly from the figures gives a seizure risk below 1 per cent

(0.6 per cent) in the second year. This is substantially different from the data of either Jennett (1998) or Annegers *et al.* (1998) and would, if applied, enable aeromedical licensing considerably earlier than has been the case until now.

In the study by Christensen *et al.* (2009), the classification of traumatic brain injury was based on retrospective coding using the *International Classification of Diseases* (World Health Organization, 2007). However, better-grade patients may have been over-included in the severe categories as the data were based on the initial information on admission.

The relative risk between mild (two times) and severe groups (seven times) versus traumatic brain injury without seizures in terms of seizure risk is comparable with other studies. The diagnosis of epilepsy, as always, has difficulties, but there is no reason to suggest that this is different from other studies. The study was reviewed by Shorvon and Neligan (2009), and welcomed as 'of value in helping to determine epilepsy risks for medico-legal purposes'. The criticism of this approach is the use of the international classification, which widens and increases the proportion of otherwise moderate head injuries that fall into the categories of severe (or mild). In addition, the risk stratification from having only two levels of categorical description may have led, unintentionally, to considerable overlap. This may slant the figures in favour of early licensing.

There is a clear issue for discussion on how precisely the initial risk in any individual can be assessed with the current tools – *The International Classification of Diseases* (World Health Organization, 2007) and clinical data. The level of initial risk is crucial in determining the subsequent pattern of *annual seizure* risk as revealed by the comparator plots (Figure 16.2). One element that might still be of value is using a combination of factors rather than a categorical threshold (Table 16.2). The stratification of subsequent risk is clearly seen with this approach in the data from Jennett (1998). Nonetheless, Christensen *et al.* (2009) have clarified the risks for interpretation of the 20 and 2 per cent thresholds. Their finding that the risk of epilepsy was increased for at least ten years after injury begs the question as to whether the 1 per cent level is robust enough in the face of this new information. This issue is also raised in the *Manual of Civil Aviation Medicine* (International Civil Aviation Organization, 2008).

These considerations bring out a number of issues that have, hitherto, been unclear. The pattern of seizure occurrence after post-traumatic brain injury is not as predictable as had been thought. The rate of development is greatest in the first few years, as expected, but there is excess risk continuing for well beyond ten years after mild and severe brain injury, longer than in other studies. The data from Christenson *et al.* (2009) are derived from a population of children and young adults, and this is of some relevance to the population likely to apply anew for medical licensing.

The relative risk of epilepsy is higher in women (2.9) than in men (2.01). The incidence of epilepsy is greater in those injured who have a family history (first-degree relatives) than in those without a family history of epilepsy: a sixfold effect in mild head injury and tenfold in severe head injury. In some cases, this may be useful information to derive from a patient's history. Christensen *et al.* (2009) also provide data for epilepsy risk for skull fracture, which remains above the relative risk of epilepsy in those without brain injury at between 1.55 and 2.06 from the fifth year to beyond ten years. The apparent *annual risk* from fracture falls below 1 per cent (0.29 per cent) at six months for all severities, but stays greater than those without fracture beyond ten years. To date, as far as aeromedical licensing at the 1 per cent level is concerned, traumatic brain injury remains a disqualifying factor for all classes. However, in view of the above data, this may well require revision.

Implications to Aircrew

The implications of traumatic brain injury may be considered in two broad groups. These are cases originally described as severe, and so originally completely excludable, and cases that would allow licensing as long as there were no compounding factors.

Severe and Excludable

It seems likely that a number of applicants with the conditions listed below – except, perhaps, those with a penetrating injury, intracerebral abscess or subdural empyema – may ultimately be in a position to apply for licensing:

- cerebral contusions shown on CT scanning without other evident injury
- parenchymal haematoma, petechial haemorrhage of any sort
- true intracerebral haematoma
- depressed fracture with a dural tear
- depressed fracture without dural tear, but with signs of brain contusion
- any penetrating injury (high risk)
- intracerebral abscess/subdural empyema (high risk).

No Compounding Factors

It is considered that these conditions may allow certification if there are no other compounding factors.

Extradural haematoma

Surgically removed extradural haematoma with no sign of associated brain contusion and early (within 24 hours) return of normal conscious level. Some young patients develop non-surgical extradural collections after head injury. These usually settle spontaneously but may be associated with prolonged headache for up to six weeks.

Subdural haematoma

Those requiring surgical removal will almost certainly have been unlikely to achieve a risk status below 1 per cent with the new approach and will need reassessment. There are, however, many instances in which small acute subdural collections confirmed by CT scan can arise where there is no obvious sign of brain contusion and when the level on the Glasgow Coma Scale is normal without focal signs. Patients such as these will have bled either from a torn cerebral bridging vein or from an undetermined contusion, possibly arising from subtemporal or subfrontal injury, which is less easily diagnosed on CT scans than vault or parenchymal injury.

These patients are often managed symptomatically for their headache and do not require surgery. The tendency is to determine whether the patient has indeed had a significant head injury in terms of the level on the Glasgow Coma Scale, post-traumatic amnesia and focal signs (parietal drift), and how well they have recovered. Using the approach described above, it might be estimated that the annual risk of seizure occurrence in the ensuing years would not drop below 2 per cent before the end of two years and would remain above 1 per cent until five years.

Post-traumatic hydrocephalus

Hydrocephalus arises from traumatic subarachnoid haemorrhage which usually occurs in the context of severe head injury or extensive skull base fracturing. The prospective risk from the underlying condition/trauma must be considered. Few patients will require ventriculoperitoneal shunts. These may, if uncomplicated, be considered low risk for seizure activity after six months.

Skull fracture

Linear skull fracture alone (simple, non-compound depressed fracture with no underlying contusion) was shown in the series by Annegers *et al.* (1998) to elevate the risk ratio (relative risk) for delayed seizures overall by 1.9 and 2. As mentioned, recent data has drawn attention to the impact of skull fracture as an isolated independent variable on epilepsy risk, with a statistically significant elevation of relative risk above 1.5 to 2.0 for up to ten years, although recent data suggests the annual risk is less than 1 per cent after six months. However, these data include an impracticably wide range of fracture severity and require careful interpretation where an applicant is otherwise well.

Intracranial pressure monitoring

Severe neurotrauma patients may be monitored for intracranial pressure using fine intraparenchymal probes introduced through twist drill bolts or burr holes. The risk of these causing local damage or bleeding sufficient to exert a greater impact on risk of sequelae than the severity of the underlying condition is very small. In cases of multiple trauma where stabilization and transport of patients is urgent, as by helicopter, patients may be intubated and ventilated. Clearly, this is unsatisfactory for more than immediate purposes where intracranial injury is at all uncertain.

Early introduction of an intracranial pressure monitor may allow investigation and stabilization of a patient, providing vital knowledge of intracranial status. A number of patients may turn out not to have had a head injury. In these patients, there is no evidence that such catheters carry an excess risk of seizures. However, as the cortical mantle is breached, as in the placement of ventricular catheters,

there is an argument for considering a six-month period of observation.

Microdialysis

In a similar way to intracranial pressure catheters, similarly sized catheters that sample parenchymal extracellular fluid can be used in the intensive care situation. They monitor the metabolic status of the injured brain by using indices such as pyruvate, lactate and glucose levels. There are no additional risks from this technique. Their use reflects the need for such investigative monitoring in the more severe head injuries and is unlikely to feature in the history of an applicant for a pilot's licence.

Extraventricular drain

These may be inserted via burr holes to measure the intracranial pressure or to drain cerebrospinal fluid to control the pressure. They are used more commonly in children. Regulatory bodies recommend a six-month period off driving a vehicle, but it is likely in aeromedical practice that the issue will only arise in a *de novo* applicant who had a head injury as a child.

Chronic subdural haematoma

These tend to occur in older people, with an incidence of 25 per cent in those over 65 years, and hence will not generally become an issue for aeromedical licensing. Simple incidental collections not requiring evacuation would not appear to carry any particular risk of seizures. However, checking for resolution with scans would allow a period of observation before consideration for licensing. A percentage (2.2 per cent) of patients with chronic subdural haematoma present with seizures. Those that need drainage can develop post-operative epilepsy with a 6 per cent incidence observed in a series of 1,000 cases. Although cortical lesions or old haematomas have not been observed in CT studies, the capsule which is left *in situ* may be responsible for late epilepsy.

Sabo *et al.* (1995) analyzed the role of prophylactic anticonvulsive medication in patients with chronic subdural haematoma, and concluded that patients receiving prophylactic phenytoin demonstrated a significant decrease in the occurrence of seizure, and recommended its use for six months following diagnosis and treatment. The duration of observation before the risk of seizure falls below 1 per cent is unknown and, again, would have to be considered against the general status of a patient. Particular risks for chronic subdural haematoma include patients requiring warfarin or who are susceptible to aspirin. A number may be otherwise well or may have comorbidity such as cardiac or thrombotic that elevates their overall risk status.

Traumatic subarachnoid haemorrhage

Vespa *et al.* (1999) showed that in patients with acute head injury the coincidence of traumatic subarachnoid haemorrhage was associated with some increase in the risk of acute seizures. This may be because traumatic subarachnoid haemorrhage reflects a greater severity of injury alone. The outcome, overall, for patients with traumatic subarachnoid haemorrhage is worse for their particular presenting level on the Glasgow Coma Scale. There is, however, little evidence that allows for definition of the longer-term risk of seizures after traumatic subarachnoid haemorrhage. For patients presenting with non-traumatic subarachnoid haemorrhage (no aneurysmal bleed – so-called perimesencephalic bleeds),

the risk of seizures seems small. In a series of 293 cases reported over a five-year period, there were no patients with seizures. However, traumatic subarachnoid haemorrhage is relatively rare except in severe trauma.

Posterior fossa or infratentorial collections

These may usefully be divided into those that have a parenchymal component that may affect the cerebellum, its peduncles or the brainstem, and those that are truly extra-axial such as subdural or extradural (5 per cent of all extradural haemorrhages). Cerebellar signs are surprisingly absent in most extradural cases. Surgical evacuation is carried out for symptomatic lesions and alone carries a very good prognosis. Parenchymal injury usually impacts on neurology and may lead to significant long-term problems with balance and coordination, fine motor control and mobility under low-light conditions where visual input to balance is crucial. Cranial nerve involvement is an additional risk, either from parenchymal damage to cranial nerve nuclei or from pressure or injury to the free nerve within the cerebellopontine angle or from fracturing to the skull base.

Extra-axial collections can arise from tears to transverse or sigmoid venous sinuses, giving rise usually to extradural collections, although subdural collections from this source also occur. There are rare reports of petrosal vein damage giving rise to lateral subdural collections. Such collections of traumatic origin imply a serious cranial impact and may well be a component of a more complex pattern including supratentorial and neck injury. Any mass effect within the confines of the posterior fossa/infratentorium can give rise to obstructive hydrocephalus which may need ventricular drainage. If a patient makes a successful recovery from posterior fossa trauma, whether requiring direct surgery or not, their risk of seizures in the absence of other pathology or intervention is generally low, and application for aeromedical licensing should be considered favourably, assuming no other debarring issues or conditions.

Provoked seizures

A review of a seizure event could permit licensing. Applicants should have no previous history of seizures. In the absence of any previous cerebral pathology, but in the context of head injury, some seizures can be considered provoked and hence not carry a risk of recurrence. These include seizures within seconds of head injury, a seizure occurring in the first week following a head injury which is not associated with any damage on the CT scan or with post-traumatic amnesia of longer than 30 minutes, and during intracranial surgery or in the ensuing 24 hours.

Post-Concussion Syndrome

Post-concussion symptoms are well recognized by those who have the responsibility to care generally or specially for patients who have had a traumatic brain injury. The spectrum of complaints is broad and includes headache, dizziness, sleeplessness and disturbed sleep patterns, behavioural changes, poor concentration, short-term memory problems, and mood swings including irritability and anxiety. The post-concussion syndrome has been defined as a clinical state in which three or more symptoms persist for more than three months. Importantly, neurological examination and CT scans should be normal.

Post-mortem examination of patients with relatively mild head injury (as indicated by levels on the Glasgow Coma Scale and the incidence of post-traumatic amnesia), who have died from other causes, has shown striking evidence of subfrontal and subtemporal contusions. These were not obviously apparent on CT scans due to their apposition and haemorrhagic nature close to the dense skull base. Some authorities have taken this and other evidence, such as the persistence of electroencephalographic changes in mild head injuries, to mean that any episode of traumatic loss of consciousness, however brief, probably involves some direct brain damage. Delayed magnetic resonance imaging of mild traumatic brain injury with apparently normal CT scans has also pointed to hippocampal cell loss and frontal cortical thinning.

In a group of 100 successive minor head injuries, 40 per cent were demonstrated three months after the injury to have the post-concussion syndrome (Ingebrigsten *et al.*, 1998) The group was categorized by four criteria: head injury with loss of consciousness, a level of less than 13–15 on the Glasgow Coma Scale on admission, absence of a neurological deficit and no abnormalities on the CT scan. Loss of consciousness was defined by witness confirmation or as amnesia for the trauma event. This contrasts with the much looser definition in the post-deployment screening form used by the US Forces that asks service members and veterans to recall whether they were 'dazed' or 'confused' at the time of an injury or blast 'experience'. Positive responses to this single unvalidated question have accounted for two-thirds of all reported cases of concussion/mild traumatic brain injury, and hence an overestimate of need (Hoge *et al.*, 2009) that strays into the realm of post-traumatic stress disorder. There may have been some self-benefit to have diagnostically completed this form in a way that those seeking aeromedical licensing would attempt to avoid.

Headaches are the most frequent complaint in the post-concussion syndrome, followed by memory, fatigue, dizziness, poor concentration, sleep disturbance, irritability, low tolerance for noise and depression. The literature on psychological sequelae emphasizes the greater likelihood of finding a premorbid history of psychiatric depression and symptoms in those for whom these are the major elements of post-concussion. At one year, only 10 per cent will continue to have sufficient symptoms to support the diagnosis. It thus appears to have a self-limiting course.

Whilst this may seem satisfactory and expected, there are increasing concerns that many of these patients, together with their more chronic symptoms, go unheeded. Indeed, Whitnall *et al.* (2006), who analyzed 475 survivors at one year, found that 115 (24 per cent) had died by seven years. From five to seven years, disability remained frequent (53 per cent), and the rate was similar to that found at one year (57 per cent). Based on survivors over the period of seven to five years, 63 (29 per cent) had improved, but 55 (25 per cent) had deteriorated. The persistence of disability and its development after previous recovery each showed stronger associations with indices of depression, anxiety and low self-esteem than with initial severity of injury or persisting cognitive impairment. They concluded that admission to hospital after head injury is followed, five to seven years later, by disability in a high proportion of survivors. Persistence of disability and development of new disability are strongly associated with psychosocial

factors that may be open to remediation, even late after injury.

In the Norwegian study (Ingebrigsten *et al.*, 1998), the authors concluded that the persistence of the syndrome appears to be influenced by cognitive, emotional, personality and motivational factors. Therapeutic measures aimed at symptomatic treatment are variously effective, but management of the underlying residual issues may take more detailed coupling of psychological paradigms with, for example, functional magnetic resonance imaging to determine the substrates of damage and to monitor interventional therapies. Headache and disturbed sleep are significant symptoms.

Headache

The impact of post-concussional headache on patient performance is largely unrecorded per se. The headaches may take many forms short of syndromic migraine or facial pain. In patients who have undergone any scalp injury or surgery, close examination and attention to the site and nature of the headache may point to local causes such as nerve injury, scalp adherence to dura through areas of skull deficit and other areas of scalp-related scarring. Local nerve blocks may thus be more effective than multiple oral analgesics. Indeed, an important issue to explore is analgesic use and dependency, with respect to overuse. This latter issue may have important considerations when considering risks from other factors in patients otherwise suitable for medical licensing. Increasingly, in these cases, patients will be encouraged to try more prophylactic analgesics such as gabapentin or carbamazepine. Care must be taken to inform the patient, the medical practitioner and the aeromedical examiner that the drug is intended for this use and not as an anticonvulsant.

Sleep disturbance

This is not uncommon after traumatic brain injury. It is most often characterized by insomnia, replacing night for day, hypersomnia and excessive daytime sleepiness. Few studies have examined the impact of these disturbances on the performance of these patients. It is estimated that 30 per cent may develop this problem. A recent study (Baumann *et al.*, 2007) concluded that sleep disturbances in 43 per cent were attributable to the injury. There was an association between the severity of the injury and hypersomnia, but not between sleep disturbance and depression. The clearest correlate was with the impact on quality of life measured using the SF-36 questionnaire. It is proposed that this may manifest itself over time in impaired social functioning. Again, these symptoms are generally self-limiting but can, on rare occasions, give rise to narcolepsy and hallucinations. Most patients recover an adequate sleep pattern within one year.

Focal Neurological Deficits

Patients are unlikely to present for an aeromedical assessment after a head injury with an obviously limiting functional deficit. Most in this position are recovering from a neurological deficit such as hemiparesis or reported dysphasia and will have responded and returned to premorbid status within several weeks of the injury. For those who require a longer period than six months, the recovery will be prolonged and they are unlikely to be fit for several years. Some features of focal change

will clearly pose significantly greater concerns than others.

Sense of Smell

Impairment of smell is not an infrequent accompaniment of an injury to the anterior fossa, though in traumatic brain injury there is rarely complete loss, often no worse than that noted in heavy smokers. Total loss of smell is more likely to occur in situations where intricate repair of the anterior fossa floor has been required to prevent or abolish resistant leakage of the cerebrospinal fluid. The capacity to smell smoke, fumes or other olfactory warning signs is naturally of importance in aircrew. However, the requirements of commercial flying are unclear when there is a co-pilot. Sense of smell very seldom recovers to normal and, if absent, will not return.

Unilateral Deafness

Unilateral deafness can occur after a head injury that involves significant skull fracturing through temporal bone. On occasion, this may have included a transient facial weakness, and assessors should explore this possibility by assessments of vestibular and cochlear function such as balance, tinnitus and pain. Hearing loss will not recover. Useful hearing usually exists up to a loss of 50 dB in intensity, but below this can be troublesome for the individual, particularly where speech discrimination is less than 50 per cent. Unilateral hearing is not uncommon and is discussed in detail in regulatory manuals (International Civil Aviation Organization, 2008).

Facial Deficit

Persisting facial deficit is remarkably rare. Patients with deficits involving the ninth, tenth and twelfth cranial nerves are likely to have had a severe injury involving the posterior fossa, and, whilst unlikely to suffer seizures, may harbour other deficits that need specialist assessment before licensing. Problems are usually manifested as trigeminal pain or dysaesthesias and will often settle over a six-month period. Trigeminal pain is best treated with drugs such as carbamazepine, and a clear distinction of their use for such treatment should be made from their use as anticonvulsants.

Cerebellar Dysfunction

Cerebellar dysfunction heralds itself as either unilateral incoordination, past-pointing or hypotonia. When the vermis is involved, posture control is impaired, with difficult midline rotational movements and poor general balance, particularly in poor light conditions where visual compensation is diminished. Speech phonation may be affected in more severe cases. Patients presenting at six months after such injuries will need a longer period of recovery and will need specialist consideration or counselling about their chances of full recovery.

Cognitive Residual Sequelae

Even a mild injury with concussion can be associated with subtemporal and subfrontal injury that is likely to impact on memory and intellect. The assessor must explore what cognitive issues may lie deeper and may be related to a level on the Glasgow Coma scale as low as 9 at presentation or to a post-traumatic period exceeding 24 hours.

Where individuals have suffered a severe injury, they might be expected to display evident cognitive sequelae that would impede them from flying safely. This would be expected to be especially true for individuals with deficits in visual scanning, visuospatial abilities, divided attention, reaction time, cognitive and behavioural control and, importantly, risk assessment and decision making. In this context, lack of awareness of impairment in cognition is the main reason why some have no qualms about returning to complex anticipatory tasks such as driving.

There is evidence that a number of patients with post-traumatic brain injury return to driving after discharge from hospital despite their licence status, though the situation is much less likely to occur in the aviation setting. Most patients with mild head injury will improve back to safe levels of performance with appropriate insight within six months. Those who have clearly suffered more than simple concussion, particularly those with any evidence of brain injury per se, such as focal deficits, intracranial haemorrhage or imaging changes, may well need neuropsychological assessment to determine the pattern of change. This not only records the baseline for later comparison but enables a tailoring of support therapy so that the most effective programme is provided. Patients with a more severe head injury will benefit from assessment, not least to provide some objective assessment of cognitive ability in the doubtful scenario of a post-traumatic period.

Many of the above neuropsychological characteristics can be individually assessed with established tools, but high-level rationality and abstraction crucial to performance under pressure is much more complex to determine. Fortunately, there is a growing body of information in cognitive science that not only is able to test paradigms of behaviour and decision making, but can also relate functional magnetic resonance imaging to these paradigms in terms of areas of cortical brain functioning and to areas of damage.

The classic case of Phineas Gage who suffered transfixion of his frontal skull from a tamping iron is well described (MacMillan, 2008). The brain area damaged included the ventromedial and orbital surfaces of the frontal lobes and was associated with profound lack of insight, inability to make decisions and change in moral capacity. A recent study reported in *Nature* (Koenigs *et al.*, 2007) has shown that patients with brain injury are much more likely to behave expediently in moral situations, such as deciding who should be sacrificed in a lifeboat survivor situation. Ventromedial and subfrontal cortex are at particular risk in head injury and together with subtemporal damage (short-term memory) represent accessible areas for assessment by functional magnetic resonance imaging and other new testing techniques.

Evidence for Recovery

The Glasgow Outcome Scale is a five-point score given to victims of traumatic brain injury at some point in their recovery, and is used in research to quantify the level of recovery that patients have achieved (Teasdale *et al.*, 1998; King *et al.*, 2005). It is a rather coarse scale, with only five levels, and it has been argued that this scale is not ideal for research purposes. Other more specific, complex and detailed grading systems have been developed.

The Glasgow Outcome Scale is a five-level score:

1. Dead

2. Vegetative state (meaning the patient is unresponsive, but alive; a 'vegetable' in lay language)
3. Severely disabled (conscious, but the patient requires others for daily support due to disability)
4. Moderately disabled (the patient is independent, but disabled)
5. Good recovery (the patient has resumed most normal activities, but may have minor residual problems).

Other scales have sought to refine measures of recovery; these include the extended Glasgow Outcome Scale (Teasdale *et al.*, 1998; Wilson *et al.*, 1997) and modifications to the Rankin Scale (Rankin, 1957; van Swieten *et al.*, 1988; Farrell *et al.*, 1991).

The overall outcome after a severe head injury has been investigated in patients admitted to the neurosurgery service at one of four centres participating in the National Institutes of Health Traumatic Coma Data Bank (Ruff *et al.*, 1993). Of 300 eligible survivors, the quality of recovery one year after injury was assessed by, at least, the Glasgow Outcome Scale in 263 patients (87 per cent), whereas complete neuropsychological assessment was performed in 127 (42 per cent). The capacity of the patients to undergo neuropsychological testing one year after injury was a criterion of recovery, as reflected by a significant relationship to neurological indices of acute injury and the score on the Glasgow Outcome Scale at the time of discharge from hospital. The neurobehavioural data were generally comparable across the four samples of patients and characterized by impairment of memory and slowed information processing. In contrast, language and visuospatial ability had recovered to within the normal range.

The lowest post-resuscitation score on the Glasgow Coma Scale was predictive of the one-year score and neuropsychological performance. The lowest presenting score was especially predictive of neuropsychological performance one year post-injury. Notwithstanding limitations related to the scope of the data bank and attrition in follow-up material, the results indicate a characteristic pattern of neurobehavioural recovery from severe head injury and encourage the use of neurobehavioural outcome measurements in clinical trials to evaluate interventions for head-injured patients

Research in neuropsychology suggests that the aetiology of a neurological injury determines the neuropathological and neuropsychological changes. A study compared neuropsychological outcome in subjects who had traumatic brain injury with that in subjects who had anoxic brain injury who were matched for age, gender and ventricle-to-brain ratio (Shah *et al.*, 2007). There were no group differences for morphological or neuropsychological measures. Both groups exhibited impaired memory, attention, and executive function, as well as slowed mental processing. Intelligence correlated with whole brain volume, and measures of memory correlated with hippocampal atrophy. There was no unique contribution of hippocampal atrophy to neuropsychological outcome between the groups. In the absence of localized lesions, the amount of neural tissue loss, rather than aetiology, may be the critical factor in neuropsychological outcome.

There continues to be debate about the long-term neuropsychological impact of mild traumatic brain injury. A meta-analysis of the relevant literature has been carried out to determine the impact of mild injury across nine cognitive domains (Belanger *et al.*, 2005). The analysis was based on 39 studies involving 1,463 cases and 1,191 control cases. The overall effect of injury on neuropsychological functioning was moderate (d = .54). However, findings were moderated by cognitive domain, time since injury, patient characteristics and sampling methods. Acute effects (less than three months post-injury) were greatest for delayed memory and fluency (d = 1.03 and .89, respectively). In unselected or prospective samples, the overall analysis revealed no residual neuropsychological impairment by three months post-injury (d = .04). In contrast, clinic-based samples and samples including participants in litigation were associated with greater cognitive sequelae (d = .74 and .78, respectively at three months or greater).

However, there are contrary views. One hundred and eighty-two individuals with complicated mild to severe traumatic brain injury were assessed in a longitudinal cohort study with inclusion criteria based on the availability of neuropsychological data at one and five years after injury (Millis *et al.*, 2001). Significant variability in outcome on neuropsychological tests was found five years after injury that ranged from no measurable impairment to severe impairment. Improvement from one year after injury to five years was also variable. Using the reliable change index, 22.2 per cent improved, 15.2 per cent declined and 62.6 per cent were unchanged on test measures. Clearly, neuropsychological recovery after injury is not uniform across individuals and neuropsychological domains. For a subset with moderate to severe injury, neuropsychological recovery may continue for several years with substantial recovery. For others, measurable impairment remains for five years after injury. Improvement was most apparent on measures of cognitive speed, visuoconstruction and verbal memory.

An explanation of these findings may, in part, be the disproportional impact of those with residual difficulties on the analysis. Between 80 and 90 per cent of all patients with mild injury have favourable outcomes, whereas 10 to 20 per cent do not. The latter subgroup, largely from the more severe groups, presented with a plethora of persistent physical, emotional and cognitive symptoms. Indeed, a dichotomy has emerged in the literature interpreting these post-concussional symptoms as being psychogenic or neurogenic. Increasingly, therapy, including cognitive behavioural therapy, is aimed at identifying and helping patients in areas of their life where changes, as a result of injury, appear to be limiting.

There is little information to help understand the relative risks for patients with unrecognized cognitive problems returning to complex activities. In a small study, León-Carrión et al. (2005) described an assessment of 17 patients of mixed injury severity, in whom six had returned to driving against advice. Three of the six reported incidents such as disorientation, mistaken pedal function and driving performance severally affected by excess emotional response to trivial matters. Whilst this report is of note, it is important to add that the authors achieved marked improvement in these subjects with the effect of targeted behavioural therapy and (of course) time passing. Perhaps more thought-provoking is the concept that whereas, given the discussion on epilepsy risk, these subjects may have been debarred based on seizure risk, they may now need a further stratification of cognitive ability, if this is in question.

Psychological interventions commonly used in the management of anxiety and certain types of psychological treatments, such as cognitive behavioural therapy, are well suited to the needs of individuals with traumatic brain injury. An advantage of these interventions is that, given their highly structured content, they are amenable to specialized adaptation for memory, attention and problem-solving impairments, reflecting the difficulties people often experience. A Cochrane review (Soo and Tate, 2007) identified three randomized controlled trials in the area of psychological treatments for anxiety after injury. Some evidence was found for the effectiveness of cognitive behavioural therapy for the treatment of acute stress after mild injury, and combining cognitive behavioural therapy and neurorehabilitation for the treatment of general anxiety symptoms in people with mild to moderate injury (Wilson, 2010).

The ability to make strong conclusions on the effectiveness of these approaches is limited by the small number of trials available for pooling of data, especially trials with similar conditions and participants (Shames et al., 2007).

The medical examiner addressing individuals with cognitive and other issues after injury is apt to be 'risk averse' in less familiar areas. Increasingly, specialist skills will be needed to support formal licensing assessments where their expertise and developing knowledge outweigh available and outdated evidence in a rapidly changing area. It seems likely that such objectivity will be facilitated by improved classification of injury coupled with both anatomic and functional imaging.

Addendum

Glasgow Coma Scale

The level on the Glasgow Coma Scale (3–15) is obtained from adding the scores that relate to eye opening and the motor and verbal responses (Teasdale and Jennett, 1974).

Eye opening

None: 1 — Even to supraorbital pressure

To pain: 2 — Pain from sternum/limb/supraorbital pressure

To speech: 3 — Non-specific response, not necessarily to command

Spontaneous: 4 — Eyes open, not necessarily aware

Motor response

None: 1 — To any pain; limbs remain flaccid

Extension: 2 — Shoulder adducted and shoulder and forearm internally rotated

Flexor response: 3 — Withdrawal response or assumption of hemiplegic posture

Withdrawal: 4 — Arm withdraws to pain, shoulder abducts

Localizes pain: 5 — Arm attempts to remove supraorbital/chest pressure

Obeys commands: 6 — Follows simple commands

Verbal response

None: 1 — No verbalization of any type

Incomprehensible: 2 — Moans/groans, no speech

Inappropriate: 3 — Intelligible, no sustained sentences

Confused: 4 — Converses but confused, disoriented

Oriented: 5 — Converses and oriented

Recreational Flying

Those flying light planes within the United Kingdom or involved in other air sports such as ballooning or gliding can seek a National Private Pilot Licence in which their medical practitioner has to countersign a self-declaration of fitness. The practitioner uses criteria provided by the UK Driver and Vehicle Licensing Agency: Group 1 criteria (equivalent to car driving) for solo-flying and Group 2 criteria (equivalent to driving heavy goods vehicles) for flying with passengers. These procedures are run by the relevant air sports governing bodies and overseen by the Civil Aviation Authority. The risk level for Group 1 is set at 20 per cent and for Group 2 at 2 per cent, based on actuarial approaches to initial risk and seizure-free period and the estimate therefrom of residual risk.

This concept has been clarified so that, for Group 2, the most stringent level for driving, the applicant may be able to drive 'when the risk of seizure has fallen to no greater than 2 per cent per year and with no debarring residual impairment likely to affect safe driving' and if they are not taking anti-epileptic medication. It is important to distinguish between residual risk and annual risk, and it is the latter that has been taken more recently as the criterion for percentage risk definition. The advisory panels to the regulatory authority differentiate between the several subgroups as defined in a guide concerned with fitness to drive. These are under continuous expert review and updated in the *At a Glance Guide to the Current Medical Standards of Fitness to Drive* (Driver and Vehicle Licensing Agency, 2011). Interpretation of the rules for recreational flying is also given.

References

Annegers, J.F., Hauser, W.A., Coan, S.P. and Rocca, W.A. 1998. A population-based study of seizures after traumatic brain injuries. *New England Journal of Medicine*, 338, 20–24.

Battle, W.H. 1890. Three lectures on some points relating to injuries to the head (Lecture II). *British Medical Journal*, 2, 75–81.

Baumann, C.R., Werth, E., Stocker, R., Ludwig, S. and Bassetti, C.L. 2007. Sleep–wake disturbances 6 months after traumatic brain injury: A prospective study. *Brain*, 130, 1873–83.

Belanger, H.G., Curtiss, G., Demery, J.A., Lebowitz, B.K. and Vanderploeg, R.D. 2005. Factors moderating neuropsychological outcomes following mild traumatic brain injury: A meta-anaylsis. *Journal of the International Neuropsychological Society*, 11, 215–27.

Bonnett, L.J., Tudur-Smith, C., Williamson, P.R. and Marson, A.G. 2010. Risk of recurrence after a first seizure and implications for driving: Further analysis of the Multicentre study of early Epilepsy and Single Seizures. *British Medical Journal*, 341, c6477.

Brown, A.W., Malec, J.F., McClelland, R.L., Diehl, N.N., Englander, J. and Cifu, D.X. 2005. Clinical elements that predict outcome after traumatic brain injury: A prospective multicenter recursive partitioning (decision-tree) analysis. *Journal of Neurotrauma*, 22, 1040–51.

Cantu, R.C. 2006. An overview of concussion consensus statements since 2000. *Neurosurgical Focus*, 21, 4, E3.

Christensen, J., Pedersen, M., Pedersen, C., Sidenius, P., Olsen, J. and Vestergaard, M. 2009. Long-term risk of epilepsy after traumatic brain injury in children and young adults: A population-based cohort study. *Lancet*, 373, 1105–10.

Driver and Vehicle Licensing Agency. 2005. Minutes of the Secretary of State's Honorary Medical Advisory Panel on Driving and Disorders of the Nervous System. 19 October 2005.

Driver and Vehicle Licensing Agency: Drivers Medical Group. 2011. *At a Glance Guide to the Current Medical Standards of Fitness to Drive*. Swansea: Driver and Vehicle Licensing Agency. Dunn, L.T., Fitzpatrick, M.O., Beard, D. and Henry, J.H. 2003. Patients with a head injury who 'talk and die' in the 1990s. *Journal of Trauma*, 54, 497–502.

Farrell, B., Godwin, J., Richards, S. and Warlow, C. 1991. The United Kingdom transient ischaemic attack (UK-TIA) aspirin trial: Final results. *Journal of Neurology, Neurosurgery and Psychiatry*, 54, 1044–54.

Hoge, C.W., Goldberg, H.M. and Castro, C.A. 2009. Care of war veterans with mild traumatic brain injury – flawed perspectives. *New England Journal of Medicine*, 360, 1588–91.

Ingebrigsten, T., Waterloo, K., Marup-Jensen, S., Attner, E. and Romner, B. 1988. Quantification of post-concussion symptoms three months after head injury in 100 consecutive patients. *Journal of Neurology*, 245, 609–12.

International Civil Aviation Organization. 2008. *Manual of Civil Aviation Medicine: Preliminary Edition Part III. Medical Assessment*. Montreal, QC: International Civil Aviation Organization.

Jennett, B. 1998. Epidemiology of head injury. *Archives of Disease in Children*, 78, 403–6.

Jennett, B. and Teasdale, G. 1977. Aspects of coma after severe head injury. *Lancet*, 1(8017), 878–81.

Joint Aviation Authorities. 2006. *Joint Aviation Requirements: Flight Crew Licensing 3 (Medical)*. The Netherlands: Joint Aviation Authorities.

King, J.T. Jr, Carlier, P.M. and Marion, D.W. 2005. Early Glasgow Outcome Scale scores predict long-term functional outcome in patients with severe traumatic brain injury. *Journal of Neurotrauma*, 22, 947–54.

Koenigs, M., Young, L., Adolph, R., Tranel, D., Cushman, F., Hauser, M. and Damasio, A. 2007. Damage to the prefrontal cortex increases utilitarian moral judgements. *Nature*, 446, 908–9.

Leon-Carrion, J., Dominguez-Morales, M.R. and Martin, J.M. 2005. Driving with cognitive deficits: Neurorehabilitation and legal measures are needed for driving again after severe traumatic brain injury. *Brain Injury*, 19, 213–9.

London Trauma Office. 2010. *Mid-year report April to September 2010*. Available at: www.londontraumaoffice.nhs.uk

Maas, A.I., Stocchetti, N. and Bullock, R. 2008. Moderate and severe traumatic brain injury in adults. *Lancet Neurology*, 7, 728–41.

MacMillan, M. 2008. Phineas Gage – Unravelling the myth. *The Pychologist*, 21, 828–31.

Miller, J.I., Chou, M.W., Capocelli, A., Bolognese, P., Pan, J. and Milhorat, T.H. 1998. Continuous intracranial multimodality monitoring comparing local cerebral blood flow, cerebral perfusion pressure, and microvascular resistance. *Acta Neurochirurgica Supplement*, 71, 82–4.

Millis, S.R., Rosenthal, M., Novack, T.A., Sherer, M., Nick, T.G., Kreutzer, J.S. *et al*. 2001. Long-term neuropsychological outcome after traumatic brain injury. *The Journal of Head Trauma Rehabilitation*, 16, 343–55.

National Confidential Enquiry into Patient Outcome and Death. 2007. *Trauma: Who Cares?* London: NCEPOD.

Pompucci, A., De Bonis, P., Pettorino, B., Petrella, G., Di Chirico, A. and Anile, C. 2007. Decompressive craniectomy for traumatic brain injury: Patient age and outcome. *Journal of Neurotrauma*, 24, 1182–8.

Rankin, J. 1957. Cerebral vascular accidents in patients over the age of 60: Prognosis. *Scottish Medical Journal*, 2, 200–215.

Ruff, R.M., Marshall, L.F., Crouch, J., Klauber, M.R., Levin, H.S., Barth, J. *et al.* 1993. Predictors of outcome following severe head trauma: Follow-up data from the Traumatic Coma Data Bank. *Brain Injury*, 7, 101–11.

Sabo, R.A., Hanigan, W.C. and Aldag, J.C. 1995. Chronic subdural hematomas and seizures: The role of prophylactic anticonvulsive medication. *Surgical Neurology*, 43, 579–82.

Schrader, H., Mickeviciene, D., Gleizniene, R., Jakstiene, S., Surkiene, D., Stovner, L.J. and Obelieniene, D. 2009. Magnetic resonance imaging after most common form of concussion. *Biomed Central Medical Imaging*, 9, 11–16.

Shah, M., Carayannopoulos, A., Burke, D. and Al-Adawi, S.A. 2007. A comparison of functional outcomes in hypoxia and traumatic brain injury: A pilot study. *Journal of the Neurological Sciences*, 260, 95–9.

Shames, J., Treger, I., Ring, H. and Giaquinto, S. 2007. Return to work following traumatic brain injury: Trends and challenges. *Disability and Rehabilitation*, 29, 1387–95.

Shores, E.A., Marosszeky, J.E., Sandanam, J. and Batchelor, J. 1986. Preliminary validation of a clinical scale for measuring the duration of post-traumatic amnesia. *Medical Journal of Australia*, 144, 569–72.

Shorvon, S. and Neligan, A. 2009. Risk of epilepsy after head trauma. *Lancet*, 373, 1060–61.

Teasdale, G. and Jennett, B. 1974. Assessment of coma and impaired consciousness: A practical scale. *Lancet*, 13, 2(7872), 81–4.

Soo, C. and Tate, R. 2007. Psychological treatment for anxiety in people with traumatic brain injury. *Cochrane Database of Systematic Reviews*, 3, CD005239.

van Swieten, J.C., Koudstaal, P.J., Visser, M.C., Schouten, H.J. and van Gijn, J. 1988. Interobserver agreement for the assessment of handicap in stroke patients. *Stroke*, 19, 604–7.

Teasdale, G. and Jennett, B. 1978. Assessment of coma and severity of brain damage. *Anesthesiology*, 49, 225–6.

Teasdale, G.M., Pettigrew, L.E., Wilson, J.T., Murray, G. and Jennett, B. 1998. Analyzing outcome of treatment of severe head injury: A review and update on advancing the use of the Glasgow Outcome Scale. *Journal of Neurotrauma*, 15, 587–97.

Vespa, P.M., Nenov, V. and Nuwer, M.R. 1999. Continuous EEG monitoring in the intensive care unit: Early findings and clinical efficacy. *Journal of Clinical Neurophysiology*, 16, 1–13.

Whitnall, L., McMillan, T.M., Murray, G.D. and Teasdale, G.M. 2006. Disability in young people and adults after head injury: 5–7 year follow up of a prospective cohort study. *Journal of Neurology, Neurosurgery and Psychiatry*, 77, 640–45.

Wilson, B.A. 2010. Brain injury: Recovery and rehabilitation. *Cognitive Science*, 1, 108–18.

Wilson, J.T.L., Pettigrew, L.E.L. and Teasdale, G.M. 1997. Structured interviews for the Glasgow Outcome Scale and the Extended Glasgow Outcome Scale: Guidelines for their use. *Journal of Neurotrauma*, 15, 573–85.

World Health Organization. 2007. *International Classification of Diseases and Related Health Problems – Tenth Revision*. Geneva: World Health Organization Press.

Chapter 17

NEURO-OPHTHALMOLOGY

Gordon T. Plant

The discipline of neuro-ophthalmology is concerned with disorders of vision that primarily result from dysfunction of the nervous system as opposed to the eye itself. Neuro-ophthalmology begins and ends with visual function, but it is primarily concerned with disorders of the optic nerve, the visual pathways in the brain and the ocular motor system. The eye is developmentally a part of the nervous system and there is, therefore, much commonality in the spectrum of conditions that affect the eye and the brain. The techniques of examination and the relevant special investigations have developed to a large extent independently in ophthalmology on the one hand and in the clinical neurosciences on the other, and there are few practitioners who are well schooled in both disciplines. It is essential that there are physicians who can sit comfortably with a foot in each camp; otherwise, patients with neurological disorders that affect vision cannot be managed in a coherent manner, having to attend one clinic to have the eye examined and another for the neurological assessment. In the United Kingdom ophthalmology is largely practised by ophthalmologists trained in surgery, whereas in other parts of the world most ophthalmologists

do not undertake surgery, although the training is the same. An ophthalmic physician with a sound background in medicine who is as competent as surgical colleagues in the diagnosis of eye disease has become a rarity.

Medical ophthalmology aims to produce physicians who are competent in the diagnosis and management of ophthalmic disorders, but who are also trained in internal medicine to the same standard as would be, for example, a rheumatologist or gastroenterologist. Neuro-ophthalmology comes under the general umbrella of medical ophthalmology, but the latter also encompasses inflammatory eye disease and non-surgical disorders of the retina ('medical retina') where there are considerable overlaps with other disciplines such as rheumatology and genetics. This chapter is concerned with visual disorders that arise as a result of disease of the central nervous system where some understanding of ophthalmology is essential for diagnosis and management. The neurologist cannot provide comprehensive care for patients without a knowledge of how the eye and vision are affected, and as long as patients with visual symptoms come first to see an ophthalmologist, it is essential that training involves a sound knowledge of the many and diverse visual manifestations of disorders of the nervous system.

In aviation medicine a knowledge of neuro-ophthalmic conditions is essential for the interpretation of tests of visual function such as visual acuity, colour vision and visual fields (perimetry) and also for the examination of ocular movements and the pupil. However, it is unlikely that the practitioner will be required to carry through to a diagnosis a new presentation of, for example, unilateral optic nerve disease. It is more likely that the practitioner will encounter individuals with a pre-existing neuro-ophthalmic disorder, or one that develops whilst working in the aviation industry. This chapter is aimed at providing the background required to understand the implications of such conditions, beginning with measurement of the parameters of visual function and the techniques of examination.

Visual Acuity

Visual acuity is defined as the *minimum separabile*, that is to say the minimum separation of two points that can be resolved by the visual system. In practice, visual acuity charts have been designed which utilize letters or other symbols, the recognition of which depends upon one or more gaps between lines. The advantage of using standard letters is that the subjects do not need to be instructed beforehand as to the nature of the symbols, provided that the subject is literate in the script. Charts using a single symbol at different orientations, such as the Landolt 'C' or 'broken rings' charts and the tumbling 'E' charts, are available. They are psychophysically purer in that there is a consistent gap to be resolved and they can also be used without prior knowledge of any particular alphabet.

The advantage of the letter charts such as the Snellen (1862) is that the subject is forced to choose from a large set of stimuli, thus reducing the probability of a correct response occurring by chance. In fact, the set of letters used is not taken from the entire alphabet (even fewer if intended to be read in a mirror). Snellen himself realized that he would need to design his own square formatted letters for the purpose (therefore known as optotypes) rather than using existing fonts (Figure 17.1).

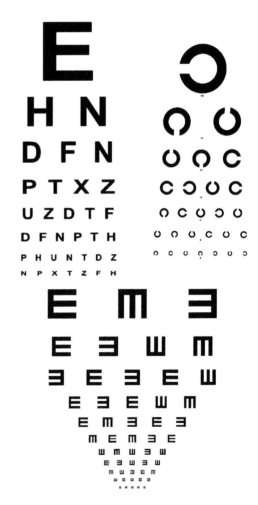

Figure 17.1 Typical visual acuity charts: Snellen, Landolt C and Tumbling E

More recently, Sloan (1959) has refined the set and design (using only C, D, H, K, N, O, R, S, V and Z) to achieve results comparable with the Landolt test. As long as the subject is not informed that the set no longer includes the entire alphabet, they will continue to confuse 'C' with 'G', 'H' with 'M', and 'O' with 'Q', and the power of the test is not much diminished. The most recent development has been the design of the LogMAR chart. This involves two innovations: one is the LogMAR unit of measurement (logarithm of the minimal angle of resolution), the second is the arrangement of the ten Sloan letters chosen in equal lines of five on the chart. There are consequently 252 possible line combinations. Each of the chosen lines has been designed to give a near equal score of difficulty (Figure 17.2).

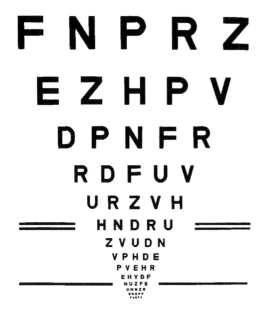

Figure 17.2 LogMAR visual acuity charts using the Sloane letters

Charts which also use LogMAR scaling have been designed which use the Tumbling E and Landolt C optotypes and for near vision.

In a LogMAR chart, the progression of letter height/width (and hence the dimension of the *minimum separabile*) is such that any line is 1.2589 times greater than the line below. Thus, there is a parametric set, with the dimension increasing in steps by a factor that is the root of ten or 0.1 log unit. A three-line worsening of visual acuity is equal to a doubling of the visual angle regardless of the initial acuity, and furthermore is based on tests of comparable difficulty. The charts are designed for use at a distance of 4 metres. This configuration was designed by Bailey and Lovie (1976) and will in time replace the Snellen chart, as it has already done so for research. The Snellen charts cannot be used for parametric analysis as the steps from one line to the next are not equivalent and the lines themselves are not of equal difficulty because the number of letters and the spacing of the letters differs from one line to the next. According to the LogMAR protocol, three charts should be used, one for refraction and one for testing each eye so that the subject cannot become familiar with any of the lines. In situations where precise measurement of visual acuity can have a major impact on an individual's career – as is the case with aviation – the most accurate and reproducible methods should be employed.

So far we have discussed the measurement of visual acuity for distance, by which is meant beyond 1 metre where accommodation of the lens will not be involved in the process. In practical terms the distance used tends to be between 3 and 6 metres. However, an estimation of near vision is important from the occupational point of view where there is a need to know that vision is adequate within 1 metre radius. Traditionally, subjects are given blocks of text to read using standard fonts at a set viewing distance, commonly 40 centimetres. In the United Kingdom the measurement is usually made using the Times New Roman font and the 'N' notation corresponds to the font size. Hence, a near vision of N10 indicates that the subject could read the 10-point font size at whatever viewing distance. Near vision charts based on the LogMAR principle (Bailey and Lovie, 1976) have been developed using carefully selected single optotypes rather than text.

Reading text requires more than just adequate acuity, and impairment of language processing (acquired alexia) will impair reading. Furthermore, *fluent* reading requires an intact visual field. Specifically, the parafoveal region in the right hemifield (for left to right readers) must be intact: fluent reading requires 'advance warning' of what is coming up along the line of text.

Visual Acuity in Neuro-Ophthalmology

A record of the best corrected visual acuity in each eye is essential to the assessment of a neuro-ophthalmic disorder. It is also essential to know what correction was used to obtain that acuity measurement. There are many aspects of the neuro-ophthalmic examination that are much influenced by the shape of the eye, such as the appearance of the optic disc, and many aspects of subjective visual complaints that cannot be understood without reference to the refractive state. Correctly, measurements should refer to foveal visual acuity because acuity can be measured at any point in the visual field, though by convention acuity is measured at the fovea. This is the only measure that is of value in refraction and it turns out to be very sensitive to impairment in a wide range of ophthalmic and neurological disorders – but by no means in all of

them. Accordingly, it is of great value in detecting and monitoring disease.

Visual acuity is exquisitely dependent upon the refractive state of the eye and the integrity of the ocular media. It is also dependent on the condition of the fovea itself, and on the integrity of the retinal ganglion cells that subserve the fovea. It is also, therefore, dependent on the integrity of the axons of those ganglion cells which project in the retinal nerve fibre layer, via the optic disc to the optic nerve itself, and subsequently to the optic chiasm and the optic tracts. Foveal vision is of great functional importance because this is the region of the visual field that provides the best acuity and the maximum ability to resolve detail in the image. For this reason the major function of the ocular motor system can be seen to be foveation, that is to say ensuring that the object of principal interest is brought into foveal vision and then held there.

Visual acuity will be affected in optic nerve disease if there is involvement of the foveal projection of nerve fibres. This will be the rule with genetically determined, compressive or inflammatory disorders of the retrobulbar optic nerve because in most cases there will be diffuse involvement of the axonal population of the optic nerve. There is some evidence that the foveal projection of fibres might even be more vulnerable than the fibres originating in peripheral retina. Furthermore, in the optic nerve there is considerable intermingling of retinal ganglion cell axons, and it is not possible to generate damage to discrete bundles of axons that could result in discrete defects in the visual field. However, if the pathology is at the optic disc, the situation is different because discrete bundles of optic nerve fibres can be damaged as they traverse the optic disc, resulting in specific 'optic disc related' defects in the visual field that can potentially spare the foveal fibres. There is, indeed, some evidence that, in a number of disorders that impact on the optic disc itself, the foveal fibres may be relatively spared until late in the disease (glaucoma, papilloedema and optic disc drusen are examples) or are commonly spared, as in anterior ischaemic optic neuropathy.

On reaching the chiasm, the situation is different again because the foveal fibres are rearranged as the four separate projections of each hemifovea at the decussation. Selective damage to the decussating fibres alone will not affect visual acuity because, although there will be a bitemporal hemianopia, acuity can be subserved by the projections of the two temporal hemifoveas in the surviving nasal hemifields. Similarly, damage to one optic tract, optic radiation or visual cortex will give rise to a homonymous hemianopia, but with no impairment of visual acuity subserved by the surviving homonymous field. It is essential to be aware that, in the case of neuro-ophthalmic disease, foveal visual acuity may be a useful screening tool, together with tests of colour vision and visual fields.

Colour Vision

The assessment of colour vision is of considerable importance in neuro-ophthalmology because in many optic nerve disorders chromatic processing seems to be especially vulnerable. The standard tests used in the clinic are simple judgements of colour saturation and the Ishihara isochromatic plates. One perceptual consequence of impaired functioning of chromatic mechanisms is that colours will appear less saturated, that is to say closer to white. Patients will usually describe this as a 'washed out' or 'faded' appearance. A coloured stimulus

that is already desaturated may appear to have no colour and to be white or grey. Small coloured targets can be used to probe the visual field looking for areas of desaturation or the degree of saturation can be compared between the two eyes in monocular or asymmetric disease.

To assess colour vision, it is necessary to devise tests which isolate chromatic mechanisms. It is a simple matter to isolate achromatic mechanisms as it is only necessary to produce an achromatic target (one that is black and white, or shades of grey). It is problematic, on the other hand, to design a stimulus that isolates colour mechanisms because it is difficult to remove all the luminance differences that may also delineate the target. One way around this is to break up the image into areas which jump randomly in luminance, masking any of the much smaller differences in luminance between the symbol or pattern to be identified and the background. Hence, as the Ishihara plates are *pseudo*-isochromatic, there may be small luminance differences between the figure and the background, but it is masked by the random variation in luminance of the component spots and the subject will not be able to utilize luminance differences in performing the task.

The plates developed by Ishihara (1917) assessed Daltonism (congenital colour anomaly: deuteranopia and protanopia), but there was no test for tritanopia (Dalton, 1766–1844). An alternative set of pseudo-isochromatic plates, referred to as the 'HRR' set (Hardy, Rand and Rittler, 1954) contains a test for tritanopia. In neuro-ophthalmic practice, an understanding of congenital colour anomalies is necessary so that they can be identified and distinguished from acquired anomalies that may be indicative of neuro-ophthalmic disease. Pseudo-isochromatic plates are extremely useful as screening tools for acquired dyschromatopsia because they are quick and easy to use. They include a set of illiterate plates and are available in most eye clinics (Figure 17.3).

The plates can be used in a non-parametric fashion to monitor changes in colour vision simply by recording the number of plates correctly identified. Where errors are made, it is worthwhile recording them. For example, a subject who consistently misses the right-hand digit on the dual-digit plates may have a right hemifield defect in that

eye. Daltonism can be distinguished from an acquired defect because of the pattern of errors. Some of the plates (the 'alternative number' plates) have two hidden numbers, one that will be read by a trichromat and the other by a deuteranope or protanope (dichromat). There are also plates ('hidden number') where the number is camouflaged for trichromats and is only read by dichromats. Subjects with acquired dyschromatopsia will not show either of these patterns. Another distinguishing feature is that in Daltonism the same

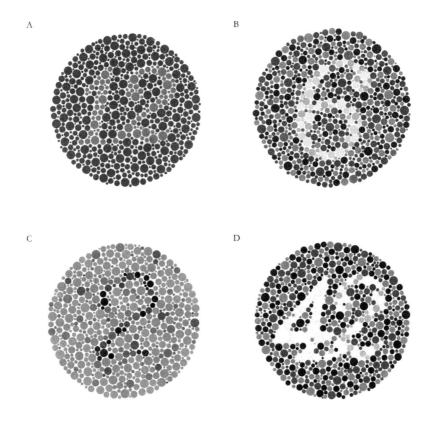

Figure 17.3 Examples of plates found in the Ishihara test book (see colour section)

A.   This is a control plate. No colour vision is required to read the '12' but the subject needs adequate visual acuity and be able to distinguish the 'Figure' (dots making up the number) from the "ground" (dots making up the background).

B.   A trichromat will read '6' whereas a dichromat may see nothing or read a different number.

C.   A trichromat cannot read a number. A dichromat may or may not read a number '2'.

D.   A trichromat will read '42'. A protanope will not see the '4' and a deuteranope will not see the '2' errors will be made in each eye, whereas this may not be the case in an acquired syndrome.

Both Ishihara and HRR plates contain a 'control' plate where no colour vision is required to read the number. This provides an assurance that the subject has adequate visual acuity to perform the task (an acuity of 6/60 or worse is not sufficient and the task is meaningless). Some patients with visual impairment due to visual cortex disorders are unable to carry out the 'figure–ground' aspect of the task. The visual system is required to group together the dots making up the figure and the dots making up the background before the number can be read. Such subjects will not be able to read the control plate and are often mistakenly thought to have an acquired dyschromatopsia.

In inflammatory and compressive optic nerve disease, it is typically found that dyschromatopsia is disproportionate to the loss of acuity because of the more diffuse involvement of the retinal projections in the optic nerve. In acquired retinal disorders, on the other hand, impairment of colour vision will only be present when there is involvement of the macula and there will be proportionate loss of acuity and colour vision. There are rare exceptions to this in retinopathy where tiny central islands of vision adequately subserve acuity while parafoveal retina is damaged and performance on the Ishihara plates is poor.

'Arrangement' tests are designed to assess hue discrimination in a more systematic manner than is possible with pseudo-isochromatic plates. The best known is the Farnsworth–Munsell 100-hue test (Farnsworth, 1943) (Figure 17.4) with its little cousin, the dichotomous D15. The subject is required to arrange a series of coloured chips in colour order which is, of course, only possible if the

subject can discriminate the small steps in colour difference. The significance of '100' hues is that this is at about the limit of discriminable colours at the saturation and brightness used, but in practice there are only 88 in the test. In view of the large number of chips and the fact that the entire colour circle is represented, the 100-hue test can be used to characterize colour deficits other than Daltonism. The D15 panel is specifically designed to categorize congenital anomalies by limiting the set to the colours required for that purpose. Lanthony (1978) has devised a desaturated version of the D15 which is more useful in acquired disease. It has a smaller set of hues, but they are desaturated and therefore more likely to be confused by patients with, for example, optic nerve disease. In other words, it is a compromise between the ease of use of the D15 and the sensitivity of the 100-hue test.

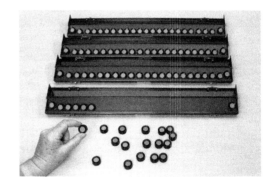

Figure 17.4 The Farnsworth–Munsell 100-hue test (see colour section)

It should be added that all of the tests mentioned so far use surface colours and the spectral content of the test colours will vary with the illumination. All the tests are standardized using a standard white illumination known as 'luminance C' at photopic levels, and with a spectral content equivalent to the light coming through a north-facing window in the northern hemisphere on an overcast day. It is rare to find this specific illumination being used in clinical practice and the accuracy of the tests suffers as a result. Increasingly, these tests are being made available for computer monitors where calibration of the monitor is crucial. Copies of the Ishihara test accessed on the internet or as iPhone apps cannot be considered to be accurate.

Colour vision requirements for pilots are defined in a behavioural context. Pilots need to have whatever colour vision is necessary for them to be able to perform their function in the cockpit. Issues will arise mostly with minor degrees of congenital colour anomaly rather than with the clear-cut 20 cases of deuteranopia and protanopia. Acquired colour vision deficiencies can be extremely varied, particularly when mild, and can be different in the two eyes, and these again are problematic in deciding whether the subject is safe to fly an aeroplane. It is very difficult to extrapolate from the colour vision tests described above to performance-based judgements of occupational relevance. For this reason, tests which can be specifically related to the occupational tasks have been developed.

Holmgren (1876) suggested that the Lagerlunda rail disaster in Sweden of the previous year (a head-on collision on a single-track railway) occurred because one of the drivers suffered from deuteranopia. This remained no more than a theory because the driver was killed in the accident and could not be tested, but Holmgren was able to show that the expected proportion of engine drivers already employed had congenital colour anomalies. Concern spread rapidly internationally and soon tests of colour vision were being used in potential recruits by railways across the globe. Holmgren devised a test

using the naming of coloured wools which became an international standard, but lantern tests were also developed because, at least superficially, they seemed more appropriate for the occupations concerned, where it is the identification of various types of illuminated signal lights that is under scrutiny. It is, needless to say, unfortunate that red and green are so often used for signalling. Other colours could be chosen which would not disadvantage Daltonists, but there is no real likelihood of a change in practice.

A number of lantern type tests are in use. These have the advantage of using stimuli that most resemble the various types of signalling lights that pilots may come across in terms of size and brightness. There is also the ability to test in dim (mesopic) conditions with minimal distortion resulting from the spectral content of the ambient lighting. Squire *et al.* (2005) have studied normal and Daltonist observers using the Ishihara plates and the Holmes–Wright Type A, Spectrolux, and Beyne aviation colour vision lanterns. The pass/fail criteria for the tests set out by the Joint Aviation Requirements were compared with the results obtained on the Nagel anomaloscope. The findings in dichromats are straightforward, but in anomalous trichromats there are discrepancies in all directions, with some failing one lantern test and passing another, some failing the Nagel test but passing one or more of the lantern tests and vice versa. Acquired colour vision deficits have not been studied in such detail on a range of tests but, given the greater variability in such anomalies, at least the same degree of inconsistency might be expected.

This same group has studied the nature of warning and information signals used by commercial pilots using colour and classified the signals and displays according to their importance for safety. At the same time a new computer-based test has been developed for assessing colour vision, the colour assessment and diagnosis (CAD) test. The results of the test can be related to the colour discriminations identified as significant for pilots. Some of the colour critical instrument displays such as the precision approach path indicator (PAPI) have been replicated as a separate section of the assessment. These developments have been the subject of a report from the United Kingdom Civil Aviation Authority (2009).

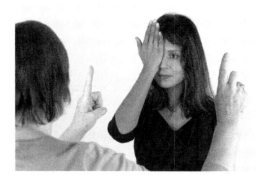

Figure 17.5 Confrontation perimetry
The visual field of the patient is compared with that of the examiner.

Perimetry

Assessment of the visual fields is an essential part of every neuro-ophthalmological examination. As pointed out above, although visual acuity and colour vision can be used as screening and monitoring tests, there are many situations in which these tests are normal, and perimetry is therefore necessary for detection and diagnosis. Confrontation perimetry (Figure 17.5) is a useful skill to acquire because it can be performed in a few minutes and will detect most neurological visual field defects. Monitoring of fixation is straightforward (during the test the subject fixes the examiner's eye) and it is possible to move from a large kinetic stimulus (the examiner's hand) to an assessment of peripheral acuity (counting fingers), to a small achromatic target for probing scotomas (a white pinhead), to a coloured target to detect localized regions of colour desaturation (a red pinhead) and, lastly, to a two-alternative forced-choice colour discrimination test using a white and a green pinhead. However, for the purposes of documentation and monitoring quantitative methods must be used.

Tangent versus Bowl Perimetry

In the 1850s von Graefe (1828–1870) introduced the ophthalmoscope into clinical use, following its invention by von Helmholtz (1821–1894). Helmholtz had suggested using a screen marked with a series of fixation points so that when viewing the fundus the subject could be instructed to move the eye in a controlled manner. Helmholtz adapted this screen to record the limits of the peripheral field and so also introduced a method of plotting the field of vision. The earliest perimetric techniques were 'tangent' perimeters of this type, so called because the test surface was a flat screen positioned at a tangent to the visual field, which is, of course, a circle with the eye at its centre. This came to be known as campimetry, to distinguish it from perimetry in which measurements were made using a spherical bowl (or a curved arm which was moved to describe a sphere) designed to maintain the stimulus at a constant distance from the eye.

The popularity of campimetry and perimetry waxed and waned, and the distinction is important today because the bowl-type of tangent screen has the advantage of extending to the extreme periphery of the visual field, but must of necessity be close to the eye – around 50 centimetres to be of practical use –which reduces the resolution. The tangent screen, on the other hand, can be positioned at any desired distance. The further away it is, the smaller the area of field tested, but the greater the resolution. It was using a large tangent screen at a viewing distance of 1 or 2 metres that Bjerrum (1851–1920) showed the world the importance of plotting the central field at high resolution in the detection of arcuate scotomas (later known as Bjerrum scotomas) in glaucoma (Bjerrum, 1889).

The general method used was the plotting of isoptres (lines of equal sensitivity) by moving the target across the screen or bowl from areas where it was not seen to the limit of visibility (kinetic perimetry). A later development was the finding that central defects could be plotted accurately by presenting a stimulus statically and varying the brightness to plot a detection threshold. This depended upon an illuminated target and was best achieved with bowl perimeters. The most sophisticated bowl perimeters (the Goldmann and Tübingen perimeters), developed in the twentieth century, permitted both kinetic plotting of the peripheral field and static testing in central field. The poor resolution of the bowl arrangement was compensated by the more precise localization afforded by the static method.

The Goldmann perimeter was adapted in the design of the first automated perimeters (Octopus and Humphrey), which are bowl perimeters relying on automated static testing and using sophisticated and well-validated psychophysical test strategies permitting comparison of the results with a normal population (Figure 17.6). This has been revolutionary in permitting quantitative and reproducible results. The

techniques were developed principally for the detection and monitoring of glaucomatous visual field defects, and as such are not well suited to some neurological defects (Wong and Sharpe, 2000). Testing outside the central 30 degrees is possible, but the system is over-engineered for this part of the field. In the last few years, automated kinetic perimetry has been introduced to emulate the older techniques using the new technology.

With all types of perimetry it is important to become familiar with the practical aspects of carrying out the tests. There are many potential pitfalls and artefacts in the results that need to be identified. They relate to the appropriate correction being used for the particular viewing distance of the test, the subject not being correctly positioned, observer errors, the subject not cooperating and forgetting to patch the other eye. It is unwise to treat perimetric charts as if they are some kind of objective analysis of the visual field. It takes two human beings to achieve the result and there are numerous possible errors on either side.

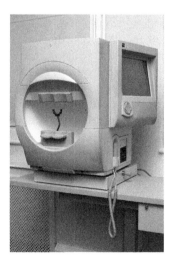

Figure 17.6 The Humphrey visual field analyzer
Automated visual field testing using a bowl perimeter.

Binocular Testing

An additional refinement for occupational use is binocular testing, which is of very little value in diagnosis and monitoring. It was promoted by Esterman (1982) for assessing the disability resulting from the totality of visual field loss. That could be a complex distribution of heteronymous defects where only the components overlapping in the two eyes contribute to disability in everyday life. Esterman proposed a particular grid of static testing points using the Goldman apparatus which he regarded as giving appropriate weight to the more and less significant regions of the visual field. For example, there is a higher density of points in the lower field because loss of field below the horizontal meridian is more likely to affect mobility in a person who is spending most of their time on two legs. The test provides a number which is simply the number of points on the grid which were missed – all the stimuli are shown at maximum brightness.

It is not necessarily the case that these are the appropriate weightings for occupational decisions or for driving and aviation safety. Nonetheless, the Esterman binocular visual field test (now carried out as a built-in paradigm using the Humphrey automated perimeter) has become the gold standard for the United Kingdom Department of Transport in assessing fitness to drive. It has the advantages that it is quick and universally available, and, although it might be possible to design a test with theoretically more appropriate weightings for visual requirements of driving, there is very little scientific evidence on which to base the judgements. Binocular visual field testing is problematic because, particularly with the viewing distance of 50 centimetres, it is necessary for the subject to make a vergence effort to fix on the target, which can lead to inconsistencies in performance.

None of the systems in place to monitor fixation can be used under binocular viewing conditions. The video system on the Humphrey perimeter is only effective under monocular viewing because the set-up for binocular testing involves positioning the bridge of the nose where the eye would otherwise be. Also the 'fixation monitoring' paradigm depends upon testing within the physiological blind spot, which is no longer a possibility. The Esterman binocular test should never be viewed in isolation but always in the context of the results of threshold testing in each eye. The binocular results can be predicted from the monocular results on the simple assumption that the eye with the higher sensitivity will determine the threshold at any particular point in the visual field (Crabb and Viswanathan, 2005). This exercise should be undertaken at least to a first approximation to ensure that the monocular results are consistent with the binocular test.

Examination of the Pupils

Examination of the pupils should never be neglected. First, the size should be noted in the ambient lighting and whether the pupils are the same size (isocoria) or differ in size (anisocoria). If there is anisocoria, the pupil diameter should be measured again in as bright and as dim ambient lighting as possible. If the smaller pupil is the abnormal one, then there is a sympathetic defect and the anisocoria will be greater in the dark; the opposite will be the case if it is the larger pupil that is abnormal (parasympathetic defect). The pupil circumference should be circular, and any irregularity is likely to be a sign of disease. Next, the pupil reaction to light should be examined. For this it is necessary to have a good-quality light source as one of the commonest reasons that an abnormality is missed is that the light source is not bright enough. Care must be taken to examine the direct and consensual responses of each eye and then the response to near using an accommodative target (that is to say one that encourages the near response such as a small image printed on the near target).

In the past few years, a class of retinal ganglion cells subserving the pupil light reflex has been identified as having the unique property of being intrinsically photosensitive due to the presence of the photopigment melanopsin (Zaidi et al., 2007). Exactly the role played by this photo-pigment is not clear as the ganglion cells also receive input from the rod and cone photoreceptors. There are only a few thousand of these ganglion cells covering the retina and they act as the visual system's light meters subserving not only the pupil light reflex but also circadian rhythmicity (see Figure 2.5 Cellular structure of the retina, Chapter 2: Circadian System and Diurnal Activity). They are not involved in image formation.

If loss of vision is entirely due to abnormalities of the ocular media (dense cataract, corneal opacity), then the pupil light reflex will be unaffected because the quantity of light reaching the retina will not be affected. If, on the other hand, an eye has no vision due to retinal or optic nerve disease, there will be no direct pupil response to light (amaurotic pupil), but the consensual response will be present. When there is partial loss of vision, the pupil light reflex becomes very helpful in distinguishing retinal from optic nerve disease, because in retinal disease the impairment of the pupil light reflex will be in proportion to the area of retina damaged, and a subject with a visual acuity of 6/60 due

to maculopathy will have a pupil light reflex indistinguishable from normal on bedside testing. A subject with optic nerve disease, particularly if it is inflammatory, compressive or ischaemic in origin, will have an obvious abnormality of the pupil light reflex. Some disorders may spare the melanopsin ganglion cells, in particular mitochondrial cytopathies, and the pupil light reflex may therefore be less affected in, for example, the hereditary optic neuropathy described by Leber (1840–1917).

The amplitude of the pupil response to light diminishes with age and has a considerable variance in the population in any given age group. Therefore, even with the help of quantitative pupillometry, it is not possible to identify a pupil light response as outside the normal range unless it is very severely affected. For this reason the relative afferent pupil defect, or Marcus Gunn (1850–1909) pupil, has become one of the most valuable signs in neuro-ophthalmology. It allows comparison of the strength of the pupil light reflex between the two eyes as the variance of the *inter-ocular* difference in the pupil light reflex is very low. The test depends upon the pupil light reflex being rather slow (120 milliseconds), which allows time to transfer the light stimulus from one eye to the other without the pupils having the time to dilate back to the size corresponding to the ambient light levels (Figure 17.7). If the test is positive, both pupils will be seen to dilate as the light source is introduced to the affected eye and to constrict as it is returned to the unaffected eye. The reduced number of functioning photosensitive ganglion cells in the affected eye will result in the *effective* luminance of the stimulus being reduced, exactly as if a neutral density filter (sunglasses) were placed in front of the eye. This is a sensitive test, but one that takes some practice. There are commercially available pupillometers that can quantify relative afferent pupillary defects (Volpe *et al.*, 2009). Problems arise if there is a *bilateral* optic neuropathy. If the deficit is symmetrical, then there will be no difference between the pupil light reflex in each eye and the test will be negative. It can be used only to detect unilateral or substantially asymmetric deficits.

Eye Movements

In the assessment of ocular motility disorders, it is necessary to establish the ocular alignment. The principal function of the oculomotor system is to ensure that the object of regard is imaged on the fovea of each eye so that the visual system can devote maximal resolution and binocular fusion giving stereopsis to that object. Diplopia is a common consequence of acquired misalignment of the eyes from whatever cause, but if the subject does not have normal binocular function (for example, if they have had a strabismus in childhood), then there may be no diplopia as the subject has developed the facility to suppress the image from one eye.

The first task is to decide whether or not there is a misalignment of the eyes, and to do this the subject is required to fix on a light source such as a small torch held by the examiner. The reflection of the light source from each cornea will immediately indicate whether both eyes are fixing on the target. If the reflection is off-centre at the cornea in one eye, then it is misaligned and the subject has a tropia; that is to say one eye is fixing on the target and the other is pointing in another direction. This will most often be associated with diplopia if due to an acquired defect. It is necessary to check for a tropia for near and distance, and in all nine positions of gaze (primary position, left gaze, right gaze, elevation from each of those three positions, depression from each of those three positions) as it may not be present in all positions.

The cover/uncover test will also check for a tropia (Figure 17.8). Check that the subject has good vision in each eye, then require the subject to fix on a distant target. Cover an eye with a suitable occluder and watch to see if there is any movement of the fellow eye to take up fixation. If so, then that eye was deviated and there is a tropia, and the direction can be deduced from the direction of movement made by the eye as it takes up fixation. In some situations either eye may take up fixation and retain

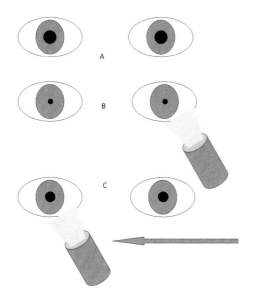

Figure 17.7 Right relative afferent pupillary defect (Marcus Gunn pupil)

A.   Observe the pupils in the ambient lighting. They are equal.

B.   The normal left eye is illuminated, both pupils constrict.

C.   The light source is moved quickly across to the right eye which has a damaged optic nerve, both pupils dilate. It is as if the light source is dimmer as it moves across to the right eye – but here it is the damaged optic nerve that signals a dimmer light.

Note: If the right eye were stimulated first (move from A to C in the Figure) both pupils constrict, but less than moving from A to B. This difference is difficult to judge without carrying out the 'swinging flash-light' test

Source: Plant, G.T. 2008. Visual disturbances. *Medicine*, 36, 520–525. Reproduced with permission from Elsevier.

it, but usually one eye will be preferred, and so if the occluder is now removed from the previously fixing eye, it will take up fixation once again. If there is a tropia and the non-fixing, deviated eye is covered, there will be no movement of the fixing eye.

If there is no evidence of a tropia, then a phoria must be sought (Figure 17.9). Here the eyes are aligned binocularly, but the stimulus for fusion of images is necessary to maintain the alignment. When the eye is covered, it will deviate under the cover; that this has occurred will be revealed when the cover is removed and the eye takes up fixation again. As before, it is this movement of redress that shows how the eye was deviated under the cover. Once again, phorias may vary for near and distance

and with gaze position. Sometimes it may be difficult to break down a phoria, and in this situation the alternate cover test is used – the occluder is moved from one eye to the other and back again without allowing the subject to fuse. In this way a controlled phoria can be broken down over time as the subject is not permitted to fuse the image. As each eye is exposed, it will be seen to take up fixation, often with an increasing angle of deviation.

In establishing a cause of diplopia, it is useful to examine the range of movements of the eyes with both eyes fixing the target (ocular versions) and with each eye viewing monocularly (ductions). If the examiner understands the actions of the 12 extraocular muscles, it is often possible to decide which

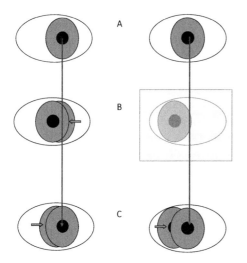

Figure 17.8 Cover/uncover test (right esotropia due to a right lateral rectus paresis)

A. The subject is fixing the target with the left eye the right eye is turned in. The patient cannot correct this by fusing the image because of the weak lateral rectus muscle.

B. When the left eye is covered the right eye takes up fixation and there is overaction of the left medial rectus muscle causing a left esotropia which is greater than the original right esotropia.

C. On removing the cover the left eye takes up fixation again and the right eye reverts to esotropia.

Source: Plant, G.T. 2008. Visual disturbances. *Medicine*, 36, 520–525. Reproduced with permission from Elsevier.

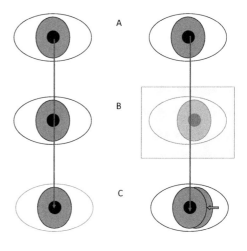

Figure 17.9 Cover/uncover test (left esophoria)

A. The eyes are fixed on a target which the patient has fused, the eyes are straight.

B. When the left eye is covered the patient can no longer fuse the image and the left eye drifts outwards.

C. What the observer sees is the eye taking up fixation again when the cover is removed.

Source: Plant, G.T. 2008. Visual disturbances. *Medicine*, 36, 520–525. Reproduced with permission from Elsevier.

muscles are affected. It is important to examine ductions as well as versions. If there is a tropia, then what happens when examining versions will depend upon which eye the subject chooses to fix. In the case of neurological disorders affecting ocular movements, there may also be a need to examine specifically pursuit eye movements, saccades and vergence movements.

Aeromedical Considerations

Restricted visual fields, blurred vision and/or diplopia, impaired visual acuity, defective colour vision and poorly coordinated eye movements may be encountered by aeromedical practitioners as such events are as likely to occur in aircrew as in the general population. The issues that are of paramount importance for the practitioner are the implications to immediate employment and the prognosis with respect to the future. In the latter context, optic nerve head drusen with progressive visual field loss is a particularly difficult problem in an occupation that demands high visual standards. In a series of aircrew with the diagnosis of optic nerve head drusen, Davis *et al.* (2010) observed that two-thirds had visual field loss at the initial consultation and that subsequent examinations revealed that in two-fifths the situation was progressive, though visual acuity and stereopsis were preserved. They emphasized that it is important to be aware of the progressive nature of visual field loss in this condition.

Very rarely, visual loss can be rapid, probably because of haemorrhage at, or ischaemia of, the optic nerve head. The visual loss in disc drusen is 'disc related' and in that respect similar to the situation in glaucoma where arcuate field loss is not noticed by the patient because it affects the mid-periphery, sparing acuity, and is extensively non-overlapping in the two eyes. Disc drusen may be visible if superficial on the optic disc, but they can also be 'buried', where it is the appearance of the optic disc that gives clues to their presence. The disc lacks a normal cup and the vessels emerge from the centre of the disc and are anomalous. Ultrasound is a very useful screening test.

Blurred vision and/or diplopia may be the initial presentation of myasthenia gravis, though the practitioner has to bear in mind that the differential diagnosis of myasthenia gravis is extensive, including thyroid eye disease and ocular motor palsies. Myopathies and motor neuron disease also cause limb weakness but rarely present with ocular symptoms other than ptosis in some myopathies (mitochondrial myopathy and myotonic dystrophy in particular). Myasthenia gravis is characteristically a condition showing variability. This applies to minute-to-minute variation with activity – such as when the examiner looks for fatigue of a ptosis – diurnal variation with worsening of symptoms towards the end of the day and a tendency over weeks and months to spontaneous remission and relapse. It is also typical for different muscles to be involved during the course of the disease.

Karmon *et al.* (2010) described two cases in aircrew, emphasizing the need for compliance, awareness of symptoms and gradual progression of ocular myasthenia in the event of return to flying. A 47-year-old fighter pilot complained of blurred vision that tended to resolve with prednisone, as did subsequent episodes. The pilot continued to fly fighter aircraft over the ensuing 15 years. In another case, a 27-year-old helicopter navigator complaining of diplopia was found to have a ptosis with weakness of the right superior oblique and lateral rectus muscles. Over a 13-year period, with active treatment, the navigator continued to be involved, from time to time, with flying. Guliuzza (2005) described the history of a 26-year-old female aircrew member with blurred vision and left-sided ptosis over ten days that worsened as each day progressed. However, the symptoms resolved without treatment, and in due course she returned to flying duties.

It must also be borne in mind that aircrew can be subjected to unusual stresses and the clinical presentation may therefore be atypical. The possibility that such pathology may be linked to a decompression must always be considered. Steigleman *et al.* (2003) described a case of retro-orbital pain during aviation training that involved exposure to 25,000 feet for nine minutes in a hypobaric chamber, with the possibility of another episode some three weeks previously. The pain resolved, but two days later it recurred with blurred vision. On examination, there were deficits in colour vision and restricted visual fields. The clinical picture was complicated by concomitant sinusitis that raised the possibility of a parainfectious aetiology which resolved with antibiotic therapy, and by mild hypothyroidism which was also treated. As far as the differential diagnosis was concerned, it was considered that the presentation was consistent with optic neuritis and that also raised the question of multiple sclerosis. However, the response to hyperbaric treatment strongly supported decompression sickness as the precipitating event.

Decompression was also suspected as the cause of mild vision loss in a 25-year-old pilot after operating a high-performance aircraft (Pokroy *et al.*, 2009) with a suspected depressurization at 30,000 feet. On examination, three days after the event, the left optic disc was swollen with haemorrhages. Five days post-flight the patient commenced treatment with hyperbaric oxygen, with immediate improvement in vision. In due course the pilot returned to high-performance flying, and there was no recurrence of loss of vision over the ensuing three-year period. The history suggested that the episode was related to the decompression event, but, as with the case described by Steigleman *et al.* (2003), due consideration was given to optic neuritis with its implications of multiple sclerosis, which is the commonest cause of spontaneous vision loss in the age group of the pilot.

Overall, the literature suggests that optic neuropathy is not a common manifestation of decompression sickness. A recent high-altitude study in the Himalayas revealed a remarkably high incidence of optic disc swelling in over half of the mountaineers (Bosch *et al.*, 2008). However, there were no visual symptoms and this likely represents papilloedema due to raised intracranial pressure and is entirely reversible. This will take time to develop and may not be relevant to the effects of acute decompression.

References

Bailey, I.L. and Lovie, J.E. 1976. New design principles for visual acuity letter charts. *American Journal of Optometry and Physiological Optics*, 53, 740–45.

Bjerrum, B.J. 1889. An addition to the usual visual field examination and the visual field in glaucoma. *Nordisk Ofthalmologisk Tidsskrift.*

Bosch, M.M., Barthelmes, D., Merz, T.M., Bloch, K.E., Turk, A.J., Hefti, U. *et al.* 2008. High incidence of optic disc swelling at very high altitudes. *Archives of Ophthalmology*, 126, 644–50.

Crabb, D.P. and Viswanathan, A.C. 2005. Integrated visual fields: A new approach to measuring the binocular field of view and visual disability. *Graefes Archives for Clinical and Experimental Ophthalmology*, 243, 210–16.

Davis, R.E., Rubin, R.M., Gooch, J.M., Ivan, D.J. and Tredici, T.J. 2010. Optic nerve head drusen (OHND) in United States Air Force aircrew: A retrospective review. *Aviation, Space, and Environmental Medicine*, 81, 281.

Esterman, B. 1982. Functional scoring of the binocular field. *Ophthalmology*, 89, 1226–34.

Farnsworth, D. 1943. The Farnsworth-Munsell 100-hue and dichotomous tests for color vision. *Journal of the Optical Society of America*, 33, 568–78.

Guliuzza, R.J. 2005. You're the flight surgeon: Myasthenia gravis. *Aviation, Space, and Environmental Medicine*, 76, 406–7.

Hardy, L.L., Rand, G. and Rittler, M.C. 1954. H-R-R polychromatic plates. *Journal of the Optical Society of America*, 44, 509–21.

Holmgren, A.F. 1876 and 1877. Om färgblindheten i dess förhållande till järnvägstrafiken och sjöväsendet. *Upsala Läkareförenings Förhandlingar*, 12, 171–251 and 267–358. Uppsala: Almqvist & Wiksell. (English translation: *Annual Report of the Smithsonian Institution for the year 1877*. 1878. Washington, DC: Smithsonian Institute, 131–200.)

Ishihara, S. 1917. *Tests for Colour-Blindness*. Tokyo: Hongo Harukicho.

Karmon, Y., Blum, S., Levite, R., Barenboim, E. and Gadoth, N. 2010. Myasthenia gravis and return to flying status. *Aviation, Space, and Environmental Medicine*, 81, 69–73.

Lanthony, P. 1978. The desaturated panel D-15. *Documenta Ophthalmologica*, 46, 185–9.

Pokroy, R., Barenboim, E., Carter, D., Assa, A. and Alhalel, A. 2009. Unilateral optic disc swelling in a fighter pilot. *Aviation, Space, and Environmental Medicine*, 80, 894–7.

Sloan, L.L. 1959. New test charts for the measurement of visual acuity at far and near distances. *American Journal of Ophthalmology*, 48, 807–13.

Snellen, H. 1862. *Optotypi ad visum determinandum*. Utrecht: P.W. van de Weijer.

Squire, T.J., Rodriguez-Carmona, M., Evans, A.D.B. and Barbur, J.L. 2005. Color vision tests for aviation: Comparison of the anomaloscope and three lantern types. *Aviation, Space, and Environmental Medicine*, 76, 421–9.

Steigleman, A., Butler, F., Chhoeu, A., O'Malley, T., Bower, E. and Giebner, S. 2003. Optic neuropathy following an altitude exposure. *Aviation, Space, and Environmental Medicine*, 74, 985–9.

United Kingdom Civil Aviation Authority. 2009. Minimum Colour Vision Requirements for Professional Flight Crew. Recommendations for new colour vision standards. Available at: http://www.caa.co.uk/docs/33/200904.pdf

Volpe, N.J., Dadvand, L., Kim, S.K., Maguire, M.G., Ying, G.S., Moster, M.L. and Galetta, S.L.

2009. Computerized binocular pupillography of the swinging flashlight test detects afferent pupillary defects. *Current Eye Research*, 34, 606–13.

Wong, A.M.F. and Sharpe, J.A. 2000. A comparison of tangent screen, Goldmann, and Humphrey perimetry in the detection and localization of occipital lesions. *Ophthalmology*, 107, 527–44.

Zaidi, F.H., Hull, J.T., Peirson, S.N., Wulff, K., Aeschbach, D., Gooley, J.J. *et al.* 2007. Short-wavelength light sensitivity of circadian, pupillary, and visual awareness in humans lacking an outer retina. *Current Biology*, 17, 2122–8.

Chapter 18

VESTIBULAR
AND
RELATED OCULOMOTOR
DISORDERS

Nicholas J. Cutfield and Adolfo M. Bronstein

Vertigo is a common complaint of the general population, and aircrew, though subject to frequent periodic examinations, are equally susceptible. Additionally, in this group, it can be a cause of in-flight problems, and the incapacitating nature of severe vertigo is prohibitive of operating an aircraft. Some practitioners can be disconcerted on facing the presenting complaint of 'dizziness' or 'vertigo' and uneasy if they are unable to provide the diagnosis. Others may not feel confident in assessing eye movements, especially when nystagmus can appear 'complicated', changing with gaze and head position.

The accurate diagnosis of vertigo, usually due to vestibular disorders, is vital to determine prognosis and make informed decisions about returning to flying. Some causes of attacks of vertigo can respond to treatment, such as simple mechanical repositioning manoeuvres to treat benign paroxysmal positional vertigo, although there remains the risk of recurrence. It is, of course, also important to differentiate peripheral disorders of the vestibular nerve or organ from central nervous system disorders requiring expedient brain imaging and other investigations. Familiarity with symptoms encountered in vestibular syndromes can help differentiate these from episodes of spatial disorientation during flight where there is a normally functioning peripheral and central vestibular system. Loud sounds and pressure changes are intrinsic to aviation and, in some patients, they can induce vertigo and nystagmus, as in the recently recognized Tullio phenomenon.

In this chapter a basic understanding of the anatomy and physiology of the vestibular system is assumed, though the reader is referred to Chapter 4 (Spatial Orientation and Disorientation) for a brief summary. As with spatial disorientation in flight, motion sickness usually involves the normal functioning of the visual and vestibular systems in an abnormal environment, and is also not covered here. This chapter will cover the pathological conditions of the peripheral and central vestibular system. After an introduction to clinical assessment, vestibular and balance disorders are considered on the basis of their presenting symptoms in three groups. These are a single attack of prolonged vertigo, episodic (or recurrent) dizziness and vertigo, and chronic dizziness and unsteadiness. Key aspects of the clinical features, major differential diagnoses, prognostic features and treatments are given. Finally, a summary of the clinical assessments and investigations are given for quick reference, followed by a discussion of the implications of disorders of the vestibular system to aircrew.

Part 1:
CLINICAL ASSESSMENT

Symptomatology

Complaints of 'dizziness', 'vertigo', 'off-balance' and 'lightheadedness' can be, and often are, used interchangeably by patients. It is, therefore, important to explore exactly the sensation that is being experienced, regardless of the particular term used, and determine the circumstances in which it appears. Is the sensation one of spinning or rotation, and so likely to be vestibular in origin? Is the 'vertigo' better described as lightheadedness suggestive of a presyncopal attack? Does it only occur on standing up, suggesting orthostatic hypotension? Is it more a sensation of imbalance when walking, suggesting a neurological gait disorder? Enquiring about the trigger factors for dizziness and vertigo can bring important diagnostic clues. Does it happen when

looking up quickly or on lying down and turning over in bed, as occurs in positional vertigo? Is it triggered by certain foods such as alcohol, chocolate and red wine, or by sleep deprivation or menstruation, as in migraine? Is it only present when changing from the sitting to the standing position, as in orthostatic hypotension?

Vertigo and Oscillopsia

Vertigo is the inappropriate perception of self-motion. It is usually used to describe a rotatory or spinning sensation, and the visual world is often seen as spinning too. This rotatory sensation is most indicative of a vestibular cause of dizziness, but motion without continuous spinning can be perceived with vestibular dysfunction, such as 'rocking' back and forth or as if 'on a boat'. Vertigo, even of a brief duration such as ten seconds, can be accompanied by severe nausea and vomiting. Oscillopsia is the illusion of motion of the visual surroundings, often 'jumping' or 'wobbly'. Some people, surprisingly, do not report oscillopsia despite having vigorous nystagmus, and that raises the possibility of congenital nystagmus.

Headache, Lightheadedness and Unsteadiness

Headache with vertigo may suggest a migrainous cause, but a secondary headache can also result from recurrent attacks of vertigo. It is important to differentiate both of these from a sudden onset of occipital headache preceding the vertigo that might indicate a haemorrhage in the posterior fossa. Lightheadedness or presyncope is the commonest cause of non-specific 'dizziness'. In the course of a syncopal faint, some individuals experience 'true' rotatory vertigo for a few seconds. The diagnosis of a presyncopal or syncopal event is still secure, despite the presence of vertigo, when it is based on typical features such as the provoking situation, lightheadedness, pallor, sweatiness, greying out of vision and recovery of hearing before vision. There are also important non-vestibular causes of dizziness. Continuous lightheadedness may accompany anaemia, and hypoglycaemia in diabetic patients, usually due to insulin or sulfnonylureas, and can cause dizziness among other neurological symptoms (Service, 1995). Unsteadiness and imbalance can be a result of peripheral vestibular disease but also of a neurological disorder. Imbalance of gait is a feature of peripheral neuropathy, Parkinsonism, cerebral white matter and cerebellar disease.

Orthostasis

Orthostatic hypotension is common with increasing age and is exacerbated by medications such as medication used for hypertension. Checking postural blood pressure, lying and standing, must be routine, even when the history suggests that the dizziness sounds vestibular in origin, as the two causes are common enough to coexist. The patient must be lying flat and relaxed, for at least five minutes, before taking the blood pressure. The standing blood pressure is taken immediately on standing, three minutes later. A drop of 20 mm Hg is significant. A postural change in blood pressure may not be evident if measured later in the day than when the symptoms occur, as many are only symptomatic early in the morning. Cardiac investigations and referral may be required when there

is the suspicion of an arrhythmia or an abnormal electrocardiogram.

Anxiety and Panic

Dizziness, vertigo or imbalance may be prominent symptoms of anxiety disorders or panic attacks. Patients often recognize the provoking situations, such as flying, themselves. Other features of panic attacks may include trembling, shortness of breath with hyperventilation, chest discomfort, nausea, fear of dying or illness, distal and perioral paraesthesias, and chills or hot flushes. Vestibular pathology causing chronic dizziness can provoke a high rate of secondary anxiety. This may be especially so when a diagnosis has not yet been made, and in this situation the secondary anxiety can become a problem in itself, requiring intervention such as counselling. Therefore, a high level of anxiety, in itself, does not distinguish between an anxiety disorder and a vestibular disorder causing anxiety, and it is important to assess the patient thoroughly for vestibular disease. If the conclusion is reached that the dizziness is a symptom of a panic disorder, it must be communicated to the patient in a sensitive manner. This will help appropriate measures to address the problem to be seen in a more positive light. Dismissal of the problem is usually most unhelpful.

The Examination

The clinical examination is secondary only to the taking of the history of the dizziness or unsteadiness: examination of the eye movements and observation of the gait are the most important aspects. With a little practice, examination of the major types of eye movements can take just a few minutes and differentiate between a 'peripheral' (including the vestibular nerve) and a 'central' neurological vestibular disorder.

Nystagmus

Nystagmus, of the most common 'jerk' type (Figure 18.1), has a 'fast' and a 'slow' phase. It is defined by the direction of the fast phase, although the primary disorder is the slow-phase abnormality. A few beats of unsustained nystagmus on extreme lateral gaze, if the fast phase is in the direction of the gaze, and symmetrical bilaterally, is normal. Nystagmus due to both recent onset peripheral and central vestibular disorders is invariably associated with oscillopsia or vertigo. Nystagmus that is long-standing, congenital or due to ocular disease from an orbital restriction of the gaze of one eye may not be symptomatic. However, individuals with congenital nystagmus can become symptomatic later in life or may decompensate acutely after a minor head injury or illness. Emergence of symptoms can be due to a reduced ability to suppress the nystagmus or to the discovery of the nystagmus resulting from increased self-awareness.

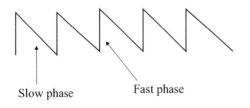

Slow phase   Fast phase

Figure 18.1 Horizontal unidirectional jerk nystagmus may be of peripheral or central origin

Source: Reproduced from Bronstein, A.M., and Lempert, T. 2006. *Dizziness: A Practical Approach to Diagnosis and Management.* Cambridge, Cambridge University Press.

When the patient is examined in the conventional head-up position, spontaneous nystagmus that is vertical, torsional or in more than one direction is central in origin. If the nystagmus is 'pendular' or 'bobs' back and forth rather than jerking with fast and slow phases, it is also always central in cause. Recent-onset central causes require imaging (magnetic resonance) with attention to the brainstem, cerebellum and the foramen magnum. Horizontal nystagmus in one direction can be peripheral or central in origin. The clinical context is then important. For example, horizontal nystagmus with acute vertigo, a positive head impulse test (see below), normal eye movements, intact hearing and no other neurological signs is likely to be due to a 'peripheral' vestibular neuritis or labyrinthitis. On the other hand, a horizontal nystagmus with abnormal eye movements such as broken pursuit and over-shooting saccades (also discussed below), limb ataxia and facial weakness will be central in origin. Both peripheral and central nystagmus can increase in intensity when looking to the direction of the fast phase, and decrease when looking away from the fast-phase direction. When due to a unilateral vestibular lesion, this is known as Alexander's Law (Jeffcoat *et al.*, 2008). Downbeat nystagmus due to midline cerebellar disease can sometimes only be seen in certain head postures, such as with the head facing down. Therefore, if the patient complains of 'jumping vision' or vertigo on looking down, it can be revealing to examine the eyes in whatever symptomatic head posture the patient describes. The origin of nystagmus whether peripheral of central is considered in Table 18.1.

Table 18.1   Nystagmus: Central or peripheral in origin?

Nystagmus	Origin
Vertical or multidirectional	Central
Torsional (head still in upright posture)	Central
Pendular or bobbing	Central
Jerking nystagmus to the left or right	Peripheral or central
Asymptomatic	Congenital or chronic
Additional features	
Sudden-onset deafness	Central, especially vascular
Other neurological signs	Central
New headache	Assume central, may be migraine
Abnormal VOR, unilateral horizontal nystagmus, no other neurological signs	Peripheral
Aural fullness, tinnitus, deafness	Peripheral, consider Ménière's

Vestibulo-Ocular Reflex

The vestibulo-ocular reflex stabilizes vision with head movement in all directions. If the head rotates left in 'yaw', the eyes respond to the right with the same angular magnitude as the head movement. If the head elevates, the eyes depress. If the head rolls, the eyes roll in the opposite direction, subject to mechanical restrictions. The reflex operates continuously, unnoticed as we move our heads, and guarantees clear vision during a large range of head movements. It is a fast reflex using only three neurons – the vestibular nerve, an interneuron from the vestibular nuclei to the oculomotor nuclei of the third, fourth or sixth cranial nerves, and the relevant efferent oculomotor nerve. A problem with the reflex is likely if fast head movements or riding in a car result in 'wobbly' vision (oscillopsia), or if, after turning the head quickly, the vision seems to 'catch up'. When visually tracking a moving object while the head is moving, the reflex is suppressed (see below).

The horizontal vestibulo-ocular reflex is assessed by asking the patient to fix their gaze on the bridge of the examiner's nose and passively rotate the head in yaw, either slowly at low acceleration, the doll's manoeuvre, or by quicker high-acceleration movements by the Halmagyi 'head impulse' or 'head thrust' test (Halmagyi and Curthoys, 1988) (Figure 18.2). The head impulse test involves low-amplitude, unpredictable fast head rotations. It has been used for three decades without reports of adverse effects, but common sense dictates avoiding the test in cases of unstable structural neck pathology or suspected arterial dissection. Failure of smooth fixation of the eyes during the doll's manoeuvre or failure of maintenance of the gaze during the head thrust test requiring a visible 'catch-up' saccade to refixate, in the absence of other signs, indicate a peripheral vestibular deficit on the side in the direction the nose is moved. The presence of a 'catch-up' refixation saccade cannot be determined if the patient blinks or looks away during the test. However, as it takes only a few seconds to do the head thrust manoeuvre, it should be repeated several times in both directions until consistent results are obtained.

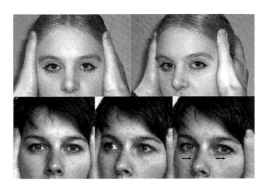

Figure 18.2 Doll's head and head thrust (see colour section)

Suppression of the vestibulo-ocular reflex

The reflex allows visual fixation of an object that moves together with the subject, as when reading a book on a bus or looking at a wristwatch whilst walking. It can be tested by asking the subject to fixate on their thumbs, held together with arms outstretched, feet held off the ground, and passively rotating the subject in a chair. Any failure to maintain fixation on their thumbs visible to the clinician as nystagmus indicates a central disorder, most commonly affecting the cerebellum.

Eye Movements That Require Intact Central Pathways

Pursuit allows fixation of objects moving slowly in the visual field. Smooth execution of this requires the input of multiple regions in the brain, including the cerebellum. Abnormal pursuit is a sensitive sign of a central neurological problem, but not specific. When testing pursuit, the target must be held far enough away so that there is minimal convergence; a slow movement should be used and extremes of gaze avoided.

Saccades

Saccades are fast refixation eye movements. They can be tested in the horizontal and vertical planes by simply asking the patient to look quickly to targets, usually the examiner's fingers. They can be reflexive to an unexpected sound or visual object, or under voluntary control when willingly shifting one's gaze. As with pursuit, the controlling pathways are widespread, but, if there is no restriction of gaze due to eye muscle disorders, slow-velocity horizontal saccades suggest lesions in the pontine reticular formation, while vertical saccades suggest a lesion in the midbrain. Saccades that overshoot a target before correcting are associated with cerebellar disease, while undershoot is less specific.

Summary

It is worth emphasizing other aspects of the clinical examination. The practitioner should look for any squint or nystagmus, with the patient looking straight ahead in 'primary gaze'. Retracting one of the eyelids a little is useful because scleral blood vessels can be easier to see when moving, especially with torsional nystagmus. Each eye should be covered alternately, as a 'latent', often congenital, squint or nystagmus may be present. It is useful to check for any restriction of gaze such as an external ophthalmoplegia due to eye complications of thyroid disease, which can produce a nystagmus when attempting to move the eye in the direction of the restricted gaze. If there is limited upgaze, convergence should be checked, as the combination suggests a midbrain lesion; the elderly, however, can have limited upgaze and convergence as part of the physiological ageing process.

Pursuit and saccades in the horizontal and vertical planes should be elicited, and the horizontal vestibulo-ocular reflex checked by the doll's manoeuvre and by head impulse testing, and then by suppression of the reflex. The Hallpike manoeuvre (Cawthorne *et al.*, 1956) checks for positioning nystagmus and must be carried out in all patients with dizziness, vertigo and unsteadiness (see Benign Paroxysmal Positional Vertigo). Peripheral vestibular disorders have an abnormal vestibulo-ocular reflex, but other eye movements are normal. Central disorders of eye movements may produce any combination of pathological nystagmus, impaired visual pursuit, suppression of the vestibulo-ocular reflex and saccades. Neurological examination in the context of dizziness and imbalance should include inspection of the gait, Romberg's test and the postural reflexes, as well as eliciting the possibility of cerebellar signs such as limb ataxia by finger–nose testing. Postural blood pressure recording is usually useful, as orthostatic hypotension can coexist with vestibular pathology.

Part 2:
CONDITIONS AND THEIR PRESENTING SYMPTOMS

I. Prolonged Vertigo: Isolated or First Episode

This is the first group of conditions to be considered on the basis of their presenting symptoms. It includes vestibular neuritis (labyrinthitis) and acute stroke with its differential diagnoses.

Vestibular Neuritis (Labyrinthitis)

The most common cause of an acute episode of vertigo is 'vestibular neuritis', 'labyrinthitis' or 'acute idiopathic unilateral peripheral vestibulopathy': these terms are used interchangeably. The incidence is 3.5 per 100,000 of the general population per year (Sekitani *et al.*, 1993), and it is commonly seen in emergency departments and in general practice. Typically, there can be increasingly intense horizontal vertigo over minutes to several hours, with spontaneous recovery over days to weeks. Nausea and vomiting are usually prominent. There is a preceding history of a probable upper respiratory tract infection in about 50 per cent of cases. There should be no deafness or prominent headache. On examination there is spontaneous horizontal nystagmus, fast phase away from the affected ear. There may be a small torsional component to the nystagmus, fast phase at the top of the eye in the same direction as the horizontal component (Figure 18.3). The nystagmus increases, with gaze directed towards the fast phase. Gait is unsteady and veers towards the affected ear, but there is no limb ataxia on heel–shin or finger–nose testing. The head impulse test should be positive on head rotation towards the affected ear, but there should be no other neurological signs. An asymmetric vestibulo-ocular reflex can be confirmed using caloric irrigations.

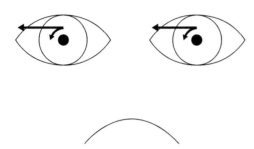

Figure 18.3 Nystagmus in left vestibular neuritis

Vestibular neuritis usually affects the superior division of the vestibular nerve that carries signals from the superior and horizontal semicircular canals. The head impulse test and caloric irrigations both test primarily horizontal semicircular canal function via the vestibulo-ocular reflex. Less commonly, the inferior division of the vestibular nerve can be affected, innervating the posterior (also called the inferior) semicircular canal and the saccule. Caloric testing may be normal, but if there is doubt, vestibular evoked myogenic potentials (VEMP) should be recorded. This procedure involves loud clicks that produce an electromyographic response in neck rotator muscles. The response will be reduced or absent when the function of the inferior division of the vestibular nerve is lost (Jiang, 2008; Halmagyi *et al.*, 2002).

Treatment in the acute phase may involve intravenous hydration and antiemetics. Studies have suggested some improvement in vestibular function by caloric testing with early use of oral steroids (Strupp *et al.*, 2004; Kitahara *et al.*, 2003), but no clear long-term benefit is apparent (Shupak *et al.*, 2008). Two-thirds of patients make an excellent recovery,

and recurrence of the prolonged vertigo is extremely rare. Imbalance is a much more common persisting symptom than vertigo for the 20 to 30 per cent who have persisting symptoms. Prognostic factors determining outcomes are being researched. Head and eye movement exercises and physical therapy by an experienced audiologist or physiotherapist can promote the restoration of balance.

For those who, after the acute vertigo phase, are left with a unilateral peripheral vestibular deficit, it is possible to compensate well for this for everyday life. The contralateral healthy vestibular organ can function adequately for many head movements, especially when at relatively low accelerations. For aircrew, however, the recovery may not be adequate. Trying to maintain an aircraft attitude during turbulence with oscillations of high acceleration and asymmetric detection of high accelerations could reduce the ability to maintain a stable attitude (European Aviation Safety Agency, 2006).

Acute Stroke

The important and immediate differential diagnosis of vestibular neuritis is stroke as an acute cerebellar or brainstem lesion can mimic vestibular neuritis. Stroke should be suspected with an acute onset and a neurological examination must be carried out. Apart from nystagmus, which may be the 'central or peripheral' horizontal jerk type, other signs to look for include recent deafness, Horner's syndrome (ptosis, constricted pupil, loss of sweating of the face on the side of the affected eye), facial paralysis or numbness, loss of sensation on one side of the body, gait ataxia and limb ataxia. Occasionally, there can be an isolated infarction of the labyrinthine artery, causing acute vertigo and deafness without other signs. Spontaneous labyrinthine haemorrhage is a rare cause of sudden-onset vertigo and deafness, and can be diagnosed by magnetic resonance imaging (Shinohara *et al.*, 2000).

In young individuals without standard vascular risk factors, cardiac embolism and vertebral artery dissection, often associated with a history of neck pain or trauma, should be considered. As with all acute strokes, urgent referral is required, as, although intravenous stroke thrombolysis is not routinely used in cases involving the posterior fossa, other interventions can help prevent the recurrence of the event. An acute vertigo has been reported in a fighter pilot during flight (Grossman *et al.*, 2004) due to a cerebellar stroke caused by embolism from a posterior circulation aneurysm. The authors speculated that the G forces during flight may have promoted growth of the aneurysm, although recurrent aneurysm growth is the natural history in many individuals who are not exposed to abnormal accelerations.

The question arises of how detailed should be the investigation of acute vertigo. If the presentation is typical for vestibular neuritis, an immediate referral for brain imaging can be deferred and improvement expected over the following days. If there are any central features, or anything atypical for vestibular neuritis, then brain imaging is urgently needed (Seemungal and Bronstein, 2008). Magnetic resonance imaging is preferable as computerized axial tomography is only adequate for demonstrating a cerebellar haemorrhage

in the context of occipital headache and acute vertigo. The indications for urgent brain imaging with an acute onset of persisting vertigo are the recent onset of occipital headache, any central neurological signs or symptoms, an acute deafness and an intact vestibulo-ocular reflex by the head impulse test.

There are several differential diagnoses. Inflammatory demyelination, either parainfectious or most commonly due to multiple sclerosis, can present with a brainstem syndrome including vertigo and nystagmus. As with posterior circulation strokes, there will usually be additional neurological symptoms or signs and positive findings on imaging. More common causes include the first attack of migrainous vertigo or Ménière's disease. Alcohol toxicity also causes vertigo with spontaneous nystagmus (Fetter *et al.*, 1999), but usually the cause will be apparent from the overall presentation. Suppurative inner ear infection (bacterial labyrinthitis) can extend from the middle ear. A history of chronic middle ear infection or otoscopy that is suggestive of active middle ear infection, combined with recent vestibular dysfunction in that ear, needs specialist attention. Computerized axial tomography of the temporal bones may be required to determine the extent of the infection and the need for surgical intervention. Acoustic neuromas presenting with vertigo alone, and without deafness, facial numbness or weakness, are very rare. If suspected, magnetic resonance imaging is indicated, specifying views of the VIII nerve and cerebellopontine angles. Other rare causes include a perilymphatic fistula (Table 18.2).

Table 18.2   Differential diagnosis of vestibular neurritis (labyrinthitis)

Vestibular neuritis	Vertigo, nausea, imbalance, nystagmus fast phase away from affected ear, impaired VOR with head movement to the affected ear
	No deafness, tinnitus, other neurological signs
Brainstem/cerebellar stroke or demyelination	Nystagmus central-type
	Cerebellar, brainstem, or other neurological signs
First attack migrainous vertigo*	Nystagmus usually central-type, photosensitivity and other migrainous features emerge
First attack Ménière's disease*	With recurrence will have deafness, tinnitus or aural fullness
Labyrinthine stroke	Acute deafness and vertigo
Bacterial labyrinthitis	Middle ear infection
Perilymph fistula*	Precipitated by pressure or sound
Alcohol toxicity	Familiar presentation
Acoustic neuroma	Preceding progressive hearing loss

* Discussed in later section

II. Episodic or Recurrent Vertigo

This is the second group of conditions to be considered on the basis of their presenting symptoms. This group includes benign paroxysmal positional vertigo, migrainous vertigo, Ménière's disease, benign recurrent vertigo, perilymphatic fistula, the Tullio phenomenon and paroxysmal recurrent vertigo. However, there are other possible causes of recurrent vertigo. Transient ischaemic attacks, as with strokes as a cause of an acute single attack of vertigo, usually present with additional neurological signs such as limb ataxia, facial paralysis or numbness, unilateral tinnitus or deafness, and long-tract signs including hemiparesis. They are attributable to lesions of the vertebrobasilar arterial territories. Complex partial seizures are also cited as a cause of recurrent vertigo, but, in the absence of any other perceptual abnormalities or alterations in consciousness, a complex partial seizure

as a cause of vertigo is a vanishingly rare event.

Positional Vertigo

It may require further questioning in patients who report 'episodic vertigo' to determine that the vertigo is positional. Positional vertigo is provoked by certain head positions. Common provocative situations are lying down, sitting up, rolling over to one side in bed, tilting the head to one side and bending the neck forward or back.

Benign Paroxysmal Positional Vertigo

Benign paroxysmal positional vertigo is the commonest vestibular disorder and usually involves the (anatomically lower) posterior semicircular canal. It is caused by dislodged otoconia from the utricle that aggregate in the canal. This effect is termed 'canalo-lithiasis'. Trauma, age and prior inner ear disease are predisposing. Patients complain of brief (less than 30 seconds), intense episodes of vertigo, usually rotatory. They occur in clusters with any number of episodes a day for days to months. Rolling over in bed can provoke an attack, fully awakening the patient. Frequent attacks throughout the day can result in continuous imbalance, nausea and malaise, and the experience is that these patients can report persistent dizziness or vertigo. Care when taking the history reveals that the duration of the actual rotational vertigo is very short. At rest, the eye movements are normal. The diagnosis is confirmed by a provocative manoeuvre which moves the head in the plane of the posterior semicircular canal, such as the Hallpike manoeuvre as shown in Figure 18.4 (Cawthorne *et al.*, 1956).

Positional vertigo is extremely unpleasant, so to elicit the nystagmus the patient must be warned and cooperate with the procedure, avoiding closing the eyes at all costs. If the positional manoeuvre is positive, the nystagmus appears after a latency of a few seconds, and lasts for 5 to 20 seconds. It is torsional if the upper pole of the eyes beats to the undermost ear. There is often a smaller vertical upbeating component (Figure 18.5).

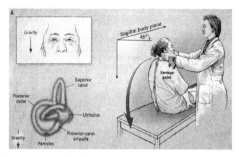

Figure 18.4 Hallpike manoeuvre: from Furman and Cass (1999) (see colour section)

Source: Reproduced with permission: Furman J.M. and Cass S.P. 1999. Benign Paroxysmal Positional Vertigo. *New England Journal of Medicine*, 1999, 341, 1590–1596.

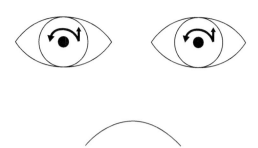

Figure 18.5 Nystagmus in right BPPV in the right ear down position

Source: Reproduced from Bronstein, A. 2005. Benign Paroxysmal Positional Vertigo (BPPV): Diagnosis and Physical Treatment. *Advances in Clinical Neuroscience and Rehabilitation*, 5, 12–14.

The examiner should move their head into the patient's primary gaze, and ask the patient to fixate on them, as other gaze positions will modulate the nystagmus. In addition, it is helpful to open one of the patient's eyelids to view a blood vessel overlying the sclera as this will make a torsional nystagmus easier to visualize. The nystagmus and symptoms tend to fatigue with repeated testing. If examination of the other eye movements is normal and the gait is free of ataxia, then no further tests are needed. The patient is often worried about the possibility of a serious neurological origin of their symptoms and can be reassured as to the benign aetiology.

However, a central cause of positional nystagmus should be suspected if the nystagmus is atypical in its direction – such as down-beating – if there is no fatigue with repeated testing and if there is no latency before it starts or if it continues for longer than 30 seconds. Positional downbeat nystagmus can be a presenting feature of degenerative cerebellar disorders (Bertholon *et al.*, 2002; Strupp *et al.*, 2007). A neurological examination is required. Magnetic resonance imaging of the brainstem, cerebellum and cerebellopontine angle should be carried out to look for a Chiari malformation, along with various haematological investigations summarized in the section below dealing with cerebellar disease.

An alternative to the traditional Hallpike manoeuvre can be carried out with the patient sitting on the side of the couch. The head is rotated such that the nose is pointing 45 degrees in the opposite direction to the side of the ear being tested, followed by a lateral tilt of the body and head in the direction of the ear being examined. For example, when testing the right posterior semicircular canal, the head is rotated with the nose going left and then the head and body tilted laterally to the right. As with the standard Hallpike manoeuvre, a positive test will reveal torsional nystagmus with the upper pole of the eye 'fast' phase beating towards the undermost ear (the ear being tested). From this position, if the test is positive, one can continue directly into the therapeutic particle-repositioning Semont manoeuvre (Figure 18.6) (Fife *et al.*, 2008). This one-step alternative to the traditional Epley manoeuvre is quicker to perform. When performed correctly, both of these tests have a success rate of about 80 per cent in terminating the current bout.

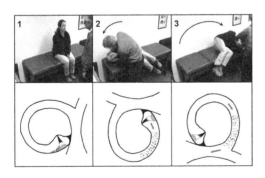

Figure 18.6 The positional manoeuvre and treatment (*Semont Manoeuvre*) (see colour section)

Source: Reproduced from Bronstein, A.M., and Lempert, T. 2006. *Dizziness: A Practical Approach to Diagnosis and Management*. Cambridge, Cambridge University Press.

Less commonly, benign paroxysmal positional vertigo can involve the horizontal or, rarely, the anterior semicircular canals. With provoking head movements, these cause nystagmus in the plane of the affected canals: horizontal nystagmus for horizontal canal vertigo and predominantly downbeat nystagmus for anterior canal vertigo. It needs to be stressed that downbeat nystagmus, even positional, should be assumed to be central, usually midline cerebellar, and imaging is indicated. Probably, because of their anatomically higher position in the labyrinth, these other types of benign vertigo tend to resolve spontaneously – more often than the much more common posterior canal vertigo. Although the therapeutic manoeuvres can terminate bouts of attacks, the condition tends to recur within a year in 40 per cent of cases, and in approximately 50 per cent of cases within five to eight years (Hain *et al.*, 2000, Brandt *et al.*, 2006). In 50 per cent, however, the prognosis is excellent, without recurrence in the medium term. Recovery is not influenced by the duration of symptoms or by age (Wolf *et al.*, 1999).

Fitness to fly after benign paroxysmal positional vertigo is debatable (Sen *et al.*, 2007; Gresty, 2008). The European Aviation Safety Authority (2006) advises that the decision concerning aeromedical status depends on the frequency of occurrences and their duration and severity. Most episodes of benign vertigo are brief, but they are intense and transiently disabling during the attack, and most of the 40 per cent risk of recurrence is in the first months. The risk is likely to decay exponentially, except when the vertigo is secondary to coexistent inner ear disease. It is difficult to decide initially who is likely to suffer a recurrence, and who will be free of a recurrence in those falling into the 50 per cent. However, given the time course of risk of recurrence, complete freedom of symptoms for a period of at least six months will significantly decrease the chances of further attacks.

Migrainous Vertigo

Typical rotatory vertigo or a 'rocking' sensation, of variable duration, in the evolution of other migrainous symptoms is a common presentation in specialist dizziness clinics. Migrainous vertigo has been reported to affect up to 23 per cent of 'migraineurs' (Vukovic *et al.*, 2007). It is not yet recognized as a distinct entity from basilar migraine by the International Headache Society. The Society requires other brainstem features to be present. Migrainous vertigo, as with migraine, can start at any age, and vertigo can become a feature even when there is a long history of migraine without vertigo.

The vertigo is of variable duration from ten minutes to several days in some cases. The vertigo can be rotatory, but can also be felt as a 'rocking' unsteadiness. During the attack, nystagmus of varying types can be seen, but the nystagmus should resolve completely after the attack. It is often worse with head movement. Suggestive features of a migrainous origin are the other migrainous symptoms evolving during the attack. These include a unilateral or retro-orbital headache, photophobia, phonophobia, mainly visual auras and triggers specific to migraine such as certain foods or hormonal changes. Triggering features, such as foods or alcohol, sleep deprivation or the menstrual cycle, and response of the vertigo to drugs used in the treatment of migraine are supportive of the diagnosis. Although the history may be suggestive, other causes should be considered, as when attributing any focal neurological symptoms to migraine. Examination of the eye movements and a neurological examination are desirable.

It should be kept in mind that other causes of vertigo can produce a secondary headache, including migraine. Indeed, an artificial vertigo induced by caloric testing has precipitated full-blown migraine with accompanying vertigo (Seemungal *et al.*, 2006). Further, though not usual practice in the context of a normal neurological examination that has included inspection for papilloedema, imaging should be considered to exclude a structural lesion with a recent onset of migraine – particularly in the elderly or when the headache has changed in nature.

Some patients with a prominent headache respond to symptomatic treatment such as simple analgesics, with or without antiemetics or triptans. However, this has not been well validated for migrainous vertigo. In many cases, the vertigo develops too quickly to be easily terminated with symptomatic treatment, and the frequency of attacks can warrant daily prophylactic treatment. The initial choice depends on the side-effect profile of the drug for the individual. Beta blockers can cause hypotension and erectile dysfunction and can trigger bronchial spasm in susceptible individuals. Tricyclic antidepressants can induce sedation and a dry mouth, and sandomigran can increase appetite and lead to weight gain. Any drug needs to be assessed for at least four to six weeks before being withdrawn on the grounds of lack of efficacy. Typical regimes are given below, but if these treatments are not tolerated or are ineffective, an anticonvulsant such as topiramate can be considered, though it carries the risk of sedation and weight loss.

Amitriptyline: 10 mg at night,
increasing by 10mg
a week up to 30–50
mg a night

Propanalol: 20 mg three times
a day, increasing to
30–40 mg, or up to
60–80 mg in males

Pizotifen: 0.5 mg, increasing to
1.5 mg

Initially, the prognosis of migrainous vertigo is unpredictable. The natural history is of attacks of a cyclical nature, and so improvement from a bad spell is always expected. A reduction in severity and frequency of attacks is common with prophylactic treatment; complete remission in severe cases is less common, but does occur. When there is freedom from attacks for several months, an attempt to wean off the prophylactic drug is appropriate. Measures other than pharmacological, such as aerobic exercise, elimination of triggers, regular sleep and psychological stress reduction, may be of help.

Ménière's Disease

The disease described by Ménière (1799–1862) typically presents between the ages of 30 and 50 years, affecting men and women equally. Endolymphatic hydrops and expansion of the endolymphatic space within the labyrinth has been found, but the causes of this are not known in most cases. Ménière's disease is characterized by recurrent vertigo associated with cochlear symptoms: a 'roaring' or 'rushing' tinnitus, a feeling of aural 'pressure' or 'fullness', and hearing loss. The vertigo increases quickly and persists for 20 minutes to several hours. Attacks can occur between twice a week and once a year. Nausea, vomiting, sweating and imbalance are associated with the condition.

Nystagmus may be present and can persist for several days, initially beating towards the affected ear in the 'irritative phase', and later beating away from the affected ear in the 'paretic phase'. A second reversal in direction is sometimes seen. For this reason, the direction of the nystagmus is not a good indicator of the affected side. Eye movements are normal between attacks, and any hearing loss must be documented by an audiogram (American Academy of Otolaryngology, 1995). In initial attacks, neither vestibular nor cochlea symptoms may be present, but both are always present after several years. For that reason, recurrent vertigo over several years, in isolation, cannot be Ménière's disease, and migrainous vertigo is often the underlying cause.

Initially, the hearing loss and tinnitus resolve fully after an attack. Audiograms may reveal a fluctuating low-frequency hearing loss – an important diagnostic parameter. Gradually, there is a permanent hearing loss, with low frequencies as characteristic. In due course the whole frequency spectrum becomes involved and affects both sides in about 40 per cent of patients. Eventually, after five to 15 years, attacks of vertigo may subside, but there is a persistent mild disequilibrium, severe hearing loss and tinnitus. A definite diagnosis of Ménière's disease can be made (when other causes are excluded) if there is evidence of two or more definitive and spontaneous episodes of vertigo of at least 20 minutes' duration, hearing loss has been demonstrated audiometrically on at least one occasion, and there is tinnitus or 'aural fullness' in the affected ear. A single 'definitive episode of vertigo' together with the other three criteria is a probable diagnosis of Ménière's disease.

Differential diagnoses are usually excluded on the clinical presentation. These include migraine, transient ischaemic attacks affecting the brainstem, perilymphatic fistula, autoimmune inner ear disease, acoustic neuromas, and otosclerosis. Ménière's disease is an overdiagnosed cause of recurrent vertigo, in favour of migraine. Acoustic neuroma more typically present with progressive rather than a fluctuating hearing loss. In some cases, the history can be difficult to disentangle, and so imaging of the cerebellopontine angles is indicated in addition to repeat audiometry.

Treatment for acute attacks involves vestibular suppressants such as prochloperazine, either intravenous or as suppositories. Betahistine is commonly prescribed chronically, but there is limited evidence that it reduces attacks. A low-salt diet, requiring a major lifestyle change, and bendrofluazide (2.5 mg in the morning) are used, based on reducing inner ear volume. Long, spontaneous remissions can occur, and that has made the evaluation of treatment difficult, but there is no evidence that treatment will delay or prevent the onset of hearing loss. With severe attacks of vertigo, invasive treatment is an option, including middle ear injections of ototoxic gentamicin. This is effective in controlling the vertigo, but carries the risk of losing the remaining hearing. Intratympanic corticosteroid injections are also used, but there is lack of evidence for this procedure. Surgical section of the vestibular nerve is also effective, but the risks are high when compared with middle ear injections.

As with the other types of recurrent and paroxysmal vertigo discussed in this chapter, it is difficult to reconcile the nature of Ménière's disease with the requirements of piloting an aircraft. Attacks have insufficient warning, as it can be seconds between onset of aural symptoms, such as pressure in the ear, to vertigo. The vertigo is disabling, preventing many ordinary daily activities, let alone flying. The attacks can last a few minutes, but usually last several hours. With time, the frequency of attacks subsides, but this is associated with progressive hearing loss and vestibular impairment. It has been suggested that if the attacks are well controlled, and that a fully operational co-pilot is available, then piloting can continue (O'Reilly, 1999). However, as attacks typically last hours, there is, in effect, a single-pilot operation. An aeromedical practitioner may feel that there are employment arrangements, such as a co-pilot, that make continued piloting possible. Due to the above factors, however, it is our opinion that the diagnosis of Ménière's disease is not compatible with piloting an aircraft.

Benign Recurrent Vertigo

Some patients have isolated recurrent episodes of vertigo that last minutes to hours, without any provoking causes and without any association with migrainous symptoms. Examination and vestibular investigations are normal. Audiometry should be carried out in case there is asymptomatic hearing loss that would suggest Ménière's disease. The syndrome is poorly understood. It is 'benign' in that it does not progress to vestibular impairment or hearing loss. Sometimes prophylaxis, as used in migraine, can be of help.

Perilymphatic Fistula

Fistulae are uncommon, but they are relevant to aircrew, given their exposure to pressure changes during flight. They can start with a 'pop' followed by vertigo, lasting seconds to days, with variable hearing loss. Individuals are sensitive to pressure changes induced by coughing, sneezing or pressing the tragus over the external ear canal. The fistula is an abnormal communication between the perilymphatic space and the middle ear due to defects in the round or oval windows or in the bone surrounding the labyrinth. The condition may be congenital, but causes include barotrauma as in childbirth and diving, surgery, erosive infection or tumour.

Examination may reveal a conductive or sensorineural hearing loss and/or a unilateral nystagmus suggestive of impaired vestibular function. These can be confirmed with an audiogram and electro-oculography. If there is the possibility of recent trauma to the tympanic membrane, caloric irrigation to investigate vestibular function may be contraindicated. Nystagmus may be provoked by inducing a pressure change by a finger over the external ear canal, a pneumatic otoscope or a Valsalva manoeuvre.

A perilymphatic fistula is a serious condition for aircrew due to the symptoms induced and the possibility of pressure changes during flight. In a series of four cabin attendants with perilymphatic fistula, none of whom was diagnosed at the primary care level, only one was able to return to flying duties (Klokker and Vesterhauge, 2005). Prior to the event, three of the four had a common cold that reduced the ability to equalize pressure in the ears during pressure changes in flight. Initial treatment is bed rest and avoidance of physical effort that may give pressure surges. Surgical repair is possible depending on the anatomy of the dehiscence.

Tullio Phenomenon

The Tullio phenomenon (Halmagyi *et al.*, 2005) is a syndrome of disequilibrium or vertigo, oscillopsia and nystagmus, and is provoked by loud sounds. Typical triggering sounds are those of an aircraft or motorcycle, but symptoms can also be provoked by the voice or playing a wind musical instrument. This syndrome was observed during the development of jet engines when engineers exposed to 150 dB had disequilibrium and tilting of their visual scenes. This did not prove to be a problem in pilots, although in an early report (Dickson and Chadwick, 1951) a pilot reported vertigo when only one ear was exposed without headphones. Many are found to have a dehiscence of a superior semicircular canal, although the symptoms of the Tullio phenomenon can also occur with a perilymphatic fistula.

Recently, high-resolution tomography of the temporal bones has shown a dehiscence of the superior semicircular canal in many but not all patients who report Tullio-type symptoms. The bone is usually 1 millimetre thick around the canal, but in 0.7 per cent of unselected autopsy cases Minor *et al.* (2001) observed a deficit. This would have allowed sounds to be transmitted directly to the canal and its fluid. The defect may be bilateral. It is often congenital, with symptoms appearing later in life for reasons not understood.

For patients who report loud sound-induced disequilibrium, oscillopsia or vertigo, the eyes should be examined for torsional nystagmus while applying a continuous loud sound (100 dB) or with a Valsalva manoeuvre. A low-amplitude torsional nystagmus can be difficult to see clinically (opening the eyelids wide to view the scleral vessels can help) and is more reliably recorded with video-oculography. However, high-resolution tomography of the temporal bones is the most important investigation. Additionally, recording muscle activity induced by applying loud clicks (vestibular-evoked myogenic potential) is easier to induce due to enhanced bone transmission (Colebatch *et al.*, 1998). Similarly, the audiogram will typically show an 'air–bone gap' at 1 kHz and below due to enhanced transmission of sound with the 'bone' stimulus, a kind of conductive hyperacusis.

Recognizing this uncommon syndrome provides relief for those whose unusual symptoms may have been thought to be psychological in cause, such as veering in response to loud sounds or 'hearing their own eyes move' (Albuquerque and Bronstein, 2004). If the symptoms are disabling, surgical repair can be attempted. Accompanying symptoms, such as the apparent increased volume of the voice or 'hearing my eyes move', can be more distressing than the Tullio phenomenon itself when, often, the diagnosis and explanation are inadequate.

Paroxysmal Recurrent Vertigo

Paroxysmal recurrent vertigo (peripheral vestibular paroxysmia) is a rare condition in medical practice, but is seen not infrequently in specialist dizziness clinics. It is a syndrome of recurrent spontaneous brief attacks of vertigo lasting only a few seconds. The attacks can occur many times a day, and there are no other symptoms. Nystagmus may be seen if an attack is witnessed. In some individuals, attacks seem to be positional, precipitated by turning the head. This, along with the finding that some have an apparent neurovascular compression of the VIII nerve, has led to speculation that vascular loops touching the VIII nerve may be responsible, but this

remains controversial. Eye movement and vestibular examinations between the brief attacks are normal. Many patients respond to low doses of carbamazepine (50–200 mg per day) which suggests a hyperexcitability of the acoustic nerve, analogous to trigeminal neuralgia which is also sensitive to carbamezapine. Diagnosis relies on the history of brief vestibular paroxysms, exclusion of other vestibular pathology and the response to treatment. The majority of patients who respond to carbamezapine have good control.

As well as irritation to the vestibular nerve, lesions in the brainstem abutting the vestibular nuclei or pathways can cause paroxysmal vertigo and oscillopsia (Radtke *et al.*, 2001; Bronstein *et al.*, 2003). These can be arteriovenous malformations, tumours or post-vascular or inflammatory events. 'Ocular flutter' is not a true nystagmus but back-to-back saccades, and is seen in brainstem and cerebellar disease (Leigh and Zee, 2006).

Superior Oblique Myokymia

A fast torsional shuddering of one eye only can cause an oscillopsia, 'shimmering' or 'shuddering' of vision. Analogous to vestibular paroxysmia (in that case, involving the VIII cranial nerve), vascular loops irritating the fourth cranial nerve are thought to be implicated, and the condition can respond to carbamazepine (Yousry *et al.*, 2002). Patients may discover that the condition is monocular by closing alternate eyes during an attack that lasts 30 seconds. If an attack occurs while being assessed, rapid use of the ophthalmoscope to visualize the retina during the attack can be required to visualize the low-amplitude torsional nystagmus.

In our opinion, paroxysmal vestibular and oculomotor disorders, such as vestibular paroxysmia and superior oblique myokimia, are not compatible with driving and flying, unless the patient has been completely symptom-free for at least 12 months.

Congenital Nystagmus

Congenital nystagmus can sometimes become symptomatic later in life, leading to concern of a recent-onset acquired brainstem problem (Gresty et al., 1991). It is suspected when the nystagmus, usually horizontal, uni- or bi-directional, is out of proportion to oscillopsia (often none at all), or when there are other neurological signs. It can often be suppressed to a degree, and a reduction in the nystagmus in a particular 'null point' of gaze direction can lead to patients holding their head turned to minimize oscillopsia. With ageing, a congenital nystagmus can 'decompensate'. Environments with reduced visual input, such as when driving at night, can precipitate oscillopsia in patients with congenital nystagmus. Visual acuity will often be reduced. Oculomotor and general neurological examination is required to rule out other pathology. Recording of eye movements can sometimes demonstrate a pathognomonic nystagmus wave form (Gresty et al., 1984).

Voluntary Nystagmus

Up to 8 per cent of people (Zahn, 1978) can voluntarily generate fast saccadic oscillations of the eyes, which can be confused for a horizontal nystagmus. It often requires the eyes to converge to some degree, and is related to other psychogenic conditions such as convergence spasm. This is regularly seen in specialist oculomotor clinics, but is not reported in the aviation literature. In many patients, voluntary nystagmus disappears on explanation and reassurance, but if it persists in a pilot, the condition should be incompatible with flying.

External Ophthalmoplegia

Chronic or slowly progressive restriction of gaze by disorders of the extraocular muscles does not usually produce vertigo or oscillopsia. For this reason, these conditions may not present early, with the first symptom often diplopia in certain gaze directions. Some causes include thyroid ophthalmopathy, chronic progressive external ophthalmoplegia due to mitochondrial disease, vasculitis, malignancy such as lymphoma, myasthenia gravis, certain muscle diseases, sarcoidosis, cavernous sinus pathology, Tolosa–Hunt syndrome (unilateral headaches with extraocular palsies) and the Miller Fisher syndrome (ataxia with ophthalmoplegia). It is important to identify the underlying cause as some causes are serious, with consideration needed of extraocular manifestations. Referral to a neuro-ophthalmologist or neurologist is required.

We believe that, in general, uncontrolled episodic or recurrent vestibular or oculomotor syndromes, as well as fixed deficits producing visual symptoms (oscillopsia, diplopia, limitations in oculomotor excursion), are incompatible with piloting aircraft.

III. Disequilibrium and Imbalance

This is the third group of conditions to be considered on the basis of their symptoms. Dizziness on standing or walking may not be true 'vertigo', but rather a sense of imbalance, unsteadiness or disequilibrium. This can be continuous under certain circumstances. Symptoms on standing up may be due to orthostatic hypotension, as described in the introductory section on non-vestibular symptoms. Imbalance only when walking may suggest a neurological cause, such as peripheral neuropathy, Parkinsonism, cerebrovascular white matter disease or a cerebellar disorder.

Bilateral Vestibular Failure

This diagnosis is often missed. It is usually a complication of gentamicin ototoxicity, and many practitioners are unaware that the vestibular organ is more susceptible than the cochlea to ototoxicity to this commonly used drug (Seemungal and Bronstein, 2007). Bilateral vestibular failure can also be post-meninigitic and associated with deafness. Not uncommonly, the cause is 'idiopathic' – a syndrome characterized by progressive loss of vestibular function with episodes of spontaneous isolated vertigo. The episodes of vertigo gradually remit over one to two years as the vestibular function completely disappears. Autoimmune and inflammatory causes of vestibular loss usually involve one side first. Ménière's disease can progress to bilateral vestibular failure, but the diagnosis should be apparent from the tinnitus and deafness, usually over many years.

Patients may present with oscillopsia during head movement such as when walking, due to absence of the vestibulo-ocular reflex. The oscillopsia may be described not as movement but as blurring of images that is worse with head movement. The oscillopsia will be worse when walking fast or riding in a car on a bumpy road. Patients may present with imbalance – an example would be patients who are slow to rehabilitate and walk after a severe sepsis for which they received gentamicin. Walking in the dark is particularly difficult when the balance system must operate mainly on proprioceptive inputs, without both visual and vestibular inputs.

Examination reveals loss of the vestibulo-ocular reflex in all directions, broken-up 'doll's eye' movements and an abnormal head impulse test. Other eye movements and the neurological examination are normal. An alternative to testing the reflex, especially if inexperienced, is to check dynamic visual acuity (Figure 18.7). Due to absence of the reflex stabilizing vision, the visual acuity is usually at least two lines worse on a Snellen chart when the head is oscillated from side to side, compared with when the head is still.

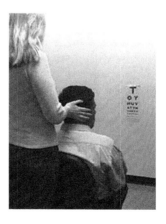

Figure 18.7 Vestibulo-ocular reflex: Clinical assessment

Source: Reproduced from Bronstein, A. 2003. Vestibular reflexes and positional manoeuvres. *Journal of Neurology, Neurosurgery and Psychiatry*, 74, 289–293.

Generally, once vestibular function is lost bilaterally, it does not recover to a meaningful degree. Treatment involves education and vestibular and physical rehabilitation. As a rule, in the months following loss of the vestibular function there is a significant improvement in balance and overall function in most patients, due to adaptation.

Neurological Disorders

Peripheral neuropathy may present, less commonly, as unsteadiness on walking, especially in the dark, rather than numbness or pain in the feet. The list of causes is long, with diabetes, alcohol and renal disease among the most commonly identified. The screening tests include glucose levels (diabetic neuropathy), haematology with sedimentation rate, erythrocyte sedimentation rate, C-reactive protein (inflammatory and haematological causes), electrolytes, liver function, serum protein electrophoresis with immunofixation (paraprotein), serum Immunoglobulins, B_{12} and folate (deficiencies), as well as thyroid function and autoimmune screening (hypothyroidism, Sjögren's syndrome and other autoimmune disorders). Referral to a neurologist or a diabetologist with a specific interest in diabetic neuropathy is appropriate, and findings can be confirmed with nerve conduction studies.

Cervical spine myelopathy can present insidiously with progressive leg and gait spasticity, before weakness, numbness or sphincter disturbance are present. Imaging of the spine is required, and if there is rapid clinical progression from some causes, such as a prolapsed disc, then urgent referral for surgical decompression is required. Parkinsonian syndromes, including typical idiopathic Parkinson's disease, can present with gait unsteadiness and loss of postural reflexes, rather than the core clinical features of rigidity, asymmetric tremor and bradykinesia (slowness and paucity of movement). Postural hypotension can be a feature contributing to dizziness, from autonomic dysfunction or as a side effect of medications for Parkinsonism.

Cerebrovascular disease, particularly of small vessels supplying the cerebral white matter, is common and can present with gait instability and Parkinsonism, and is evident on both tomography and imaging. If the distribution on imaging is atypical, or in the absence of standard vascular risk factors, then referral to a neurologist is advisable to consider other inflammatory causes.

Cerebellar disease, particularly midline, can present with an ataxic, wide-based gait, without incoordination of the limbs on finger–nose or heel–shin testing. Eye-movement examination can show overshoot or undershoot of saccades, impaired smooth pursuit and suppression of the vestibulo-ocular reflex. Alcohol, drugs (phenytoin, cisplatin, lithium), cerebrovascular and neurodegenerative disease are causes, but a proportion remain idiopathic. A syndrome of downbeat nystagmus (often with vertical oscillopsia) and moderate gait unsteadiness is relatively common in balance clinics. If the downbeat nystagmus is not clearly visible in primary gaze, lateral gaze and the positional manoeuvre are usually likely to enhance it. This is one of the reasons why positional manoeuvres should be carried out in all patients complaining of dizziness or unsteadiness, and not only in those with a typical benign vertigo history. Imaging is always indicated, taking care to inspect the craniocervical junction for the Chiari malformation.

Consideration of an underlying malignancy (paraneoplastic cerebellar syndrome) must be given, with clinical examination and imaging (chest X-ray, mammography, computerized tomography of chest, abdomen and pelvis, or proton emission tomography, if available). Screening blood tests in isolated cerebellar dysfunction include those for thyroid function and antibodies, vitamin B_{12}, vitamin E, antineuronal antibodies (paraneoplastic), autoimmune antibodies and liver function, as well as a full blood count, erythrocyte sedimentation, C-reactive protein and serum electrolytes. Apart from the specific vitamin deficiencies, other tests are done to detect predominantly autoimmune dysfunction. Coeliac disease antibodies are controversial. Genetic testing for the common spinocerebellar ataxias and episodic ataxia type 2 can be done if there is no cause on initial screening. These are usually negative in the absence of a positive family history, but *de novo* mutations do occur.

Part 3:
PROGNOSIS – THE PRACTICE OF AVIATION MEDICINE

It is evident that a pilot should not suffer from spells of vertigo, dizziness or unsteadiness of any origin, and that position is adopted by the regulatory authorities (European Aviation Safety Agency, 2006). However, many symptoms, especially when in the context of circumstances that can give rise to rapid pressure changes or exposure to accelerations, may be physiological. Indeed, an anonymous survey of Portuguese fighter pilots found a prevalence of 29 per cent of likely alternobaric vertigo due to asymmetric middle ear pressure equalization (Subtil *et al.*, 2007). However, it is emphasized that reported in-flight incapacitations due to vestibular disease are rare. In a study carried out in commercial aircrew involving 1,800 events over 20 years, only one of ten events that were incapacitating was vestibular in nature – due to labyrinthitis (Martin-Saint-Laurent *et al.*, 1990).

It has to be accepted that, as far as vestibular disorders are concerned, the prognosis in relation to the continued employment of the individual as aircrew can often present a demanding clinical decision. Indeed, in pilots who have had a history of vertigo, and even in those whose condition has 'resolved', there are difficulties in recommending appropriate stand-down times relevant to the diagnosis. The position may be complicated by the likelihood of the under-reporting of vestibular symptoms for fear of being deemed medically unfit. It could be useful to approach the problem by considering the implications of disorders that are *probably* incompatible from those that are *possibly* compatible with flying. These suggestions are based on our neurological and neuro-otological experience of these conditions (Table 18.3). However, they are not intended as regulatory guidelines, and ultimately the responsibility rests with the aeromedical practitioner in liaison with the aviation safety authority. Erring on the side of caution would always seem appropriate.

Probably Incompatible with Flying

As is evident from the current review, many vestibular and oculomotor conditions, particularly those of a paroxysmal or episodic nature, are clearly incompatible with the requirements for operating an aircraft, and an appreciation of the implications of these disorders for the task undertaken by aircrew has clearly been a significant contribution to air safety. Conditions such as Ménière's

Table 18.3 Summary of clinical assessments

Feature on history	Consider
Vertigo rotational	Vestibular origin, peripheral or central
Vertigo positional	BPPV, migraine, or cerebellar
Gait imbalance	Bilateral loss of function, or neurological
Postural light-headedness	Exclude presyncopal postural hypotension
Auditory symptoms	Ménière's disease
Headache or migrainous features	Migrainous vertigo
Pressure changes, coughing, sneezing	Perilymphatic fistula
Examination	*Implication*
Eye movement examination	May identify a central neurological sign
Head impulse test	Impaired VOR, unilateral or bilateral
Positional manoeuvres	BPPV or, rarely, cerebellar
Postural blood pressure	Exclude postural hypotension
Gait and postural reflexes	Neurological gait imbalance
Romberg test	Vestibular, cerebellar or peripheral neuropathy
Joint position and vibration perception in feet	Peripheral neuropathy
Full neurological examination	If no peripheral vestibular cause found
Investigations	*Indications*
Pure-tone audiometry	Initial fluctuating or low-frequency loss in Ménière's disease Hearing often lost unilaterally in vascular causes, e.g. posterior fossa stroke Normal in vestibular neuritis, BPPV, migraine
Caloric testing	To confirm or quantitate loss of peripheral vestibular function e.g. acute vestibular neuritis, prior vestibular injury, or to prove intact
Rotational testing with eye movement recording, e.g. electro-oculography	Can confirm central eye movement signs, and also test vestibular system asymmetry when caloric cannot be done, e.g. ruptured tympanic membrane
MRI brain, including cerebellum, cerebello-pontine angles and craniocervical junction	Central signs on examination Atypical positional nystagmus Progressive unilateral sensorineural hearing loss
MRI spine	Gait imbalance not attributable to vestibular or obvious neurological cause
Vestibular-evoked myogenic potential	Suspected inferior vestibular neuritis or in the Tullio phenomenon
Autoimmune blood tests	Asymmetric bilateral vestibular loss

disease, poorly recovered vestibular neuritis or labyrinthitis, and the relevant neurological conditions, are unlikely ever to be free from adverse symptoms. In all of the conditions causing recurrent vertigo, the timing of attacks is unpredictable, and they are therefore incompatible with flying unless there is a sustained and complete freedom from symptoms.

Possibly Compatible with Flying

Nevertheless, the majority of patients recover from vestibular neuritis or labyrinthitis, both symptomatically and functionally, even if a considerable caloric canal paresis persists in some cases. A bout of benign vertigo may resolve spontaneously or be terminated with the positional manoeuvre, and will not be followed by a recurrence in up to 50 per cent of cases. With this diagnosis, a wait of six months before return to flying is advisable, given the frequency of recurrence within this time period. With regard to migrainous vertigo, often under-recognized, there are likely to be long spells of remission, but, again, freedom from all symptoms for at least six to 12 months would seem appropriate.

Conclusion

Symptomatology in aircrew related to the vestibular system may arise from the demands of the aviation domain or from disease of the vestibular system itself, and unravelling the aetiology and predicting the prognosis remains a challenge to the practice of aviation medicine. The investigation of complaints by aircrew related to the vestibular system and determining the prognosis demand the skills of the aeromedical practitioner familiar with the physiology of orientation and the manifestations of vertigo and of disorientation in flight (Chapter 4: Spatial Orientation and Disorientation) and of the neurologist specializing in otology. The involvement of these combined disciplines is particularly necessary when the neurologist is faced with symptomatology, but the conventional clinical assessment, as described in this chapter, has proved to be normal.

References

American Academy of Otolaryngology – Head and Neck Foundation. 1995. Committee on hearing and equilibrium guidelines for the diagnosis and evaluation of therapy in Menière's disease. *Otolaryngology – Head Neck Surgery*, 113, 181–5.

Albuquerque, W. and Bronstein, A.M. 2004. 'Doctor, I can hear my eyes': Report of two cases with different mechanisms. *Journal of Neurology, Neurosurgery and Psychiatry*, 75, 1363–4.

Bertholon, P., Bronstein, A.M., Davies, R.A., Rudge, P. and Thilo, K.V. 2002. Positional down beating nystagmus in 50 patients: Cerebellar disorders and possible anterior semicircular canalithiasis. *Journal of Neurology, Neurosurgery and Psychiatry*, 72, 366–72.

Brandt, T., Huppert, D., Hecht, J., Karch, C. and Strupp, M. 2006. Benign paroxysmal positioning vertigo: A long-term follow-up (6–17 years) of 125 patients. *Acta Otolaryngologica*, 126, 160–63.

Bronstein, A.M., Pérennou, D.A., Guerrazk, M., Playford, D. and Rudge, P. 2003. Dissociation of visual and haptic vertical in two patients with vestibular nuclear lesions. *Neurology*, 61, 1260–62.

Cawthorne, T., Dix, M.R., Hallpike, C.S. and Hood, J.D. 1956. The investigation of vestibular function. *British Medical Bulletin*, 12, 131–42.

Colebatch, J.G., Day, B.L., Bronstein, A.M., Davies, R.A., Gresty, M.A., Luxon, L.M. and Rothwell, J.C. 1998. Vestibular hypersensitivity to clicks is characteristic of the Tullio phenomenon. *Journal of Neurology, Neurosurgery and Psychiatry*, 65, 670–78.

Dickson, E.D. and Chadwick, D.L. 1951. Observations on disturbances of equilibrium and other symptoms induced by jet-engine noise. *Journal of Laryngology and Otology*, 65, 154–5.

European Aviation Safety Agency. 2006. Otorhinolaryngology. In: *Joint Aviation Requirements: Flight Crew Licensing (Medical), Amendment 5*. The Netherlands: Joint Aviation Authorities.

Fetter, M., Haslwanter, T., Bork, M. and Dichgans, J. 1999. New insights into positional alcohol nystagmus using three-dimensional eye-movement analysis. *Annals of Neurology*, 45, 216–23.

Fife, T.D., Iverson, D.J., Lempert, T., Furman, J.M., Baloh, R.W., Tusa, R.J. et al. 2008. Practice parameter: Therapies for benign paroxysmal positional vertigo (an evidence-based review). Report of the Quality Standards Subcommittee: American Academy of Neurology. *Neurology*, 70, 2067–74.

Gresty, M.A. 2008. BPPV and fitness to fly – or drive. *Aviation, Space, and Environmental Medicine*, 79, 541–2.

Gresty, M.A., Bronstein, A.M., Page, N.G. and Rudge, P. 1991. Congenital-type nystagmus emerging in later life. *Neurology*, 41, 653–6.

Gresty, M., Page, N. and Barratt, H. 1984. The differential diagnosis of congenital nystagmus. *Journal of Neurology, Neurosurgery and Psychiatry*, 47, 936–42.

Grossman, A., Chapnik, L., Ulanovski, D., Goldstein, L., Azaria, B., Sherer, Y. and Barenboim, E. 2004. Acute cerebellar vertigo in a fighter pilot. *Aviation, Space, and Environmental Medicine*, 75, 913–5.

Hain, T.C., Helminski, J.O., Reis, I.L. and Uddin, M.K. 2000. Vibration does not improve results of the canalith repositioning procedure. *Archives of Otolaryngology – Head & Neck Surgery*, 126, 617–22.

Halmagyi, G.M., Aw, S.T., Karlberg, M., Curthoys, I.S. and Todd, M.J. 2002. Inferior vestibular neuritis. *Annals of the New York Academy of Sciences*, 956, 306–13.

Halmagyi, G.M. and Curthoys, I.S. 1988. A clinical sign of canal paresis. *Archives of Neurology*, 45, 737–9.

Halmagyi, G.M., Curthoys, I.S., Colebatch, J.G. and Aw, S.T. 2005. Vestibular responses to sound. *Annals of the New York Academy of Sciences*, 1039, 54–67.

Jeffcoat, B., Shelukhin, A., Fong, A., Mustain, W. and Zhou, W. 2008. Alexander's Law revisited. *Journal of Neurophysiology*, 100, 154–9.

Jiang, X.S. 2008. Inferior vestibular neuritis in a Chinese fighter pilot. *Aviation, Space, and Environmental Medicine*, 79, 256.

Kitahara, T., Kondoh, K., Morihana, T., Okumura, S., Horii, A., Takeda, N. et al. 2003. Steroid effects on vestibular compensation in human. *Neurological Research*, 25, 287–91.

Klokker, M. and Vesterhauge, S. 2005. Perilymphatic fistula in cabin attendants: An incapacitating consequence of flying with common cold. *Aviation, Space, and Environmental Medicine*, 76, 66–8.

Leigh, R.J. and Zee, D.S. 2006. *The Neurology of Eye Movements*. Oxford: Oxford University Press.

Martin-Saint-Laurent, A., Lavernhe, J., Casano, G. and Simkoff, A. 1990. Clinical aspects of inflight incapacitations in commercial aviation. *Aviation, Space, and Environmental Medicine*, 61, 256–60.

Minor, L.B., Cremer, P.D., Carey, J.P., Della Santina, C.C., Streubel, S.O. and Weg, N. 2001. Symptoms and signs in superior canal dehiscence syndrome. *Annals of the*

New York Academy of Sciences, 942, 259–73.

O'Reilly, B.J. 1999. Otorhinolaryngology. In: J. Ernsting, A.N. Nicholson and D.J. Rainford (eds) *Aviation Medicine – Third Edition*. London: Butterworth-Heinemann, Ch. 24.

Radtke, A., Bronstein, A.M., Gresty, M.A., Faldon, M., Taylor, W., Stevens, J.M. et al. 2001. Paroxysmal alternating skew deviation and nystagmus after partial destruction of the uvula. *Journal of Neurology, Neurosurgery and Psychiatry*, 70, 790–93.

Seemungal, B., Rudge, P., Davies, R., Gresty, M. and Bronstein, A. 2006. Three patients with migraine following caloric-induced vestibular stimulation. *Journal of Neurology*, 253, 1000–1001.

Seemungal, B.M. and Bronstein, A.M. 2007. Aminoglycoside ototoxicity: Vestibular function is also vulnerable. *British Medical Journal*, 335, 952.

Seemungal, B.M. and Bronstein, A.M. 2008. A practical approach to acute vertigo. *Practical Neurology*, 8, 211–21.

Sekitani, T., Imate, Y., Noguchi, T. and Inokuma, T. 1993. Vestibular neuronitis: Epidemiological survey by questionnaire in Japan. *Acta Otolaryngologica*, 503, S9–12.

Sen, A., Al-Deleamy, L.S. and Kendirli, T.M. 2007. Benign paroxysmal positional vertigo in an airline pilot. *Aviation, Space, and Environmental Medicine*, 78, 1060–63.

Service, F.J. 1995. Hypoglycemic disorders. *New England Journal of Medicine*, 332, 1144–52.

Shinohara, S., Yamamoto, E., Saiwai, S., Tsuji, J., Muneta, Y., Tanabe, M. et al. 2000. Clinical features of sudden hearing loss associated with a high signal in the labyrinth on unenhanced T1-weighted magnetic resonance imaging. *European Archives of Otorhinolaryngology*, 257, 480–84.

Shupak, A., Issa, A., Golz, A., Margalit, K. and Braverman, I. 2008. Prednisone treatment for vestibular neuritis. *Otology and Neurotology*, 29, 368–74.

Strupp, M., Zingler, V.C., Arbusow, V., Niklas, D., Maag, K.P., Dieterich, M. et al. 2004. Methylprednisolone, valacyclovir, or the combination for vestibular neuritis. *New England Journal of Medicine*, 351, 354–61.

Strupp, M., Zwergal, A. and Brandt, T. 2007. Episodic ataxia type 2. *Neurotherapeutics*, 4, 267–73.

Subtil, J., Varandas, J., Galrao, F. and Dos Santos, A. 2007. Alternobaric vertigo: Prevalence in Portuguese Air Force pilots. *Acta Otolaryngologica*, 127, 843–6.

Vukovic, V., Plavec, D., Galinovic, I., Lovrencic-Huzjan, A., Budisic, M. and Demarin, V. 2007. Prevalence of vertigo, dizziness, and migrainous vertigo in patients with migraine. *Headache*, 47, 1427–35.

Wolf, M., Hertanu, T., Novikov, I. and Kronenberg, J. 1999. Epley's manoeuvre for benign paroxysmal positional vertigo: A prospective study. *Clinical Otolaryngology*, 24, 43–6.

Yousry, I., Dieterich, M., Naidich, T.P., Schmid, U.D. and Yousry, T.A. 2002. Superior oblique myokymia: Magnetic resonance imaging support for the neurovascular compression hypothesis. *Annals of Neurology*, 51, 361–8.

Zahn, J.R. 1978. Incidence and characteristics of voluntary nystagmus. *Journal of Neurology, Neurosurgery and Psychiatry*, 41, 617–23.

Chapter 19

DISORDERS OF HEARING

Linda M. Luxon and Ronald Hinchcliffe

Hearing loss is the commonest sensory disability worldwide, with 278 million suffering from a moderate to a profound hearing loss in both ears (World Health Organization, 2006), while tinnitus affects approximately 10 per cent of developed populations (Coles, 1984), and half of those find the symptom troublesome and seek help (Davis, 1995). Disorders of the ear represent about a quarter of all disabilities in the adult population. A third of the population over 50 years old has at least a mild hearing loss (Davis, 1993), and one third of those over 60 years of age has hearing loss of 25 decibels (dB) or more (Steel, 1998). Prevalence statistics for tinnitus vary depending upon the diagnostic criteria. Based on a national study of hearing (Coles, 1984), 15 per cent of the adult population has prolonged 'spontaneous' tinnitus with no obvious trigger and a symptom duration of over five minutes, while in 8 per cent tinnitus interferes with sleep and causes moderate or severe annoyance, though only 0.5 per cent describe tinnitus as severely intrusive, affecting the ability to lead a normal life. Tinnitus prevalence is positively correlated with age (Coles, 1984) and with increasing hearing loss of all aetiologies (Coles *et al.*, 1990; Collet *et al.*, 1990).

This chapter on disorders of hearing is focused toward the practice of aviation medicine, bearing in mind that all of those involved in aviation are equally susceptible to the same causes of auditory dysfunction as the general population. Part 1 (Clinical Audiology) is concerned with auditory symptoms, the relevant anatomy and physiology of hearing, the causes of auditory symptoms in the general population and specifically in those involved in aviation, clinical assessment and investigation, and appropriate management strategies. Part 2 (Trauma to the Auditory System) includes head injury, blast and barotraumas, together with noise-induced hearing loss. In the context of noise-induced hearing loss, it is appreciated that flight personnel of commercial aircraft, under normal circumstances, are not reported to have an increased risk of hearing loss, but the exponential increase in air transport over the last 40 years, together with military activities and conflicts, requires careful consideration of risks to the hearing of aircrew and associated personnel. Part 3 (Aircraft Noise and Annoyance) deals with the problem of high noise levels and the community.

Part 1:
Clinical Audiology

Hearing loss is judged clinically by the threshold of hearing across a standard frequency range of 250 to 8,000 hertz (Hz) with threshold values better than 25 dB hearing level (dBHL) considered to be normal. Average values across the 500 to 4,000 Hz range are used by the World Health Organization to define significant to profound impairment, including deafness (see Appendix III).

Tinnitus is defined as the perception of a sound that originates from within the body rather than the external world and is described as subjective when it is perceived only by the patient, and objective when the sound may be audible externally, as a consequence of a physical source such as palatal myoclonus, an arteriovenous fistula or turbulent blood flow through a stenotic artery. A distinction is made between tinnitus 'presence' and tinnitus 'complaint'. Occasional tinnitus is an almost universal perception. Tinnitus 'complaint' and intrusiveness have been shown to have no direct correlation with psychoacoustic changes in the inner ear, but a strong correlation with psychological factors (Hinchcliffe and King, 1992; Ćeranić and Luxon, 2008).

Dysacusis refers to any deviation from normal auditory perception, and includes a variety of phenomena (Hinchcliffe, 2003). The most common dysacusis is hyperacusis, defined as a reduced tolerance to noise or an increased sensitivity to sounds in levels that would not cause discomfort in a normal individual. This distinguishes hyperacusis from loudness recruitment, which refers to oversensitivity to loud sounds. Tinnitus and hearing loss are most commonly consequent upon disordered cochlear function, but may also present as a result of central auditory pathology with normal cochlear function. Characteristically, this latter pathology presents as difficulty in hearing in conditions of poor signal-to-noise ratio, for example in listening to transmitted sound on the telephone or on a television or conversation in the presence of background noise. Above the level of the cochlear nuclei there are multiple relays and bilateral representations such that central auditory dysfunction does not usually present with hearing loss.

Anatomy and Physiology

The ear is divided into the external, the middle and the internal ears (Figure 19.1). The pinna collects sound, and loss of this structure leads to a deterioration in the hearing level of about 5 dB across the speech frequencies. The external ear canal is approximately 2.5 centimetres long, and, while there is no amplification of sound within the external canal, a redistribution of energy in the form of resonant peaks produces an enhancement over the mid-frequency range of hearing with a gain of up to 15 dB at the tympanic membrane across the 2 to 6 kHz region. The middle ear includes the tympanic membrane and the tympanic cavity (middle ear cleft) and, inferiorly, the pharyngotympanic or auditory (eustachian) tube links the middle ear to the nasopharynx.

The internal ear is embedded in the bony labyrinth filled with perilymph, and can be divided into three anatomical and functional regions: the semicircular canals, the vestibule and the cochlea. Within the bony labyrinth lies the membranous labyrinth which is filled with endolymph and contains the sensory cells of both hearing and balance. The bony cochlea resembles the shell of a snail, within which lies the cochlear duct with a flat floor known as the spiral lamina, a side wall which is comprised mainly of the stria vascularis and a sloping diagonal 'roof' known as the vestibular membrane of Reissner (1824–1878) (Figure 19.2). The spiral organ of Corti (1822–1876) is situated on the basilar membrane and contains the auditory sensory receptor cells known as hair cells. There are two types of cells, the inner and the outer hair cells, both of which have stereocilia projecting from their upper endolymphatic surface. The stereocilia are embedded in the gelatinous tectorial membrane.

Each inner hair cell is surrounded by supporting cells, with approximately ten separate afferent auditory nerve fibres making a synaptic connection with the base of the cell. The outer hair

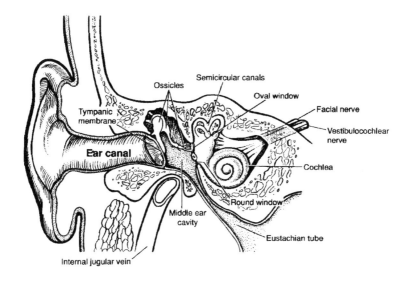

Figure 19.1 Diagram to illustrate the anatomy of the external, middle and internal ear

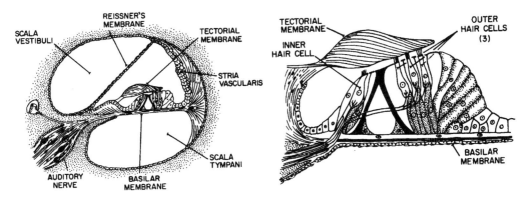

Figure 19.2 Diagrams to illustrate a cross-section through one turn of the cochlea, with magnification of the spiral organ of Corti

cells are cylindrical in shape, arranged in three parallel rows, and receive input from the efferent olivocochlear bundle, but contribute little to the afferent innervation arising from the cochlea. The stereocilia of the cochlear hair cells pivot about their insertions into the thickened upper surface of the hair cell. Each of the stereocilia of one hair cell is linked by fine bands to the adjacent stereocilia, and these links are thought to be responsible for the opening of ion channels during auditory stimulation, causing movement of the stereocilia. The flow of ions through the ion channels results in the transformation at the inner hair cells of mechanical acoustical information into electrical activity conveyed to the type 1 auditory afferent fibres. The outer hair cells, on the other hand, are thought to act as a modulator and amplifier capable of fine-tuning the receptor function of the cochlea (Santos-Sacchi, 2001).

The auditory signal generated in the inner hair cells travels through the auditory nerve to the ipsilateral cochlear nucleus, and from thence the majority of the afferent auditory fibres project to the contralateral superior olivary complex, the lateral lemniscus, the inferior colliculus, the medial geniculate body and to the auditory cortex (Figure 19.3a) (Chermak and Musiek, 1997). The auditory efferent pathway (Figure 19.3b) arises in the auditory cortex and descends parallel to the afferent tracts to the level of the cochlear nuclei (Suga et al., 2000). The anatomy of the higher efferent auditory system remains ill-defined, but within the brainstem the olivocochlear bundle projects from the superior olivary complex to the cochlea (reviewed by Warr, 1992), and has two main pathways:

○ the medial olivocochlear system that projects mainly to the contralateral cochlea and connects to the outer hair cells, and

○ the lateral olivocochlear system that projects to the ipsilateral cochlea and ends on the type 1 afferent dendrites that connect to the inner hair cells.

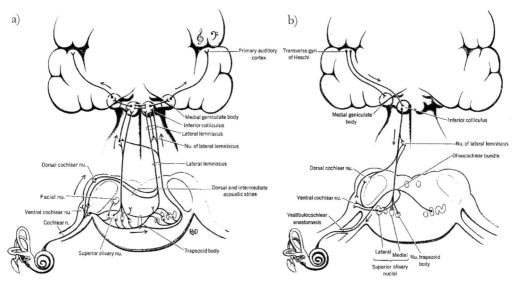

Figure 19.3 Diagrams of auditory pathways: a) ascending afferent auditory pathway and b) descending efferent auditory pathway

Source: Noback, C.R. and Demarest, R.J. 1981. *The Human Nervous System – Third Edition*. New York, McGraw Hill. With permission from R.J. Demarest.

The exact function of the efferent auditory system remains poorly understood, but it is thought that there is an autoregulatory feedback mechanism that is mainly inhibitory, but may also be excitatory at different levels, and thus adjust and improve the processing of the auditory signal (Suga *et al.*, 2000) (Figure 19.4). The efferent fibres leave the brainstem in the superior division of the vestibular nerve. The reader is referred to the detailed description of cochlear physiology and mechanics by Pickles (2007).

Conductive Hearing Loss

Pathology affecting the external and middle ear may give rise to abnormalities of the mechanical transmission of sound waves from the environment to the cochlea. This is known as conductive hearing loss (Figure 19.5a). Bone-conducted sounds are heard more efficiently than air-conducted sounds. Causes of conductive hearing loss include:

- impacted wax in the external canal
- middle ear barotraumas (otitis media with effusion, perforation)
- middle ear disease such as chronic infection
- ossicular chain dysfunction secondary to trauma or otosclerosis.

Conductive hearing loss is significantly less common than the causes of sensorineural hearing loss in the adult population, but may occur as a consequence of barotrauma with middle ear effusion and, *in extremis*, with tympanic membrane perforation. Another common cause is head injury with haemotympanum, ossicular discontinuity, temporal bone fractures and middle ear adhesions (Ishman and

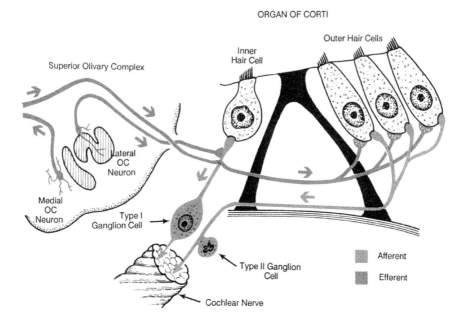

Figure 19.4 Diagram to illustrate efferent supply to inner and outer hair cells from medial and lateral olivocochlear bundles (see colour section)

Friedland, 2004; Wennmo and Svensen, 1989; Davis and Luxon, 1995). Unilateral or asymmetric conductive hearing loss in an adult with normal middle ear pressure and tympanic membrane compliance should raise the suspicion of otosclerosis, which may be genetic in origin with a typical family history (Menger and Tange, 2003) or present as a sporadic case (Holt, 2003).

In immigrants from the developing world, chronic suppurative otitis media (Acuin, 2004) and tuberculous otitis media should be considered. In the latter condition, while there may be evidence of tuberculosis elsewhere, ear disease may be the only manifestation. The diagnosis and treatment of suppurative otitis media is important because of the life-threatening intratemporal and intracranial complications (Youngs, 1998). Rarely, a vascular malformation such as a glomus tumour or a benign or malignant primary or secondary tumour may invade the middle ear and present with a conductive hearing loss, often associated with tinnitus. A mass may be seen behind the tympanic membrane, which may be white in congenital cholesteatoma, pink in middle ear adenoma, or blue in glomus tumour or an aberrant vascular structure. Computer tomography and magnetic resonance imaging are required to aid the diagnosis.

Sensorineural Hearing Loss

Pathology of the cochlea and vestibulocochlear (VIII cranial) nerve characteristically gives rise to a sensorineural hearing loss, in which there is an inability to transduce mechanical energy of sound waves into electrical activity within the cochlea or transmit the signals along the VIII nerve. In sensorineural hearing loss, as in a normal subject, air-conducted sounds

are perceived more loudly than bone-conducted sounds (Figure 19.5b). There is, in addition, an inability to perceive both bone- and air-conducted sounds, and both the intensity of sound and the frequency resolution of complex sounds are impaired. Many different conditions may result in sensorineural hearing loss (see below), but certain pathologies involving both the middle and internal ears – for example, chronic middle ear disease, otosclerosis with involvement of the ossicles and otic capsule and physical trauma – may give rise to a mixed hearing loss in which there is both a conductive and sensorineural component (Figure 19.5c).

❑ Sensorineural hearing loss may be differentiated into that of cochlear origin and that of neural origin on the basis of two pathophysiological phenomena:

❑ Loudness recruitment, as exemplified by noise-induced hearing loss, is defined as an abnormally rapid increase in loudness with an increase of intensity of stimulus. This is characteristic of disorders affecting the hair cells of the organ of Corti, but is absent in pathology of the VIII nerve and brainstem.

❑ Abnormal auditory adaptation, as exemplified by vestibular schwannoma, refers to a decline in discharge frequency with time that is observed following an initial burst of neural activity in response to an adequate continuing stimulus applied to the organ of Corti. This phenomenon is characteristic of neural dysfunction arising in both the VIII nerve and brainstem.

❑ Retrocochlear hearing loss is characterized by abnormal adaptation, and is the term used to classify hearing loss caused by

A

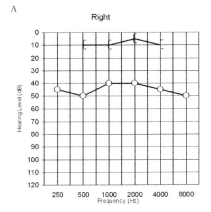

B

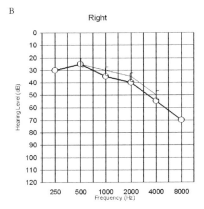

C

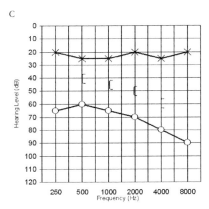

Figure 19.5 Patterns of hearing loss

a)   Right conductive hearing loss
b)   Right sensorineural hearing loss
c)   Mixed right hearing loss , normal left hearing

Key: o, x = air conduction threshold; [= masked right bone conduction threshold.

lesions more proximal to the brain than the cochlea, namely the VIII nerve and lower brainstem. Lesions above this level do not give rise to hearing loss as a result of bilateral representation and multiple commissures within the central auditory pathways.

Starr *et al.* (1996) defined the entity of auditory neuropathy, which is associated with a wide range of pure-tone audiometric findings from essentially normal to profound loss. Recent work has renamed the entity 'auditory dyssynchrony' (Berlin *et al.*, 2001), partly in recognition that it includes a heterogeneous group of conditions affecting three different auditory sites:

◌   impairment of electrical and mechanical transduction of the inner hair cells
◌   impairment of axons, cell bodies and/or myelin sheaths
◌   iteration in efferent influences through the olivocochlear efferent pathway.

Criteria for the diagnosis of auditory neuropathy or dyssynchrony include normal outer hair cell function (otoacoustic emissions and a normal cochlear microphonic), together with absent or abnormal inner hair cell/neural function (auditory brainstem-evoked responses, with absent stapedial reflexes and absent contralateral suppression of otoacoustic emissions via the efferent pathway). Auditory neuropathy is now recognized as a significant cause of hearing impairment in children, but the prevalence of auditory neuropathy in adults has not been defined. However, it may be associated with congenital and inherited disorders such as the Arnold–

Chiari malformation with elongation of the VIII nerve, the ataxia described by Friedreich (1825–1882), trauma, infection such as meningitis, the Ramsay Hunt (1872–1937) syndrome (herpes zoster viral infection of the geniculate ganglion of the facial nerve), vascular disease, neoplasia, temporal bone disorders compressing the VIII nerve, toxic disorders (such as vincristine ototoxicity, alcohol and both lead and mercury poisoning), autoimmune disorders and demyelination.

In recent years, interest in the aetiology of sensorineural hearing loss has paralleled a better understanding of the auditory system and the development of effective prosthetic, pharmacological and possible genetic interventions. Many disorders giving rise to hearing loss affect both parts of the labyrinth and/or vestibulocochlear nerve, and the clinician needs to be aware of the range of conditions and examine both auditory and vestibular function. The relevance of the vestibular system and its disorders to aviation medicine is dealt with in Chapter 18 (Vestibular and Related Oculomotor Disorders). The aetiologies of sensorineural hearing loss are listed below. Trauma- and noise-induced hearing loss are particularly relevant to the practice of aviation medicine, and are dealt with in Part 2 (Trauma to the Auditory System) of this chapter.

Aetiologies of sensorineural hearing loss are listed below:

Genetic Hearing Loss

In the last two decades, there have been enormous strides in the understanding of genetic and environmental causes of hearing loss (Nance, 2003), in addition to the demonstration of genetic factors conferring susceptibility to environmental triggers. Currently,

Genetic	Monosyndromal and syndromal		
Vascular:	Malformation		
	Cardiovascular and cerebrovascular ischaemia		
Autoimmune	Isolated inner ear disease Systemic disorders		
		For example	Systemic lupus erythematosus Polyarthritis nodosa
Infection:	Bacterial, viral and fungal		
Degenerative:	Cochlear, neuropathy and neurological		
	Drugs, surgery and radiotherapy Organic chemicals		
Trauma:	Head injury, blast and barotrauma		
	Noise-induced hearing loss		

67 loci for autosomal-recessive and 54 for autosomal-dominant inheritance of hearing loss have been reported, in addition to mitochondrial mutations and genetic aberrations giving rise to X-linked hearing loss (Hereditary Hearing Loss Homepage – see References). The majority of genes identified to date are associated with cochlear hearing loss, although auditory neuropathy may also be related to genetic abnormalities.

A number of these forms of genetic hearing impairment may present in adult life. Age-related hearing loss is the commonest cause of adult auditory impairment and has been previously attributed to a variety of factors including genetic, nutritional, socio-economic and environmental variables. However, recent work has suggested that this condition may in fact represent inherited late-onset progressive hearing loss, and that specific genes may predispose to environmental triggers affecting various molecular mechanisms underlying changes in auditory function (Seidman *et al.*, 2004; Pickles, 2004).

Autosomal-dominant sensorineural hearing loss is well recognized in families with various audiometric configurations (unilateral loss, low-frequency sensorineural hearing loss both of stable and progressive type, mid-frequency loss, high-frequency loss), differing ages of onset and differing rates of progression. Commonly, there is good correlation between phenotype and genotype, and vestibular involvement has been identified in the deafness autosomal dominants DFNA 9 and 11.

More than a hundred syndromes have been reported with associated hearing impairment, and while the majority of these present in childhood, some can progress or indeed become apparent in adult life, such as the adult condition described by Refsum (1907–1991) (Bamiou *et al.*, 2003), mitochondrial cytopathies (Majamaa-Voltti *et al.*, 2006), and neurological degenerative disorders such as multisystem atrophy (Duvoisin, 1987) and late-onset cerebellar ataxia (Harding, 1981).

Diseases and Disorders

Vascular

There is a wealth of conflicting literature on the possible relationship of vascular risk factors and sensorineural hearing loss. To date, no definitive association has been demonstrated between sensorineural hearing loss and essential hypertension, postural hypotension, hyperlipidaemias (Jones and Davies, 2001) or diabetes mellitus. Moreover, a questionnaire assessment of angina, myocardial infarction and stroke showed no association between these conditions and cochlear impairment in men (Torre *et al.*, 2006). However, women with a self-reported history of myocardial infarction were twice as likely to have cochlear impairment as women without a history of myocardial infarction.

Vascular loops are the subject of further controversy, as they are commonly a normal variant crossing the VIII nerve, but a recent study using high-resolution images (magnetic resonance imaging; constructive interference steady state) demonstrated a significantly higher number of vascular loops in the internal auditory canal of patients with pulsatile tinnitus compared with patients with non-pulsatile tinnitus (Nowé *et al.*, 2004). Moreover, a correlation between tinnitus and hearing loss was found. Sudden deafness has been reported in a number of isolated cases of posterior circulation pathology, anterior-inferior cerebellar artery ischaemia and migrainous infarction, but only 8 per cent of patients with vertebrobasilar insufficiency demonstrated sensorineural hearing loss commonly associated with vertigo (Lee and Baloh, 2005).

Autoimmune (Inner Ear)

Pathology of the inner ear has been associated with virtually all forms of immune-mediated disease and may be organ specific or systemic. McCabe (1979) reported several cases of sensorineural hearing loss that had been successfully treated with dexamethasone and cyclophosphamide. He coined the term autoimmune-mediated inner ear disease. The importance of this diagnosis is that it represents a treatable and thus reversible form of hearing impairment, although diagnosis remains difficult as there are no uniform evidence-based diagnostic criteria and assessment methods remain to be established (Agrup and Luxon, 2006). The presentation of autoimmune inner ear disease is characteristically bilateral sequential or simultaneous auditory and/or vestibular loss. Fluctuation in symptomatology may occur, but, untreated, there is relentless deterioration in both auditory and vestibular function.

Systemic disorders that may present with autoimmune hearing impairment include the syndrome described by Cogan (1908–1993) (Schuknecht, 1994), granulomatosis described by Wegener (1907–1990) (Stephens et al., 1982; McDonald and DeRemee, 1983), rheumatoid arthritis, systemic lupus erythematosus, polyarthritis nodosa, systemic sclerosis and dermatomyositis (Ruckenstein, 2004). Sarcoidosis is a common multi-system disease presenting with mild to profound, fluctuant hearing loss and vestibular abnormalities (Colvin, 2006). A similar review of patients with the syndrome described by Behçet (1889–1948) showed hearing loss in approximately one-third of patients.

Infection

With increased international travel for business and leisure, infections commonly encountered and tropical infections are relevant to aircrew. Bacterial, viral and myototic infections may give rise to hearing impairment by direct invasion, blood-borne transmission or by transfer along the nerves from the cerebrospinal compartment. In adults, sudden sensorineural hearing loss is usually attributed to viral or vascular pathology. Westmore et al. (1979) reported the detection of mumps virus in the perilymph after sudden-onset deafness, and there is circumstantial evidence to suggest that sudden hearing loss may be associated with a variety of viruses.

The commonest infective condition is the Ramsay Hunt syndrome, characterized by facial palsy, hearing loss and herpetic vesicles around the pinna and in the external auditory meatus. Sensorineural hearing loss occurs in between a quarter and two-thirds of cases (Wayman et al., 1990) and may be the result of cochlear or retrocochlear involvement (Kuhweide et al., 2002). A variety of auditory abnormalities have been reported in Aids (acquired immune deficiency syndrome). These range from conductive to sensorineural hearing loss, with mild audiometric changes, abnormalities in the brainstem-evoked response and central auditory dysfunction, but hearing loss may be attributable to opportunistic infections, such as otosyphilis, cyclomegalovirus or streptococcal meningitis, or treatment for the human immunodeficiency virus (Khoza and Ross, 2002).

Labyrinthine involvement is more common in late-acquired syphilis than congenital syphilis. Various presentations have been observed including sudden sensorineural hearing loss and an audiovestibular presentation suggestive of the disease described by Ménière (1799–1862). The recently reported increase in sexually transmitted diseases emphasizes the need to check syphilitic serology in a patient with unexplained sensorineural hearing loss, and this is particularly the case with an increase in opportunistic infections in patients with Aids. Importantly, this is one form of treatable progressive sensorineural hearing loss (Darmstadt and Harris, 1989), with penicillin and corticosteroid treatment reported to bring about improvement in hearing, tinnitus and vertigo in a quarter of a small group of patients with otosyphilis (Linstrom and Gleich, 1993).

Sensorineural hearing loss in association with bacterial meningitis is well documented, and treatment with antibiotics and adjuvant corticosteroids results in lower rates of mortality, long-term neurological sequelae and severe hearing loss (Van de Beek *et al.*, 2003). Tuberculous meningitis is now rare in Western societies, but should be considered in immigrant, debilitated, alcoholic and immunologically suppressed populations (Kotnis and Simo, 2001). Lyme disease is a tic-borne infection with the spirochaete *Borrelia burgdorferi*. Elevated antibodies to borrelia antigen were found in 17 per cent of patients with a unilateral sudden or fluctuating sensorineural hearing loss, and approximately one-third improved with intravenous penicillin (Hanner *et al.*, 1989). This is a treatable cause of sensorineural hearing loss (Peltomaa *et al.*, 2000).

Metabolic

There is no clear evidence linking diabetes mellitus with auditory and/or vestibular abnormalities as a consequence of neuropathy, angiopathy or of both pathologies (Maia and Campos, 2005). However, recent genetic studies have defined the relationship of diabetes and hearing loss in mitochondrial mutations (Maassen, 2002) and in mutations of the WFS1 gene in the Wolfman syndrome (generalized congenital hypertrichosis) of non-syndromic hearing impairment, diabetes mellitus and psychiatric disease (Cryns *et al.*, 2003). Hearing loss is a common finding in patients with renal failure. The disease process, ototoxic drugs and axonal uraemic neuropathy have all been suggested as possible factors, while dialysis and renal transplantation have been reported to be associated with recovery of hearing impairment (Anteunis and Mooy, 1987). Recently, an underlying neuropathy with retrocochlear involvement has been suggested (Küstel *et al.*, 1993).

Neoplasia

Vestibular schwannomas (Schwann, 1810–1882) are rare, but account for 10 per cent of intracranial tumours and more than three-quarters of cerebellopontine angle lesions (Gonzalez-Revilla, 1948). The most common presenting features are unilateral hearing loss and tinnitus (Pulec *et al.*, 1971), considered to be due to compression or ischaemia of the auditory division of the VIII nerve. However, a review of patients with vestibular schwannoma revealed that less than half demonstrated a classical retrocochlear hearing impairment (Johnson, 1968), while brainstem-evoked responses are reported to be abnormal in 95 per cent of surgically proven cases (Josey *et al.*, 1980).

In all patients with a unilateral or asymmetric bilateral sensorineural hearing impairment, or unilateral tinnitus, it is mandatory to consider and exclude the presence of a small vestibular schwannoma, the gold standard being magnetic resonance imaging. However, a vestibular schwannoma may not be an absolute contraindication to flying. In a review of ten cases, Pons *et al.* (2010) judged that two were fit to fly as transport aircrew. In each case, the decision took into consideration the size of the tumour, the nature of their hearing loss, the integrity of their balance and the complications that may have arisen with treatment.

Tumours other than schwannomas account for a quarter of all cerebellopontine angle lesions, and include meningiomas, epidermoid cysts, neuromas of the fifth and seventh cranial nerves, and brainstem gliomas. In addition, the eighth cranial nerve may be compressed by schwannomas on the fifth, seventh, ninth or eleventh cranial nerves. Metastatic tumours within the temporal bone are relatively common and include secondary deposits from the breast, kidneys, lungs, stomach, larynx, prostate and thyroid gland. In addition, leukaemic infiltrates (Paparella *et al.*, 1973), carcinomatous meningitis (Zeller *et al.*, 2002) and paraneoplastic syndromes (Gulya, 1993) of the eighth cranial nerve may give rise to auditory symptoms, and may manifest with auditory loss. Treatment of malignancy may also give rise to post-radiation and drug-induced ototoxicity with hearing loss (Low *et al.*, 2006a; van der Putten *et al.*, 2006) Cochlear implantation may result in good hearing outcomes in some patients with iatrogenic loss (Low *et al.*, 2006b).

Toxic disorders

Drugs, alcohol and chemicals have all been reported to give rise to auditory dysfunction. Lead and mercury poisoning may affect the auditory and vestibular systems, although the underlying pathophysiology is unclear. Early work in animals demonstrated segmental demyelination and axonal degeneration of the eighth cranial nerve in three-quarters of animals receiving intraperitoneal injections of 1 per cent lead acetate solution, and human temporal bone studies in lead and mercury poisoning have reported eighth nerve pathology (Gozdzick-Zolnierkiewicz and Moszynski, 1969).

Quinine, loop diuretics and aminoglycosides are the commonest drugs associated with ototoxicity (Shine and Coates, 2005). Platinum-based chemotherapeutic agents, in addition to the aminoglycosides, damage the hair cells of the inner ear as a result of the production of reactive oxygen species in the cochlea, while vincristine sulphate has been shown to produce bilateral cochlear nerve damage (Mahajan *et al.*, 1981). Salicylates, which are highly concentrated in the perilymph, may interfere with the enzymatic activity of the hair cells or the cochlear neurons, or both (Silverstein *et al.*, 1967). Thalidomide has been demonstrated to produce aplasia of the eighth cranial nerve in association with the aplasia described by Michel (1863) of the inner ear (Jørgensen *et al.*, 1964). Extensive degeneration of both myelinated and unmyelinated nerve fibres in the cochlear and the vestibular division of the eighth cranial nerve have been reported in a chronic alcoholic patient with a marked peripheral neuropathy (Ylikoski *et al.*, 1981), although whether this is a direct toxic effect or neuropathy related to malnutrition is unclear.

The molecular and biological mechanisms of ototoxic effects and other forms of cochlear damage have been the subject of extensive scientific investigation. The formation of reactive oxygen metabolites (ROM), including free oxygen radicals and other metabolites, is thought to be central to damage of cochlear tissue, as these highly reactive compounds can oxidize a wide variety of targets, such as proteins, mitochondrial deoxyribonucleic acid (mtDNA) or lipids. An understanding of these mechanisms has led to a series of studies evaluating administration of antioxidants, or ROM (reactive oxygen metabolites) scavengers. For example, iron chelators were found to reduce gentamicin ototoxicity (Schacht, 1998), and calorie restriction, vitamins C (L-ascorbic acid) and E (α-tocopherol) supplementation and melatonin treatment were reported to attenuate age-related hearing loss (Seidman, 2000). These findings herald an exciting future, with the potential identification of pharmacological strategies for prevention of ototoxicity and different forms of cochlear degeneration.

Ménière's Disease

The disease described by Ménière (1799–1862) is a clinical diagnosis based on the triad of hearing loss that is frequently fluctuant in the early stages of the disorder, acute episodes of vertigo and ipsilateral tinnitus. Commonly, aural pressure or fullness in the affected ear is an associated feature. It is considered that endolymphatic hydrops is the underlying pathophysiological abnormality, although many pathophysiological mechanisms have been proposed, and endolymphatic hydrops may be an epiphenomenon or result. Despite an extensive literature on Ménière's disease, the diagnosis, pathology and aetiology remain poorly understood (Semaan *et al.*, 2005; Gates, 2006).

The diagnosis of Ménière's disease should be based on the criteria of the American Academy of Otolaryngology and Head and Neck Surgery (1995). The early hearing loss is characteristically a low-tone, sensorineural loss, but over time the loss may become plateau in configuration or 'tent-shaped' with preservation of the mid-frequencies. Occasionally, sensorineural hearing loss may progress for some months or years before the onset of acute vertiginous episodes. Treatment options remain empirical rather than evidence-based (Bamiou and Luxon, 2003), in view of the diagnostic difficulties and the natural history of relapses and remissions over many months or years. The condition is also dealt with in Chapter 18 (Vestibular and Related Oculomotor Disorders).

Demyelination

Sudden, unilateral sensorineural loss is an unusual initial presentation of demyelination, and may also occur in the course of the disease (de Seze *et al.*, 2001). The natural history of both presentations is frequently complete resolution. The pathology is thought to be in the intramedullary auditory nerve or cochlear nucleus (Barratt *et al.*, 1988) and enhanced magnetic resonance has demonstrated imaging lesions at the route entry zones in a patient with multiple sclerosis (Miller *et al.*, 1988). More rarely, the involvement of midline brainstem plaques may give rise to auditory processing deficits.

Auditory Processing Disorder

This is defined as difficulty in processing non-speech sounds and is attributed to abnormal function within the central nervous system. A variety of aetiologies, including trauma, neoplasia, degenerative disease, metabolic dysfunction, neurotoxicity, infection and/or iatrogenic lesions, have been implicated in adults. The prevalence of auditory processing disorders in adults is unknown but is likely to be underestimated because of lack of professional knowledge and resources.

Brainstem Dysfunction

Hearing loss associated with brainstem pathology is rare because of the multiplicity of pathways and decussations above the cochlear nuclei, and the symmetrical tonotopic organization subserved by the auditory nuclei at all levels. The asymmetrical low-frequency loss has been demonstrated in animals with focal brainstem lesions and has been confirmed in a study of well-defined midline brainstem lesions in humans (Cohen *et al.*, 1996).

The most effective tests in identifying brainstem auditory pathology include auditory brainstem-evoked responses, acoustic reflex thresholds and masking level difference. These techniques are highly sensitive in the absence of a peripheral auditory deficit, but their application may be limited if there is significant cochlear or eighth nerve pathology. Efferent auditory function may also be impaired in brainstem pathology. Hyperacusis may be a prominent symptom in lesions of the floor of the fourth ventricle, with dysfunction of the olivocochlear bundle and release of the outer hair cells from normal inhibitory influences. Recent work has demonstrated a lack of efferent suppression of transient-evoked otoacoustic emissions with contralateral masking in demyelination (Coelho et al., 2007) and in head injury.

Cortical Hearing Impairment

Cortical hearing loss is rare, but is most commonly associated with vascular disease (Kaga et al., 2000) or trauma (Wirkowski et al., 2006), affecting both temporal lobes (Musiek and Lee, 1998). Additional and more severe neurological signs, such as hemiparesis and dysphasia, are the rule. The primary auditory cortex lies in the anterior/posterior transverse temporal gyrus of Heschl (1824–1876). Each ear has bilateral representation in the auditory cortex, and it is possible to remove the non-dominant hemisphere in humans without significant effect on either the pure-tone audiogram or the discrimination of distorted speech. Auditory deficits due to cerebral pathology can be divided into auditory agnosias (Pan et al., 2004), in which pure-tone audiometry is normal or only minimally affected, and cortical deafness, in which there is a severe if not total hearing loss (Leussink et al., 2005). Recent work has demonstrated subtle auditory deficits in patients with insular strokes (Bamiou et al., 2006).

Tinnitus

Tinnitus is associated with otological, neurological, systemic and psychological pathologies. In a Swedish study, approximately two-thirds of patients with tinnitus presenting to an otorhinolaryngological clinic suffered ear disease, although almost 6 per cent suffered neurological disease (Axelsson, 1992). A variety of different mechanisms have been suggested in the pathophysiology of tinnitus:

❑ Abnormal afferent excitation at the cochlea level: based on spontaneous cochlear oscillations
  – glutamate neuro-excitotoxicity
  – enhanced sensitivity of N-methyl-D-Aspartic Acid (NMDA) and non-NMDA receptors
  – abnormal ion channel conductance or calcium channel dysfunction
❑ Efferent dysfunction/reduction of γ-Aminobutyric Acid (GABA) effect
❑ Stress and psychological disorders
❑ Damaged hair cells or primary neurons
❑ Ephaptic transmission (Møller, 1984)
❑ Decoupling of the stereocilia of the hair cells (Holgers and Barrenäs, 2003)
❑ Misinterpretation of auditory neural activity in higher auditory centres (Jastreboff, 1990)
❑ Self-sustaining oscillation of the basilar membrane (Ćeranić and Luxon, 2002).

All these hypotheses are postulated to lead to an alteration in the spontaneous activity, arising from an alteration in the balance between excitation and inhibition, within the auditory system. Following the discovery by Kemp (1978) of otoacoustic emissions from within the human auditory system, it was thought that spontaneous otoacoustic emissions might provide an explanation for many cases of tinnitus. However, despite the demonstration of such a link, the association has proved to be uncommon (Penner, 1990). Atherley and Noble (1971) showed that tinnitus was not a prominent feature of occupational noise-induced hearing loss – at least in drop forgers.

Lindgren *et al.* (2009) mailed a self-administered tinnitus questionnaire to over 500 pilots of a Swedish airline for information on age, gender, smoking habits and employment date. Audiometric test results were obtained from the medical records. The prevalence of tinnitus was no greater than in the general Swedish population. Moreover, there was a significant negative correlation between years of employment and the presence of tinnitus. However, pilots with tinnitus were more likely to report being disturbed by noise in the cockpit. No measures of operational efficiency were obtained. Tinnitus in the pilots was significantly correlated with exposure to impulse noise, as in hunting. The authors conceded that the study suffered from selection factors that plague other sub-experimental studies of this type.

It must be emphasized that the majority of patients who suffer from tinnitus do not find the symptom intrusive. Psychological factors are highly significant in patients with tinnitus complaint, as noted above, and the onset of tinnitus has been related to negative life events such as retirement, redundancy, bereavement and divorce (Holgers and Barrenäs, 2003). In the clinical context, studies of the 'loudness' and the 'annoyance' of tinnitus have shown these to be two distinct dimensions. 'Annoyance' is important as it is the primary complaint of tinnitus patients. Fortunately, annoyance is the measure that responds to appropriate treatment (Jakes *et al.*, 1986). This suggests an approach to ameliorating community annoyance towards aircraft noise by using the social cognitive theory of Bandura (2009).

Hearing Loss

In adults, the clinical presentation of both hearing loss and tinnitus may be of value in raising the suspicion of the underlying aetiology. Sudden hearing loss is most commonly sensorineural in type, and is associated with trauma, infection, vascular pathology or autoimmune disease. Hearing loss associated with autoimmune disease is often fluctuant, lacks concordant vestibular symptoms and is asymmetric. There are no internationally accepted criteria for sudden sensorineural hearing loss, and thus the literature abounds with studies of heterogeneous groups of patients, making comparison of aetiology and configurations of auditory loss difficult (Hughes *et al.*, 1996). Nonetheless, the majority of cases of sudden sensorineural hearing loss defy precise aetiological diagnosis, and about two-thirds recover spontaneously, with maximal improvement in the first few weeks after onset (Mattox and Simmons, 1977).

Slowly progressive hearing loss is most commonly associated with so-called 'presbyacusis'. However, recent work has led to the view that presbyacusis merely represents a genetic predisposition (Garringer *et al.*, 2006), together with the cumulative effects of multiple otological insults over a lifetime. Specific risk factors for cochlear damage include hazardous noise exposure, barotrauma, head injury, ototoxic drugs and infections such as syphilis. More rapidly progressive hearing loss causes alarm for both the patient and physician, and may represent autoimmune disease, a congenital defect or genetic hearing loss (Martini and Prosser, 2003).

The audiometric configuration may also confer valuable diagnostic information, although no configuration is uniquely associated with any one specific diagnosis. Fluctuating low-frequency hearing loss is the hallmark of Ménière's disease, mid-frequency losses are characteristic of congenital/genetic hearing loss, while 4 kHz notched are associated with noise-induced hearing loss and high-frequency losses are common with so called 'presbyacusis', trauma and ototoxicity.

The asymmetry between the hearing threshold levels in the left and right ears in a random sample (n = 3,487) of the general population has been analyzed by Pirila et al. (1992). Males and females of age groups 5–10 years, 15–50 years and over 50 years were analyzed separately. A significant average inferiority of the hearing in the left ear was found at high frequencies, especially at 3–6 kHz, among adult males and females but not among children. A slight superiority of the left ear at low frequencies was noted in all age groups. At 4 kHz, the average inferiority of the left ear in the male population was greater among subjects aged 15–50 years than among older subjects. In conclusion, the inferiority of hearing in the left ear at 4 kHz seems to be associated more with noise damage than with presbyacusis. Further analyses of the epidemiological data indicated that handedness cannot be responsible for the average inferiority of the hearing

in the left ear at 4 kHz or for the average slight superiority of the left ear at 0.125–0.5 kHz (Pirila et al. 1991).

It must be emphasized that a detailed general medical history may convey crucial information regarding past medical, family, occupational and drug history, as well as information about concurrent medical symptoms, and that a detailed medical examination should include the eyes, cardiovascular and neurological systems, in addition to the ears.

Clinical Examination

The head and anatomy of the external ear should be carefully examined to define visible signs of congenital ear disease such as pits, tags, nodules or malformations and evidence of craniofacial features, which may suggest the presence of a syndrome associated with hearing impairment. Wax or debris obstructing the external auditory meatus should be removed manually or by suction. Syringing should not be undertaken in the presence of an infection, if it is unknown whether the tympanic membrane may be perforated or if an atelectatic area of the drum appears fragile. A detailed examination of the tympanic membrane is required, to note the presence of a light reflex from the lower tympanic membrane, scarring, the ossicular chain, and any obvious abnormalities from within the middle ear, for example tumours or fluid levels.

Tuning fork tests are a valuable clinical tool, enabling a clinician to distinguish a conductive loss from a sensorineural hearing loss (Figure 19.6) and, on rare occasions, to identify a non-organic hearing loss. Tuning fork tests rely on two physiological phenomena: first, the inner ear is normally more sensitive to sound conducted by air, as a consequence of the redistribution of frequencies in the external canal and the amplification of sound through the middle ear mechanism; and second, in the presence of a purely conductive hearing loss, the affected ear is subject to less environmental noise, making it more sensitive to bone-conducted sound.

Auditory Investigations

The aim of auditory investigations is to define the presence and site of pathology in the auditory system. A battery of audiological tests is required to:

- quantify the audiometric threshold at each frequency
- differentiate a conductive from a sensorineural hearing loss
- differentiate a cochlear from a retrocochlear abnormality

- identify central auditory dysfunction in the brainstem, mid-brain or auditory cortex
- identify a non-organic hearing impairment.

Tests may be either subjective, depending upon patient cooperation, or objective in that they do not rely on patient cooperation. In the differentiation of a sensorineural hearing loss of cochlear origin from that of VIII nerve dysfunction or neurological impairment, loudness recruitment and abnormal auditory adaptation are important.

Pure-tone audiometry is the standard auditory test to document the threshold of hearing (British Society of Audiology, 1981). The technique, performed in a sound-proofed room according to standardized protocols, allows the severity, symmetry and configuration of any hearing loss to be defined across frequencies between 125 and 8,000 Hz

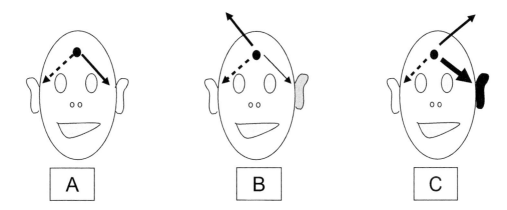

Figure 19.6 Diagram illustrating the results observed during the Weber test

a) in a normal subject, the perceived sound is heard in the middle of the head

b) in a patient with a left sensorineural hearing loss, the perceived sound is heard towards the better i.e. right ear;

c) in a patient with a left conductive hearing loss, the perceived sound is heard towards the left, i.e. the affected side.

────────▶ Reduced perception by cochlea secondary to sensorineural loss

- - - - - ▶ Normal perception of tuning fork by cochlea

────▶ Direction of perceived sound

━━━━▶ Enhanced perception of bone conducted sound as a consequence of reduction of air conducted environmental sound due to conductive hearing loss

▨ Conductive hearing loss   ■ Sensorineural hearing loss

in each ear. Electrically generated pure-tones are delivered by headphones, and the subject is required to respond to the quietest tone. Sound may be delivered by air conduction or by bone conduction via a bone vibrator on the mastoid process. In this latter condition, because the intra-aural attenuation for a bone-conducted sound is negligible, the ear which is not being tested must be masked with narrow-band noise centred on the test frequency. Bone-conduction thresholds, which are significantly better than air-conduction thresholds, indicate a disorder affecting the transmission of sound waves through the middle ear into the inner ear – that is, conductive hearing loss – whereas similar bone-conduction and air-conduction thresholds imply a sensorineural hearing loss (Figure 19.5). The determination of normal auditory thresholds was considered to be sufficiently important to aircrew to merit investigation. The results (Wheeler and Dickson, 1952) formed the basis for a standard (1954: British Standard 2497), and this evolved to the current International Organization Standards concerned with the effect of noise on auditory thresholds. These are dealt with in detail in Part 2 of this chapter.

Acoustic impedance measurements (Figure 19.7a) provide information about the middle and internal ears in addition to the eighth cranial nerve and brainstem function. Passive measurements are made of the change in acoustic impedance or immitance of the tympanic membrane as a function of the pressure in the sealed external acoustic meatus (British Society of Audiology, 1992). Dynamic changes resulting from the contraction of the stapedius muscle, acoustic reflex thresholds (Figure 19.7b), in response to stimuli of 500, 1,000, 2,000 and 4,000 Hz, at intensities of 70 to 100 dB sound pressure level, are also measured.

These values provide objective evidence of recruitment and abnormal auditory adaptation, and allow an assessment of middle ear, cochlea, VIII nerve and brainstem auditory function (Figure 19.7c).

Otoacoustic emissions represent weak signals generated by the contractile properties of the outer hair cells in the cochlea in response to acoustic stimuli (Figure 19.8). They are time locked and averaged using computer analysis. These responses are measured in the external auditory canal and provide direct objective information about the integrity of the outer hair cells. Efferent auditory function can be assessed by suppression of otoacoustic emissions by the application of noise to the contralateral ear (Figure 19.9). Speech audiometry (Figure 19.9) is concerned with the assessment of auditory discrimination as opposed to the assessment of auditory acuity. The test is subjective and requires the subject to repeat standard lists of words delivered at varying intensities through headphones. The responses are scored and provide an assessment of auditory discrimination which, together with other tests, may be of value in distinguishing conductive, sensory and neural hearing impairment, but this test is of particularly value in assessing the efficacy of hearing aid provision.

Speech-in-noise tests were developed many years ago for assessing the operational efficiency of aircrews and have subsequently been further developed (Nilsson et al., 1994). Speech intelligibility/perception-in-noise tests have now been standardized (Kalikow et al., 1977; Bilger et al., 1984), and recent work has advocated the use of insert earphones for hearing-in-noise tests as opposed to supra-aural earphones (Ribera, 2007).

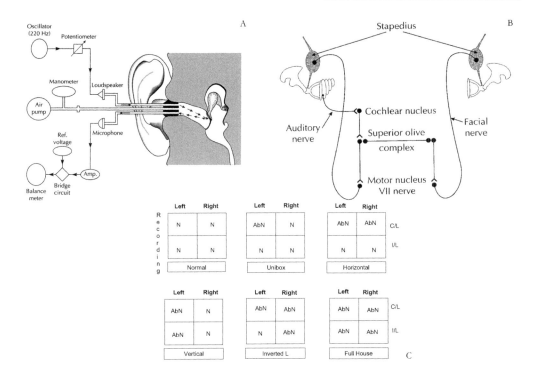

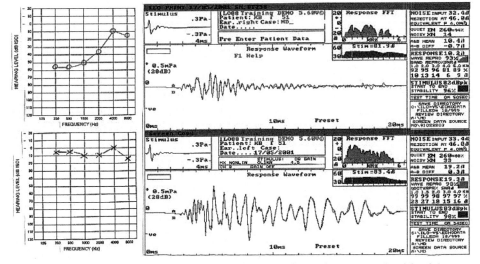

Figure 19.7 Diagrams to illustrate acoustic impedance measurements

a) and b)   Components of electroacoustic impedance bridge and Anatomical pathway of the bilateral acoustically-induced stapedius reflex.
Source: Ludman, H. 1998. Basic acoustics and hearing tests. In: H. Ludman and T. Wright (eds.) *Diseases of the Ear*- Sixth Edition. Arnold, London, pp 58–86. Reproduced by permission of Hodder Education.

c)   Diagram to illustrate anatomical pathway of the bilateral acoustically-induced stapedius reflex.

Key: N = normal; AbN = abnormal; C/L = contralateral; I/L = Ipsilateral; Unibox = small unilateral brainstem lesion medial to cochlear nucleus; Figure horizontal = midline brainstem lesion; vertical = left VIIIth nerve lesion; Inverted L= intra-axial brainstem lesion plus extension to the cochlear nucleus or VIIIth nerve on the affected side (NB, a conductive lesion may also present in this way); Full-house = a midline brainstem lesion with extension to involve the cochlear nuclei and/or VIIIth nerves (a bilateral conductive disorder requires exclusion).

Figure 19.8 Otoacoustic emissions recorded from each ear in a normal subject (see colour section)

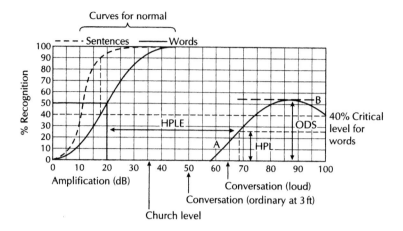

Figure 19.9 Speech audiogram

AB = speech audiogram of a sensorineural hearing loss; HPL = half-peak level; HPLE = half-peak level elevation; ODS = optimal discrimination score.

Source: Ludman, H. 1998. Basic acoustics and hearing tests. In: H.Ludman and T. Wright (eds.) *Diseases of the Ear*- Sixth Edition. Arnold, London, pp 58–86. Reproduced by permission of Hodder Education.

Electrophysiology

These tests provide an objective assessment of auditory function and facilitate the identification of the site of pathology in the auditory system. Electrocochleography is the measurement of the electrical output of the cochlea and eighth cranial nerve in response to auditory stimulation. It is most commonly used in the diagnosis of Ménière's disease, when the ratio of the summating potential and the action potential is greater than 30 per cent, whereas in the normal population it is significantly smaller (Gibson, 2009). Brainstem-evoked responses (Figure 19.10a) are a series of neurogenic potentials which are recorded using surface electrodes in response to click stimuli, in the ten milliseconds immediately after the stimulus. As a diagnostic tool, brainstem auditory evoked responses are of particular value in discriminating between cochlear and VIII nerve/brainstem dysfunction. Analysis of the waveform (Figure 19.10b)

must be undertaken in the knowledge of pure-tone audiometric thresholds, if appropriate, and valid conclusions are to be drawn.

Prolongation of the I–III interval can be seen in auditory nerve and cochlear nucleus pathology. Prolongation of the III–V is usually indicated when pathology is sited above the level of the cochlear nucleus, while absent IV and/or V waves are found in cases with involvement of the mid/upper pons. In severe brainstem pathology, waves III–V may be absent. Interaural latency comparisons of wave V are of value in diagnosis of acoustic neurinoma (Figure 19.10c), but may not be useful in detecting brainstem involvement (Weinstein, 1994). In general, while the abnormality in brainstem lesions may be ipsilateral, with respect to the acoustic stimulus, or bilateral, contralateral findings are rare (Musiek and Lee, 1995). The sensitivity and specificity of the auditory brainstem response in identifying brainstem lesions depends on the site of lesion. More caudal intra-axial structured brainstem

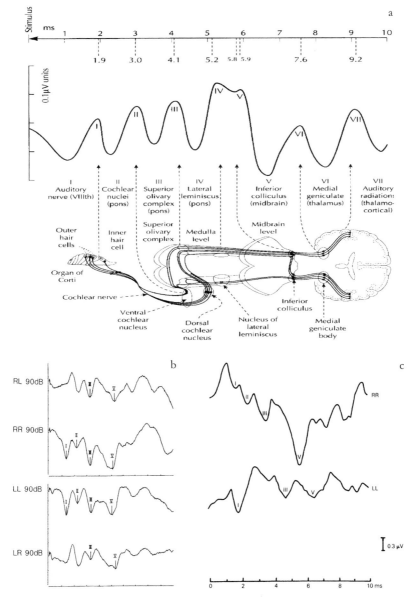

Figure 19.10   Brainstem auditory-evoked responses

a) Anatomical correlates of the waves I-VII observed in auditory brainstem-evoked responses. *Source*: Duane, D.D. 1977. A Neurologic Perspective of Central Auditory Dysfunction. New York, Grune & Stratton. With permission from Elsevier and D.D. Duane.

b) Diagram to illustrate auditory brainstem-evoked responses in a normal subject.

c) Diagram to illustrate delay of wave III and wave V in a small left acoustic neuroma compared with normal response from the right ear.

Key: LL = ipsilateral left recording; RR = ipsilateral right recording.
    LR =Left stimulation ,right recording RL = Right stimulation, left recording

lesions are identified, but the auditory brainstem response is only moderately sensitive to degenerative disorders or a rostral lesion involving the brainstem. Overall, the sensitivity/specificity of the auditory brainstem response for a variety of brainstem lesions is around 80 per cent, which is less than that noted for acoustic tumours (Musiek and Lee, 1995).

The middle latency response generator sites are thought to be in the thalamocortical pathway in the auditory cortex (Kraus *et al.*, 1994). There is much intersubject variability in both latency and amplitude measurements of the middle latency response, but in general the most effective measurements are intrasubject comparisons of the electrode effect and the ear effect (Musiek *et al.*, 1994). Maturation of the middle latency response is relatively long, and very variable, such that this test cannot be applied reliably to children under the age of ten years. The sensitivity and specificity of the middle latency response for central auditory pathology is reasonably good, and it is therefore a valid objective test in the assessment of central auditory dysfunction (Musiek *et al.*, 1999; Kileny *et al.*, 1987), but sleep and/or sedation may affect the response. Cortical- or late-evoked auditory responses are the most effective method of defining auditory threshold at each frequency (Figure 19.11) in a patient who is unable or unwilling to cooperate, and are essential in legal cases in which non-organic loss should always be excluded.

Future Measurements

Almost all the measures of auditory function reported in earlier work have been obtained by conventional manual pure-tone audiometry – the

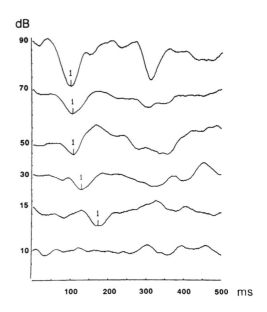

Figure 19.11   Tracings of cortical-evoked responses recorded to threshold in a normal subject

Source: Luxon, L.M. and Cohen, M. 1997. Central Auditory Dysfunction In: A.G. Kerr (ed.) *Scott Brown's Diseases of the Ear Nose and Throat – Sixth Edition*. S.D.G Stephens (ed.) *Adult Audiology*. Volume 2: Butterworths. With permission from Elsevier and L. Luxon.

determination of hearing sensitivity at selected frequencies by a psychophysical procedure (see above). However, clinicians are now investigating hearing, particularly with reference to noise hazards, using more sophisticated psychophysical methods as well as the physiological methods mentioned in the main body of this chapter. The temporal fine structure (TFS) test, a fast, sophisticated psychoacoustical test for determining the temporal fine structure of hearing, has become available (Moore and Sęk, 2009). This should prove to detect noise damage to hearing at an earlier stage than is currently possible with conventional tonal threshold audiometry.

Otoacoustic emissions are characterized by a high sensitivity in detecting subtle changes of the outer hair cells, and this property makes them very valuable in identifying early noise-induced change, even before there is any notable shift in the audiometric thresholds. Although there is a high inter-individual variability, they display remarkable intra-individual stability. They are, therefore, useful in the monitoring of intra-individual otoacoustic emissions of subtle changes in cochlear integrity following noise exposure (Ćeranić, 2007). A longitudinal study of soldiers, beginning prior to their basic training and continuing for two years, showed a decrease in transient-evoked otoacoustic emissions over time, but their relationship with auditory thresholds were complex (Duvdevany and Furst, 2007).

Management of Hearing Impairment

Management of hearing impairment may be divided into three aspects:

○ prevention to ensure protection from ototoxic agents including both hazardous noise (occupational and leisure-related) and ototoxic drugs
○ medical management of systemic medical conditions which may be impacting, causing or exacerbating auditory dysfunction
○ auditory rehabilitation which is a problem-solving exercise centred on the needs of the individual, assessing both the auditory disability and the relevance of this to the patient's lifestyle and other important people in their life. Auditory impairment, communication skills, including lip-reading ability, the use of visual cues, and the level of speech and language, together with psychological and sociological factors, must all be considered.

Prevention and Hearing Protection

All employed personnel exposed to a noise hazard, including aviators, should be recruited into a hearing conservation programme (HCP) that should include:

○ noise monitoring
○ engineering controls
○ administrative controls
○ use of appropriate hearing protection devices.

Periodic auditory evaluation and worker education are key elements, while engineering controls refer to the steps taken to mitigate against hazardous noise exposure, using engineering solutions such as barriers and enclosures. Administrative controls refer to organizational regulation by limiting shift duration and thus exposure to noise, and the introduction of guidelines for specification of equipment to reduce noise dose. A recent questionnaire study conducted on Canadian military personnel including aviation staff (Abel, 2005) suggested that 'training on noise hazard and selection and use of hearing protection were inadequate. Hearing protection was reported to be incompatible with other gear, uncomfortable and an impediment to communication.' Thus, improved hearing protection programmes are required.

Although Owen (1995) concluded that, in the past, the level of hearing protection had been inadequate, more recent studies have shown that noise-induced hearing loss in aircrew is becoming less marked, principally due to improved helmet design and awareness of the need to comply with hearing protection measures. Under actual working conditions, the sound attenuation provided by the helmets worn by aircrew has been reported to be in the range 10 to 22 dB. The attenuation provided by the ear muffs worn by ground engineers is somewhat more – up to 27 dB (Pääkkönen and Kuronen, 1996, 1997).

Over the past 20 years, active noise-control techniques have been developed to supplement the passive techniques used in the classical hearing protectors ('ear defenders'). Active noise reduction (ANR) consists of continuously sampling the noise in the earshell of the protector using a miniature microphone. This signal is then inverted in phase and reintroduced into the shell by the earphone. The noise levels within the shell are, thereby, reduced. In an example given by Rood (1988), the average cabin noise level in a jet aircraft flying at high speed at low altitude was measured as 117.6 dB. The average noise level at the ear was measured as 92.5 dB, and with active noise reduction the noise level at the ear was 81.5 dB. In contrast with the passively acting hearing protectors, ANR is particularly effective at low frequencies.

Pääkkönen et al. (2001) measured the effect of active noise reduction during a military jet trainer test flight. Cockpit noise measurements were carried out in a two-seat jet trainer. For the continuous time and frequency analyses, a two-channel tape-recording system was constructed of two miniature microphones connected through an amplifier to a digital tape-recorder. The analyzed and averaged noise exposure, including radio communication, was 80 to 81 dB with the ANC system and 84 to 89 dB without the ANC system. For the conventional flight helmet, the same noise exposure was 86 dB, and the noise exposure in the cockpit was 104 to 106 dB. The effect of the ANC system on the averaged noise exposure (L (Aeq8min)) was an improvement of 4 to 8 dB over the noise attenuation of the same helmets when the ANC system was off. Both ANC systems worked properly during the test flights. No severe ringing or voice circulation was found except during extreme vibration.

A study by Brungart et al. (2003) compared different forms of single hearing protection (earplugs, earmuffs) and a combination of both forms of hearing protection on auditory localization in the horizontal plane. The results demonstrate optimal attenuation with the combination of plugs and muffs, but maximal impairment of right–left localization. In contrast, plugs or muffs alone had little effect on localization.

Medical Standards

Each country establishes medical standards for the hearing of various skill groups. The most stringent standards apply to aircrew; less stringent standards to ground crews. The International Civil Aviation Organization (ICAO) sets rules and regulations for 189 contracting states. These are published as Standards and Recommended Practices (SARPs) for international civil aviation. They are concerned with medical provisions that also cover hearing, and are contained in Annex 1 to the Convention on International Civil Aviation, ICAO. They are minimum requirements to which contracting states must abide unless they file a 'difference' with ICAO, which is available to other states. If a state chooses not to apply such standards and instead imposes a lower national standard, another state may, if it wishes, prevent an aircraft operating to such reduced requirements from entering its own airspace. A state, however, may set higher (stricter) national standards without any penalty.

The principal responsibilities of the International Civil Aviation Organization (ICAO) as far as medicine is concerned are:

○ monitoring the developments within the field of medicine and aviation medicine and adjusting the appropriate Annex 1 provisions as necessary to ensure they remain up-to-date
○ reviewing and maintaining current the Manual of Civil Aviation Medicine (Doc. 8984), the Manual on Prevention of Problematic Use of Substances in the Aviation Workplace (Doc. 9654) and the Manual on Laser Emitters and Flight Safety (Doc. 9815)
○ developing appropriate Standards and guidance material to ensure that the aviation community contributes to reducing the risk of transmitting communicable diseases by air
○ providing guidance to licensing authorities in contracting states on medical standards; medical problems relevant to flight operations; the effect of working conditions on health; biological and psychological problems relating to passengers and crew; first aid and survival equipment; and the medical aspects of accident investigation and prevention
○ conducting and participating in regional seminars on aviation medicine, conducting ICAO educational sessions at international aviation medicine scientific meetings and presenting papers at such meetings.

The European Aviation Safety Agency (2010) establishes implementing rules for the licensing and medical certification of pilots, including decisions on acceptable means of compliance.

Rehabilitation and Management

Although hearing aids play a pivotal role in audiological rehabilitation, a detailed description of their prescription is outside the scope of this chapter (review by Gatehouse, 2003). Conventional aids may be divided into those that are body- and head-worn, which may be in or around the ear or within spectacles. The primary advantage of body-worn aids is the high gain and maximum output which can be achieved, whereas the disadvantages are the unsightly nature of the device and the poor microphone placement.

The general principles of hearing aid provision include:

○ the fitting of a comfortable ear mould to provide a secure mounting for the aid
○ a good acoustic connection between the aid and the ear canal
○ hearing aid selection – matching the amplification at specific frequencies with that required by the user.

The major complaint of hearing-impaired users is difficulty in hearing speech in the presence of background noise. Programmable digital processing devices are of some help in this situation, but conventional analogue aids provide selective amplification across speech frequencies with minimal amplification at the peak frequencies of background noise. For the majority of patients, post-aural, in-the-ear or in-the-canal hearing aids are highly effective, but some patients will also require additional environmental aids, such as assistive listening devices (amplification systems attached to televisions or telephones) and/or alerting warning devices (flashing lights connected to a door bell or an alarm clock) (Stephens, 2003).

The value of counselling for the hearing-impaired subject cannot be overemphasized, as simple hearing tactics, such as light on a speaker's face, placement of the better ear towards the speaker, sitting close to a sound source and minimizing background noise can improve communication significantly. The need for psychological, social and occupational support should not be overlooked.

Conductive Hearing Loss

In the management of conductive loss, clear transmission of sound through the external ear from the pinna to the tympanic membrane should be checked and foreign bodies, wax, polyps, tumour or infection should be treated appropriately. Acute otitis externa requires suction clearance under microscopy, culture and sensitivity of the organism, and appropriate medication, with or without steroids (Rosenfeld et al., 2006).

The treatment of acute otitis media requires pain relief, re-establishment of eustachian tube function using nasal drops, inhalations or decongestants, mucolytics and the prescription of systemic antibiotics. The drug of choice is amoxycillin or, in cases of sensitivity to penicillin, erythromycin. Myringotomy is indicated if the drum is bulging. In recurrent acute otitis media, a focus of infection within the upper respiratory tract should be sought, while persistent otitis media with effusion requires the exclusion of naspharyngeal malignancy (Ho et al., 2008). The aim of treatment of chronic suppurative otitis media is to eliminate infection using antibiotics, and, when the ear is healthy, repair aural damage such as a perforated ear drum or damage to the ossicles, which may prevent reinfection and improve sound

transmission (Robinson, 1998; Raglan, 2003). Conductive hearing loss caused by otosclerosis or the hereditary osseous dysplasias may be managed conservatively using hearing aids, or surgically by stapedectomy. The procedure carries a small risk of complication of late sudden sensorineural hearing loss, and for this reason stapedectomy has historically not been undertaken in both ears, although recent work has shown more promising results (Kujala et al., 2008).

Sensorineural Hearing Loss

The management of sensorineural hearing loss is determined by the time course of the loss, be it sudden, progressive or chronic. Sudden hearing loss is a medical emergency requiring hospital admission, bed rest and investigation of possible causes. There is no consensus on the accepted form of treatment and a variety of different interventions have been proposed, including treatment with rapidly decreasing high-dose steroids. A spontaneous recovery rate for sudden unilateral sensorineural hearing loss in about two-thirds of patients has been reported (Haberkamp and Tanyeri, 1999). In the case of bilateral hearing loss, midline brainstem lesion, trauma and autoimmune inner ear disease should all be considered, and psychological and aggressive auditory rehabilitation are required. This latter condition requires urgent management with steroids and/ or immunosuppressives following diagnosis (Agrup and Luxon, 2006).

Progressive hearing impairment may be the result of a range of pathologies which may be treatable medically or surgically, with subsequent rehabilitation to reduce disability. Syphilitic labyrinthitis requires treatment with steroids and penicillin, while large or rapidly growing acoustic neurinoma require surgical intervention or laser therapy. However, there is now a consensus that small tumours can be managed with a 'watch, wait and monitor' policy, which avoids surgery for many extremely slowly progressive benign tumours (British Association of Otorhinolaryngologists – Head and Neck Surgeons, 2002).

There is a plethora of treatments for Ménière's disease, but no definitive therapy has been supported by a double-blind control trial. Strupp et al. (2008) have recently reported efficacy with high-dose betahistine. Trials of therapy in this condition are particularly difficult, because of the lack of diagnostic certainty, the relapsing and remitting nature of the disorder, and the variability of frequency and severity of the different symptoms within the diagnostic triad between and within patients. Medical therapy includes lifestyle changes, diet, drugs (including diuretics, vestibular sedatives, vasodilators and immunosuppressives), psychological support, physiotherapy and auditory rehabilitation (James and Thorp, 2004; Cohen-Kerem et al., 2004; Doyle et al., 2004; Minor et al., 2004).

A recent low-pressure pulse generator (Meniett device) has been advocated as a non-invasive effective treatment for Ménière's disease, but there is no definite evidence available (Gates, 2005). Chemical labyrinthectomy using intratympanic gentamicin has been popularized as a method of controlling severe vestibular symptoms, although no clear treatment protocol has been established and cochleotoxicity is a significant risk (Sajjadi and Paparella, 2008). Surgical treatment is considered when medical management has failed to control vertigo and is not an intervention advocated for control of progression of hearing impairment. 'Therapeutic' procedures such as endolymphatic

sac decompression continue to be undertaken despite the lack of evidence of efficacy, while destructive procedures may control vertigo by section of the vestibular nerve if good hearing is preserved, or, in cases of severe/profound hearing loss, labyrinthectomy may be undertaken (Van de Heyning et al., 2005). Chronic symptoms of dizziness due to vestibular dysfunction and hearing impairment may be treated with auditory and vestibular rehabilitation.

Chronic sensorineural hearing impairment may be managed using specific treatment to rectify or halt the progression of the underlying causative condition, followed by audiological rehabilitation. The aims are to minimize disablements and facilitate optimal physical, mental and social potential, as outlined by Goldstein and Stephens (1981). The selection and fitting of hearing aids is a key element of rehabilitation for the majority of patients with hearing impairment (Luxon and Raglan, 2006). Hearing aid benefit may be assessed by a number of questionnaires, of which the Glasgow Hearing Aid Benefit Profile (Gatehouse, 2000) is of particular value and well validated. Cochlear implants, either in one or both ears, have revolutionized the rehabilitation of profound hearing impairments in adults secondary to such disorders as meningitis and head trauma (Das and Buchman, 2005). As with all hearing aid provision, the patient requires long-term auditory training. Middle ear implants (vibrators on one of the ossicles or on the tympanic membrane) may be used with all types of hearing loss, although their value is not yet clearly defined (Magnan et al., 2005).

Part 2:
TRAUMA TO THE AUDITORY SYSTEM

Hearing loss may result from impulsive noise as with gunfire, from blast and barotrauma and from head injury and whiplash. Noise-induced hearing loss may also be considered to be traumatic in origin, and that is a cause of hearing disorder of particular relevance to the practice of aviation medicine. Exposure to high-level impulsive sounds (as from gunfire) forms a greater threat to hearing than does exposure to the high-level continuous sound which is responsible for the chronic acoustic trauma of occupational noise-induced hearing loss. Many, especially those involved in military aviation, are subject to such exposure, although a recent study has highlighted that within the military the 'combat group' is more at risk of elevated hearing thresholds than the 'aviation group' (Barney and Bohnker, 2006).

Acute Acoustic Trauma (Impulsive Noise)

Coles *et al.* (1968) reported that a 7.62 mm rifle produced a 161 dB peak level at the firer's ear. The authors pointed out the need to measure the complete impulse (waveform, rise-and-decay times, peak pressure) and give correction factors to be applied where necessary to allow, for example, for reverberation, orientation of the head to the noise source and the number of shots fired. With the passage of time, peak levels of impulsive sounds in the military environment have increased. Levels as high as 185 dB sound pressure level (SPL) have been reported (Dancer *et al.*, 1998). Ylikoski (1987) analyzed the pure-tone audiograms of individuals who suffered acute acoustic trauma during military service. In more than three-quarters of the ears, the hearing loss was found in the high-frequency region (above 2 kHz). In the remaining quarter, the speech-frequency range was also affected. The main threshold shift started at 1 kHz in 8 per cent, at 2 kHz in 49 per cent, at 4 kHz in 19 per cent and at 6 kHz in 6 per cent of the ears. Impulse noise from large-calibre weapons and explosions appeared to cause low-tone hearing loss slightly more often than small arms fire. No aetiological differences were apparent between the ears with dip-type hearing loss and ears with more abrupt-like hearing loss.

The hazardous nature of gunfire was also highlighted by Tschopp and Probst (1989). Most individuals had been exposed to a single rifle shot. Both ground crews and aircrews who service or fly in military aircraft are obliged to undergo annual firearms practice, and this would be a source of noise damage even though it may be claimed that hearing protectors have always been worn. Indeed, in spite of strict safety regulations concerning firearm shooting in the armed forces, acute acoustical trauma may result in tinnitus and/or hearing impairment. However, careful planning of training exercises could probably prevent some but not all acute acoustic traumas (Mrena *et al.*, 2004b).

It was stated formerly that 'there is no rule superior to the energy rule for dealing with impulse noise' (von Gierke *et al.*, 1982), and this concept is still frequently adopted. However, animal experiments (Henderson *et al.*, 1982; Danielson *et al.*, 1991) and clinical observations (Borchgrevink *et al.*, 1986) provide no support for the equal energy hypothesis. Experimental exposure of animals to impact noise demonstrated that the magnitude of the hearing loss was more dependent on the peak sound level of the impulse than on the total energy level of the noise exposure. Duration, repetition rates and peak level were adjusted to ensure each experimental exposure had the same total sound energy. Marked permanent shifts were produced by peak levels above 125 dB SPL. This was associated with substantially greater loss of hair cells (Henderson *et al.*, 1991). Observations after known variations of impulse noise exposure have indicated a critical peak level for impulse noise which lies between 160 dB and 170 dB linear. Models to predict the damaging effect of impulse noise will need to take into account one or more of the following factors: peak pressure, duration, energy spectrum and number of impulses. Appropriate models have been proposed by Price and Kalb (1991) and by Smoorenburg (1992).

Blast Injury

Blast noise is probably the main source of injury in the armed services (Attias *et al.*, 2007), and it was the report by Wilson (1917) on the effects of high explosives that drew attention to what has become known as otic blast injury. Zajtchuk and Phillips (1989) edited a multi-authored contribution to the clinical and experimental aspects of otic blast injury, though a more detailed clinical picture (Kerr, 2007) has developed from studies on civilian populations of the effects of blast stemming from either terrorist activities (Kerr and Byrne, 1975; Pahor, 1981; Mrena *et al.*, 2004a) or accidental explosions (Bruins and Cawood, 1991). Kerr and Byrne (1975) reported the remarkable recovery commonly noted after blast injuries:

> Almost everyone experienced temporary severe deafness … In most instances, this severe deafness was short-lived and recovered fairly quickly … Almost all complained of severe tinnitus immediately after the blast.

Bruins and Cawood (1989) have also reported the nature of ear and hearing injuries following an explosion. There were ear symptoms with some perforations and some healed within four months. Some individuals had immediate hearing loss, and, of those with symptoms, there were abnormal audiograms. Many complained of tinnitus. However, Goh (2009) has pointed out that the presence of a tympanic membrane perforation is not a reliable indicator of the presence of a blast injury in the other air-containing organs elsewhere. Radiological imaging of the head, chest and abdomen helps with the early identification of blast lung injury, head injury, abdominal injury, eye and sinus injuries, as well as any penetration by foreign bodies. In addition, it must be borne in mind that bomb blasts could also be used to disperse radiological and chemical agents.

Barotrauma

Reduced pressurization during air travel (Mirza and Richardson, 2005), explosions (Persaud *et al.*, 2003) and diving (Newton, 2001; Shupak *et al.*, 2003) may give rise to tympanic membrane haemorrhage into the middle ear with a conductive hearing loss, or a perilymph fistula commonly associated with vestibular symptoms. The first recorded episode of otic barotrauma was when the French physicist Jacques Alexandre Charles took his first (and only) balloon flight in 1783 (O'Reilly, 1999). Otic barotrauma results from a failure to equalize the pressure in the middle ear cavity with that of the external environment. It is characterized by pain in the affected ear, impaired hearing and, sometimes, vertigo.

The primary factors involved in the production of otic barotraumas are the expansion and contraction of gases under alteration of atmospheric pressure, and the collapsible nature of the proximal two-thirds of the pharyngotympanic tube (Dickson *et al.*, 1947a and 1947b; McGibbon, 1947a and 1947b). Severe cases may result in perforation of the tympanic membrane and even rupture of the secondary tympanic membrane (King, 1979, 1988). The condition may affect both the crews and passengers of civilian aircraft (Rosenkvist *et al.*, 2008; Mirza and Richardson, 2005). Individuals with acute otic barotraumas who return to flying before resolution of the condition is complete are likely to sustain further episodes. The condition is then termed chronic otic barotrauma (King, 1979; 1988). A diagnosis of delayed otic barotraumas is made when the subject begins to suffer from aural pain and impairment of hearing several hours after a trouble-free flight. This condition follows long flights in which 100 per cent oxygen was breathed (King, 1979, 1988).

In a study of the hearing of military pilots aged 30 and 40 years, the subjects were 'interviewed by the ear-nose-throat specialist with a standardized questionnaire' (Raynal *et al.*, 2006). Question 2 was 'Otitis due to air pressure' (Yes/No). A positive answer to this item meant that subjects had been cured after a painful ear and/or sensation of hearing loss due to pressure during a flight mission with an inflammatory eardrum or perforated eardrum. The subsequent analysis failed to show that impaired hearing was associated with a history of 'pressure trauma otitis, but

the statistical p-value was close to the significance limit (χ^2 = 2.3, df = 1, p = 0.09)'. Ashton and Watson (1990) have reported the use of tympanometry in predicting otic barotraumas, while Karahatay *et al.*, (2008) have reported the therapeutic role for hyperbaric oxygen, together with the predictive value of the nine-step inflation/deflation test.

Physical Trauma

Head injury may lead to middle ear, inner ear, VIII nerve and central auditory loss, and give rise to various pathologies such as labyrinthine concussion with or without fracture, and fractures of the temporal bone. The fractures may be longitudinal, extending through the middle ear cavity with concomitant conductive hearing loss, or transverse fractures, which may result in section of the VIII nerve accompanied by facial paralysis and haemotympanum. Frequently, there is a profound sensorineural loss and acute vertigo.

Labyrinthine concussion may result from all degrees of head trauma and produce both auditory and vestibular symptoms, without any obvious clinical neurological signs. Severe closed head trauma may give rise to auditory processing disorders, with cortical deafness or auditory agnosia being the most extreme presentations, though difficulty in hearing degraded speech or in background noise or in localization is more common. Over one-third of patients with mild and moderate head injuries complain of hearing loss and/ or tinnitus (Davies and Luxon, 1995), whereas the prevalence of auditory abnormalities attributed to trauma on detailed testing is around a half.

The commonest configuration of sensorineural hearing loss without a fracture is a bilateral high-tone sensorineural hearing loss (Toglia and Katinsky, 1976; Davies and Luxon, 1995), although a variety of other configurations, including asymmetric and unilateral loss, may be observed. A notch-shaped hearing loss at 4 Hz has been reported by Schuknecht (1969) and confirmed by subsequent workers (Wennmo and Svensson, 1989). A recent study has shown progression of sensorineural hearing loss after closed head injury in three-quarters of cases (Bergemalm, 2003). Moreover, tinnitus is a common sequela of head injury (Ćeranić *et al.*, 1998).

Following whiplash injury, auditory symptoms and tinnitus are common, although the mechanism and aetiology remain obscure. A recent study has identified subtle auditory abnormalities, but no correlation has been established between objective auditory deficits and tinnitus (Tjell *et al.*, 1999).

Noise-Induced Hearing Loss

Noise is a major aviation hazard, affecting the operational efficiency of air and ground crews by interference with communication and by damaging their hearing and impacting upon community health. Hearing in a noisy environment is a particularly relevant issue in aviation medicine, and in military aircrew involves not only the possible effects of the day-to-day exposure to noise inherent in the aviation environment but also the potential exposure to impulsive hazards as with gunfire and explosions. The nature, sources and effects of the problem of noise and what measures could be taken to mitigate the hazard were addressed, initially, many years ago. The Committee on the Problem of Noise (1963) defined noise as sound which is undesired by the recipient. It accepted that nearly all activity results in

the production of noise of one kind or another, but limited its concern to noise that gave rise to substantial complaints. Chief amongst these were the noises from aircraft and motor vehicles.

As far as noise-induced hearing loss is concerned, the aeromedical practitioner must be familiar with hearing standards and understand how hearing is assessed. The aeromedical practitioner may also become involved with the effects of noise on the equanimity of the community at large, and that issue is also addressed. It is, therefore, necessary to have some familiarity with the measurement of noise and of hearing, and in this context the reader may find it helpful to refer to the glossary of terms relevant to measurement of noise and of the effects of noise on hearing. The international bodies involved in acoustics are the International Organization for Standardization (ISO) and the International Electrotechnical Commission (IEC). In this chapter their deliberations will be referenced as the year and the number of the standard provided by the respective body. For example, the reference (1997: ISO 10843) would refer to a publication in 1997 from the International Organization for Standardization, numbered 10843.

Measurement of Noise

The use of the term 'level', as in 'sound pressure level', indicates that a value is being expressed on a decibel scale. A value given as a 'sound pressure' would be in pascals. Similarly, sound energy values are stated in joules, sound exposure values are in pascal-squared seconds, and sound exposure levels are in decibels. The International Organization for Standardization (1997: ISO 10843) defines the peak sound pressure for any specified time interval as the maximum absolute value of the instantaneous sound pressure (expressed in pascals) that occurs during that specified time interval. The same standard defines peak sound pressure level as ten times the common logarithm of the square of the ratio of peak frequency weighted sound pressure to the reference sound pressure (expressed in decibels).

A-weighted sound pressure level (L_{pA}): the sound pressure level in decibels, is determined by using frequency-weighting A (IEC 651) from the equation (1999: ISO 1999):

$$L_{pA} = 10 \lg (p_A / p_0)^2$$
where p_A = A-weighted sound pressure in pascals

Following the suggestion of Botsford (1967), A-weighted sound level expressing noise levels as dB (A) should be used as a measure of the degree of hazard posed by sound to hearing. Frequency-weighting A is designed to give the same frequency response as the human ear at the 40-phon equal-loudness contour.

Psychoacoustics

Since the middle of the nineteenth century, psychophysicists have studied the relationship between the subjective magnitude of a sensation, loudness, and its physical magnitude, in this case the physical intensity of the sound. The psychophysical function has been expressed as a power function $\psi = k (\phi - \phi_0)^n$

where ψ = subjective magnitude of the stimulus
ϕ = physical magnitude of the stimulus
ϕ_0 = physical magnitude of stimulus at threshold

k = a constant (scaling factor)
n = exponent (index)
so that $\log \psi = n\log (\phi - \phi_0) + \log k$

The data that conform to this power function show a straight line when the logarithm of ψ is plotted against the logarithm of $(\phi - \phi_0)$; the slope of the line is the exponent n, and the intercept is $\log k$ (Stevens, 1955).

Loudness is measured in sones. Individual differences in loudness susceptibility are reflected by differences in the exponent n of the psychophysical function (Stevens and Guirao, 1964; Barbenza et al., 1970). A scheme for quantifying the noisiness of sound (analogous to the loudness of sound), with a unit termed the noy, is used to scale human reactions to the sound, for example from aircraft (Kryter, 1959; Kryter and Pearsons, 1964). The noy, as the unit of noisiness, parallels the sone for loudness; thus a sound of 4 noys is four times as noisy as a sound of 1 noy (Kryter, 1959; Kryter and Pearsons, 1964). The noy, like the sone, is an international (IEC) unit. Experimental comparisons with the scales of loudness and noisiness show that a scale of unpleasantness is not directly related to these measures (Bowsher and Robinson, 1962)

The standard *Acoustics: Method for Calculating Loudness Level* (1975: ISO 532) specifies two procedures for calculating the loudness of sounds experienced by a typical listener. Method A, which is designed specifically for the types of broad-band spectra most commonly encountered, uses octave band analyses of sound (Stevens, 1956, 1957). Method B uses critical band analyses of sound and may be used with all types of spectra (Zwicker, 1960, 1961). Both procedures are designed for noises that are steady, rather than intermittent.

Noise and Auditory Acuity: Modelling

Eldred *et al.* (1955) enunciated the concept that the adverse effect of noise on the threshold of hearing was a function of the amount of energy in daily exposures to noises above a certain level. The proposal of the equal energy concept was to be adopted by the United States Air Force (AFR 160-3) and, subsequently, by the National Physical Laboratory (United Kingdom) in the noise immission level concept (Robinson and Cook, 1968). In an epidemiological study of noise and hearing in industry, Burns and Robinson (1970) endorsed the noise immission level concept based on equal energy hypothesis to combine level of noise exposure and duration of exposure into a single value. Working *Tables for the Estimation of Noise-Induced Hearing Loss* were subsequently provided by Robinson and Shipton (1973, 1977), and these have been used, at least in the United Kingdom, for medico-legal purposes.

However, Scheiblechner (1974) tested the validity of the noise immission level concept on data obtained from workers exposed to hazardous occupational noise. The analyses failed to endorse the concept. Robinson (1987, 1988) subsequently discarded the equal-energy hypothesis in favour of a compressive (less than additive) model for the interaction of the age and noise factors. Thus, the international standard (1990: ISO 1990) for the determination of occupational noise exposure and the estimation of noise-induced hearing impairment does not use the noise immission level concept. More specifically, the standard is as follows for exposure times between 10 and 40 years:

$$N_{0,50} = [u + v \lg (\Theta / \Theta_0)] (L_{EX,8h} - L_0)^2 \tag{1}$$

where $N_{0,50}$ = median potential NIPTS (noise-induced permanent threshold shift) at a given frequency

u = a value dependent on the audiometric test frequency

v = a value dependent on the audiometric test frequency

Θ = exposure time in years

Θ_0 = one year

$L_{EX,8h}$ = noise exposure level normalized to a nominal 8-hour working day

and L_0 = a cut-off sound pressure level defined as a function of frequency

$$H' = H + N - HN/120 \tag{2}$$

where H' = HTL associated with age and noise (HTLAN) in dB

H = HTL associated with age (HTLA) in dB

and N = actual or potential noise-induced permanent threshold shift in dB

For exposure times of less than 10 years, N is to be extrapolated from the value $N_{0,50}$ for 10 years using the equation:

$$N_{0,50; \Theta<10} = [\lg (\Theta + 1)]/[\lg (11)] N_{0,50; \Theta =10} \tag{3}$$

A Finnish development, the NoiseScan (Pyykkö *et al.*, 2000), uses factors additional to the three input parameters (age, noise exposure, sex) used by the International Organization for Standardization to predict auditory thresholds. The NoiseScan predicts better thresholds for military pilots (Kuronen *et al.*, 2004).

Measurement of Hearing

The problems inherent in epidemiological studies concerned with the hearing of military aircrew have been identified by Raynal *et al.* (2006). They are:

❍ the non-random allocation of subjects (to type of aircraft) and difficulty in ensuring exclusion of confounding factors (impulsive noise and the higher noise exposure in helicopter pilots)
❍ the self-imposed floor effect: 'If sound intensity was audible at 10 dB HL, lower intensities were not tested; subjects would be considered to have normal hearing'
❍ the 6 kHz problem: the model of the earphone was not disclosed either by the authors or by the manufacturer's technical specifications of the audiometer.

The commonest earphone to be used in audiometry is the Telephonics TDH-39, although it is known to be associated with calibration problems at 6 kHz (Hinchcliffe, 1959) due to a marked resonance at this frequency (Rudmose, 1964). The problem shows up as spurious 6 kHz notches in thresholds of hearing, for both ears and various aircraft categories. Moreover, when the graphically presented results for the 'abnormal hearing' group are compared with appropriate controls (Davis, 1995),

there appears to be little difference. To avoid the problem at 6 kHz, the Telephonics TDH-39 earphone should be replaced with the TDH-49 which is designed to have more built-in damping and a flatter frequency response to higher frequencies (Fuller, 1987). An alternative to the Telephonics TDH-39 is the Sennheiser HDA 280 supra-aural earphone, for which equivalent threshold sound pressure levels are available (Poulsen and Oakley, 2009). A further problem that is inherent in supra-aural earphones is collapse of the walls of the outermost part of the external acoustic meatus resulting from pressure of the earphone. This can produce spurious notches at 6 kHz (Coles, 1967) and at 4 kHz (Mahoney and Luxon, 1996). To avoid this problem, the supra-aural earphones should be replaced with either circumaural or insert earphones. The above, and other studies, reflect the difficulties in interpreting epidemiological studies.

There is also difficulty in assessing the damaging effect of noise in the absence of control data. Indeed, following an early study of the hearing of naval aircraft maintenance personnel, Ward (1957) concluded that it was difficult to demonstrate any permanent damaging effect of noise on the hearing of aircraft carrier flight deck personnel:

The evidence that noise exposure has produced any permanent hearing loss appears exceedingly flimsy at this point. If one uses the clinical approach, interpreting each individual audiogram in terms of what 'probably' caused that particular hearing loss, then there are cases in which one feels quite confident that aircraft noise was the responsible agent. But in the absence of pre-exposure audiograms, one cannot be sure. These results are all consistent with the hypothesis that aircraft noise was, at the time of this study, much less dangerous to the hearing of Navy personnel than was gunfire. These results emphasise the obvious: one cannot make a valid decision as to the effects of a particular noise environment unless adequate controls are employed. A causal relation between noise and hearing loss cannot be assumed simply on the basis of joint occurrence.

Clinical Aspects

High-level noise can produce a temporary reduction of hearing sensitivity, referred to as a noise-induced temporary threshold shift (NITTS), which may be a protective mechanism (Salvi *et al.*, 1986), before it produces a noise induced permanent threshold shift (NIPTS). It is possible to conduct a range of studies on the noise–hearing relationship (Ewing and Littler, 1935; Hirsh and Ward, 1952). Under certain conditions, the hearing does not recover gradually after a temporary 'deafening' effect, but bounces (Bronstein's bounce) up and down before settling into a steady recovery pattern (Hirsh and Ward, 1952). Other studies have sought to identify the minimum noise level capable of producing an asymptotic temporary threshold shift (Stephenson *et al.*, 1980).

Studies on the effects of aircraft noise on the auditory acuity of aircrew were carried out initially by Dickson *et al.* (1939). Much of this was in respect of temporary shifts, but later King and Gannon (1958) reported that the temporary noise-induced impairment of hearing does not betoken a noise-induced permanent threshold shift. After adequate rest, hearing returns to normal, despite 40 dB noise-induced temporary threshold shifts at 1 kHz being produced by long flights. Kuronen *et al.* (2003) have also studied temporary

shifts military aircrew. The test subjects flew missions on one of five aircraft that included a turboprop basic trainer, a turbofan combat aircraft and turbojets. The duration of noise exposure was one flight mission, which varied from 30 to 60 minutes. Noise doses and levels were measured using a miniature microphone at the entrance to the external acoustic meatus, and a second microphone was located at the level of the shoulder. Hearing thresholds were measured before each flight using conventional (0.125 to 8.0 kHz) and extended high-frequency (8 to 20 kHz) audiometry. The measurements were repeated as soon as possible after the flight.

In the study by Kuronen *et al.* (2003) the pre-flight threshold levels were good, and both conventional and extended high-frequency audiometry revealed temporary shifts in threshold at several frequencies and with all aircraft types involved. The changes were, however, minor. The authors concluded that the risk of noise-induced hearing impairment at the studied exposure levels is, in all probability, rather small. The study suggests that it could be worthwhile using extended high-frequency audiometry for flying personnel upon entering service and periodically thereafter.

The left–right asymmetry in the human response to experimental noise exposure has been studied by Pirila (1991a and 1991b). Non-shooting healthy young adults were exposed binaurally to symmetrical broad-band noise for a maximum of eight hours. The hearing thresholds at 4 kHz of each individual were monitored alternately in the left and the right ears during short interruptions in the exposure. A significant positive correlation between temporary threshold shifts in the left and in the right ear was found. The average interaural hearing threshold difference was significant during the exposure, the left ear being worse than right. The negative correlation found between the pre-exposure threshold level and the temporary threshold shift was more marked in the left than in the right ear. The author concluded that a good hearing threshold level in the right ear seems to be better protected from noise-induced temporary threshold shift than a good hearing threshold in the left ear.

Noise-induced permanent threshold shift is one of the commonest and most preventable causes of sensorineural hearing loss, and that is highly relevant in aviation medicine as it is one of the most important sensory deficits that could affect the performance of aircrew (Antunano and Spanyers, 2008). It is commonly the consequence of hazardous occupational exposure to noise, but it may also be associated with acoustic trauma, for example gun fire and explosions. The studies by Barr (1886), by Perlman (1941), by Johnston (1953) and by Burns and Robinson (1970) have all helped to define the clinical and audiometric features of what is termed 'occupational noise-induced hearing loss'. However, as Coles (1975)

has pointed out, 'The diagnosis of noise deafness is difficult. There is nothing positive about it: it is done by exclusion of other factors.'

Characteristically, noise-induced hearing loss demonstrates the maximal loss at 4,000 Hz, with a notched configuration to the audiogram (Figure 19.12), but, with the passage of time, the adjacent frequencies gradually deteriorate. Individuals complaining of hearing difficulties and diagnosed as having occupational noise-induced hearing loss all have hearing thresholds at 2 kHz of at least 30 dB (Chadwick, 1971). The threshold level at which workers perceive that they have difficulties hearing (a positive response to the question 'Do you have hearing difficulties?') corresponds to 48 dB hearing threshold level at 4 kHz, by which time the 4 kHz loss would be pulling down the lower frequencies (Tsalighopoulos *et al.*, 1986).

It is rare for a hearing loss greater than 70 db to be the result of occupational noise exposure. The diagnosis of noise-induced hearing loss is by exclusion of other causes, but as the aetiology cannot be established in up to two-thirds of

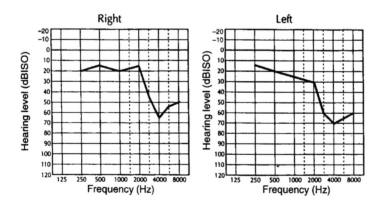

Figure 19.12   Diagram to illustrate characteristic configuration of noise-induced hearing loss with a 'notch' at 4 kHz

Source: Luxon, L.M. 1998. Clinical Diagnosis of Noise Induced Hearing Loss. In: *Advances in Noise Research: Volume I:-Biological Effects*. In: D.K. Prasher and L.M. Luxon, (eds.) London, Whurr Publishers, p. 96. With permission of John Wiley & Sons Ltd.

patients with sensorineural hearing loss, this presents a diagnostic dilemma. The American College of Occupational Medicine (1989) has devised clear diagnostic criteria for occupational noise-induced hearing loss. A variety of factors should be considered in making this diagnosis, but in all cases of high-frequency sensorineural hearing loss, a history of noise exposure should be sought (Luxon, 1998).

The noise of military aircraft is experienced as particularly intrusive by both operators and those on the ground. 'We flew out from the operating base (in a transport aircraft). There was too much noise for talking. I put on a pair of ear defenders and got my head down.' 'All the time, there was the deafening zsh, zsh, zsh of the rotor blades. Not much was said between ourselves because of the noise. I could tell by the grind of the blades that the helicopter was manoeuvring close to the ground... the noise was deafening' (McNab, 1996).

The potentially hazardous noise levels from military helicopters has been described by Rood and Glen (1977), while Owen (1995), quoting average sound levels at 'ear level' of 99.8 dB (A) and 100 dB (A) for two types of helicopter, has reviewed the evidence for noise-induced hearing loss in military helicopter aircrews. Gasaway (1986) has also measured the average noise levels inside the cockpit, for a range of aircraft, and these are listed below:

- tail-mounted turbojet/fan-powered aircraft   85.5 dB
- all fixed-wing aircraft   95.0 dB
- single-rotor turbine helicopters 97.6 dB
- single-rotor reciprocating engine-powered helicopters   101.8 dB
- dual-rotor reciprocating or turbine powered helicopters   105.0 dB

However, there is the additional hazard of the acoustic communication system, and acoustic signals and extraneous background noises associated with communication systems must also be considered a potential threat to the hearing of many flyers. In addition, Kuronen et al. (2004) have pointed out that the noise level in the cockpit depends not only on the particular aircraft, but also on the engine power settings required in different flight conditions and on aerodynamic noise.

Importantly, communication systems may also present a noise hazard, either occupationally or in everyday use, and such a possibility must be borne in mind by the aeromedical practitioner. Palva (1957) reported the occurrence of mid-frequency audiometric notches due to noise trauma in telephone exchange workers. Four out of 28 employees with impaired hearing had 1.5 kHz notches. Further, Singleton et al. (1984), Orchik et al. (1987) and Gerling and Jerger (1985) have reported damage to hearing resulting from use of cordless phones. Spectral analysis of the ring signal indicates sound-pressure levels of approximately 140 dB, with a fundamental frequency near 750 Hz. The most severe hearing loss was found at 500 Hz and 1000 Hz, where the mean threshold difference in the injured ear was 20 dB and 29 dB, respectively. All the patients described a painful sensation in the ear associated with exposure to the ring. They were immediately aware of a hearing loss and experienced the onset of tinnitus of varying degrees. Unlike regular cord-type telephones, these devices have no automatic gain control in the receiver circuit.

It is reported that commercial airline pilots are exposed to an equivalent continuous noise level of less than 78 dB(A) for an assumed eight-hour working day (Lindgren et al., 2009).

This value is well below the limit of 85 dB(A) and the risk of noise damage to hearing amongst commercial pilots would appear to be low (Kronoveter and Somerville, 1970). However, a study of commuter air carrier and air taxi pilots has identified a significant prevalence of hearing deficits which increase with age (Qiang *et al.*, 2008). Similar studies have been carried out in helicopter pilots (Wagstaff and Årva, 2009). Aircraft passengers are not at risk of hearing deficits under normal circumstances, but comfort/discomfort is dependent on both noise and vibration levels that interact with one another (Stephens and Powell, 1980).

Part 3:
AIRCRAFT NOISE AND ANNOYANCE

The early study by McKennell (1963) that introduced the issue of annoyance to the community by the noise of aircraft is of interest:

> From the physical measurements carried out (in a social survey around Heathrow Airport), 14 different variables could be picked out as characterising the noise climate, and 58 socio-psychological variables could be found from the answers to the questionnaires … all the significant correlations with the physical variables could be reduced to two, namely those with the average peak noise level (in PNdb) of the aircraft and the number heard per day … Average annoyance could be considered to be a function of one composite physical variable only – the noise and number index (the sum of the individual noise levels in PNdb and 15 log N, where N is the number of aircraft per day) … When 1% of people had complained about noise, 10% felt like complaining; when the noise was such

that 10% had complained, 40% felt like complaining. The percentage of people who are highly annoyed by aircraft noise is a curvilinear function of people who complain about the noise. (Connor and Patterson, 1973)

The noise and number index (NNI) has been followed by a curve designed by Schultz (1978). The curve relates the DNL (day–night level: L_{dn}) to the percentage of highly annoyed people. It has been endorsed by Fidell and Barber (1991) and by Finegold *et al.* (1994) in respect of general transportation noise, and by the United States Federal Interagency Committee on Noise (1992) in respect of airport noise. The L_{dn} noise measurement procedures involve the addition of a 10-dB penalty to noises occurring during typical hours of sleep (22:00 to 07:00). The metric, the 'community noise exposure level', is used in the State of California. The 'weighted equivalent perceived noise level' (PN_{dB}, or dB_A) is recommended internationally and used in Japan and elsewhere. For noise-assessment purposes, it involves, in addition to the 10-dB 22:00–07:00 penalty, a 5-dB penalty to aircraft noise exposures between 19:00 and 22:00. These penalties are based on a mixture of laboratory and field research and the general experience of acoustical consultants working on community noise problems (Kryter, 1994).

Further studies on the annoyance arising from aircraft noise have been undertaken since the study by McKennell (1963). These include the *United Kingdom Aircraft Noise Index Study* (ANIS) (Brooker *et al.*, 1985) and the *Attitudes to Noise from Aviation Sources* (ANASE). The 'equivalent continuous sound level' (L_{eq}) to describe noise and community annoyance was adopted, and it was decided that a value of 57 should mark the approximate onset of significant community annoyance from aircraft noise. The value of 57 is considered to indicate the start of low community annoyance, 63 is considered to indicate medium annoyance, and 69 high annoyance. The latter study (ANASE) claimed to show that people are becoming less tolerant to aircraft noise, but Brooker (2008a) has argued that the study contained methodological flaws. The search for a good aircraft noise annoyance curve continues (Brooker, 2008b). In a review of community response to noise, Borsky (1980) concluded that the non-acoustical properties of noises, for example controllability, fears, beliefs about maleficent effects, were more important determinants of individual annoyance than the acoustical properties of the noises.

Although annoyance may be the predominant issue affecting the community, the possibility that hearing may be impaired, at least temporarily, by overflying aircraft cannot be ruled out completely. Individuals have claimed to have sustained damage to hearing (a unilateral hearing loss in each case) from exposure to the noise of low-flying jet aircraft (Kuronen *et al.*, 1999). Audiometry confirmed the hearing loss in each case, and subsequent noise measurements during such overflights have shown peak noise levels between 109 dB and 150 dB, depending on the aircraft type and the use of the afterburner. The 1-s single A-weighted exposure levels during the overflights were 95–135 dB which correspond to daily (eight hours) exposure levels of 50–90 dB. The authors concluded that there should be no risk of permanent hearing loss when the distance from an overflying jet fighter is more than 200 metres, but one wonders whether or not the conventional method of calculating the noise risk to hearing is appropriate in cases such as this.

Glossary: Terms and Definitions

A-duration (pressure-wave duration): The time (in seconds) required for the main or principal wave of a single sound impulse to reach its unweighted peak sound pressure and return momentarily to zero (1997: ISO 10843).

A-weighted sound exposure ($E_{A,T}$): The time integral of the squared A-weighted sound pressure over a specified time period, T, or event, expressed in pascal squared seconds ($Pa^2.s$). The period, T, measured in seconds, is usually chosen so as to cover a whole day of occupational exposure to noise (usually 8 h, i.e. 28,800 s) (para 3.3, ISO 1999).

A-weighted sound pressure level (L_{pA}): The sound pressure level, in decibels, determined by using frequency-weighting A (see IEC 651), from the equation

$$L_{pA} = 10 \lg (p_A / p_0)^2$$
where p_A = A-weighted sound pressure in pascals
(para 3.2, ISO 1999)

Frequency-weighting A is designed to give the same frequency response as the human ear at the 40 phon equal loudness contour.

B-duration (pressure-envelope duration): The total time that the envelope of the pressure fluctuations (positive and negative) is within 20 dB of the peak pressure level.

Loudness: The subjective dimension of the objective (physical) dimension of sound (intensity, pressure); unit is the sone. As a rule of thumb, a 1-dB increase in the SPL of a noise gives a 10 per cent increase in loudness; a 10-dB increase produces a doubling of the loudness.

Loudness level: The loudness level of a sound in phons is numerically equal to the sound pressure level in decibels (relative to a pressure of 20 μPa) of a simple tone of frequency 1 kHz which is judged by the median listener to be equivalent in loudness (BS 4198).

Noise and number index: A measure of aircraft noise annoyance that takes into account the noise levels produced by the aircraft and the number of aircraft passing in a given period (McKennell, 1963).

Noy: The unit of noisiness, equal to the noisiness of a one-third-octave band of noise centred on 1 kHz and having a sound pressure level of 40 dB (IEC 801-29-13).

Socioacusis: Nonindustrial noise-induced threshold shifts (Glorig, 1958).

Sone: The unit of loudness; equal to the loudness of a pure tone presented frontally as a plane wave of frequency 1,000 Hz and a sound pressure level of 40 dB, re 20μPa. Note: The loudness of a sound that is judged by the listener to be n times that of the 1-sone tone is n sones (IEC 801-29-04).

References

Abel, S. 2005. Hearing loss in military aviation and other trades: Investigation of prevalence and risk factors. *Aviation, Space, and Environmental Medicine*, 76, 1128–35.

Acuin, J. 2004. Chronic suppurative otitis media. *Clinical Evidence*, 12, 710–29.

Agrup, C. and Luxon, L.M. 2006. Immune-mediated inner ear disorders in neuro-otology. *Current Opinion in Neurology*, 19, 26–32.

American Academy of Ophthalmology and Otolaryngology. 1995. Committee on Hearing and Equilibrium: Guidelines for diagnosis and evaluation of therapy in Menière's disease. *Otolaryngology and Head and Neck Surgery*, 113, 181–5.

American Academy of Otolaryngology and Head and Neck Surgery. Committee of Hearing and Equilibrium (1995). Guidelines for the diagnosis and evaluation of therapy in Meniere's disease. *Otolaryngology and Head and Neck Surgery*, 113, 181–5.

American College of Occupational Medicine. 1989. Occupational noise induced hearing loss. Noise and Hearing Conservation Committee. *Journal of Occupational Medicine*, 31, 996.

Anteunis, L.J. and Mooy, J.M. 1987. Hearing loss in a uraemic patient: Indications of involvement of the VIIIth nerve. *Journal of Laryngology and Otology*, 101, 492–6.

Antunano, M.J. and Spanyers, J.P. 2008. Hearing and Noise in Aviation. Available at: http://www.faagov/pilots/safety/pilotsafetybrochures/media/hearing-brochure.pdf

Ashton, D.H. and Watson, L.A. 1990. The use of tympanometry in predicting otic barotrauma. *Aviation, Space, and Environmental Medicine*, 61, 56–61.

Atherley, G.R.C. and Noble, W.G. 1971. Clinical Picture of Occupational Hearing Loss Obtained with the Hearing Measurement Scale. In: D.W. Robinson (ed.) *Occupational Hearing Loss*. London: Academic Press, 193–216.

Attias, J., Duvdevanny, A.Y., Reshef-Haran, I., Zilberberg, M. and Nageris, B. 2007. Military Noise-Induced Hearing Loss. In: L.M. Luxon and D. Prasher (eds) *Noise and Its Effects*. London: John Wiley, Ch. 19.

Axelsson, A. 1992. Causes of Tinnitus. In: J.M. Aran and R. Dauman (eds) *Tinnitus 91. Proceedings of the IV International*

Tinnitus Seminar, Bordeaux. Amsterdam/ New York, NY: Kugler Publications, 275–7.

Bamiou, D. and Luxon, L.M. 2003. Medical Management of Vestibular Disorders and Vestibular Rehabilitation. In: L.M. Luxon, S.D.G. Stephens, A. Martini and J. Furman (eds) *Textbook of Audiological Medicine*. London: Martin Dunitz, 889–916.

Bamiou, D.E., Musiek, F.E., Stow, I., Stevens, J., Cipolotti, L., Brown, M.M. and Luxon, L.M. 2006. Auditory temporal processing deficits in patients with insular stroke. *Neurology*, 67, 614–9.

Bandura, A. 2009. Social cognitive theory goes global. *The Psychologist*, 22, 504–6.

Bamiou, D.E., Spraggs, P.R., Gibberd, F.B., Sidey, M.C. and Luxon, L.M. 2003. Hearing loss in adult Refsum's disease. *Clinical Otolaryngology and Allied Science*, 28, 227–30.

de Barbenza, C.M., Bryan, M.E., McRobert, H. and Tempest, W. 1970. Individual loudness susceptibility. *Sound*, 4, 75–9.

Barney, R. and Bohnker, B.K. 2006. Hearing thresholds for US marines: Comparison of aviation, combat arms and other personnel. *Aviation, Space, and Environmental Medicine*, 77, 53–6.

Barr, T. 1886. Enquiry into the effects of loud sounds upon the hearing of boilermakers and others who work among noisy surroundings. *Proceedings of the Glasgow Philosophical Society*, 17, 223–39.

Barratt, H.J., Miller, D. and Rudge, P. 1988. The site of the lesion causing deafness in multiple sclerosis. *Scandinavian Audiology*, 17, 67–71.

Bergemalm, P.O. 2003. Progressive hearing loss after closed head injury: A predictable outcome? *Acta Oto-Laryngologica*, 123, 836–45.

Berlin, C., Hood, L. and Rose, K. 2001. On renaming auditory neuropathy as auditory dys-synchrony. *Audiology Today*, 13, 15–17.

Bilger, R.C., Nuentzeq, J.M., Rabinowitz, W.M. and Rzeczkowski, C. 1984. Standardization of a test of speech perception in noise. *Journal of Speech and Hearing Research*, 27, 32–48.

Borchgrevink, H.M., Woxen, O. and Oftedal, G. 1986. Critical Peak Level for Impulse Noise Hazard: Permanent Hearing Threshold Shifts in Military Drill Squads Following Known Variation of Impulse Noise Exposure. In: R.J. Salvi, D. Henderson, R.P. Hamernik and V. Colletti (eds) *Basic and Applied Aspects of Noise-Induced Hearing Loss*. New York, NY: Plenum Press, 433–9.

Borsky, P.N. 1980. Review of Community Response to Noise. In: J.V. Tobias, G. Jansen and W.D. Ward (eds) *Noise as a Public Health Problem: Proceedings of the Third International Congress, Freiburg 1978*. Rockville, MD: American Speech-Language-Hearing Association, Report No. 10, 453–74.

Botsford, J.H. 1967. Simple method for identifying acceptable noise exposures. *Journal of the Acoustical Society of America*, 42, 810.

Bowsher, J.M. and Robinson, D.W. 1962. On scaling the unpleasantness of sounds. *British Journal of Applied Physics*, 13, 179–85.

British Association of Otolaryngologists – Head and Neck Surgeons. 2002. *Clinical Effectiveness Guidelines: Acoustic Neuroma (Vestibular Schwannoma)*. London: British Association of Otolaryngologists – Head and Neck Surgeons, Document 5.

British Society of Audiology. 1981. Recommended procedure for pure-tone audiometry using a manually operated instrument. *British Journal of Audiology*, 15, 213–6.

British Society of Audiology. 1992. Recommended procedure for tympanometry. *British Journal of Audiology*, 26, 255–7.

Brooker, P. 2008a. Attitudes to noise from aviation sources in England: Measuring aircraft noise annoyance very unreliably. *Significance*, 5, 18–24.

Brooker, P. 2008b. Finding a good aircraft noise annoyance curve. *Acoustics Bulletin*, 33, 36–40.

Brooker, P., Critchley, J.B., Monkman, D.J. and Richmond, C. 1985. *United Kingdom Aircraft Noise Index Study*. London: Civil Aviation Authority, Report 8402.

Bruins, W.R. and Cawood, R.H. 1991. Blast injuries of the ear as a result of the Peterborough lorry explosion: 22 March 1989. *Journal of Laryngology and Otology*, 105, 890–95.

Brungart, D.S., Kordik, A.J., Simpson, B.D. and McKinley, R.L. 2003. Auditory localization in the horizontal plane with single and double hearing protection. *Aviation, Space, and Environmental Medicine*, 74, 937–46.

Burns, W. and Robinson, D.W. 1970. *Hearing and Noise in Industry*. London: Her Majesty's Stationery Office.

Ćeranić, B. 2007. The value of otoacoustic emissions in the investigation of noise damage to hearing. *Audiological Medicine*, 5, 10–24.

Ćeranić, B. and Luxon, L.M. 2002. Disorders of the Auditory System. In: A. Asbury, G. McKhann, W.I. McDonald et al. (eds) *Diseases of the Nervous System – Third Edition*. Cambridge: Cambridge University Press, 658–77.

Ćeranić, B. and Luxon, L.M. 2008. Tinnitus and Other Dysacuses. In: M. Gleeson (ed.) *Scott Brown's Otolaryngology – Seventh Edition*. London: Hodder.

Ćeranić, B.J., Prasher, D.K., Raglan, E. and Luxon, L.M. 1998. Tinnitus after head injury: Evidence from otoacoustic emissions. *Journal of Neurology, Neurosurgery and Psychiatry*, 65, 523–9.

Chadwick, D.L. 1971. The behaviour of the pathological ear in noise. *Acta Oto-Rhinolaryngologica Belgica*, 15, 113–26.

Chermak, G.D. and Musiek, F.E. 1997. Neurobiology of the Central Auditory Nervous System Relevant to Central Auditory Processing. In: G.D. Chermak and F.E. Musiek (eds) *Central Auditory Processing Disorders: New Perspectives*. San Diego, CA: Singular Publishing Group, 27–70.

Coelho, A, Ćeranić, B., Prasher, P., Miller, D. and Luxon, L.M. 2007. Auditory efferent function in multiple sclerosis. *Ear and Hearing*, 28, 593–604.

Cohen, M., Luxon, L.M. and Rudge, P. 1996. Auditory deficits and hearing loss associated with focal brainstem haemorrhage. *Scandinavian Audiology*, 25, 133–41.

Cohen-Kerem, R., Kisilevsky, V., Einarson, T.R., Kozer, E., Koren, G. and Rutka, J.A. 2004. Intratympanic gentamicin for Menière's disease: A meta-analysis. *Laryngoscope*, 114, 2085–91.

Coles, R.R.A. 1967. External meatus closure by audiometer earphone. *Journal of Speech and Hearing Disorders*, 32, 296–7.

Coles, R.R.A. 1975. Medico-legal aspects of noise hazards to hearing. *Medico-Legal Journal*, 43, 3–19.

Coles, R.R.A. 1984. Epidemiology of tinnitus: (1) Prevalence and (2) Demographic and clinical features. *Journal of Laryngology and Otology*, Suppl. 9, (1) 7–15, (2) 195–202.

Coles, R.R.A., Davis, A. and Smith, O. 1990. Tinnitus: Its Epidemiology and Management. In: J.H. Jensen (ed.) *Proceedings XIV Danavox Symposium*. Copenhagen: Danavox Jubilee Foundation, 377–402.

Coles, R.R.A., Garinther, G.R., Hodge, D.C. and Rice, C.G. 1968. Hazardous exposure to impulse noise. *Journal of the Acoustical Society of America*, 43, 336–43.

Collet, L., Kemp, D.T., Veuillet E., Duclaux, R., Molulin, A. and Morgon, A. 1990. Effect of contralateral auditory stimuli on active cochlear micromechanical properties in human subjects. *Hearing Research*, 43, 251–62.

Colvin, I.B. 2006. Audiovestibular manifestations of sarcoidosis: A review of the literature. *Laryngoscope*, 116, 75–82.

Committee on the Problem of Noise. 1963. *Expansion of Heathrow Airport*. London: Her Majesty's Stationery Office, Cmnd 2056.

Connor, W.K. and Patterson, H.P. 1973. Cited by K.D. Kryter 1994.

Cryns, K., Sivakumaran, T.A., van dem Ouweland, J.M., Pennings, R.J., Cremers, C.W., Flothman, K. et al. 2003. Mutational spectrum of the WFS1 gene in Wolfram syndrome, nonsyndromic hearing impairment, diabetes mellitus, and psychiatric disease. *Human Mutations*, 22, 275–87.

Dancer, A., Buck, K., Hamery, P. and Parmentier, G. 1998. The specific problem of noise in military life. *Scandinavian Audiology*, 48 (Suppl.), 123–30.

Danielson, R., Henderson, D., Gratton, M.A., Bianchi, L. and Salvi, R. 1991. The importance of 'temporal pattern' in traumatic impulse noise exposures. *Journal of the Acoustical Society of America*, 69, 209–18.

Darmstadt, G.L. and Harris, J.P. 1989. Luetic hearing loss: Clinical presentation, diagnosis and treatment. *American Journal of Otolaryngology*, 10, 410–21.

Das, S. and Buchman, C.A. 2005. Bilateral cochlear implantation: Current concepts. *Current Opinion in Otolaryngology and Head and Neck Surgery*, 13, 290–93.

Davies, R.A. and Luxon, L.M. 1995. Dizziness following head injury: A neuro-otological study. *Journal of Neurology*, 242, 222–30.

Davis, A. 1993. The Prevalence of Deafness. In: J. Ballantyne, A. Martin and M. Martin (eds) *Deafness*. London: Whurr.

Davis, A. 1995. *Hearing in Adults*. London: Whurr.

Dickson, E.D.D., Ewing, A.W.G. and Littler, T.S. 1939. The effects of aeroplane noise on the auditory acuity of aviators: Some preliminary remarks. *Journal of Laryngology and Otology*, 54, 531–48.

Dickson, E.D.D., McGibbon, J.E.G. and Campbell, A.C.P. 1947a. Acute Otitic Barotrauma – Clinical Findings, Mechanism and Relationship to the Pathological Changes Produced Experimentally in the Middle Ears of Cats by Variations of Pressure. In: E.D.D. Dickson (ed.) *Contributions to Aviation Otolaryngology*. London: Headley Brothers, Ch. IX.

Dickson, E.D.D., McGibbon, J.E.G., Harvey, W. and Turner, W. 1947b. An Investigation into the Incidence of Acute Otitic Barotrauma amongst 1,000 Aircrew Cadets during a Decompression Test. In: E.D.D. Dickson (ed.) *Contributions to Aviation Otolaryngology*. London: Headley Brothers, Ch. XI.

Doyle, K.J., Bauch, C., Battista, R., Beatty, C., Hughes, G.B., Mason J. et al. 2004. Intratympanic steroid treatment: A review. *Otology and Neurotology*, 25, 1034–9.

Duvdevany, A. and Furst, M. 2007. The effect of longitudinal noise exposure on behavioral audiograms and transient-evoked otoacoustic emissions. *International Journal of Audiology*, 46, 119–27.

Duvoisin, R.C. 1987. The Olivopontocerebellar Atrophies. In: C.D. Marsden and S. Fahn (eds) *Movement Disorders II*. London: Butterworth, 249–71.

Eldred, K.M., Gannon, W.J. and von Gierke, H. 1955. *Criteria for Short Time Exposure of Personnel to High Intensity Jet Aircraft Noise*. Ohio, USA: Wright Air Force Base Aerospace Medical Laboratory, Report WADC-TN-355.

European Aviation Safety Agency. 2010. Medical certification of pilots and medical fitness of cabin crew. Opinion 07/2010 dated 14 December 2010.

Ewing, A.W.G. and Littler, T.S. 1935. Auditory fatigue and adaptation. *British Journal of Psychology*, 25, 284–307.

Federal Interagency Committee on Noise (FICON). 1992. *Federal Agency Review of Selected Airport Noise Analysis Issues.* Washington, DC: US Government Printing Office.

Fidell, S. and Barber, D. 1991. Updating a dosage effect relationship for prevalence of annoyance due to general transportation noise. *Journal of the Acoustical Society of America*, 89, 221–33.

Finegold, L.S., Harris, C.S. and von Gierke, H.E. 1994. Community annoyance and sleep disturbance: Updated criteria for assessing the impacts of general transportation noise on people. *Noise Control Engineering Journal*, 42, 25–30.

Fuller, H. 1987. Equipment for Speech Audiometry and its Calibration. In: M. Martin (ed.) *Speech Audiometry.* London: Taylor and Francis, Ch. 4.

Garringer, H.J., Pankratz, N.D., Nichols, W.C. and Reed, T. 2006. Hearing impairment susceptibility in elderly men and the DFNA18 locus. *Archives of Otolaryngology and Head and Neck Surgery*, 132, 506–10.

Gasaway, D.C. 1986. Noise levels in cockpits of aircraft during normal cruise and considerations of auditory risk. *Aviation, Space, and Environmental Medicine*, 57, 103–12.

Gatehouse, S. 2000. The Glasgow Hearing Aid Benefit Profile and what it measures and how to use it. *The Hearing Journal*, 53, 10–18.

Gatehouse, S. 2003. Auditory Amplification in Adults. In: L.M. Luxon, A. Martini, J. Furman and S.D.G. Stephens (eds) *A Textbook of Audiological Medicine.* London: Martin Dunitz, 533–53.

Gates, G.A. 2005. Treatment of Menière's disease with the low-pressure pulse generator (Meniett device). *Expert Review of Medical Devices*, 2, 533–7.

Gates, G.A. 2006. Menière's disease review 2005. *Journal of the American Academy of Audiology*, 17, 16–26.

Gerling, I.J. and Jerger, J.F. 1985. Cordless telephones and acoustic trauma: A case study. *Ear and Hearing*, 6, 203–5.

Gibson, W.P. 2009. A comparison of two methods of using transtympanic electrocochleography for the diagnosis of Menière's disease: Click summating potential/action potential ratio measurements and tone burst summating potential measurements. *Acta Oto-Laryngolica*, Suppl. 560, 38–42.

von Gierke, H.E., Robinson, D.W. and Karmy, S.J. 1982. Results of a workshop on impulse noise and auditory hazard. *Journal of Sound and Vibration*, 83, 579–84.

Glorig, A. 1958. *Noise and Your Ear.* New York, NY: Grune & Stratton.

Goh, S.H. 2009. Bomb blast mass casualty incidents: Initial triage and management of injuries. *Singapore Medical Journal*, 50, 101–6.

Goldstein, D. and Stephens, S.D.G. 1981. Audiological rehabilitation: Management model. *Audiology*, 20, 432–52.

Gonzalez-Ravilla, A. 1948. Differential diagnosis of tumours at the cerebellar recess. *Bulletin of the Johns Hopkins Hospital*, 83, 187–212.

Gozdzick-Zolnierkiewicz, T. and Moszynski, B. 1969. VIII nerve in experimental lead poisoning. *Acta Oto-Laryngologica*, 68, 85–9.

Gulya, A.J. 1993. Neurologic paraneoplastic syndromes with neurotologic manifestations. *Laryngoscope*, 103, 754–61.

Haberkamp, T.J. and Tanyeri, M. 1999. Management of idiopathic sensorineural hearing loss. *American Journal of Otology*, 20, 587–93.

Hanner, P., Rosenhall, U., Edström, S. and Kaijser, B. 1989. Hearing impairment in patients with antibody production against Borrelia burgdorferi antigen. *Lancet*, 7, 13–15.

Harding, A.E. 1981. 'Idiopathic' late onset cerebellar ataxia: A clinical and genetic study of 36 cases. *Journal of the Neurological Sciences*, 51, 259–71.

Health Survey for England: Department of Health. 1997. London: Her Majesty's Stationery Office.

Henderson, D., Salvi, R.J. and Hamernik, R.P. 1982. Is the equal energy rule applicable to impact noise? *Scandinavian Audiology*, Suppl. 16, 83–8.

Henderson, D., Subramaniam, M., Gratton, M.A and Saunders, S.S. 1991. Impact noise: The importance of level, duration, and repetition rate. *Journal of the Acoustical Society of America*, 89, 1350–57.

Hereditary Hearing Loss Homepage. Available at: http://www.heriditaryhearingloss.org/

Hinchcliffe, R. 1959. The threshold of hearing of a random sample rural population. *Acta Oto-Laryngologica*, 50, 411–22.

Hinchcliffe, R. 2003. Aspects of Paracuses. In: L.M. Luxon (ed.) *Textbook of Audiological Medicine*. London: Martin Dunitz, 271–87.

Hinchcliffe, R. and King, P. 1992. Medico-legal aspects of tinnitus. I: Medico-legal position and current state of knowledge. *Journal of Audiological Medicine*, 1, 38–58.

Hirsh, I.J. and Ward, W.D. 1952. Recovery of the auditory threshold after strong acoustic stimulation. *Journal of the Acoustical Society of America*, 24, 131–41.

Ho, K.Y., Lee, K.W., Chai, C.Y., Kuo, W.R., Wang, H.M. and Chien, C.Y. 2008. Early recognition of nasopharyngeal cancer in adults with only otitis media with effusion. *Journal of Otolaryngology and Head Neck Surgery*, 37, 362–5.

Holgers, K.-M. and Barrenäs, M.-L. 2003. The Pathophysiology and Assessment of tinnitus. In: L.M. Luxon, J.M. Furman, A. Martini and S.D.G. Stephens (eds) *Textbook of Audiological Medicine*. London: Martin Dunitz, 555–70.

Holt, J.J. 2003. Cholesteatoma and otosclerosis: Two slowly progressive causes of hearing loss treatable through corrective surgery. *Clinical Medicine Research*, 1, 151–4.

Hughes, G.B., Freedman, M.A., Haberkamp, T.J. and Guay, M.E. 1996. Sudden sensorineural hearing loss. *Otolaryngological Clinics of North America*, 29, 393–405.

International Organization for Standardization. 1990. *Acoustics – Determination of Occupational Noise Exposure and Estimation of Noise-Induced Hearing Impairment*. Geneva: International Organization for Standardization, ISO 1999.

Ishman, S.L. and Friedland, D.R. 2004. Temporal bone fractures: Traditional classification and clinical relevance. *Laryngoscope*, 114, 1734–41.

Jakes, S.C., Hallam, R.S., Rachman, S. and Hinchcliffe, R. 1986. The effect of reassurance, relaxation training and distraction on chronic tinnitus sufferers. *Behavioural Research and Therapy*, 24, 497–507.

James, A. and Thorp, M. 2004. Menière's disease. *Clinical Evidence*, 12, 742–50.

Jastreboff, P.J. 1990. Phantom auditory perception (tinnitus): Mechanisms of generation and perception. *Neuroscience Research*, 8, 221–54.

Johnson, E.W. 1968. Auditory findings in 200 cases of acoustic neuromas. *Archives of Otolaryngology*, 88, 598–604.

Johnston, C. 1953. A field study of occupational deafness. *British Journal of Industrial Medicine*, 10, 41–50.

Jones, N.S. and Davis, A. 2001. A prospective case-control study of 50 consecutive patients presenting with hyperlipidaemia. *Clinical Otolaryngology and Allied Sciences*, 26, 189–96.

Jørgensen, M.B., Kristensen, H.K. and Buch, N.H. 1964. Thalidomide-induced aplasia of the inner ear. *Journal of Laryngology and Otology*, 78, 1095–101.

Josey, A.F., Jackson, C.G. and Glasscock, M.E. 1980. Brainstem evoked response audiometry in confirmed eighth nerve tumors. *American Journal of Otolaryngology*, 1, 285–90.

Kaga, K., Shindo, M., Tanaka, Y. and Haebara, H. 2000. Neuropathology of auditory agnosia following bilateral temporal lobe lesions: A case study. *Acta Oto-Laryngologica*, 120, 259–62.

Kalikow, D.N., Stevens, K.N. and Elliot, L.L. 1977. Development of a test of speech intelligibility in noise using sentence materials with controlled word predictability. *Journal of the Acoustical Society of America*, 61, 1337–51.

Karahatay, S., Yilmaz, Y.F., Birkent, H., Ay, H. and Satar, B. 2008. Middle ear barotrauma with hyperbaric oxygen therapy: Incidence and the predictive value of the nine-step inflation/deflation test and otoscopy. *Ear, Nose and Throat Journal*, 87, 684–8.

Kemp, D.T. 1978. Stimulated acoustic emissions from within the human auditory system. *Journal of the Acoustical Society of America*, 64, 1386–91.

Kerr, A.G. 2007. The Effects of Blast on the Ear. In: L.M. Luxon and D. Prasher (eds) *Noise and its Effects*. London: John Wiley, Ch. 13.

Kerr. A.G. and Byrne, J.E.T. 1975. Concussive effects of bomb blast on the ear. *Journal of Laryngology and Otology*, 89, 131–43.

Khoza, K. and Ross, E. 2002. Auditory function in a group of adults infected with HIV/AIDS in Gauteng, South Africa. *South African Journal of Communication Disorders*, 49, 17–27.

Kileny, P., Paccioretti, D. and Wilson, A.F. 1987. Effects of cortical lesions on middle latency auditory evoked responses (MLR). *Electroencephalography and Clinical Neurophysiology*, 66, 108–20.

King, P.F. 1979. The eustachian tube and its significance in flight. *Journal of Laryngology and Otology*, 93, 659–78.

King, P.F. 1988. Otorhinolaryngology. In: J. Ernsting and P. King (eds) *Aviation Medicine – Second Edition*. London: Butterworths, Ch. 50.

King, P.F. and Gannon, R.P. 1958. The problem of noise in the Royal Air Force. *Proceedings of the Royal Society of Medicine*, 51, 45–52.

Kotnis, R. and Simo, R. 2001. Tuberculous meningitis presenting as sensorineural hearing loss. *Journal of Laryngology and Otology*, 115, 491–2.

Kraus, N., Kileny, P. and McGee, T. 1994. Middle Latency Auditory Evoked Potentials. In: J. Katz (ed.) *Handbook of Clinical Audiology – Fourth Edition*. Baltimore: Williams & Wilkins, 487–505.

Kronoveter, K.J. and Somerville, G.W. 1970. Airplane cockpit noise levels and pilot hearing sensitivity. *Archives of Environmental Health*, 20, 495–9.

Kryter, K.D. 1959. Scaling human reactions to the sound from aircraft. *Journal of the Acoustical Society of America*, 31, 1415–29.

Kryter, K.D. 1994. *The Handbook of Hearing and the Effects of Noise*. San Diego, CA: Academic Press.

Kryter, K.D. and Pearsons, K.S. 1964. Modification of noy tables. *Journal of the Acoustical Society of America*, 36, 394–7.

Küstel, M., Büki, B., Gyimesi, J., Makó, J., Komora, V. and Ribári, O. 1993. Auditory brainstem potentials in uraemia. *Journal of Otorhinolaryngology and Related Specialties*, 55, 89–92.

Kuhweide, R., Van de Steene, V., Vlaminck, S. and Casselman, J.W. 2002. Ramsay Hunt syndrome: Pathophysiology of cochleovestibular symptoms. *Journal of Laryngology and Otology*, 116, 844–8.

Kujala, J., Aalto, H., Ramsay, H. and Hirvonen, T.P. 2008. Simultaneous bilateral stapes surgery. *Acta Oto-Laryngologica*, 128, 347–51.

Kuronen, P., Pääkönen, R. and Savolainen, S. 1999. Low-altitude overflights of fighters and the risk of hearing loss.

Aviation, Space, and Environmental Medicine, 70, 650–55.

Kuronen, P., Sorri, M.J., Pääkönen, R. and Muhli, A. 2003. Temporary threshold shift in military pilots measured using conventional and extended high-frequency audiometry after one flight. *International Journal of Audiology*, 42, 29–33.

Kuronen, P., Toppila, E., Starck, J., Pääkönen, R. and Sorri, M.T. 2004. Modelling the risk of noise-induced hearing loss among military pilots. *International Journal of Audiology*, 43, 79–84.

Lee, H. and Baloh, R.W. 2005. Sudden deafness in vertebrobasilar ischemia: Clinical features, vascular topographical patterns and long-term outcome. *Journal of the Neurological Sciences*, 228, 99–104.

Leussink, V., Andermann, P., Reiners, K., Shehata-Dieler, W., Gunthener-Lengsfeld, T. and Naumann, M. 2005. Sudden deafness from stroke. *Neurology*, 64, 1817–8.

Lindgren, T., Wieslander, G., Dammström, B.-G. and Norbäck, D. 2009. Tinnitus among airline pilots: Prevalence and effects of age, flight experience, and other noise. *Aviation, Space, and Environmental Medicine*, 80, 112–6.

Linstrom, C.J. and Gleich, L.L. 1993. Otosyphilis: Diagnostic and therapeutic update. *Journal of Otolaryngology*, 22, 401–8.

Low, W.K., Gopal, K., Goh, L.K. and Fong, K.W. 2006a. Cochlear implantation in post-irradiated ears: Outcomes and challenges. *Laryngoscope*, 116, 1258–62.

Low, W.K., Toh, S.T., Wee, J., Fook-Chong, S.M. and Wang, D.J. 2006b. Sensorineural hearing loss after radiotherapy and chemoradiotherapy: A single, blinded, randomized study. *Journal of Clinical Oncology*, 24, 1904–9.

Luxon, L.M. 1998. The Clinical Diagnosis of Noise-Induced Hearing Loss. In: D.K. Prasher and L.M. Luxon (eds) *Advances in Noise Research Volume 1: Biological Effects*. London: Whurr.

Luxon, L.M. and Raglan, E. 2006. Deafness and Tinnitus. In: J.H. Noseworthy (ed.) *Neurological Therapeutics: Principles and Practice – Second Edition*. Abingdon: Informa Healthcare, 2157–81.

Maassen, J.A. 2002. Mitochondrial diabetes: Pathophysiology, clinical presentation, and genetic analysis. *American Journal of Medical Genetics*, 115, 66–70.

McCabe, B.F. 1979. Autoimmune sensorineural hearing loss. *Annals of Otology, Rhinology and Laryngology*, 88, 585–90.

McDonald, T.J. and DeRemee, R.A. 1983. Wegener's granulomatosis. *Laryngoscope*, 93, 220–31.

McNab, A. 1996. *Bravo Two Zero*. London: Corgi Books.

McGibbon, J.E.G. 1947a. Aviation Pressure Deafness. In: E.D.D. Dickson (ed.) *Contributions to Aviation Otolaryngology*. London: Headley Brothers, Ch. VI.

McGibbon, J.E.G. 1947b. The Nature of the Valvular Action (Passive Opening) of the Eustachian Tube in Relation to Changes of Atmospheric Pressure and to Aviation Pressure Deafness. In: E.D.D. Dickson (ed.) *Contributions to Aviation Otolaryngology*. London: Headley Brothers. Ch. VI.

McKennell, A.C. 1963. *Aircraft Noise Annoyance round London Heathrow Airport*. London: Central Office of Information.

Magnan, J., Manrique, M., Dillier, N., Snik, A. and Häusler, R. 2005. International consensus on middle ear implants. *Acta Oto-Laryngologica*, 125, 920–21.

Mahajan, S.L., Ikeda, Y., Myers, T.J. and Baldini, M.G. 1981. Acute acoustic nerve palsy associated with vincristine therapy. *Cancer*, 47, 2404–6.

Mahoney, C.F. and Luxon, L.M. 1996. Misdiagnosis of hearing loss due to ear canal collapse: A report of two cases. *Journal of Laryngology and Otology*, 110, 561–6.

Maia, C.A. and Campos, C.A 2005. Diabetes mellitus as etiological factor of hearing loss. *Review Brazilian Otorhinolaryngologica*, 71, 208–14.

Majamaa-Voltti, K.K., Wingvist, S., Remes, A.M., Tolonen, U., Pyhtinen, J., Uimonen, S. et al., 2006. A 3-year clinical follow-up of adult patients with 3243A>G in mitochondrial DNA. *Neurology*, 66, 1470–75.

Martini, A. and Prosser, S. 2003. Disorders of the Inner Ear in Adults. In: L.M. Luxon, A. Martini, J. Furman and S.D.G. Stephens (eds) *A Textbook of Audiological Medicine*. London: Martin Dunitz, 451–75.

Mattox, D.E. and Simmons, F.B. 1977. Natural history of sudden sensorineural hearing loss. *Annals of Otology, Rhinology and Laryngology*, 86, 463–80.

Menger, D.J. and Tange, R.A. 2003. The aetiology of otosclerosis: A review of the literature. *Clinical Otolaryngology and Allied Science*, 28, 112–20.

Michel, P. 1863. Mémoire sur les anomalies congénitales de l'oreille interne. *Gazette Médicale de Strasbourg*, 23, 55–8.

Miller, D.H., Rudge, P., Johnson, G., Kendall, B.E., Macmanus, D.G., Moseley, I.F. et al. 1988. Serial gadolinium enhanced magnetic resonance imaging in multiple sclerosis. *Brain*, 111, 927–39.

Minor, L.B., Schessel, D.A. and Carey, J.P. 2004. Menière's disease. *Current Opinion in Neurology*, 17, 9–16.

Mirza, S. and Richardson, H. 2005. Otic barotrauma from air travel. *Journal of Laryngology and Otology*, 119, 366–30.

Møller, A.R. 1984. Pathophysiology of tinnitus. *Annals of Otology, Rhinology and Laryngology*, 93, 39–44.

Moore, B.C.J. and Sęk, A. 2009. Development of a fast method for determining sensitivity to temporal fine structure. *International Journal of Audiology*, 48, 161–71.

Mrena, R., Paakkonen, R., Back, L., Pirvola, U. and Ylikoski, J. 2004a. Otologic

consequences of blast exposure: A Finnish case study of a shopping mall bomb explosion. *Acta Oto-Laryngologica*, 124, 946–52.

Mrena, R., Savolainen, S., Pirvola, U. and Ylikoski, J. 2004b. Characteristics of acute acoustical trauma in the Finnish Defence Forces. *International Journal of Audiology*, 43, 177–81.

Musiek, F.E., Baran, J.A. and Pinheiro, M.L. 1994. *Neuroaudiology: Case Studies*. San Diego, CA: Singular Publishing Group.

Musiek, F.E., Charette, L., Kelly, T., Lee., W.W. and Musiek, E. 1999. Hit and false-positive rates for the middle latency response in patients with central nervous system involvement. *Journal of the American Academy of Audiology*, 10, 124–32.

Musiek, F.E. and Lee, W.W. 1995. The auditory brainstem response in patients with brainstem and cochlear pathology. *Ear and Hearing*, 16, 631–6.

Musiek, F.E. and Lee, W.W. 1998. Neuroanatomical correlates to central deafness. *Scandinavian Audiology*, 27, 18–25.

Nance, W.E. 2003. The genetics of deafness. *Mental Retardation and Developmental Disabilities Research Reviews*, 9, 109–19.

Newton, H.B. 2001. Neurologic complications of scuba diving. *American Family Physician*, 63, 2211–8.

Nilsson, M., Soli, S.D. and Sullivan, J.A. 1994. Development of the Hearing in Noise Test for the measurement of speech reception thresholds in quiet and in noise. *Journal of the Acoustical Society of America*, 95, 1085–99.

Nowé, V., de Ridder, D., Van de Heyning, P.H., Wang, X.L., Gielen, J., Van Goethem, J. et al. 2004. Does the location of a vascular loop in the cerebellopontine angle explain pulsatile and non-pulsatile tinnitus? *European Radiology*, 14, 2282–9.

Orchik, D.J., Schmaier, D.R., Shea, J.J. Jr, Emmett, J.R., Moretz, W.H. and Shea, J.J. III. 1987. Sensorineural hearing loss in cordless telephone injury. *Otolaryngology – Head and Neck Surgery*, 96, 30–33.

O'Reilly, B.J. 1999. Otorhinolaryngology. In: J. Ernsting, A.N. Nicholson and D.J. Rainford (eds) *Aviation Medicine – Third Edition*. Oxford: Butterworth Heinemann, Ch. 24.

Owen, J.P. 1995. Noise-induced hearing loss in military helicopter aircrews: A review of the evidence. *Journal of the Royal Army Medical Corps*, 141, 98–101.

Pääkkönen, R. and Kuronen, P. 1996. Noise exposure of fighter pilots and ground technicians during flight rounds. *Acta Acustica*, 83, 1–6.

Pääkkönen, R. and Kuronen, P. 1997. Noise attenuation of helmets and headsets worn by Finnish Air Force pilots. *Applied Acoustics*, 49, 373–82.

Pääkkönen, R., Kuronen, P. and Korteoja, M. 2001. Active noise reduction in aviation helmets during a military jet trainer test flight. *Scandinavian Audiology*, Suppl. 52, 177–9.

Pahor, A.L. 1981. The ENT problems following the Birmingham bombings. *Journal of Laryngology and Otology*, 95, 399–406.

Palva, T. 1957. Occupational deafness in telephone exchange workers. *Acta Oto-Laryngologica*, 47, 510–19.

Pan, C.L., Kuo, M.F. and Hsieh, S.T. 2004. Auditory agnosia caused by a tectal germinoma. *Neurology*, 63, 2387–9.

Paparella, M.M., Berlinger, N.T., Oda, M. and el-Fiky, F. 1973. Otological manifestations of leukemia. *Laryngoscope*, 83, 1510–26.

Peltomaa, M., Pyykko, I., Sappala, I. and Viljanen, M. 2000. Lyme borreliosis, an etiological factor in scnsorineural hearing loss? *European Archives of Otorhinolaryngology*, 257, 317–22.

Penner, M.J. 1990. An estimate of the prevalence of tinnitus caused by spontaneous otoacoustic emissions. *Archives of Otolaryngology and Head and Neck Surgery*, 116, 418–23.

Perlman, H.B. 1941. Acoustic trauma in man: Clinical and experimental studies. *Archives of Otolaryngology*, 34, 429–52.

Persaud, R., Hajioff, D., Wareing, M. and Chevretton, E. 2003. Otological trauma resulting from the Soho nail bomb in London, April 1999. *Clinical Otolaryngology and Allied Sciences*, 28, 203–6.

Pickles, J.O. 2004. Mutation in mitochondrial DNA as a cause of presbyacusis. *Audiology and Neurotology*, 9, 23–33.

Pickles, J.O. 2007. Physiology of the Auditory System. In: M. Gleason (ed.) *Scott Brown's Otolaryngology – Seventh Edition*. London: Hodder.

Pirila, T. 1991a. Left-right asymmetry in the human response to experimental noise exposure. I. Interaural correlation of the temporary threshold shift at 4 kHz frequency. *Acta Oto-Laryngologica*, 111, 677–83.

Pirila, T. 1991b. Left-right asymmetry in the human response to experimental noise exposure. II. Pre-exposure hearing threshold and temporary threshold shift at 4 kHz frequency. *Acta Oto-Laryngologica*, 111, 861–6.

Pirila, T., Jounio-Ervasti, K. and Sorri, M. 1991. Hearing asymmetry among left-handed and right-handed persons in a random population. *Scandinavian Audiology*, 20, 223–6.

Pirila, T., Jounio-Ervasti, K. and Sorri, M. 1992. Left-right asymmetries in hearing threshold levels in three age groups of a random population. *Audiology*, 31, 150–61.

Pons, Y., Raynal, M., Hunkemöller, I., Lepage, P. and Kossowski, M. 2010. Vestibular schwannoma and fitness to fly. *Aviation, Space, and Environmental Medicine*, 81, 961–4.

Poulsen, T. and Oakley, S. 2009. Equivalent threshold sound pressure levels (ETSPL) for Sennheiser HAD 280 supra-aural audiometric earphones in the frequency range 125 Hz to 8000 Hz. *International Journal of Audiology*, 48, 271–6.

Price, G.R. and Kalb, J.T. 1991. A new approach to a damage risk criterion for weapons impulses. *Scandinavian Audiology*, 34 (Suppl.), 21–37.

Pulec, J.L., House, W.F. and Britten, B.H. 1971. A system of management of acoustic neuroma based on 364 cases. *Transactions of the American Academy of Ophthalmology and Otolaryngology*, 75, 48–55.

van der Putten, L., de Bree, R., Plukker, J.T., Langendijk, J.A., Smits, C., Burlage, F.R. and Leemans, C.R. 2006. Permanent unilateral hearing loss after radiotherapy for parotid gland tumors. *Head and Neck*, 28, 902–8.

Pyykkö, I., Toppila, E., Starck, J., Juhola, M. and Auramo, Y. 2000. Database for a hearing conservation program. *Scandinavian Audiology*, 29, 52–8.

Qiang, Y., Rebok, G.W., Baker, S.P. and Li, G. 2008. Hearing deficit in birth cohort of US male commuter air carrier and air taxi pilots. *Aviation, Space, and Environmental Medicine*, 79, 1051–5.

Raglan, E. 2003. Otitis Media with Effusion in Children. In: L.M. Luxon, A. Martini, J. Furman and S.D.G. Stephens (eds) *A Textbook of Audiological Medicine*. London: Martin Dunitz, 381–92.

Raynal, M., Kossowski, M. and Job, A. 2006. Hearing in military pilots: One-time audiometry in pilots of fighters, transports, and helicopters. *Aviation, Space, and Environmental Medicine*, 77, 57–61.

Ribera, J.E. 2007. Functional hearing in noise: Insert earphones vs supra-aural headphones. *Aviation, Space, and Environmental Medicine*, 78, 1159–61.

Robinson, D.W. 1987. *Noise Exposure and Hearing: A New Look at the Experimental Data*. London: Health and Safety Executive, Research Report No. 1/1987.

Robinson, D.W. 1988. *Tables for the Estimation of Hearing Impairment due to Noise for Otologically Normal Persons and for a Typical Unscreened Population as a Function of Age and Duration of Exposure*. London: Health and Safety Executive, Research Report No. 2/1988.

Robinson, D.W. and Cook, J.P. 1968. *The Quantification of Noise Exposure*. Teddington: National Physical Laboratory, Aero Report Ac 31.

Robinson, D.W. and Shipton, M.S. 1973. *Tables for the Estimation of Noise-Induced Hearing Loss*. Teddington: National Physical Laboratory, Acoustic Report Ac 61 (First Edition).

Robinson, D.W. and Shipton, M.S. 1977. *Tables for the Estimation of Noise-Induced Hearing Loss*. Teddington: National Physical Laboratory, Acoustic Report Ac 61 (Second Edition).

Robinson, J. 1998. Reconstruction of the Middle Ear. In: H. Ludman and A. Wright (eds) *Diseases of the Ear – Sixth Edition*. London: Arnold, 429–38.

Rood, G.M. 1988. Noise and Communication. In: J. Ernsting and P. King (eds) *Aviation Medicine – Second Edition*. London: Butterworth, Ch. 24.

Rood, G.M. and Glen, M.C. 1977. *A Survey of Noise Doses Received by Military Aircrew*. London: Her Majesty's Stationery Office, Technical Report 77080.

Rosenfeld, R.M., Singer, M., Wasserman, J.M. and Stinnett, S.S. 2006. Systematic review of topical antimicrobial therapy for acute otitis externa. *Otolaryngology and Head and Neck Surgery*, 134, Suppl., 24–48.

Rosenkvist, L., Klokker, M. and Katholm, M. 2008. Upper respiratory infections and barotraumas in commercial pilots: A retrospective survey. *Aviation, Space, and Environmental Medicine*, 79, 960–63.

Ruckenstein, M. 2004. Autoimmune inner ear disease. *Current Opinion in Otolaryngology and Head and Neck Surgery*, 12, 426–30.

Rudmose, W. 1964. Concerning the problem of calibrating the TDH-39 earphones at 6 kHz with a 9A coupler. *Journal of the Acoustical Society of America*, 36, 1049(A).

Sajjadi, H. and Paparella, M.M. 2008. Ménière's disease. *Lancet*, 372, 406–14.

Salvi, R.J., Henderson, D. and Hamernik, R.P. (eds). 1986. *Basic and Applied Aspects of Noise-Induced Hearing Loss*. New York, NY: Plenum Press.

Santos-Sacchi, J. 2001. Cochlear Physiology. In: A.F. Jahn and J. Santos-Sacchi (eds) *Physiology of the Ear*. Australia: Singular, 357–91.

Schacht, J. 1998. Aminoglycoside ototoxicity: Prevention in sight? *Otolaryngology and Head and Neck Surgery*. 118, 674–7.

Scheiblechner, H. 1974. The validity of the 'energy principle' for noise-induced hearing loss. *Audiology*, 13, 93–111.

Schuknecht, H.F. 1969. Mechanisms of inner ear injury from blows to the head. *Annals of Otology*, 78, 253–62.

Schuknecht, H.F. 1994. Temporal bone pathology in a case of Cogan's syndrome. *Laryngoscope*, 104, 1135–42.

Schultz, T.J. 1978. Synthesis of social surveys and noise annoyance. *Journal of the Acoustical Society of America*, 64, 377–405.

Seidman, M.D. 2000. Effects of dietary restriction and antioxidants on presbyacusis. *Laryngoscope*, 110, 727–38.

Seidman, M.D., Ahmad, N., Joshi, D., Seidman, J., Thawani, S. and Quirk, W.S. 2004. Age-related hearing loss and its association with reactive oxygen species and mitochondrial DNA damage. *Acta Oto-Laryngologica*, Suppl. 552, 16–24.

Semaan, M.T., Alagramam, K.K. and Megerian, C.A. 2005. The basic science of Ménière's disease and endolymphatic hydrops. *Current Opinion in Otolaryngology Head and Neck Surgery*, 13, 301–7.

de Seze, J., Assouad, R., Stojkovic, T., Desaulty, A., Dubus, B. and Vermersch, P. 2001. Hearing loss in multiple sclerosis: Clinical, electrophysiologic and radiological study. *Revue Neurologique (Paris)*, 157, 1403–9.

Shine, N.P. and Coates, H. 2005. Systemic otoxicity: A review. *East African Medical Journal*, 82, 536–9.

Shupak. A., Gil, A., Nachum, Z., Miller, S., Gordon, C.R. and Tal, D. 2003. Inner ear decompression sickness and inner ear barotrauma in recreational divers: A long-term follow-up. *Laryngoscope*, 113, 2141–7.

Silverstein, H., Bernstein, J.M. and Davies, D.G. 1967. Salicylate ototoxicity: A biochemical and electrophysiological study. *Annals of Otology, Rhinology and Laryngology*, 76, 118–28.

Singleton, G.T., Whitaker, D.L., Keim, R.J. and Kemker, F.J. 1984. Cordless telephones: A threat to hearing. *Annals of Otology, Rhinology and Laryngology*, 93, 565–8.

Smoorenburg, G.F. 1992. Damage Risk for Low Frequency Impulse Noise: The Spectral Factor in Noise-Induced Hearing Loss. In: A. Dancer, D. Henderson, R.J. Salvi and R.P. Hamernik (eds) *Noise-Induced Hearing Loss*. St Louis, MO: Mosby, 313–24.

Starr, A., Picton, T.W., Sininger, Y., Hood, L.J. and Berlin, C.I. 1996. Auditory neuropathy. *Brain*, 119, 741–53.

Steel, K.P. 1998. New interventions in hearing impairment. *Science*, 279, 1870–71.

Stephens, D.G. and Powell, C.A. 1980. Laboratory and Community Studies of Aircraft Noise Effects. In: J.V. Tobias, G. Jansen and W.D. Ward (eds) *Noise as a Public Health Problem: Proceedings of the Third International Congress, Freiburg 1978*. Rockville, MD: American Speech-Language-Hearing Association Report 10, 488–94.

Stephens, S.D.G. 2003. Audiological Rehabilitation. In: L.M. Luxon, A. Martini, J. Furman and S.D.G. Stephens (eds) *A Textbook of Audiological Medicine*. London: Martin Dunitz, 451–75.

Stephens, S.D.G., Luxon, L.M. and Hinchcliffe, R. 1982. Immunological disorders and auditory lesions. *Audiology*, 21, 128–48.

Stephenson, M.R., Nixon, C.W. and Johnson, D.L. 1980. Identification of the minimum noise level capable of producing an asymptotic temporary threshold shift. *Aviation, Space, and Environmental Medicine*, 51, 391–6.

Stevens, S.S. 1955. The measurement of loudness. *Journal of the Acoustical Society of America*, 27, 815–29.

Stevens, S.S. 1956. Calculation of the loudness of complex noise. *Journal of the Acoustical Society of America*, 28, 807–32.

Stevens, S.S. 1957. Calculating loudness. *Noise Control*, September, 11–22.

Stevens, J.C. and Guirao, M. 1964. Individual loudness functions. *Journal of the Acoustical Society of America*, 36, 2210–13.

Strupp, M., Hupert, D., Frenzel, C., Wagner, J., Hahn, A., Jahn, K. et al. 2008. Long-term prophylactic treatment of attacks of vertigo in Menière's disease: Comparison of a high with a low dosage of betahistine in an open trial. *Acta Oto-Laryngologica*, 128, 520–24.

Suga, N., Gao, E., Zhang, Y., Ma, X. and Olsen, J.F. 2000. The corticofugal system for hearing: Recent progress. *Proceedings of the United States of America National Academy of Sciences*, 97, 11807–14.

Tjell, C., Tenenbaum, A. and Rosenhall, U. 1999. Auditory function in whiplash-associated disorders. *Scandinavian Audiology*, 28, 203–9.

Toglia, J.U. and Katinsky, S. 1976. Neuro-Otological Aspects of Closed Head Injury. In: P.J. Vinken and G.W. Bruyn (eds) *Handbook of Clinical Neurology. Injuries of the Brain and Skull – Volume 24*. Amsterdam: North Holland, 119–40.

Torre, P., Cruickshanks, K.J., Klein, B.E., Klein, R. and Nondahl, D.M. 2006. The association between cardiovascular disease and cochlear function in older adults. *Journal of Speech Language and Hearing Research*, 48, 473–81.

Tsalighopoulos, M., Mavridis, M., Themelis, C., Harisopoulos, I., Dagilas, A., Kafkias, V. et al. 1986. Screening of the workers hearing in a cannery. *Helleniki Iatriki*, 52, 311–9.

Tschopp, K. and Probst, R. 1989. Acute acoustic trauma. *Acta Oto-Laryngologica*, 108, 378–84.

Department of the Air Force, United States of America. 1956. *Hazardous Noise Exposure*. Washington, DC: Department of the Air Force Report, 160–63.

Van de Beek, D., de Gans, J., McIntyre, P. and Prasad, K. 2003. Corticosteroids in acute bacterial meningitis. *Cochrane Database Systematic Review*, 3, No. CD004405.

Van de Heyning, P.H., Wuyts, F. and Boudewyns, A. 2005. Surgical treatment of Menière's disease. *Current Opinion in Neurology*, 18, 23–8.

Wagstaff, A.S. and Årva, P. 2009. Hearing loss in civilian airline and helicopter pilots compared to air traffic control personnel. *Aviation, Space, and Environmental Medicine*, 80, 857–61.

Ward, W.D. 1957. Hearing of naval aircraft maintenance personnel. *Journal of the Acoustical Society of America*, 29, 1289–301.

Warr, W.B. 1992. Organization of the Olivocochlear Efferent Systems in Mammals. In: D.B. Webster, A.N. Popper and R.R. Fay (eds) *Mammalian Auditory Pathway: Neuroanatomy*. New York, NY: Springer-Verlag, 410–48.

Wayman, D.M., Pham, H.N., Byl, F.M. and Adour, K.K. 1990. Audiological manifestations of Ramsay Hunt syndrome. *Journal of Laryngology and Otology*, 104, 104–8.

Weinstein, B.E. 1994. Presbycusis. In: J. Katz (ed.) *Handbook of Clinical Audiology – Fourth Edition*. Baltimore, MD: Williams & Wilkins, 553–67.

Wennmo, C. and Svensson, C. 1989. Temporal bone fractures. *Acta Oto-Laryngologica* (Suppl.), 468, 379–83.

Westmore, C.A., Pickard, B.H. and Stern, H. 1979. Isolation of mumps virus from the inner ear after sudden deafness. *British Medical Journal*, 6155, 14–15.

Wheeler, L.J. and Dickson, E.D.D. 1952. The determination of the threshold of hearing. *Journal of Laryngology and Otology*, 66, 379–95.

Wilson, J.G. 1917. Injury to the ear from high explosives. *Transactions of the American Otolaryngology Society*.

World Health Organization. 2006. Available at: http://www.who.int/mediacentre/factsheets/fs300/en/index.html

Wirkowski, E., Echausse, N., Overby, C., Ortiz, O. and Radler, L. 2006. I can hear you yet cannot comprehend: A case of pure word deafness. *Journal of Emergency Medicine*, 30, 53–5.

Ylikoski, J. 1987. Audiometric configurations in acute acoustic trauma caused by firearms. *Scandinavian Audiology*, 16, 115–20.

Ylikoski, J.S., House, J.W. and Hernandez, I. 1981. Eighth nerve alcoholic neuropathy: A case report with light and electron microscopic findings. *Journal of Laryngology and Otology*, 95, 631–42.

Youngs, R. 1998. Complications of Suppurative Otitis Media. In: H. Ludman and T. Wright (eds) *Diseases of the Ear – Sixth Edition*. London: Arnold, 394–416.

Zajtchuk, J.T. and Phillips, Y.Y. (eds). 1989. Effects of blast overpressure on the ear. *Annals of Otology, Rhinology and Laryngology*, 98, Supplement 140, 5.

Zeller, J.A., Zunker, P., Witt, K., Schlueter, E. and Deuschl, G. 2002. Unusual presentation of carcinomatous meningitis: Case report and review of typical CSF findings. *Neurological Research*, 24, 652–4.

Zwicker, E. 1960. Ein Verfahren zur Berechnung der Lautstärke. *Acustica,* 10, 304–8.

Zwicker, E. 1961. Subdivision of the audible frequency range into critical bands (Frequenzgruppen). *Journal of the Acoustical Society of America*, 33, 248.

Further Reading

Luxon, L.M. and Prasher, D. (eds). 2007. *Noise and Its Effects*. London: John Wiley.

Hinchcliffe, R. and Śliwińska-Kowalska, M. (eds). 2007. Noise damage to hearing. *Audiological Medicine*, 5, 2–80.

Appendix I

A BIBLIOGRAPHY OF CASE REPORTS OF NEUROLOGICAL DISORDERS IN AIRCREW

This bibliography is concerned with accounts of neurological disorders in individual aircrew published over recent years in the pages of *Aviation, Space, and Environmental Medicine*. The references are listed alphabetically with respect to the first author in broad clinical categories. Many of the cases have been cited in the chapters in the present book. The diagnosis or proposed diagnosis of each condition is given after the reference if it is not clear from the title of the paper.

The bibliography does not indicate the likely incidence of neurological disorders in a cohort of individuals that has been carefully screened and then periodically reviewed. However, it demonstrates the need for the aeromedical practitioner to be alert to the possibility of a wide variety of neurological disorders in aircrew, even at routine examinations.

Editor

Degenerative Diseases

Branch, L.S. 2005. You're the flight surgeon. *Aviation, Space, and Environmental Medicine*, 76, 697–8. (Multiple sclerosis)

Brooks, K.E. and Hopkins, E.W. III. 1997. An aviator with an unusual gait: A rare disease teaches some everyday lessons. *Aviation, Space, and Environmental Medicine*, 68, 147–51. (Muscular dystrophy)

Carter, D., Azaria, B. and Goldstein, L. 2005. Diabetes mellitus type 1 in five military aviators: Flying with insulin. *Aviation, Space, and Environmental Medicine*, 76, 861–2.

Christensen, D.E. 2005. You're the flight surgeon. *Aviation, Space, and Environmental Medicine*, 76, 802–4. (Neurodegenerative condition)

Critchley, E.P. 2004. Multiple sclerosis: Initially presenting as facial palsy. *Aviation, Space, and Environmental Medicine*, 75, 1001–4.

Ma, K.-W. 2008. You're the flight surgeon: Transient global amnesia. *Aviation, Space, and Environmental Medicine*, 79, 1117–8.

Zinger, H., Grossman, A., Assa, A., Barel, O., Barenboim, E. and Levite, R. 2011. Return to flight with multiple sclerosis: Aeromedical considerations. *Aviation, Space, and Environmental Medicine*, 82, 61–4.

Intracranial Tumours, Ischaemic Lesions and Aneurysms

Hopkins, E.W. 1994. Stroke in the young aviator. 1994. *Aviation, Space, and Environmental Medicine*, 65, 367–8. (Ischaemic lesion of left caudate nucleus with atrial septal defect and aneurysm)

Jackson, M. 2008. Unruptured intracranial cerebral aneursyms in aviation. *Aviation, Space, and Environmental Medicine*, 79, 62–4.

Johnson, J.M. 2009. You're the flight surgeon: Incidentaloma. *Aviation, Space, and Environmental Medicine*, 80, 424–5.

Little, J.R. 1996. You're the flight surgeon. *Aviation, Space, and Environmental Medicine*, 67, 1002–4. (Pituitary mass)

Serkowski, R.J. 2010. You're the flight surgeon: Colloidal cyst of the third ventricle. *Aviation, Space, and Environmental Medicine*, 81, 797–8.

Storms, P.R. 2004. You're the flight surgeon. *Aviation, Space, and Environmental Medicine*, 75, 918–9. (Parieto-occipital tumour)

Impaired Consciousness, Syncope and Seizures

Bisges, J. and Baldwin, P. 2009. You're the flight surgeon: Concussion and post-concussion syndrome. *Aviation, Space, and Environmental Medicine*, 80, 906–8.

Feeks, E.F., Murphy, G.L. and Porter, H.O. 1997. Laughter in the cockpit: Gelastic seizures – A case report. *Aviation, Space, and Environmental Medicine*, 68, 66–8.

Fitzsimons, M.G. 1998. Case report: Cough syncope in a U.S. Army aviator. *Aviation, Space, and Environmental Medicine*, 69, 515–6.

Friend, R. 2004. You're the flight surgeon. *Aviation, Space, and Environmental Medicine*, 75, 818–9. (Syncope)

Gould, R.K. 2010. Syncope as the first sign of complete heart block in a military aviator. *Aviation, Space, and Environmental Medicine*, 81, 431–2.

Kupke, M.J. 2005. You're the flight surgeon. *Aviation, Space, and Environmental Medicine*, 76, 151–3. (Closed head injury)

Kupke, M.J. 2006. Traumatic subdural haematoma and medical certification. *Aviation, Space, and Environmental Medicine*, 77, 870–72.

Manen, O., Parrier, E. and Généro, M. 2011. Ground vasovagal presyncopes and fighter pilot fitness: Aeromedical concerns. *Aviation, Space, and Environmental Medicine*, 82, 917–20.

Sharma, S. and Agarwal, A. 2005. Algorithm for evaluation and disposition of a single episode of loss of consciousness. *Aviation, Space, and Environmental Medicine*, 76, 863–8.

Wright, S.C. 1998. Case report: Postconcussion syndrome after minor head injury. *Aviation, Space, and Environmental Medicine*, 69, 999–1000.

Neuro-Ophthalmology

Anderson, W. 2006. You're the flight surgeon: Aniscoria. *Aviation, Space, and Environmental Medicine*, 77, 987–8. (Benign episodic pupillary dilatation)

Clinton, C.D. 2008. You're the flight surgeon: A painful eye. *Aviation, Space, and Environmental Medicine*, 79, 442–3. (Tolosa-Hunt syndrome: Inflammation of the superior orbital fissure or anterior cavernous sinus)

Cohen, M.W. 1995. You're the flight surgeon. *Aviation, Space, and Environmental Medicine*, 66, 285–6. (Optic neuritis)

Davis, R.E., Rubin, R.M., Gooch, J.M., Ivan, D.J. and Tredici, T.J. 2010. Optic nerve head drusen (ONHD) in United States Air Force aircrew: A retrospective review. *Aviation, Space, and Environmental Medicine*, 81, 281.

Guliuzza, R.J. 2005. You're the flight surgeon. *Aviation, Space, and Environmental Medicine*, 76, 406–7. (Ocular myasthenia gravis)

Ivan, D.J., Tredici, T.J., Burroughs, J.R., Pasquale, A., Hickman, J.R. Jr, Cuervo, H. and Gooch, J. 1998. Primary idiopathic optic neuritis in U.S. Air Force aviators. *Aviation, Space, and Environmental Medicine*, 69, 158–65.

Karmon, Y., Blum, S., Levite, R., Barenboim, E. and Gadoth, N. 2010. Myasthenia gravis and return to flying status. *Aviation, Space, and Environmental Medicine*, 81, 69–73.

Morrissette, K.L. 1998. You're the flight surgeon. *Aviation, Space, and Environmental Medicine*, 69, 1116. (Ophthalmic migraine)

Pokroy, R., Barenboim, E., Carter, D., Assa, A. and Alhalel, A. 2009. Unilateral optic disc swelling in a fighter pilot. *Aviation, Space, and Environmental Medicine*, 80, 894–7. (Decompression sickness-related papillophlebitis)

Steigleman, A., Butler, F., Chhoeu, A., O'Malley, T., Bower, E. and Giebner, S. 2003. Optic neuropathy following an altitude exposure. *Aviation, Space, and Environmental Medicine*, 74, 985–9.

Sleep Disorders

Alan, M. 2003. Sleep apnea: A case report. *Aviation, Space, and Environmental Medicine*, 74, 288–90.

Grossman, A., Barenboim, E., Azaria, B., Sherer, Y. and Goldstein, L. 2004. The maintenance of wakefulness test as a predictor of alertness in aircrew members with idiopathic hypersomnia. *Aviation, Space, and Environmental Medicine*, 75, 281–3.

Kucik, J., Husak, J.P. and Porter, H.R. 2002. You're the flight surgeon: Somnambulism (sleep walking). *Aviation, Space, and Environmental Medicine*, 73, 156–7.

Marks, F.A. 2006. You're the flight surgeon: Restless leg syndrome. *Aviation, Space, and Environmental Medicine*, 77, 1094–5.

Panton, S., Norup, P.W. and Videbaek, R. 1997. Case report: Obstructive sleep apnea – An air safety risk. *Aviation, Space, and Environmental Medicine*, 68, 1139–44.

Parker, P.E. 2000. You're the flight surgeon: Uvulopalatoplasty. *Aviation, Space, and Environmental Medicine*, 71, 1159–60.

Smart, L.T. and Singh, B. 2006. Excessive daytime sleepiness in a trainee military pilot. *Aviation, Space, and Environmental Medicine*, 77, 753–7.

Withers, B.G., Loube, D.I. and Husak, J.P. 1999. Idiopathic hypersomnia in an aircrew member. *Aviation, Space, and Environmental Medicine*, 70, 797–801.

Wygnanski, T., Kokia, E., Barak, P., Terlo, L. and Caine, Y.G. 1996. The sleeping aviator – Aeromedical disposition of Kleine-Levin syndrome. *Aviation, Space, and Environmental Medicine*, 67, 61–2.

Toxicology

Casbon, J.M. 2007. You're the flight surgeon: Carbon monoxide poisoning. *Aviation, Space, and Environmental Medicine*, 78, 911–3.

Clint, D. 2008. You're the flight surgeon: Tetrodotoxin. *Aviation, Space, and Environmental Medicine*, 79, 714–5.

Headache

Bradley, K.R. 2007. Migraine headaches and cerebrovascular accident secondary to patent foramen ovale. *Aviation, Space, and Environmental Medicine*, 78, 530–31.

Butler, J.W. 1997. You're the flight surgeon. *Aviation, Space, and Environmental Medicine*, 68, 350–51. (Cluster headaches)

Hattrup L.M. 1995. You're the flight surgeon. *Aviation, Space, and Environmental Medicine*, 66, 1015–6. (Migraine with aura)

Vestibular and Related Oculomotor Disorders, Disorders of Hearing and Facial Paralysis

Day, R.S. 2006. You're the flight surgeon. *Aviation, Space, and Environmental Medicine*, 77, 462–3. (Conductive hearing loss)

Grossman, A., Chapnik, L., Ulanovski, D., Goldstein, L., Azaria, B., Sherer, Y. and Barenboim, E. 2004. Acute cerebellar vertigo in a fighter pilot. *Aviation, Space, and Environmental Medicine*, 75, 913–5.

Grossman, A., Ulanovski, D., Barenboim, E., Azaria, B. and Goldstein, L. 2004. Facial nerve palsy aboard a commercial aircraft. *Aviation, Space, and Environmental Medicine*, 75, 1075–6. (Facial baroparesis)

Ildiz, F. and Dündar, A. 1994. A case of Tullio phenomenon in a subject with oval window fistula due to barotrauma. *Aviation, Space, and Environmental Medicine*, 65, 67–9.

Jiang, X.S. 2008. Inferior vestibular neuritis in a Chinese fighter pilot. *Aviation, Space, and Environmental Medicine*, 79, 256.

Klingenberger, J.K. 2011. You're the Flight Surgeon: Labyrinthine Dysfunction. *Aviation, Space and Environmental Medicine*, 82, 926–7.

Koda, E.K. 2008. You're the flight surgeon: Sinus barotrauma. *Aviation, Space, and Environmental Medicine*, 79, 805–6.

Lezama, N.G. 2003. You're the flight surgeon. *Aviation, Space, and Environmental Medicine*, 74, 1110–11. (Bell's palsy)

Pons, Y., Raynal, M., Hunkemöller, I., Lepage, P. and Kossowski, M. 2010. Vestibular schwannoma and fitness to fly. *Aviation, Space, and Environmental Medicine*, 81, 961–4.

Sen, A., Al-Deleamy, L.S. and Kendirli, T.M. 2007. Benign paroxysmal positional vertigo in an airline pilot. *Aviation, Space, and Environmental Medicine*, 78, 1060–63.

Tran, D.A. 2010. You're the flight surgeon: Alternobaric vertigo. *Aviation, Space, and Environmental Medicine*, 81, 896–7.

Wood, R.L. 2007. You're the flight surgeon: Dizziness. *Aviation, Space, and Environmental Medicine*, 78, 1172–3.

Appendix II

INTERNATIONAL STANDARDS FOR HEARING MEASUREMENTS, AIRCRAFT NOISE AND VIBRATION CONTROL

International Organization for Standardization and International Electrotechnical Commission Guide 98-3: 2008

Uncertainty of Measurement – Part 3: Guide to the Expression of Uncertainty in Measurement (http://www.iso.org/sites/JCGM/JCGM-introduction.htm)

International Organization for Standardization

Acoustics

1974: Assessment of noise with respect to its effect on the intelligibility of speech (ISO/TR 3352) (Withdrawn 2008)

1975: Method for calculating loudness level (ISO 532)

1978: Procedure for describing aircraft noise heard on the ground (ISO 3891)

1979: Guide to International Standards on the measurement of airborne acoustical noise and evaluation of its effects on human beings (ISO 2204) (Withdrawn 1997)

1983: Pure tone air conduction threshold audiometry for hearing conservation purposes (ISO 6189)

1987: Description and measurement of environmental noise

Part 3: Application to noise limits (ISO 1996-3) (Withdrawn 2007)

1990: Determination of occupational noise exposure and estimation of noise-induced hearing impairment (ISO 1999)

1993: Determination of sound power levels of noise sources using sound intensity

Part 1: Measurement at discrete points (ISO 9614-1)

1996: Determination of sound power levels of noise sources using sound intensity – Part 2: Measurement by scanning (ISO 9614-2)

1997: Methods for the description and physical measurement of single impulses or series of impulses (ISO 10843)

1997: Guidelines for the measurement and assessment of exposure to noise in a working environment (ISO 9612) (Withdrawn 2009)

2000: Statistical distribution of hearing thresholds as a function of age (ISO 7029)

1999: Requirements for the performance and calibration of reference sound sources used in the determination of sound power levels (ISO 6926)

2001: Measurement of sound pressure levels in the interior of aircraft during flight (ISO 5129)

2002: Determination of sound power levels of noise sources using sound intensity – Part 3: Precision method for measurement by scanning (ISO 9614-3)

2003: Normal equal-loudness-level contours (ISO 226).

2003: Description, measurement and assessment of environmental noise – Part 1: Basic quantities and procedures (ISO 1996-1)

2005: Noise from shooting ranges – Part 1: Determination of muzzle blast by measurement (ISO/DIS 17201-1)

2006: Noise from shooting ranges – Part 2: Estimation of muzzle blast and projectile sound by calculation (ISO/DIS 17201-2)

2006: Noise from shooting ranges – Part 4: Prediction of projectile sound (ISO/DIS 17201-4)

2008: Preferred reference values for acoustical and vibratory levels (ISO 1683)

Mechanical Vibration and Shock

1988: Hand-held portable power tools – Measurement of vibrations at the handle – Part 1: General (ISO 8662-1)

1989: Evaluation of human exposure to whole-body vibration – Part 2: Continuous and shock-induced vibrations in buildings (1 Hz to 80 Hz) (ISO 2631-2)

1996: Hand-arm vibration – Method for the measurement and evaluation of the vibration transmissibility of gloves at the palm of the hand (ISO 10819)

1997: Evaluation of human exposure to whole-body vibration – Part 1: General requirements (ISO 2631-1)

1997: Human exposure: Vocabulary (ISO 5805)

2001: Measurement and evaluation of human exposure to hand-transmitted vibration – Part 1: General requirements (ISO 5349-1)

2001: Measurement and evaluation of human exposure to hand-transmitted vibration – Part 2: Practical guidance for measurement at the workplace (ISO 5349-2)

2001: Range of idealized values to characterize seated-body biodynamic response under vertical vibration (ISO 5982)

2005: Human response to vibration – Measuring instrumentation (ISO/DIS 8041)

Audiometric Test Methods

1989: Audiometric test methods
Part 1: Basic pure tone air and bone conduction threshold audiometry (ISO 8253-1)

1996: Audiometric test methods Part 3: Speech audiometry (ISO 8253-3)

Hearing Protectors

1990: Part 1: Subjective method for the measurement of sound attenuation (ISO 4869-1)

1994: Part 2: Estimation of effective A-weighted sound pressure levels when hearing protectors are worn (ISO 4869-2)

2007 Part 3: Measurement of insertion loss of ear-muff type protectors using an acoustic test fixture (ISO 4869-3)

1998: Part 4: Measurement of effective sound pressure levels for level-dependent sound-restoration ear-muffs (ISO/TR 4869-4)

2006: Part 5: Method for estimation of noise reduction using fitting by inexperienced test subjects (ISO/TS 4869-5)

Calibration of Audiometric Equipment (Reference Zero)

1994: – Part 2: Reference equivalent threshold sound pressure levels for pure tones and insert earphones (ISO 389-2)

1994) – Part 3: Reference equivalent threshold force levels for pure tones and bone vibrators (ISO 389-3)

1998: Part 1: Reference equivalent threshold sound pressure levels for pure tones and supra-aural earphones (ISO 389-1; Cor 1: 1995)

1994 Part 4: Reference levels for narrow-band masking noise (ISO 389-4)

2006: Part 5: Reference equivalent threshold sound pressure levels for pure tones in the frequency range 8 kHz to 16 kHz (ISO 389-5)

1996 Part 7: Reference threshold of hearing under free-field and diffuse-field listening conditions (ISO 389-7)

2004: Part 8: Reference equivalent threshold sound pressure levels for pure tones and circumaural earphones. ISO 389-8

International Electrotechnical Commission

1994: International Electrotechnical Vocabulary: Acoustics and electroacoustics (IEC 60050-801)

Simulators of Human Head and Ear (60318-1, 3, 4 and 6)

2009: Part 1: Ear simulator for the calibration of supra-aural Earphones

1998: Part 3: Acoustic coupler for calibration of supra-aural earphones used in audiometry

Part 4: Occluded ear simulator for the measurement of earphones coupled to the ear by ear inserts

2007: Part 6: Mechanical coupler for measurements on bone vibrators

Audiological Equipment (IEC 60645 1-5)

2001: Part 1: Pure tone audiometers

1993: Part 2: Equipment for speech audiometry

2007: Part 3: Test signals of short duration

1994: Part 4: Equipment for extended high-frequency audiometry (Specifies requirements for 2009: equipment in the frequency range 8 kHz to 16 kHz)

Part 5: Instruments for the measurement of aural acoustic impedance/admittance

Electroacoustics

1995: Instruments for measurement of aircraft noise – Performance requirements for systems to measure one-third-octave band sound pressure levels in noise certification of transport-category aeroplanes (IEC 61265)

1997: Sound calibrators (IEC 60942)

2002: Specifications for personal sound exposure meters (IEC 61252)

2003: Sound level meters

Part 1: Specifications (IEC 61672 – 1)

Part 2: Pattern evaluation tests (IEC 61672 – 2)

WORLD HEALTH ORGANIZATION DESCRIPTORS OF HEARING IMPAIRMENT

Grade of impairment	Corresponding audiometric ISO value	Performance	Recommendations
0 – No impairment	25 dB or better (better ear)	No or very slight hearing problems. Able to hear whispers.	
1 – Slight/mild impairment	26–40 dB (better ear)	Able to hear and repeat words spoken in normal voice at 1 metre.	Counselling. Hearing aids may be needed.
2 – Moderate impairment	41–60 dB (better ear)	Able to hear and repeat words spoken in raised voice at 1 metre.	Hearing aids usually recommended.
3 – Severe impairment	61–80 dB (better ear)	Able to hear some words when shouted into better ear.	Hearing aids needed. If no hearing aids available, lip-reading and signing should be taught.
4 – Profound impairment including deafness	81 dB or greater (better ear)	Unable to hear and understand even a shouted voice.	Hearing aids may help understanding words. Additional rehabilitation needed. Lip-reading and sometimes signing essential.

Grades 2, 3 and 4 are classified as 'disabling hearing impairment'.
The audiometric ISO values are averages of values at 500, 1,000, 2,000, 4,000 Hz.

INDEX

❖

THE
NEUROSCIENCES
AND THE
PRACTICE OF AVIATION MEDICINE

Comments on the Text

The Editor is indebted to

Charles Berry, Houston, Texas
Yehezkel Caine, Jerusalem, Israel
Jean-Pierre Crance, Nancy, France
Gábor Hardicsay, Budapest, Hungary
David Powell, Auckland, New Zealand
Jarnail Singh, Singapore
Claude Thibeault, Montréal, Canada
Zuoming Zhang, Xi'an, China

Physicians distinguished by their Practice in Aviation Medicine

The Editor and the assembled authors have accomplished a masterful task in relating the neurosciences to the practice of aviation medicine. This volume lays out the anatomical and functional basis in the nervous system for most of the neurological diagnoses which may be encountered in the care and qualification of those who would fly. From the neurological examination through common problems such as headache, vision and hearing reduction, hypoxia and disorientation, to the more complicated states of sleep, wakefulness, consciousness and awareness of the airman, the causes are outlined and then the reader is led to the qualification decision. This volume should be a welcome addition to the library of all the disciplines involved in Aviation Medicine, and particularly to physicians in the practice of aviation medicine.

Charles Berry
Past President
Aerospace Medical Association
Houston, Texas

The Editor has brought together a very distinguished group of some seventeen co-authors, and, from a vantage point of over fifty years in defining the arena of neurosciences in aviation medicine, has created a volume that spans the field in its entirety, as known today. It will surely join the pantheon of major textbooks in both of these fields. The chapters cover the basics of neuroscience, the physiology and clinical applications to flight. It is copiously referenced and well illustrated with figures and tables to help clarify technical points. Of special interest to the clinician are the chapters dealing with neurological disorders and their application to the aeromedical disposition of all those who fly, and will be the definitive reference for many years to come.

Yehezkel (Geoff) Caine
Past President
International Academy of Aviation and Space Medicine
Jerusalem, Israel

This textbook provides the highest level of current knowledge in aviation-related human physiology and physiopathology involving the neurosciences. It reviews the classical stresses associated with flight and brings up to date the neurological and sensory disorders in an aeromedical context. Authored by the most eminent British experts in these fields, this book will be a classic, an essential companion to students training for higher qualifications, and to practitioners in charge of the care of aircrew and the medical assessment of fitness to fly.

Jean-Pierre Crance
Emeritus Professor of Physiology and Aerospace Medicine
University of Nancy
Nancy, France

The Neurosciences and the Practice of Aviation Medicine is a must document for the aviation medicine practitioner, adviser and the specialist in human factors. It brings best scientific knowledge to the aeromedical examiner as well as to regulatory bodies and managers of scientific programmes. The book provides an excellent scientific basis to safety related topics such as flight and duty time regulations. It is highly recommended reading for non-medical human factors specialists involved in research, teaching and accident investigation with its state of the art information on aircrew alertness, wakefulness and disorientation.

Gábor Hardicsay
Chief Medical Officer
Civil Aviation Authority
Budapest, Hungary

The Neurosciences and the Practice of Aviation Medicine departs from the traditional approach to aviation medicine, delving more into where neurology and the special senses interact with the flight environment. This text will serve both as a valuable information source for students and practitioners wishing to read at a deeper level, and as a reference for those undertaking more specialized research.

David Powell
Chief Medical Officer
Air New Zealand
Auckland, New Zealand

This textbook presents the neurosciences in simple language thus making a subject that is often perceived as confusing and complex, easy to understand. The approach of highlighting the operational implications and aeromedical significance of each topic is particularly valuable to the aviation medicine practitioner. Incorporating the historical element in literature and scientific review provides a holistic coverage of the subject matter discussed.

Jarnail Singh
Chairman
Civil Aviation Medical Board
Singapore

The Neurosciences and the Practice of Aviation Medicine is a well-written, properly illustrated and practical textbook. The aeromedical practitioner will find in the same book the impairments of neurological function that may arise from the interaction of aircrew with the air domain as well as the clinical information necessary to properly look after aircrew with neurological disorders. Add an extensive bibliography of case reports of neurological disorders in aircrew to this information and it makes this book a must in any aeromedical library

Claude Thibeault
Past President
International Academy of Aviation and Space Medicine
Montréal, Canada

A very interesting book on clinical neurology and operational aviation medicine. The book is focused on neurological problems in aviation medicine from clinical to operational practice, but is not limited to these issues. Basic knowledge in visual, vestibular and hearing function and their aeromedical considerations are included. It also covers topics, such as sleep, circadian rhythmicity, hypoxia, hypotension and hypoglycaemia and their relation to aviation safety. Adhering to a consistent style, the authors pay attention to background and basic knowledge and provide detailed references. It should be a very useful reference book for those who are interested in aviation medicine and aviation safety.

Zuoming Zhang
Professor of Clinical Aerospace Medicine
Medical University
Xi'an, China

Printed and bound by CPI Group (UK) Ltd, Croydon, CR0 4YY

21/10/2024

01777046-0002